HERBAL MEDICINE

EXPANDED
COMMISSION E MONOGRAPHS

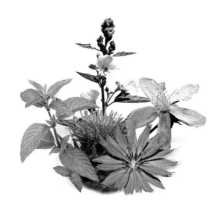

HERBAL MEDICINE

EXPANDED
COMMISSION E MONOGRAPHS

*Herb Monographs, Based on Those Created by a Special
Expert Committee of the German Federal Institute for
Drugs and Medical Devices*

Senior Editor

Mark Blumenthal
Founder and Executive Director
American Botanical Council

Associate Editor
Alicia Goldberg

Assistant Editor
Josef Brinckmann

Photographs by
Steven Foster

With Foreword by
Varro E. Tyler, Ph.D., Sc.D.
Dean and Distinguished Professor of Pharmacognosy Emeritus
School of Pharmacy and Pharmacal Sciences, Purdue University

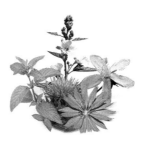

© 2000 American Botanical Council
Published by Integrative Medicine Communications.
All Rights Reserved. Neither this book nor any part may be stored, reproduced, or transmitted in any form or by any means, mechanical or electronic, without prior permission from the publisher and the copyright holder.

First edition 2000
Printed in the United States of America
03 02 01 00 99

ISBN 0-9670772-1-4

Library of Congress Catalog Card Number: 99-73645

Design by Williams Artworks Graphic Studio, Inc.
Electronic production by Leslie Anne Feagley.

American Botanical Council
P.O. Box 144345
Austin, TX 78714-4345
www.herbalgram.org
abc@herbalgram.org

Publisher:
Integrative Medicine Communications
1029 Chestnut Street
Newton, MA 02464
1-877-426-6633
www.onemedicine.com

TABLE OF CONTENTS

"QUICK-LOOK" CROSS-REFERENCES

APPENDICES

FOREWORD

Varro E. Tyler, Ph.D., Sc.D.

Dean and Distinguished Professor of Pharmacognosy Emeritus
School of Pharmacy and Pharmacal Sciences, Purdue University

In publishing these expanded monographs on America's most commonly used herbs, the authors have worked to address perceived deficiencies in the original *The Complete German Commission E Monographs—Therapeutic Guide to Herbal Medicines*. Practically all of the criticism of that initial, pioneering work centered on what the monographs did not say. One heard the cry, "No references!" by those who overlooked the fact that the drug standards monographs in *The United States Pharmacopeia* (USP) and *The National Formulary* (NF) are also without references. Probably some of the critics are familiar with the high scientific standards of the committee members who developed the USP and NF monographs, so the lack of references in those volumes does not bother them. I am personally acquainted with many of the scientists who have served on the German Commission E, and, knowing their high standards, the lack of references in their work does not bother me.

As explained in the introduction of the previous book, references were not included because the Commission's monographs were intended primarily as package inserts for herbal preparations sold as drugs in German pharmacies. Also, some of the information provided to the Commission was proprietary in nature and not subject to public disclosure. Omitting this material would have made any reference list incomplete, so none was included.

One also heard, "The monographs are too brief. They are just summaries of the essential points regarding the herbs." Of course, that is exactly what they were intended to be. As summaries of professional judgments regarding safety and efficacy of the botanicals, clarity, not verbosity, was considered to be the primary objective.

A further criticism was that German science and medicine were not up to our high American standards, rendering the Commission E judgements defective. When I heard this, I would think of Germans like Professor Otto Wallach, whose outstanding work with the chemistry of volatile oil constituents not only earned him the title "messiah of the terpenes," but a Nobel prize as well. For many years, our best chemists and physicians received their advanced education in Germany. A visit to any of the great German universities will convince the skeptic that science and medicine are not only alive and well, but thriving there. I spent one sabbatical year at the Institut für Biochemie der Pflanzen in Halle/Saale and another at the Georg-August-Universität in Göttingen, and have attended scores of scientific meetings in Germany. I can attest to the fact that the study of phytotherapy is much further advanced there than in the United States. German expertise in the area is, without question, the best in the world.

Although the pioneering judgments rendered by the Commission E on the safety and efficacy of over 380 herbs remain generally the best available, there is, of course, always room for improvement. The medicinal potential of herbs has become the focus of more and more scientific and clinical studies in the field in recent years. New information has provided additional insights and, in some cases, modified previous judgments. That is only to be expected in such a dynamic field.

Therefore, Mark Blumenthal, Alicia Goldberg, and Josef Brinckmann have performed a substantial service to all those interested in herbal medicine by expanding the content in the Commission E herb monographs of the most widely used herbs in America to include updated, detailed information on their botany, history, composition, safety, efficacy, and therapeutic use. And for those who lamented its initial absence, an extensive list of published references is provided, each of which is appropriately keyed to a specific statement in the monograph. This listing is followed by a compilation of additional literature resources for those who want still more background information on a particular botanical.

In short, these expanded versions of selected original Commission E monographs would seem to fulfill all of the desires of those who felt that the original version did not meet their expectations, or that its large size and price did not allow for its widest distribution and use. I am quite certain that this volume will meet and even exceed those expectations and wishes. It is destined to occupy a prominent position on the shelf of useful herbal literature for the foreseeable future.

PREFACE

Mark Blumenthal

Founder and Executive Director, American Botanical Council

Editor, *HerbalGram*

Senior Editor, *The Complete German Commission E Monographs*

Alittle more than a year has passed since the publication of *The Complete German Commission E Monographs—Therapeutic Guide to Herbal Medicines.* This book is based on that original work, which we produced to provide the American public authoritative information on the therapeutic benefits and potential risks of herbs and herbal medicine products (phytomedicines). The German Commission E (henceforth referred to as the Commission E) is generally acknowledged as the leading regulatory model of the industrialized nations for its evaluation of the therapeutic activities of herbs being prescribed and sold for medicinal purposes.

When we published *The Complete German Commission E Monographs*, there was a paucity of authoritative data on herbal medicines, at least insofar as a government-sponsored expert review is concerned. Although our book was designed primarily for healthcare professionals, we were gratified by the large response we received from consumers who found the book a useful guide to understanding more about the many herbal medicines now popular in the United States marketplace. Further, we were extremely honored when *Doody's Medical Book Review Journal* ranked our publication as one of the top three books published in the medical and allied healthcare professions in 1998. *The Complete German Commission E Monographs* is the first "alternative medicine" title to receive such a high ranking.

We are publishing this follow-up book in response to the public's interest in having access to more scientific information documenting the efficacy of the herbs most commonly used medicinally in America today. The original book detailed 380 monographs; for this publication, we have focused our attention on more than 100 of the herbs commonly sold in the United States. All of these herbs were approved by the Commission E for nonprescription drug use, with the exception of the following six: echinacea angustifolia herb and root/pallida herb, echinacea purpurea root (component characteristic), hawthorn berry, hawthorn flower, hawthorn leaf, and yohimbe bark. We have included these last six due to their relative importance in the U.S. market and/or because they are part of the "cluster" of herbs that make up a popular category (e.g., echinacea, hawthorn).

Several sections included in *The Complete German Commission E Monographs* do not appear in this book: a 65-page introduction providing an extensive discussion of the herbal market and regulatory situation in the United States and Germany, monographs from the *German Pharmacopoeia* on herb standards, and monographs from the *Pharmacopoeia Europa* on methods for formulation of leading dosage forms.

The Commission E began to publish its monographs in a new format in 1992 and we have standardized all of the monographs in this book to more closely match the revised Commission E format. The majority of the monographs in this book were published by the Commission E between 1983 and 1992 (prior to the revised format)—to these we have added new information to bring the monographs up-to-date and to make them concordant with the new format. The additional material in these monographs was obtained mostly from the General

References listed on pages 495–497, plus specific references cited in each monograph. The following 19 monographs were published by the Commission E since 1992 and, therefore, did not require as much revision or supplemental information: bromelain, buckthorn bark, cascara sagrada bark, chaste tree fruit, dandelion herb, echinacea angustifolio herb and root/pallida herb, echinacea pallida root, echinacea purpurea root, ginkgo biloba leaf extract, hawthorn berry, hawthorn flower, hawthorn leaf, hawthorn leaf with flower, horse chestnut seed extract, senna leaf, senna pod (fruit), soy phospholipid, uva ursi leaf, brewer's yeast/Hansen CBS 5926.

EXPLANATION OF MONOGRAPH SECTIONS

Each monograph contains the following:

Color Photograph: Supplied by Steven Foster, America's pre-eminent photographer of medicinal plants. In some cases, the plant part pictured does not reflect the part used medicinally and described in the monograph.

Common Name: We have chosen the common name most widely used in the United States. For most of the herbs we relied on the American Herbal Product Association's *Herbs of Commerce*. This self-regulatory book is accepted by the Food and Drug Administration (FDA) and establishes uniform common names for the most popular herbs sold in the United States (Foster, 1992; FDA, 1997).

Latin Name: As listed by the Commission E.

Pharmacopeial Name: As listed by the Commission E. Pharmacopeial names (sometimes called pharmaceutical names) provide a convenient system for pharmacists, physicians, and botanists to identify a substance used as materia medica by referring to its Latin name plus the plant part and/or type of preparation being used. (Note regarding the spelling of pharmacopeia: We prefer the modern spelling of pharmacopeia and have used this when referring to pharmacopeias in general. However, whenever we cite the actual title of a foreign pharmacopeia, we spell it as it is done in the country of origin, usually pharmacopoeia. Older versions of the *United States Pharmacopeia* are also spelled with the more archaic spelling, using the silent *o*.)

Other Names: The primary source we used was *Herbs of Commerce;* additional sources may be found in the General References list on pages 495–497.

Overview: This section contains general information on the herb's history, distribution, cultivation, commerce, safety issues, and quality standards, as well as comments on the original Commission E monograph and summaries of clinical studies. Some herbs contain several plant parts that have distinct therapeutic uses; for these herbs we have written one combined overview followed by separate monographs for each part. The following 12 monographs appear in this format: dandelion (dandelion herb/dandelion root with herb); echinacea (echinacea augustifolia herb and root, pallida herb/echinacea pallida root/echinacea purpurea herb/echinacea purpurea root); eucalyptus (eucalyptus leaf/eucalyptus oil); fennel (fennel oil/fennel seed); hawthorn (hawthorn berry/hawthorn flower/hawthorn leaf/ hawthorn leaf with flower); marshmallow (marshmallow leaf/marshmallow root); peppermint (peppermint leaf/peppermint oil); psyllium (psyllium seed, black/psyllium seed, blonde/psyllium seed husk, blonde); senna (senna leaf/senna pod (fruit); soy (soy lecithin/soy phospholipid); stinging nettle (stinging nettle herb and leaf/stinging nettle root); and brewer's yeast (brewer's yeast/brewer's yeast, Hansen CBS 5926).

Description: This section identifies the therapeutic properties of the herb: the specific part of the plant that is used medicinally, its botanical name, its plant family, some of its primary chemical constituents, and its required time of harvest, if applicable. It is identical to the section entitled "Composition of Drug" in *The Complete German Commission E Monographs*.

Chemistry and Pharmacology: This section first details the primary constituents of the plant and then lists its pharmacological actions, as indicated by the Commission E. The pharmacological actions were determined by laboratory experiments carried out either *in vitro* or *in vivo* using test animals. These actions do not represent the results of human clinical trials; they are provided only to better indicate the *potential* activity of the herbal preparation in humans.

Uses: This section lists the uses that have been approved by the Commission E followed by the uses that we have collected from other sources that may be found in the General References list. External and internal uses are listed separately. Most of the uses pertain to the following 11 medical groupings:

- the cardiovascular system
- dermatology
- endocrinology, obstetrics/gynecology, the reproductive system, and the prostate gland
- the gastrointestinal system
- hematology, the lymphatic system, and cancer
- immunology, AIDS, and infectious diseases
- the liver and gallbladder
- neurology and psychiatry
- ophthalmology
- the respiratory system (the lower and upper respiratory tract, including ears, nose, throat, and sinuses)
- the urinary tract system (the kidneys, ureter, and bladder)

A key for these categories is given in the Uses cross-reference on pages 435–437. This section is one of the most important sections of the monograph: in Germany, where the labels on licensed phytomedicines indicate the uses approved by the Commission E, it is the official guide for patients and healthcare practitioners; outside of Germany, it serves not only as a usage indicator but also as a model for the rational evaluation and regulation of the therapeutic uses of herbs. This section is an expanded version of the "Uses" section in *The Complete German Commission E Monographs*.

Contraindications: This section lists any conditions with which the herb should not be used. Contraindications listed include allergies to particular constituents, restrictions for children and infants, and restrictions related to diabetes. Also listed are contraindications to conventional medications. Contraindications are arranged in a separate index according to the 11 medical groupings listed in the "Uses" description. This section is an updated version of the "Contraindications" section in *The Complete German Commission E Monographs*.

Side Effects: This section lists any potential side effects that may be experienced when administering the herb. Examples of side effects associated with the use of approved herbs include ocular accommodation disturbances, albuminuria, allergic reactions, cramps, diarrhea, fever, gastrointestinal disturbances, headaches, hematuria, intestinal sluggishness associated with stimulant laxatives, nausea, photosensitization, and vomiting. Some of the side effects are noted to occur only in "rare cases" or in "sensitive individuals"; this indicates a possible adverse effect that is not typical of the herb but has been documented in literature or is based on theoretical presumptions. Side effects are arranged in a separate index according to the 11 medical groupings listed in the "Uses" description. This section is an updated version of the "Side Effects" section in *The Complete German Commission E Monographs.*

Use During Pregnancy and Lactation: This section contains information taken from both the "Contraindications" section of *The Complete German Commission E Monographs* and the herb's listing in the American Herbal Product Association's *Botanical Safety Handbook.*

Interactions with Other Drugs: This section lists any potential interactions between the herb and pharmaceutical drugs. It is based on information from the Commission E, the *Botanical Safety Handbook*, plus additional data from ESCOP (European Scientific Cooperative on Phytotherapy) monographs, World Health Organization (WHO) monographs, and other sources. This section is an updated version of the "Interactions with Other Drugs" section in *The Complete German Commission E Monographs.*

Dosage and Administration: This section is a combination of the "Dosage," "Mode of Administration," and "Duration of Administration" sections in *The Complete German Commission E Monographs.*

This section lists dosage equivalents for other applicable types of preparations for the herb. For example, a dosage of 2 g may be expanded upon as follows:

Unless otherwise prescribed: 2 g per day of [powdered, crushed, cut, or whole] [plant part]
Infusion: 2 g in 150 ml of water.
Fluidextract 1:1 (g/ml): 2 ml.
Tincture 1:5 (g/ml): 10 ml.

The Commission E occasionally cites "Erg.B.6" (the supplemental volume to the *German Pharmacopoeia*, 6th edition) as a source for certain dosage recommendations. The official pharmacopoeias of other countries are the source for any dosage information added to this book.

The Mode of Administration describes the method of preparation and the form in which the herb should be taken. The Commission E indicates Duration of Use for herbs to address safety concerns or to acknowledge the minimum amount of usage time required for therapeutic results. For example, in order to be effective, *Ginkgo biloba* leaf extract must be taken for a minimum of six to eight weeks, depending on the indication, and licorice root preparations with a content of 300 mg glycyrrhizin should not be taken for more than four to six weeks. The Commission E also stipulates that the popular herb uva ursi, which is used as a urinary tract antiseptic, should not be taken for more than one week or more than five times per year. Of particular safety concern is limiting the use of stimulant laxative herbs (aloe, buckthorn bark and berry, cascara sagrada, senna leaf and pod, and rhubarb root) to one to two weeks. The monographs for the herbs used to treat diarrhea strongly recommend a physician consultation if the diarrhea persists for more than three to four days.

References: This section lists the sources from which the information used in the monograph text was derived. This list includes primary medical and pharmacy journal articles as well as authoritative herbal books and pharmacopeias from around the world. We have chosen to repeat the references that appear in most monographs—rather than abbreviate them and list them elsewhere in the book, as is frequently done in books of this type. We chose to list each reference used in each monograph in recognition of the common practice of many researchers of copying individual monographs for filing or faxing purposes (copyright laws notwithstanding). Thus, while the repeated mention of general references requires more space, we trust the reader will find this format beneficial in the long-term. For convenience, we have also listed these general references on pages 495–497.

Additional Resources: This section provides further articles and books to refer to for more information on the herb.

Footnote: The footnote provides a brief summary of which sections are excerpted from the Commission E.

THE COMMISSION E MONOGRAPHS

Over about sixteen years the Commission E evaluated more than three hundred herbs and herb combinations for their safety and efficacy. The results were published in the form of monographs in the *Bundesanzeiger,* which is the German equivalent to the *Federal Register* in the United States. Monographs were published to be used as package inserts in phytomedicines sold in German pharmacies. The monograph format was proposed and reviewed by all of the Commission E members, and other scientists, scientific associations, universities, and herbal experts. All comments were reviewed by the Commission E and changes were incorporated in its final monograph format (Schilcher, 1997). Three types of monographs were published by the Commission E: "Approved" monographs permit the use of the herb as a nonprescription drug; "Unapproved" monographs do not permit the herb to be sold for general use because the documented risks were deemed too great; and "Neutral" monographs permit the sale of the herb but indicate that the documentation was inadequate to prove therapeutic benefit but at the same time did not present any safety concerns. We chose to label both unapproved and neutral monographs as "Unapproved" in *The Complete German Commission E Monographs.* Since 1995 the Commission E has not issued any new monographs. Their focus instead has been on the registration and registration extension process of phytomedicines currently being sold as drugs in Germany.

Of considerable interest to regulators and industry alike, there is a strikingly close parallel between the approved uses for almost all of the herbs that have been evaluated by the European Scientific Cooperative on Phytotherapy (ESCOP), a pan-western-European group of medicinal plant experts, and published in 60 monographs to date, as well as the 28 monographs published by the World Health Organization (WHO) and the approved uses and dosages for the same herbs in the Commission E monographs. Commission E members point out that this frequent similarity in approvals by ESCOP and WHO, who both based their monographs on the same research reviewed by Commission E plus new data published since the publication of the Commission E monographs, validates overall accuracy of the work produced by the Commission E (Schilcher, 1999).

THE COMMISSION E EVALUATION METHODS AND CRITERIA

Bibliographic Review

The members of the Commission E actively collected and assessed bibliographic data on the herbal preparations being reviewed to determine their safety and efficacy. This is in accordance with applicable European drug laws and with Section 26 of the Second German Medicines Act. Members use from one to two hundred sources from around the world to evaluate each herb (Schilcher, 1997). This work was supported from 1992 to 1995 by an industry and scientific coalition group called *Kooperation Phytopharmaka* (Steinhoff, 1997). Regarding the production of the monographs, the Commission E's referee, Dr. K. Keller of *Bundesinstitut für Arzneimittel und Medizinprodukte* (the Federal Institute for Drugs and Medical Devices), or BfArM, writes, "Due to the great number of individual drugs, the work of the committee was concentrated on the evaluation of active constituents. The evaluation is based on bibliographic data presented by manufacturers or organizations of manufacturers of herbal medicinal products. These documents are completed by data obtained from literature search, for example, online research in EMBASE, MEDLARS, and TOXALL, and other data available to our office" (Keller, 1992).

Following are some of the types of sources from which data was collected and reviewed:

1. **Traditional use.** Historical literature often reveals long-term use of a botanical substance and may indicate relative safety and presumed efficacy.

2. **Chemical data.** Herbs have been analyzed to determine their chemical composition, especially the main constituents. These chemical constituents may indicate the potential activity and/or toxicity of a botanical substance, depending on the known range of compounds and their relative quantities.

3. **Experimental, pharmacological, and toxicological studies.** Laboratory/experimental (*in vitro*) and pharmacological/toxicological (*in vivo*) studies on whole plant extracts or on individual constituents of medicinal plants are conducted worldwide. These studies provide documentation of potential uses of a particular plant, which is particularly helpful when clinical studies are lacking.

4. **Clinical studies.** In many European countries, clinical studies on leading medicinal plants and phytomedicines are routinely conducted in accordance with strict scientific controls. These studies suggest and often confirm the safety and efficacy of herbs and their preparations. Many recently conducted clinical studies adhere to the Good Clinical Practice (GCP) guidelines.

5. **Field and epidemiological studies.** The known use of a medicinal plant by a particular population over an extended period of time is helpful when evaluating safety and efficacy. The Commission E reviews any such available information.

6. **Patient case records submitted from physicians' files.** Case reports about individual patients under physician care in clinical practice, although not as indicative as controlled clinical studies, are nevertheless useful in obtaining information on the efficacy of herbal preparations and phytomedicines.

7. **Additional studies, including unpublished proprietary data submitted by manufacturers.** Some phytomedicinal preparations have undergone extensive chemical, toxicological, pharmacological, and clinical testing conducted by a manufacturer. Because these are commercial preparations, some of these studies are proprietary and have not been published. Although the Commission did review some of this type of data, it was not instrumental in the final evaluations made by the members on the relative safety and efficacy of the herb or preparation being reviewed. The Commission relied only on published reports and studies in making its assessments. Nevertheless, when it was submitted, the Commission E maintained the confidentiality of proprietary information.

Conclusion

One of the most important issues facing integrative medicine today is the need to access information about clinical research on herbal products. The Commission E process has helped to bring to light an abundance of clinical research on herbs. The editors have attempted to provide in this publication some documentation of clinical and pharmacological research studies, as well as other relevant data, which in turn may serve to encourage the responsible use and clinical integration of phytomedicines in the United States. To assist the reader in understanding which products have undergone clinical testing, we have frequently mentioned those products in the respective monographs, and we have included in the Appendix a table to show which of the top-selling herbs in Germany have been the subject of the most clinical research and are most prescribed by physicians. The brand names in the United States that correspond to some of these preparations are also provided. (Please see Table 5 on page 479.)

The Commission E process provides an excellent model of regulatory reform for the United States and other countries seeking to develop a system to review herbs and phytomedicines for safety and efficacy. The Commission E monographs provide the most rational science-based example of an evaluation process for the development of phytomedicine regulations in the United States. A process like this would provide U.S. healthcare practitioners and consumers with reliable and authoritative information on the therapeutic benefits and risks of herbal medicines. The Commission E model should not, however, be viewed as an endpoint of herbal regulatory scheme. Instead, it should be seen as a point of departure, a baseline upon which new data can be reviewed with respect to the herbs used in the United States today. Using an expert panel system similar to the Commission E to review herbal literature could offer substantial benefits to the American healthcare system and to American consumers.

References

Foster, S. (ed.). 1992. *Herbs of Commerce.* Austin, TX: American Herbal Products Association.

Keller, K. 1992. Results of the revision of herbal drugs in the Federal Republic of Germany with a special focus on risk aspects. *Zeitschrift Phytother* 13:116–120.

Schilcher, H. 1999. Personal communication to M. Blumenthal, Aug. 5.

Schilcher, H. 1997. Personal communication to M. Blumenthal, Dec. 30.

Steinhoff, B. 1997. Personal communication to M. Blumenthal, Dec. 12.

FDA. Food and Drug Administration. 1997. *Code of Federal Regulations 21*, (CFR 21) Part 51 and 5 U.S.C. 552(a). Washington DC: Office of the Federal Register National Archives and Records Administration.

Editor's Notice

This work is based on *The Complete German Commission E Monographs—Therapeutic Guide to Herbal Medicines*, which consists of translations of the original monographs published by the Commission E after an extensive peer review process. The editors have consulted a variety of authoritative sources in these "expanded" monographs and have added them to the "skeleton" of the monographs produced by Commission E, thereby creating a new format. These expanded monographs are based on references that include primary literature (original studies) plus a wide variety of secondary literature, including books by authoritative authors, pharmacopeial monographs, review articles and meta-analyses, etc. Many of these primary and secondary references most likely form the basis of some of the research consulted by the Commission E in its deliberations when they evaluated an herb. However, much the reference material was published since the respective Commission E monograph was published, thereby adding new material to document (or in some cases, contradict) the Commission's evaluations.

In an effort to respond quickly to the public's rapidly growing demand for trustworthy information on phytomedicines, the editors have prepared this volume on an accelerated schedule, and have employed a streamlined peer review process. The reader should note that the additional information added by the editors to the original monographs has not been subjected to the extensive level of expert peer review as was conducted by the Commission E in the development of its original monographs. Thus, neither the editors nor the publisher are suggesting that the publication of this work is tantamount to the work produced by the Commission.

A revision of this book will incorporate additional primary references and reflect a more extensive peer review. That book will also include new research and related data that has been published since this first edition.

Editorial Acknowledgments

A book of this nature requires a significant amount of editorial attention, research, organization, editing, re-editing, peer-review, and numerous other tasks. The book you are currently holding would not be in existence were it not for the excellent organizational and editorial talents and execution of Alicia Goldberg, one of the principal authors of this work. For many months, she labored with various iterations of draft manuscripts of each of the monographs and coordinated the research and editing that has resulted in this book. She is also one of the principal assoc. editors of the previous work, *The Complete German Commission E Monographs—Therapeutic Guide to Herbal Medicines*, upon which much of this book is based. In addition, she is also one of the editors of the American Herbal Product Association's *Botanical Safety Handbook*, a review of about 550 of the most popular herbs in the U.S. market and their ranking via safety according to numerous authoritative sources, including the Commission E monographs. We are also indebted to our good friend and assoc. editor, Josef Brinckmann, Dir. of Product Dev. at Traditional Medicinal Herb Teas in Sebastapol, CA. Josef's knowledge of the original German literature, his extensive experience in the botanical mfg. industry, as well as his access to numerous German and English sources, have provided an invaluable resource for much of the information that we have added to the original framework provided by the Commission E.

Additional editorial contributions to some of the overviews was provided by Helen Batchelder. Stephanie Gray offered her valuable research and organizational skills to the production of the book. Amanda Long selected the medical terminology for the database of therapeutic cross-references. Dawnelle Malone of the American Botanical Council efficiently provided the retrieval of clinical studies. We are also deeply grateful to George Stamathis at Integrative Medicine Communications, for his conceptual ideas in helping to structure this publication and for his persistent follow up in pushing this project forward. Syndi Bowab and Charissa Lyons provided their excellent copyediting and proofreading skills.

The editors offer their thanks to the following peer reviewers for their expert critiques on specific herb monographs: Dennis Awang, Ph.D., Pres. of MediPlant; Prof. Ruldolf Bauer, Ph.D., of Heinrich Heine Univ. Inst. for Pharmaceutical Biology in Dusseldorf; Don Brown, N.D., Dir. of Natural Products Research Consultants; Werner Busse, Ph.D., head of Regulatory and Scientific Affairs for Willmar Schwabe Gmbh & Co.; Jerry Cott, Ph.D., Chief, Adult Psychopharmacology Research Program of Nat. Inst. of Mental Health; Prof. Gerhard Franz, Univ. of Regensburg and Commission E member; Claus Gehringer of CamoCare®/ABKIT, Inc.; Christopher Hobbs, L.Ac.; Timothy Kostelecky, Tech. Svc. Mgr. at John I. Haas, Inc.; Larry Lawson, Ph.D., Research Dir. of Murdock Madaus Schwabe; Albert Leung, Ph.D., Pres. of AYSL Corp.; Gail Mahady, Ph.D., of the Dept. of Medicinal Chemistry and Pharmacognosy, College of Pharmacy at the Univ. of Illinois; Muhammed Majeed, Ph.D., of Sabinsa Corp.; Prof. Heinz Schilcher, VP of Commission E; Michael Murray, N.D.; Matt Schueller of Enzymatic Therapy; Fabio Soldati, Ph.D., VP, Research and Dev., Pharmaton SA, Switzerland; Subhuti Dharmananda, Ph.D., Dir. of the Inst. for Traditional Medicine; Meir Tenne, D.Sc., of Dalidar Pharma Ltd.; Varro E. Tyler, Ph.D., Sc.D., Dean and Distinguished Prof. Emeritus at Purdue University; and Dana Ullman, M.P.H., of Homeopathic Ed. Services.

Also, we offer our appreciation to the following persons who read the manuscript and provided quotes for the back cover and promotional literature: Thomas Kurt, M.D., M.P.H., Clinical Prof., Dept. of Internal Medicine at the Univ. of Texas Southwestern Medical Center; Jean Carper, author and syndicated columnist; and Joe and Terry Graedon, Ph.D., People's Pharmacy. We extend our deep appreciation for the writing of the foreword to Varro E. Tyler, Ph.D., Sc.D., a leader in providing information on the responsible and appropriate use of herbs.

ACKNOWLEDGMENT OF CONTRIBUTORS

The ongoing educational and research work of the American Botanical Council is supported by foundations, organizations, businesses and individuals. The American Botanical Council would like to thank the following for their support of ABC's role in this project:

CORPORATE PARTNERS

Enzymatic Therapy
Nature's Way
PhytoPharmica
Rexall Sundown
Stryka Botanics Co., Inc.

CORPORATE FRIENDS

Botanicals International
Capsugel
Emil Flachsmann AG
Herbalife International, Inc.
Lichtwer Pharma U.S., Inc.
MW International
NBTY, Inc.
Triarco Industries, Inc.

GENERAL NOTICE AND DISCLAIMER

The editors have attempted to exercise the utmost care in providing accurate translations of the monographs as published by Commission E of the German Institute for Drugs and Medical Products in the *Bundesanzeiger,* the German equivalent of the U.S. *Federal Register.* As is the case with any work that is based on translations, there may be some latitude in choosing English terminology for German words, either common or technical. Also, the editors have made every possible attempt to verify the accuracy of the indexes, cross-references, and other materials presented in this volume.

It should be noted by the reader that constant changes in information resulting from ongoing research and clinical experience, differences in opinions among authorities, unique individual circumstances, and the possibility of human error in compiling this publication require that the reader use judgment and other resources when making decisions based on this material.

The information contained in the monographs was originally intended as package insert information for physicians, pharmacists, other health professionals, and consumers in Germany. Accordingly, the publication of this material in English is intended primarily to help provide English-speaking health professionals with much-needed therapeutic information on botanicals.

However, this book is not intended as a guide to self-medication by consumers. The lay reader is advised to discuss the information contained herein with a physician, pharmacist, nurse or other authorized health care practitioner. Neither the editors nor the publisher accepts any responsibility for the accuracy of the information itself or the consequences from the use or misuse of the information in this book.

HERB MONOGRAPHS

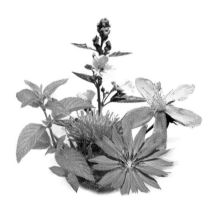

Lapland

Lapland

Lapland

Lapland

Lapland

Lapland

Lapland

Lapland

Lapland

Angelica Root

Latin Name:
Angelica archangelica

Pharmacopeial Name:
Angelicae radix

Other Names:
European angelica

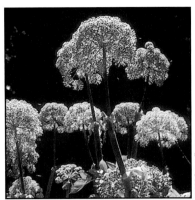

©1999 Steven Foster

Overview

European angelica is a biennial or perennial herb native to northern and eastern Europe (Leung and Foster, 1996) and parts of Asia (Budavari, 1996; Wichtl and Bisset, 1994). Its natural habitat includes Iceland, Scotland, Holland, and Lapland (Grieve, 1979; Leung and Foster, 1996). In Germany, it is cultivated in the states of Bavaria and Thüringen (Lange and Schippmann, 1997). The material of commerce is obtained from northern Europe, including the United Kingdom (BHP, 1996), almost entirely from plants cultivated in the Netherlands, Poland, and Germany, and to a lesser extent from Belgium, Italy, and the Czech Republic (Wichtl and Bisset, 1994).

Angelica has been used for centuries in European medicine as an expectorant for bronchial illnesses, colds and coughs, and also as a digestive aid for stomach disorders (Leung and Foster, 1996; Wren, 1988). By the fifteenth century it was in popular use. In the English herbal entitled *Paradisus Terrestris*, published in 1629 C.E. by John Parkinson, angelica was reported to be one of the most important medicinal herbs of that time (Bown, 1995; Grieve, 1979).

In Germany, angelica root is official in the *German Pharmacopeia* (DAB 10, 1993), listed in the *German Drug Codex* (DAC, 1986), approved in the Commission E monographs (BAnz, 1998), and the tea form is official in the German Standard License monographs (Braun et al., 1997). Clinically, it is mainly used as an aromatic and bitter tonic for the digestive system, used to stimulate the appetite, and to treat dyspepsia. It is commonly employed as a component in bitters and liqueurs such as Bénédictine, Boonekamp, and Chartreuse (Weiss, 1988; Wichtl and Bisset, 1994) and also as a component in numerous gastrointestinal, cholagogue, and biliary remedies (Wichtl and Bisset, 1994). In German pediatric medicine, angelica root is used for treatment of gastrointestinal disorders. For example, a Commission E approved "stomach tea" is composed of 20% angelica root, 40% gentian root (*Gentiana lutea* L.) and 40% caraway seed (*Carum carvi* L.) (Schilcher, 1997). In the United States, angelica root was formerly official in the *United States Pharmacopeia* and *National Formulary* (Leung and Foster, 1996).

German pharmacopeial grade angelica root consists of the whole dried rhizome and roots of *Angelica archangelica* L., carefully dried at below 40° C. It must contain not less than 0.25% (v/m) volatile oil with reference to the dried drug. It may contain no more than 5% stem and leaf fragments and no more than 5% discolored components. Botanical identity must be confirmed with thin-layer chromatography (TLC), macroscopic and microscopic examinations, and organoleptic evaluation. Additionally, a test for adulteration with lovage root (*Levisticum officinale*) is required (DAB 10, 1993). The *Austrian Pharmacopeia* requires not less than 0.3% volatile oil (ÖAB, 1983; Wichtl and Bisset, 1994). Additionally, the *British Herbal Pharmacopoeia* requires it to be harvested in Autumn and that it should contain not less than 30% water-soluble extractive (BHP, 1996). The *German Drug Codex* also requires not less than 30% extractive (DAC, 1986; Wichtl and Bisset, 1994).

Description

Angelica root consists of the dried root and rhizome of *A. archangelica* L. [Fam. Apiaceae], and their preparations in effective dosage. The root and rhizome contain essential oil, coumarin, and coumarin derivatives.

Chemistry and Pharmacology

Angelica root contains 0.35–1.9% volatile oil, of which 80–90% are monoterpene hydrocarbons such as β-phellandrene (13–28%), α-phellandrene (2–14%) and α-pinene (14–31%); sesquiterpenes (Wichtl and Bisset, 1994); 0.3% angelic acid ($C_5H_8O_2$; Mr 100.12) (Budavari, 1996; Weiss, 1988); 6% resin; sterols (e.g. sitosterol); phenolic acids such as chlorogenic and caffeic acids (Budavari, 1996); fatty acids (e.g. palmitic, oleic, and linoleic acids); coumarins (approximately 0.2% osthol) and furanocoumarins (e.g. angelicin, bergapten); sugars; and tannins (Bruneton, 1995; Leung and Foster, 1996; Wichtl and Bisset, 1994).

Note: Under proper storage conditions, angelica root still loses approximately 0.05–0.10% volatile oil content per year. Therefore, product shelf life should be determined based on this known rate of volatilization, calculating the difference between the volatile oil content on the date of packaging against the minimum amount required in the drug codex or pharmacopeial monograph (Braun et al., 1997). Shelf life for the cut or sliced root is maximum 18 months and for the powdered root only 24 hours (DAB–DDR, 1983; Meyer-Buchtela, 1999).

The Commission E reported antispasmodic and cholagogue actions, and that it stimulates the secretion of gastric juices.

The *British Herbal Pharmacopoeia* reported aromatic bitter and spasmolytic actions (BHP, 1996). *The Merck Index* reported its therapeutic category as carminative, diaphoretic, and diuretic (Budavari, 1996). In addition, animal studies using the root oil have documented antibacterial activity against *Mycobacterium avium* and antifungal activity against 14 types of fungi (Opdyke, 1975). *In vitro*, angelica root extracts of various species have demonstrated calcium-antagonist-like effects, which may be relevant for treatment of cardiovascular disease (Leung and Foster, 1996).

Some of its early uses are at least partially supported by *in vitro* studies of angelica's active coumarin and furanocoumarin constituents. One of these, angelicin, relaxes smooth muscles *in vitro*, including those in the gastrointestinal and respiratory tracts. Angelica also relaxes tracheal (Reiter and Brandt, 1985) and vascular smooth muscles *in vitro*. This latter effect is likened to calcium-antagonist mechanisms (Härmälä et al., 1992). European angelica may also increase uterine contractions, similar to the effects shown by Chinese angelica, *A. sinensis* (dong quai) in anesthetized rabbits (Harada et al., 1984).

Uses

The Commission E approved angelica for loss of appetite, peptic discomforts such as mild spasms of the gastrointestinal tract, feeling of fullness, and flatulence.

The German Standard License indicates the use of angelica root tea for treatment of complaints such as feeling of fullness, flatulence, and mild cramplike gastrointestinal disturbances, as well as stomach conditions such as insufficient formation of gastric juice (Braun et al., 1997). In India, it is used to treat anorexia nervosa and flatulent dyspepsia (Karnick, 1994).

Contraindications

None known.

Side Effects

The furanocoumarins present in angelica root sensitize the skin to light. Subsequent exposure to UV radiation can lead to inflammation of the skin. During treatment with the drug or its preparations, prolonged sun-bathing and exposure to intense UV radiation should be avoided.

Use During Pregnancy and Lactation

Not recommended during pregnancy (McGuffin et al., 1997). No restrictions known during lactation.

Interactions with Other Drugs

None known.

Dosage and Administration

Unless otherwise prescribed: 4.5 g per day of cut dried root and other oral galenical preparations.

Dried root and rhizome: 1–2 g, three times daily (BHP, 1983; Karnick, 1994; Newall et al., 1996).

Decoction: Place 1.5 g fine-cut root in 150–250 ml cold water, bring to a boil and simmer for approximately 10 minutes in a covered vessel (Meyer-Buchtela, 1999; Wichtl and Bisset, 1994). Or: Simmer 2–4 g in 150 ml boiling water for approximately 10 minutes. Drink warm, several times daily one half-hour before meal times (Braun et al., 1997; Meyer-Buchtela, 1999).

Infusion: Steep 2–4 g in 150 ml boiled water for approximately 10 minutes. Drink warm, several times daily one half-hour before meal times (Braun et al., 1997; Meyer-Buchtela, 1999).

[Note: According to the *Austrian Pharmacopeia*, the average single dose for angelica root tea infusion is 1.5 g per cup (Meyer-Buchtela, 1999; ÖAB, 1991).]

Fluidextract 1:1 (g/ml): 1.5–3 ml (Commission E); 0.5–2.0 ml, three times daily (BHP, 1983; Karnick, 1994; Newall et al., 1996).

Tincture 1:5 (g/ml): 1.5 ml (Commission E); 0.5–2.0 ml, three times daily (BHP, 1983; Newall et al., 1996). Essential oil (Oleum Angelicae): 10–20 drops (Commission E).

References

BAnz. See *Bundesanzeiger.*

Bown, D. 1995. *Encyclopedia of Herbs and Their Uses.* New York: DK Publishing, Inc. 238.

Braun, R. et al. 1997. *Standardzulassungen für Fertigarzneimittel—Text and Kommentar.* Stuttgart: Deutscher Apotheker Verlag.

British Herbal Pharmacopoeia (BHP). 1983. Keighley, U.K.: British Herbal Medicine Association.

British Herbal Pharmacopoeia (BHP). 1996. Exeter, U.K.: British Herbal Medicine Association.

Bruneton, J. 1995. *Pharmacognosy, Phytochemistry, Medicinal Plants.* Paris: Lavoisier Publishing.

Budavari, S. (ed.). 1996. *The Merck Index: An Encyclopedia of Chemicals, Drugs, and Biologicals,* 12th ed. Whitehouse Station, N.J.: Merck & Co, Inc. 109.

Bundesanzeiger (BAnz). 1998. Monographien der Kommission E (Zulassungs- und Aufbereitungskommission am BGA für den humanmed. Bereich, phytotherapeutische Therapierichtung und Stoffgruppe). Köln: Bundesgesundheitsamt (BGA).

Deutscher Arzneimittel-Codex (DAC). 1986. Stuttgart: Deutscher Apotheker Verlag.

Deutsches Arzneibuch, 10th ed., 2nd suppl. (DAB 10). 1993. Stuttgart: Deutscher Apotheker Verlag.

Deutsches Arzneibuch der Deutsche Demokratische Republik (DAB-DDR). 1983. Berlin: Akademie Verlag.

Grieve, M. 1979. *A Modern Herbal.* New York: Dover Publications, Inc.

Harada, M., M. Suzuki, Y. Ozaki. 1984. Effect of Japanese Angelica root and peony root on uterine contraction in the rabbit in situ. *J Pharmacobiodyn* 7(5):304–311.

Härmälä, P., H. Vuorela, K. Tornquist, R. Hiltunen. 1992. Choice of solvent in the extraction of *Angelica archangelica* roots with reference to calcium blocking activity. *Planta Med* 58(2):176–183.

Karnick, C.R. 1994. *Pharmacopoeial Standards of Herbal Plants,* Vol. 1. Delhi: Sri Satguru Publications. 11–12.

Lange, D. and U. Schippmann. 1997. *Trade Survey of Medicinal Plants in Germany—A Contribution to International Plant Species Conservation.* Bonn: Bundesamt für Naturschutz. 32.

Leung, A.Y. and S. Foster. 1996. *Encyclopedia of Common Natural Ingredients Used in Food, Drugs, and Cosmetics,* 2nd ed. New York: John Wiley & Sons, Inc. 32–34.

McGuffin, M., C. Hobbs, R. Upton, A. Goldberg. 1997. American Herbal Product Association's *Botanical Safety Handbook*. Boca Raton: CRC Press. 10.

Meyer-Buchtela, E. 1999. *Tee-Rezepturen—Ein Handbuch für Apotheker und Ärzte*. Stuttgart: Deutscher Apotheker Verlag.

Newall, C.A., L.A. Anderson, J.D. Phillipson. 1996. *Herbal Medicines: A Guide for Health-Care Professionals*. London: The Pharmaceutical Press. 28–29.

Opdyke, D.L.J. 1975. Angelica root oil. *Food Cosmet Toxicol* 13(suppl.):713.

Österreichisches Arzneibuch, 1st suppl. (ÖAB). 1983. Wien: Verlag der Österreichischen Staatsdruckerei.

Österreichisches Arzneibuch (ÖAB). 1991. Wien: Verlag der Österreichischen Staatsdruckerei.

Reiter, M. and W. Brandt. 1985. Relaxant effects on tracheal and ileal smooth muscles of the guinea pig. *Arnzeimforsch* 35(1A):408–414.

Schilcher, H. 1997. *Phytotherapy in Paediatrics: Handbook for Physicians and Pharmacists*. Stuttgart: Medpharm Scientific Publishers. 48.

Weiss, R.F. 1988. *Herbal Medicine*. Beaconsfield, England: Beaconsfield Publishers. 46–47.

Wichtl, M. and N.G. Bisset (eds.). 1994. *Herbal Drugs and Phytopharmaceuticals*. Stuttgart: Medpharm Scientific Publishers. 70–72.

Wren, R.C. 1988. *Potter's New Cyclopaedia of Botanical Drugs and Preparations*. Essex: The C.W. Daniel Company Ltd.

Additional Resources

British Pharmaceutical Codex (BPC). 1934. London: The Pharmaceutical Press.

Salikhova, R.A., Sh.N. Dulatova, G.G. Poroshenko. 1993. Izuchenie antimutagennykh svoistv dudnika lekarstvennogo (*Angelica archangelica* L.) mikroiadernym testom [Study of the antimutagenic properties of *Angelica archangelica* by the micronucleus test]. *Biull Eksp Biol Med* 115(4):371–372.

Salikhova, R.A. and G.G. Poroshenko. 1995. Antimutagennye svoistva dudnika lekarstvennogo [Antimutagenic properties of *Angelica archangelica* L]. *Vestn Ross Akad Med Nauk* (1):58-61.

Wichtl, M. (ed.). 1989. *Teedrogen*, 2nd ed. Stuttgart: Wissenschaftliche Verlagsgesellschaft.

This material was adapted from *The Complete German Commission E Monographs—Therapeutic Guide to Herbal Medicines*. M. Blumenthal, W.R. Busse, A. Goldberg, J. Gruenwald, T. Hall, C.W. Riggins, R.S. Rister (eds.) S. Klein and R.S. Rister (trans.). 1998. Austin: American Botanical Council; Boston: Integrative Medicine Communications.

1) The Overview section is new information.

2) Description, Chemistry and Pharmacology, Uses, Contraindications, Side Effects, Interactions with Other Drugs, and Dosage sections have been drawn from the original work. Additional information has been added in some or all of these sections, as noted with references.

3) The dosage for equivalent preparations (tea infusion, fluidextract, and tincture) have been provided based on the following example:
   Unless otherwise prescribed: 2 g per day of [powdered, crushed, cut or whole] [plant part]
   Infusion: 2 g in 150 ml of water
   Fluidextract 1:1 (g/ml): 2 ml
   Tincture 1:5 (g/ml): 10 ml

4) The References and Additional Resources sections are new sections. Additional Resources are not cited in the monograph but are included for research purposes.

ARNICA FLOWER

Latin Name:
Arnica montana or
A. chamissonis subsp. *foliosa*

Pharmacopeial Name:
Arnicae flos

Other Names:
n/a

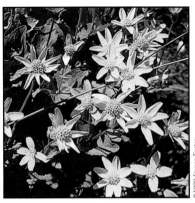

© 1999 Steven Foster

Overview

Arnica grows up to two feet in the mountainous regions of Europe and western North America (Foster, 1998; Grieve, 1979; Schulz et al., 1998). American *arnica* species include *A. fulgens, A. sororia,* and *A. cordifolia.* In Europe, *A. chamissonis* is cultivated in addition to *A. montana* to fill the demand for the estimated three hundred arnica-containing tinctures, ointments, and homeopathic remedies manufactured for the German market (Foster, 1998). Dried orange-yellow flower heads supply a therapeutic volatile oil, that contains fatty acids, aromatic terpenes, flavonoids, tannins, and sesquiterpenes of the helenalin type (Leung and Foster, 1996).

Arnica soothes sore muscles and reduces pain and inflammation. Europeans and Native Americans, who referred to arnica as mountain tobacco and leopard's bane, used it for sprains, bruises, and wounds (Grieve, 1979). Eclectic physicians, alternative medical practitioners of the late nineteenth and early twentieth centuries, recommended it for contusions and bruised muscles, mastalgia, and chronic sores or abscesses (Ellingwood, 1983). Rubbed on the head, arnica tincture was said to stimulate hair growth (Grieve, 1979). Some physicians recommended internal use for depression, dyspnea, typhoid, pneumonias, anemia, diarrhea, and cardiac weakness (Felter, 1922).

Contemporary studies demonstrate *in vitro* antimicrobial, anti-inflammatory, positive inotropic, respiratory-stimulating, and uterine activities (Schulz et al., 1998). Experimental trials suggest further potential uses. Arnica enhanced immune response in laboratory animals against *Listeria monocytogenes* and *Salmonella typhimurium* (Leung and Foster, 1996). One trial found that bile and liver enzyme levels improved when rats with carbon-tetrachloride-induced hepatic toxicity were administered phenols obtained from arnica (Marchishin, 1983). However, internal use of tinctures and fluidextracts is not recommended. Cardiac toxicity has been demonstrated, and arnica's effects on respiration and the uterus require further study. Oral administration of arnica is often accompanied by severe side effects. For this reason the monograph refers to the herb's external use only, in contrast to the comment section in the *German Pharmacopoeia* that refers to the internal use of a tea infusion of arnica for circulatory disorders of the heart and brain (DAB 8, 1978).

External use is also risky. Individuals sensitive to sesquiterpenes of the helenalin type may develop contact dermatitis from topical applications of arnica preparations. Edematous dermatosis and eczema have been reported following long-term use (Schulz et al., 1998). Arnica should not be applied to broken skin (McGuffin et al., 1997).

Arnica is a common homeopathic remedy. Arnica in a dilution of 6X is given to epileptics, and Arnica 3X may prevent seasickness (Grieve, 1979). However, its predominant place in homeopathy is now being questioned. A recent study determined that Arnica 30X was ineffective in reducing muscle soreness in long-distance runners (Vickers, 1998). Also, a literature review of available articles discussing applications of homeopathic arnica found no supportive evidence for use (Ernst, 1998).

Description
Arnica flower consists of the fresh or dried inflorescence of *A. montana* L. or *A. chamissonis* Less. subsp. *foliosa* (Nutt.) Maguiere [Fam. Asteraceae], as well as its preparations in effective dosage. It contains sesquiterpene lactones of the helenanolid type, predominantly ester derivatives of helenalin and 11,13-dihydrohelenalin. Additionally, the herb contains flavonoids (e.g., isoquercitrin, luteolin-7-glucoside, and astragalin), volatile oil (with thymol and its derivatives), phenol carbonic acid (chlorogenic acid, cynarin, caffeic acid), and coumarins (umbelliferone, scopoletin).

Chemistry and Pharmacology
The Commission E reports that when applied topically, arnica preparations have antiphlogistic (anti-inflammatory) activity. In cases of inflammation, arnica preparations also show analgesic and antiseptic activity. In animal studies, helenalin and dihydrohelenalin were found to have analgesic, antibiotic, antimicrobial and anti-inflammatory activity (Vanhaelen-Fastré, 1968; 1972; 1973). *In vitro* experiments concluded that helanalin also works as an immunostimulant (Leung and Foster, 1996).

Uses
The Commission E approved the external use of arnica flower for injuries and for consequences of accidents, e.g., hematoma, dislocations, contusions, edema due to fracture, rheumatic muscle and joint problems. It is also approved for use in inflammation of the oral and throat region, furunculosis, inflammation caused by insect bites, and superficial phlebitis.

Contraindications
Arnica allergy.

Side Effects
Prolonged treatment of damaged skin, e.g., use for injuries or ulcus cruris (indolent leg ulcers), often causes edematous dermatitis with the formation of pustules. Long use can also give rise to eczema. In treatment involving higher concentrations of the preparation, toxic skin reactions with formation of vesicles or even necroses may occur.

Use During Pregnancy and Lactation
No restrictions known.

Interactions with Other Drugs
None known.

Dosage and Administration
Unless otherwise prescribed:
Infusion: 2 g of herb per 100 ml of water.
Tincture: For cataplasm: 3–10 times dilution.
For mouth rinses: 10 times dilution.
As ointment: Not more than 20–25% tincture.
"Arnica oil": Extract of 1 part herb and 5 parts fatty oil.
Ointments with not more than 15% "arnica oil."

References
Deutsches Arzneibuch, 8th ed. (DAB 8). 1978. Stuttgart: Deutscher Apotheker Verlag.
Ellingwood, F. 1983. *American Materia Medica, Therapeutics and Pharmacognosy.* Portland, OR: Eclectic Medical Publications [reprint of 1919 original].

Ernst, E. 1998. Efficacy of homeopathic *arnica:* a systematic review of placebo-controlled clinical trials. *Arch Surg* 133(11):1187–1190.

Felter, H.W. 1922. *The Eclectic Materia Medica, Pharmacology and Therapeutics.* Portland, OR: Eclectic Medical Publications.

Foster, S. 1998. *101 Medicinal Herbs: An Illustrated Guide.* Loveland: Interweave Press.

Grieve, M. 1979. *A Modern Herbal.* New York: Dover Publications, Inc.

Leung, A. and S. Foster. 1996. *Encyclopedia of Common Natural Ingredients Used in Food, Drugs, and Cosmetics.* 2nd ed. New York: John Wiley & Sons, Inc.

Marchishin, S.M. 1983. [Efficacy of the phenol compounds of *Arnica* in toxic lesion of the liver] [In Russian]. *Farmakol Toksikol* 46(2):102–106.

McGuffin, M., C. Hobbs, R. Upton, A. Goldberg. 1997. American Herbal Product Association's *Botanical Safety Handbook.* Boca Raton: CRC Press.

Schulz, V., R. Hansel., V. Tyler. 1998. *Rational Phytotherapy: A Physician's Guide to Herbal Medicine.* New York: Springer Verlag.

Vanhaelen-Fastré, R. 1968. *Cnicus benedictus:* Separation of antimicrobial constituents. *Plant Med Phytother* (2):294–299.

———. 1972. [Antibiotic and cytotoxic activity of cnicin isolated from *Cnicus benedictus* L.] [In French]. *J Pharm Belg* 27(6):683–688.

———. 1973. [Constitution and antibiotical properties of the essential oil of *Cnicus benedictus*] [In French]. *Planta Med* 24(2):165–175.

Vickers, A.J. 1998. Homeopathic Arnica 30X is ineffective for muscle soreness after long-distance running: a randomized, double-blind, placebo-controlled trial. *Clin J Pain* 14(3):227–231.

Additional Resources

Baillargeon, L., J. Drouin, L. Desjardins, D. Leroux, D. Audet. 1993. [The effects of *Arnica montana* on blood coagulation. Randomized controlled trial] [In French]. *Can Fam Physician* (39):2362–2367.

Hausen, B.M. 1978. Identification of the allergens of *Arnica montana* L. *Contact Dermatitis* 4(5):308.

Kaziro, G.S. 1984. Metronidazole (Flagyl) and *Arnica Montana* in the prevention of post-surgical complications, a comparative placebo-controlled clinical trial. *Br J Oral Maxillofac Surg* 22(1):42–49.

Rossetti, V., A. Lombard, P. Sancin, M. Buffa. 1987. Characterization of *Arnica montana* L. flowers. *Boll Chim Farm* 126(11):458–461.

Rudzki, E. and Z. Grzywa. 1977. Dermatitis from *Arnica montana. Contact Dermatitis* 3(5):281–282.

Schroder, H. et al. 1990. Helenalin and 11 alpha, 13-dihydrohelenalin, two constituents from *Arnica montana* L., inhibit human platelet function via thiol-dependent pathways. *Thromb Res* 57(6):839–845.

Tveiten, D., S. Bruseth, C.F. Borchgrevink, K. Lohne. 1991. [Effect of Arnica D 30 during hard physical exertion. A double-blind randomized trial during the Oslo Marathon] [In Norwegian]. *Tidsskr Nor Laegeforen* 111(30):3630–3631.

Wagner, H. et al. 1991. [Immunologic studies of plant combination preparations. *In-vitro* and *in-vivo* studies on the stimulation of phagocytosis] [In German]. *Arzneimforsch* 41(10):1072–1076.

Wagner, H., S. Bladt, E.M. Zgainski. 1983. *Plant Drug Analysis.* Berlin-Heidelberg: Springer Verlag.

Willuhn, G. and H.D. Herrman. 1978. *Pharm Ztg* 123.

This material was adapted from *The Complete German Commission E Monographs—Therapeutic Guide to Herbal Medicines.* M. Blumenthal, W.R. Busse, A. Goldberg, J. Gruenwald, T. Hall, C.W. Riggins, R.S. Rister (eds.) S. Klein and R.S. Rister (trans.). 1998. Austin: American Botanical Council; Boston: Integrative Medicine Communications.

1) The Overview section is new information.
2) Description, Chemistry and Pharmacology, Uses, Contraindications, Side Effects, Interactions with Other Drugs, and Dosage sections have been drawn from the original work. Additional information has been added in some or all of these sections, as noted with references.
3) The dosage for equivalent preparations (tea infusion, fluidextract, and tincture) have been provided based on the following example:
   Unless otherwise prescribed: 2 g per day of [powdered, crushed, cut or whole] [plant part]
   Infusion: 2 g in 150 ml of water
   Fluidextract 1:1 (g/ml): 2 ml
   Tincture 1:5 (g/ml): 10 ml
4) The References and Additional Resources sections are new sections. Additional Resources are not cited in the monograph but are included for research purposes.

ARTICHOKE LEAF

Latin Name:
Cynara scolymus

Pharmacopeial Name:
Cynarae folium

Other Names:
globe artichoke

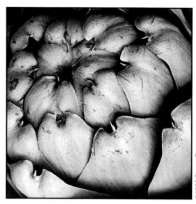

©1999 Steven Foster

Overview

Globe artichoke is a perennial herb native to Mediterranean southern Europe and northern Africa and the Canary Islands (Leung and Foster, 1996). Its cultivation in Europe dates back to ancient Greece and Rome (Grieve, 1971). It is cultivated in North Africa as well as in other subtropical regions (Iwu, 1993). The material of commerce comes as whole or cut dried leaves obtained mainly from southern Europe and northern Africa (BHP, 1996).

Artichoke leaf has been used as a choleretic and diuretic in traditional European medicine since Roman times (Bianchini and Corbetta, 1977). Traditional medicinal uses of artichoke pertain to liver function. Artichoke leaf is considered choleretic (bile increasing), hepatoprotective, cholesterol-reducing, and diuretic (Kirchhoff et al., 1994). In Germany, it is used today as a choleretic (BAnz, 1998; Meyer-Buchtela, 1999) for its lipid-lowering, hepato-stimulating, and appetite-stimulating actions (Hänsel et al., 1992–1994; Meyer-Buchtela, 1999). In German pediatric medicine, herbs with a relatively low bitter value (800–2000), such as artichoke leaf, are considered suitable for the treatment of appetite disorders (Schilcher, 1997).

Modern human studies have investigated its choleretic activity for treatment of digestive disorders (Kirchhoff et al., 1994). An article by Kraft summarized various post-marketing surveillance studies conducted on patients with dyspepsia and/or diseases of the liver or bile duct. The studies included anywhere from 417 to 557 patients and treatment duration ranged from 4 to 6 weeks. Statistically significant reduction of symptoms (e.g., abdominal pain, bloating, flatulence, and nausea) were reported for the surveillance studies referred to in this paper. Artichoke preparations were well tolerated (up to 95% of cases) with a low rate of side-effects (Kraft, 1997).

In one clinical trial, 20 men with acute or chronic metabolic disorders were separated at random into two groups. The test group was given a standardized artichoke extract (Hepar SL forte, Seturner, Germany) of 320 mg in a capsule dissolved in 50 ml water, taken intraduodenally. Results were assessed by measuring intraduodenal bile secretions, which increased 127.3% after 30 minutes, 151.5% after 60 minutes, and 94.3% after 90 minutes. The relative differences for the placebo were significant. The researchers concluded that artichoke extract can be used for the treatment of digestive disorders characterized by poor assimilation of fat due to insufficient bile secretion. No adverse side effects were observed (Kirchhoff et al., 1994).

Pharmacopeial grade artichoke leaf consists of the dried radical leaves of *Cynara scolymus* L. Botanical identification is carried out by thin-layer chromatography (TLC), macroscopic and microscopic evaluations, and organoleptic tests. The dried leaf must contain not less than 25% water-soluble extractive (BHP, 1996).

Description

Artichoke leaf consists of the fresh or dried leaf of *C. scolymus* L. [Fam. Asteraceae] and its preparations in effective dosage. The preparation contains caffeoylquinic acid derivatives such as cynarin and bitter principles.

Chemistry and Pharmacology

Artichoke leaf contains up to 2% phenolic acids, mainly 3-caffeoylquinic acid (chlorogenic acid), plus 1,5-di-O-caffeoylquinic acid (cynarin), and caffeic acid; 0–4% bitter sesquiterpene lactones of which 47–83% is cynaropicrin; 0.1–1.0% flavonoids including the glycosides luteolin-7-β-rutinoside (scolymoside), luteolin-7-β-D-glucoside and luteolin-4-β-D-glucoside; phytosterols (taraxasterol); sugars; inulin; enzymes; and a volatile oil consisting mainly of the sesquiterpenes β-selinene and caryophyllene (Hänsel et al., 1992–1994; Leung and Foster, 1996; Meyer-Buchtela, 1999; Newall et al., 1996).

The Commission E reported choleretic activity.

The *British Herbal Pharmacopoeia* reported hepatic action (BHP, 1996). *In vivo*, artichoke leaf has demonstrated hepatoprotective and hepatostimulating properties (Adzet et al., 1987; Maros et al., 1966). *The Merck Index* reported the therapeutic category of cynarin, an active principle of artichoke, as choleretic (Budavari, 1996). The *African Pharmacopoeia* reported diuretic and anti-atherosclerotic actions (Iwu, 1993). Artichoke leaf has shown cholesterol-lowering and lipid-lowering activity in rats and humans (Lietti, 1977). Human studies have validated carminative, spasmolytic, antiemetic, and choleretic actions (Kraft, 1997).

Uses

The Commission E approved artichoke leaf for dyspeptic problems.

The *African Pharmacopoeia* indicates its use for the treatment of liver dysfunction (Iwu, 1993). Preparations of artichoke have been used for bloating, nausea, and impairment of digestion (Bruneton, 1995). It is specifically indicated for "dyspeptic syndrome" though its proven lipid-lowering actions suggest that it may also be useful as a prophylactic against atherosclerosis (Kraft, 1997).

Contraindications

Known allergies to artichokes and related species (Asteraceae or Compositae).

Obstruction of bile ducts.

In case of gallstones, use only after consulting a physician.

Side Effects

None known.

Use During Pregnancy and Lactation

No restrictions known.

Interactions with Other Drugs

None known.

Dosage and Administration

Unless otherwise prescribed: 6 g per day of dried cut leaves, pressed juice of fresh plant, and other equivalent galenical preparations for internal use.
Leaf: 2 g, three times daily.
Infusion: Artichoke leaf is not typically prepared as an infusion.
Dry extract 12:1 (w/w): 0.5 g single daily dose.
Fluidextract 1:1 (g/ml): 2 ml, three times daily.
Tincture 1:5 (g/ml): 6 ml, three times daily.

References

Adzet, T. et al. 1987. Action of an artichoke extract against CC1₄-induced hepatotoxicity in rats. *Acta Pharm Jugosl* 37:183–187.
BAnz. See *Bundesanzeiger*.
Bianchini, F. and F. Corbetta. 1977. *Health Plants of the World—Atlas of Medicinal Plants*. New York: Newsweek Books.

British Herbal Pharmacopoeia (BHP). 1996. Exeter, U.K.: British Herbal Medicine Association.

Bruneton, J. 1995. *Pharmacognosy, Phytochemistry, Medicinal Plants.* Paris: Lavoisier Publishing.

Budavari, S. (ed.). 1996. *The Merck Index: An Encyclopedia of Chemicals, Drugs, and Biologicals,* 12th ed. Whitehouse Station, N.J.: Merck & Co, Inc. 467-468.

Bundesanzeiger (BAnz). 1998. Monographien der Kommission E (Zulassungs- und Aufbereitungskommission am BGA für den humanmed. Bereich, phytotherapeutische Therapierichtung und Stoffgruppe). Köln: Bundesgesundheitsamt (BGA).

Grieve, M. 1971. *A Modern Herbal.* New York: Dover Publications, Inc. 60.

Hänsel, R., K. Keller, H. Rimpler, G. Schneider (eds.). 1992–1994. *Hagers Handbuch der Pharmazeutischen Praxis,* 5th ed. Vol. 4–6. Berlin-Heidelberg: Springer Verlag.

Iwu, M.M. 1993. *Handbook of African Medicinal Plants.* Boca Raton: CRC Press. 167–168.

Kirchhoff, R. et al. 1994. Increase in choleresis by means of artichoke extract. *Phytomedicine* 1:107–115.

Kraft, K. 1997. Artichoke leaf extract—recent findings reflecting effects on lipid metabolism, liver, and gastrointestinal tracts. *Phytomedicine* 4(4):369–378.

Leung, A.Y. and S. Foster. 1996. *Encyclopedia of Common Natural Ingredients Used in Food, Drugs, and Cosmetics,* 2nd ed. New York: John Wiley & Sons, Inc. 42–44.

Lietti, A. 1977. Choleretic and cholesterol lowering properties of two artichoke extracts. *Fitoterapia* (48):153-158.

Maros T, G. Racz, B. Katonai, V.V. Kovacs. 1966. Wirkungen der *Cynara scolymus*-Extrakte auf die Regeneration der Rattenleber [Effects of *Cynara scolymus* extracts on the regeneration of rat liver. 1]. *Arzneimforsch* 16(2):127–129.

Meyer-Buchtela, E. 1999. *Tee-Rezepturen—Ein Handbuch für Apotheker und Ärzte.* Stuttgart: Deutscher Apotheker Verlag.

Newall, C.A., L.A. Anderson, J.D. Phillipson. 1996. *Herbal Medicines: A Guide for Health-Care Professionals.* London: The Pharmaceutical Press. 37–38.

Schilcher, H. 1997. *Phytotherapy in Paediatrics: Handbook for Physicians and Pharmacists.* Stuttgart: Medpharm Scientific Publishers. 45–46.

Additional Resources

Adzet, T., J. Camarasa, J.C. Laguna. 1987. Hepatoprotective activity of polyphenolic compounds from *Cynara scolymus* against CCl4 toxicity in isolated rat hepatocytes. *J Nat Prod* 50(4):612–617.

Fintelmann, V. and H.G. Menssen. 1996. Artischockenblätterextrakt - Aktuelle Erkenntnis zur Wirkung als Lipidsenker und Antidyspeptium. *Dtsch Apoth Ztg* 136(17):1405–1414.

Mills, S.Y. 1985. *The Dictionary of Modern Herbalism.* Wellingborough: Thorsons.

Mitchell, J.C. 1975. *Recent Advances in Phytochemistry,* Vol. 9. New York: Plenum.

Reynolds, J.E.F. (ed.). 1982. *Martindale: The Extra Pharmacopoeia,* 28th ed. London: The Pharmaceutical Press.

Wren, R.C. 1988. *Potter's New Cyclopaedia of Botanical Drugs and Preparations.* Essex: The C.W. Daniel Company Ltd.

This material was adapted from *The Complete German Commission E Monographs—Therapeutic Guide to Herbal Medicines.* M. Blumenthal, W.R. Busse, A. Goldberg, J. Gruenwald, T. Hall, C.W. Riggins, R.S. Rister (eds.) S. Klein and R.S. Rister (trans.). 1998. Austin: American Botanical Council; Boston: Integrative Medicine Communications.

1) The Overview section is new information.

2) Description, Chemistry and Pharmacology, Uses, Contraindications, Side Effects, Interactions with Other Drugs, and Dosage sections have been drawn from the original work. Additional information has been added in some or all of these sections, as noted with references.

3) The dosage for equivalent preparations (tea infusion, fluidextract, and tincture) have been provided based on the following example:
   Unless otherwise prescribed: 2 g per day of [powdered, crushed, cut or whole] [plant part]
   Infusion: 2 g in 150 ml of water
   Fluidextract 1:1 (g/ml): 2 ml
   Tincture 1:5 (g/ml): 10 ml

4) The References and Additional Resources sections are new sections. Additional Resources are not cited in the monograph but are included for research purposes.

Asparagus Root

Latin Name:
Asparagus officinalis

Pharmacopeial Name:
Asparagi rhizoma

Other Names:
sparrowgrass

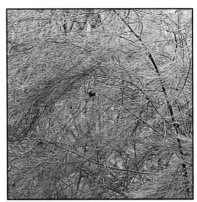

©1999 Steven Foster

Overview

Asparagus, brought to the United States by Eurasian colonists and commonly called sparrowgrass, is widely cultivated as a food crop. Its medical applications are less well known, despite Commission E approval of root use to irrigate the urinary tract. The perennial can produce edible shoots for up to 30 years (Stephens, 1994). These shoots provide fiber and vitamins A and C (Hamilton and Whitney, 1982). There is also a peculiar urinary odor following ingestion, that can be detected only in individuals who have inherited a particular autosomal dominant trait (Mitchell et al., 1987).

Shoots are harvested in the spring for a few months and then left to develop into a fern-like plant, which prepares the roots for the next year's production. Female plants produce red berries that turn black in the fall. In the United States, in which 90% of commercial production occurs in Massachusetts, New Jersey, Washington, and California, both a dark green and a light green-to-whitish variety are cultivated (Stephens, 1994). Rarely does this production result in a medicinal preparation.

In Europe and Asia, however, all parts of the asparagus plant, the shoots and in particular the roots, or crowns, as they are called, have a medicinal history. Root preparations are diuretic and laxative. Folk medicinal use of asparagus root includes treatment of heart disease, hypertension, and rheumatism (Leung and Foster, 1996; Wren, 1988). Home skin formulas reportedly employ asparagus shoots to rid the face of dirt and acne. The red berries (on female plants) were regarded as a contraceptive (Leung and Foster, 1996). India's *Asparagus* species, *A. racemosus*, or *shatavari*, which means "she who has a hundred husbands," is used to strengthen the female reproductive system, and is also administered for diuretic and anti-inflammatory purposes by traditional Ayurvedic practitioners (Lad and Frawley, 1986).

The fructo-oligosaccharides, the most frequently studied constituents in asparagus, alter fecal microflora beneficially, particularly in elderly patients (Mitsuoka et al., 1987). Shoot saponin constituents have been found to have some activity against human leukemia HL-60 cells *in vitro* (Leung and Foster, 1996; Shao et al., 1996). Immune stimulant effects of roots may benefit cancer patients receiving chemotherapy (Thatte and Dahanukar, 1988). Root constituents may be found, as were those in Chinese asparagus, *A. cochinchinensis*, to inhibit SA (Boik, 1995) and mouse S-180 leukemia cells (Huang, 1993). In other studies, Indian shatavari root was found to reduce gastric emptying time comparably to metoclopramide (Dalvi et al., 1990), an effect that may relieve heartburn. Animal studies show that shatavari increases macrophage activity and prevents intraperitoneal adhesions in laboratory animals, an effect that may prevent postoperative intraperitoneal adhesions (Rege et al., 1989).

Description

Asparagus root consists of the rhizome of *Asparagus officinalis* L. [Fam. Liliaceae], as well as its preparations in effective dosage. The rhizome contains saponins.

Chemistry and Pharmacology

The main constituents include inulin, asparagusic acid, and eight fructo-oligosaccharides (Leung and Foster, 1996). The two glycosidic bitter principles, officinalisnin-I and officinalisnin-II, are isolated from the dried root and yield β-sitosterol, sarsasapogenin, and nine steroidal glycosides (named asparagosides A to I, in order of increasing polarity) (Leung and Foster, 1996). Other constituents include asparagine, tyrosine, succinic acid, arginine, α-aminodimethyl-γ-butyrothetin (a methylsulfonium derivative of methionine), fat, and sugar (Stecher, 1968). The roots are thought to possess diuretic and hypotensive properties, and to enhance the renal elimination of water (Bruneton, 1995; Leung and Foster, 1996).

The Commission E reported a diuretic effect in animals.

Uses

The Commission E approved the use of asparagus root in irrigation therapy for inflammatory diseases of the urinary tract and for prevention of kidney stones. Traditionally, the root has been used as diuretic, laxative, and to treat neuritis and rheumatism (Leung and Foster, 1996).

Contraindications

Inflammatory kidney diseases.
Note: No irrigation therapy if edema exists because of functional heart or kidney disorders.

Side Effects

In rare cases, allergic skin reactions.

Use During Pregnancy and Lactation

No restrictions known.

Interactions with Other Drugs

None known.

Dosage and Administration

Unless otherwise prescribed: 45–60 g per day of cut rhizome.
Infusion: 45–60 g of cut herb in 150 ml water.
Fluidextract 1:1 (g/ml): 45–60 ml.
Tincture 1:5 (g/ml): 225–300 ml.

References

Boik, J. 1995. *Cancer and Natural Medicine: A Textbook of Basic Science and Clinical Research.* Princeton, Minnesota: Oregon Medical Press.

Bruneton, J. 1995. *Pharmacognosy, Phytochemistry, Medicinal Plants.* Paris: Lavoisier Publishing.

Dalvi, S.S., P.M. Nadkarni, K.C. Gupta. 1990. Effect of *Asparagus racemosus* (Shatavari) on gastric emptying time in normal healthy volunteers. *J Postgrad Med* 36(2):91–94.

Hamilton, E.M.N. and E.N. Whitney. 1982. *Nutrition: Concepts and Controversies,* 2nd ed. New York: West Publishing.

Huang, K.C. 1993. *The Pharmacology of Chinese Herbs.* Boca Raton: CRC Press.

Lad, V. and D. Frawley. 1986. *The Yoga of Herbs.* Sante Fe, N.M.: Lotus Press.

Leung, A.Y. and S. Foster. 1996. *Encyclopedia of Common Natural Ingredients Used in Food, Drugs and Cosmetics,* 2nd ed. New York: John Wiley & Sons, Inc.

Mitchell, S.C., R.H. Waring, D. Land, W.V. Thorpe. 1987. Odorous urine following *Asparagus* ingestion in man. *Experientia* 43(4):382–383.

Mitsuoka, T., H. Hidaka, T. Eida. 1987. Effect of fructo-oligosaccharides on intestinal microflora. *Nahrung* 31(5–6):427–436.

Rege, N.N. et al. 1989. Immunotherapeutic modulation of intraperitoneal adhesions by *Asparagus racemosus. J Postgrad Med* 35(4):199–203.

Shao, Y. et al. 1996. Anti-tumor activity of the crude saponins obtained from asparagus. *Cancer Lett* 104(1): 31–36.

Stecher, P.G. (ed.). 1968. *The Merck Index: An Encyclopedia of Chemicals and Drugs,* 8th ed. Rahway, N.J.: Merck & Co., Inc.

Stephens, J.M. 1994. Asparagus—*Asparagus officinalis* L. Fact Sheet HS-546, Horticultural Sciences Department, Florida Cooperative Extention Service, Institute of Food and Agricultural Sciences, University of Florida.

Thatte, U.M. and S.A. Dahanukar. 1988. Comparative study of immunomodulating activity of Indian medicinal plants, lithium carbonate and glucan. *Methods Find Exp Clin Pharmacol* 10(10):639–644.

Wren, R.C. 1988. *Potter's New Cyclopaedia of Botanical Drugs and Preparations.* Essex: The C.W. Daniel Company Ltd.

Additional Resources

Jiangsu Institute of Modern Medicine. 1977. *Zhong Yao Da Ci Dian* (Encyclopedia of Chinese Materia Medica), Vols. 1–3. Shanghai: Shanghai Scientific and Technical Publications.

This material was adapted from *The Complete German Commission E Monographs—Therapeutic Guide to Herbal Medicines.* M. Blumenthal, W.R. Busse, A. Goldberg, J. Gruenwald, T. Hall, C.W. Riggins, R.S. Rister (eds.) S. Klein and R.S. Rister (trans.). 1998. Austin: American Botanical Council; Boston: Integrative Medicine Communications.

1) The Overview section is new information.
2) Description, Chemistry and Pharmacology, Uses, Contraindications, Side Effects, Interactions with Other Drugs, and Dosage sections have been drawn from the original work. Additional information has been added in some or all of these sections, as noted with references.
3) The dosage for equivalent preparations (tea infusion, fluidextract, and tincture) have been provided based on the following example:
   Unless otherwise prescribed: 2 g per day of [powdered, crushed, cut or whole] [plant part]
   Infusion: 2 g in 150 ml of water
   Fluidextract 1:1 (g/ml): 2 ml
   Tincture 1:5 (g/ml): 10 ml
4) The References and Additional Resources sections are new sections. Additional Resources are not cited in the monograph but are included for research purposes.

BILBERRY FRUIT

Latin Name:
Vaccinium myrtillus

Pharmacopeial Name:
Myrtilli fructus

Other Names:
dwarf bilberry, European blueberry,
huckleberry, whortleberry

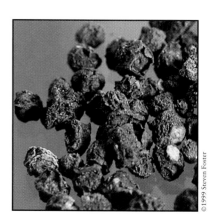

©1999 Steven Foster

Overview

Bilberry is a small deciduous shrublet found in underbrush and barren fields throughout central and northern Europe, northern Asia, and North America (Wichtl, 1996). In North America, it is found in montane and subalpine regions from British Columbia to Alberta, south to Arizona and New Mexico (Leung and Foster, 1996). The material of commerce is obtained from Albania, Poland, the former Yugoslavia, and the former U.S.S.R. (Wichtl and Bisset, 1994). The common name bilberry is derived from the Danish word *bollebar,* which means dark berry (Grieve, 1979).

Bilberry fruit has been used in traditional European medicine for nearly one thousand years (Morazzoni and Bombardelli, 1996), reported by twelfth century German herbalist Hildegarde von Bingen (1098–1179 C.E.) and later by sixteenth century herbalist Hieronymos Bock. Traditionally, strong decoctions of the dried fruit have been used as an astringent for treatment of diarrhea and dysentery (Bone and Morgan, 1997; Foster, 1996). Bilberry preparations were also administered to help stop the flow of breast milk, as well as to relieve scurvy and dysuria (Grieve, 1979). For these purposes, fruits were dried in the sun and eventually prepared as teas or syrups (Tyler, 1994).

In Germany, bilberry fruit is approved in the Commission E monographs (BAnz, 1998), listed in the *German Drug Codex* (DAC, 1986), and the tea form is official in the German Standard Licenses (Braun et al., 1997). Due to its tannin content, it is used internally to treat acute diarrhea, particularly in children, and externally to treat mild inflammation of oral mucous membranes. Bilberry is used as a component in a few astringent tea preparations (e.g., Stopftee Fides) (Wichtl and Bisset, 1994). A mother tincture (1:10) of the fresh, ripe fruit is also official in the *German Homeopathic Pharmacopoeia* (GHP, 1993). However, in other parts of Europe, particularly in Italy, fruit preparations are used to treat microcirculatory disorders, which include varicose veins, atherosclerosis, venous insufficiency, and degenerative retinal conditions, such as macular degeneration, glaucoma, and cataracts (Leung and Foster, 1996; Morazzoni and Bombardelli, 1996; Tyler, 1994). Possible mechanisms of action for its effects on ophthalmic conditions include its ability to protect against the breakdown of rhodopsin (retinal purple), a light sensitive pigment located in the rods of the retina, and its ability to regenerate rhodopsin. It may also provide vasoprotection by decreasing capillary fragility and permeability (Bone and Morgan, 1997; Regtop, 1998).

Bilberry anthocyanidins have demonstrated a variety of physiological effects. They may prevent angina episodes as exhibited by the prevention of lactate dehydrogenase liberation from cardiac isoenzymes in *in vitro* experiments (Leung and Foster, 1996). Retinal protection may be aided by anthocyanidinic retinal phosphoglucomutase and glucose-6-phosphatase inhibition (Cluzel et al., 1969). The anthocyanidins also stimulate prolonged capillary resistance, and are vasoprotective, antiedematous, and vasodilative (Lietti et al., 1976). They inhibit platelet aggregation and thrombus formation, interacting with vascular prostaglandins (Leung and Foster, 1996). In one study, an injected proprietary bilberry preparation altered the rhythmic changes in the diameter of mouse cheek pouch and terminal arterioles, which was beneficial to microvascular blood flow and interstitial fluid formation (Colantuoni et al., 1991). These findings, however, have largely employed animal or *in vitro* conditions, and have not been replicated with well-designed human trials (Tyler, 1994).

Several human clinical studies have been found in the literature investigating possible new uses for bilberry not mentioned in the Commission E monograph, particularly visual dysfunctions, including those caused by impaired microcirculation and diabetes mellitus. Bilberry fruit preparations have been investigated for their effects on vision acuity in dim light (Jayle and Aubert, 1964), on patients with pigmentary retinitis when taken with beta-carotene (Fiorini et al., 1965), on night vision in normal subjects (Jayle et al., 1965), on patients with diabetic retinopathy when taken in combination with beta-carotene (Sevin and Cuendet, 1966), on patients with significant hemeralopia (diminished vision in bright light) (Zavarise, 1968), on patients with macular degeneration, diabetic retinopathy, retinal inflammation, or retinitis pigmentosa (Neumann, 1971), and on patients with progressive myopia (Politzer, 1977). Later research investigated bilberry's capillarotropic activity in patients with venous diseases (Ghiringhelli et al., 1978), diabetic patients with microangiopathy (Lagrue et al., 1979), microcirculatory function in patients with polyneuritis due to vascular insufficiency (Pennarola et al., 1980), patients with various retinopathies (Scharrer and Ober, 1981), patients with myopia, glaucoma, or retinitis pigmentosa (Caselli, 1985), patients with diabetic and/or hypertensive retinopathy (Perossini et al., 1987), and its effects on the progression of cataract formation in patients with senile cortical cataracts when taken in combination with vitamin E (Bravetti, 1989).

German pharmacopeial grade bilberry fruit consists of the whole, dried, ripe fruit of *Vaccinium myrtillus* L. An identity test is described wherein the fruit is first extracted with water, in order to extract the invert sugars. Subsequently, the anthocyanin glycosides are extracted with methanol. The anthocyanidins are then obtained by hydrolysis with hydrochloric acid (DAC, 1986; Wichtl, 1996). Macroscopic and microscopic examinations are carried out as well as a thin-layer chromatography (TLC) test for detection of anthocyan pigments. A test for adulteration with the fruit of bog bilberry (*V. uliginosum* L.) is carried out (DAC, 1986; Wichtl and Bisset, 1994; Wichtl, 1996). As bilberry is typically used in its whole form, macroscopic verification is the most essential requirement (Wichtl and Bisset, 1994). The *Austrian Pharmacopoeia* requires that it contain not less than 50% water-soluble extractive (ÖAB, 1983; Wichtl and Bisset, 1994). Additionally, the *Swiss Pharmacopoeia* requires that it contain not less than 1.5% tannins (Ph.Helv.VII, 1987; Wichtl and Bisset, 1994).

Description

Bilberry consists of the dried, ripe fruit of *V. myrtillus* L. [Fam. Ericaceae], and its preparations in effective dosage. The fruit contains tannins, anthocyanins, and flavonoid glycosides.

Chemistry and Pharmacology

Bilberry fruit contains 5–10% catechin tannins; approximately 30% invert sugar; over 1% fruit acids (Wichtl, 1996); flavonol glycosides including astragalin, hyperoside, isoquercitrin, and quercitrin; phenolic acids (e.g., caffeic and chlorogenic acids) (Azar et al., 1987; Friedrich and Schönert, 1973);

pectins; triterpenes (0.25% ursol acid); polyphenols (0.5% anthocyans) (Hänsel et al., 1992–1994; Meyer-Buchtela, 1999), such as the procyanidins B1–B4 (Leung and Foster, 1996; Morazzoni and Bombardelli, 1996), and particularly the anthocyanidins malvidin, cyanidin, and delphinidin (Wichtl, 1996) bonded to one of three carbohydrates (e.g., glucose, galactose, arabinose) (Barrette, 1999), for example, delphinidine-3-O-arabinoside, delphinidine-3-O-galactoside, and delphinidine-3-O-glucoside. The anthocyanosides (anthocyanins) are aglycones bound to one of three glycosides (Cunio, 1993). The anthocyanoside content increases as the fruit ripens whereas the catechin tannins and dimeric proanthocyanidins (B1–B4) decrease with the progression of ripeness (Morazzoni and Bombardelli, 1996).

The Commission E reported astringent activity.

Bilberry has shown vasoprotective, antiedematous, antioxidant, antiinflammatory, and astringent actions (Bone and Morgan, 1997). It has demonstrated free radical scavenging and inhibition of cAMP phosphodiesterase actions (Bruneton, 1995; Ferretti et al., 1988). *In vitro* and *in vivo* clinical studies show platelet aggregation and stimulation of vascular prostacyclin. Preliminary human trials indicate vasoprotective properties. Bilberry anthocyanins regenerate rhodopsin and are indicated in treatment of poor night vision, macular degeneration, glaucoma, and cataracts (Bruneton, 1995).

Uses

The Commission E approved the internal use of bilberry to treat non-specific, acute diarrhea, and local therapy for mild inflammation of the mucous membranes of mouth and throat.

The German Standard License indicates the use of bilberry fruit tea as a supportive therapy in the treatment of acute, non-specific diarrhea in children and adults (Braun et al., 1997; Wichtl and Bisset, 1994). Bilberry fruit extracts may offer symptomatic relief for vascular disorders including capillary weakness, venous insufficiency, and hemorrhoids. It is also used as a secondary treatment for spasmodic colitis (Bruneton, 1995).

Contraindications

None known.

Side Effects

None known.

Use During Pregnancy and Lactation

No restrictions known.

Interactions with Other Drugs

None known.

Dosage and Administration

Unless otherwise prescribed: 20–60 g of dried ripe fruit per day for infusions or decoctions, as well as other galenical preparations for internal use.

External: 10% decoction or equivalent preparations for local application.

Internal: [Note: According to the *Austrian Pharmacopeia*, the average single dose for bilberry fruit is 5 g (Meyer-Buchtela, 1999; ÖAB, 1991).]

Dried fruit: 4–8 g taken with water, several times daily (Braun et al., 1997; Meyer-Buchtela, 1999; Wichtl and Bisset, 1994).

Decoction: Place 5–10 g crushed dried fruit in 150 ml cold water, bring to a boil for approximately 10 minutes, then strain while hot. Drink cold several times daily until the diarrhea is gone (Braun et al., 1997; Meyer-Buchtela, 1999; Wichtl and Bisset, 1994).

Cold macerate: Soak 5–10 g crushed dried fruit in 150 ml cold water for two hours, allowing the fruit to swell. Drink cold several times daily (Braun et al., 1997; Meyer-Buchtela, 1999; Wichtl and Bisset, 1994).

Fluidextract 1:1 (g/ml): 2–4 ml, three times daily (Anderhuber, 1991; Cunio, 1993).

Dry extract (25% anthocyanosides): 80–160 mg, three times daily (Foster, 1996; Pizzorno and Murray, 1992).

External: Decoction: Place 5–10 g crushed dried fruit in 150 ml cold water, bring to a boil for approximately 10 minutes, then strain while hot (Meyer-Buchtela, 1999; Wichtl and Bisset, 1994).

Gargle mouthwash: Containing 10% decoction.

Duration of administration: If diarrhea persists for more than 3 to 4 days, consult a physician.

References

Anderhuber, R. 1991. *Vaccinium myrtillus. Aust J Med Herbalism* 3:13–14.

Azar, M., E. Verette, S. Brun. 1987. Identification of some phenolic compounds in bilberry juice *Vaccinium myrtillus. J Food Sci* 52(5):1255–1257.

BAnz. See *Bundesanzeiger.*

Barrette, E.P. 1999. Bilberry fruit extract for night vision. *Alternative Medicine Alert™* 2(2):20–21.

Bone, K. and M. Morgan. 1997. Bilberry—The Vision Herb. *MediHerb Professional Review* 59:1–4.

Braun, R. et al. 1997. *Standardzulassungen für Fertigarzneimittel—Text and Kommentar.* Stuttgart: Deutscher Apotheker Verlag.

Bravetti, G. 1989. Preventive medical treatment of senile cataract with vitamin E and anthocyanosides: clinical evaluation. *Ann Ottalmol Clin Ocul* 115:109.

Bruneton, J. 1995. *Pharmacognosy, Phytochemistry, Medicinal Plants.* Paris: Lavoisier Publishing.

Bundesanzeiger (BAnz). 1998. Monographien der Kommission E (Zulassungs- und Aufbereitungskommission am BGA für den humanmed. Bereich, phytotherapeutische Therapierichtung und Stoffgruppe). Köln: Bundesgesundheitsamt (BGA).

Caselli, L. 1985. Studio clinico ed elettroretinografico sull'attivita degli antocianosidi [Clinical and electroretinographic study on activity of anthocyanosides]. *Arch Med Int (Parma)* 37:29–35.

Cluzel, C., P. Bastide, P. Tronche. 1969. [Phosphoglucomutase and glucose-6-phosphatase activities of the retina and anthocyanoside extracts from *Vaccinium myrtillus* (study *in vitro* and *in vivo*)] [In French]. *C R Seances Soc Biol Fil* 163(1):147–150.

Colantuoni, A., S. Bertuglia, M.J. Magistretti, L. Donato. 1991. Effects of *Vaccinium myrtillus* anthocyanosides on arterial vasomation. *Arzneimforsch* 41(9):905–909.

Cunio, L. 1993. *Vaccinium myrtillus. Aust J Med Herbalism* 5(4):81–85.

Deutscher Arzneimittel-Codex (DAC). 1986. Stuttgart: Deutscher Apotheker Verlag.

Ferretti, C., M.J. Magistretti, A. Robotti, P. Ghi, E. Genazzani. 1988. Vaccinium myrtillus anthocyanosides are inhibitors of cAMP and cGMP phosphodiesterases. *Pharm Res Comm* 20(11):150.

Fiorini, G., A. Biancacci, F.M. Graziano. 1965. Modificazioni perimetriche ed adattometriche dopo ingestione di mirtillina associata a beta-carotene [Perimetric and adaptometric modifications after ingestion of myrtillin associated with beta-carotene]. *Ann Ottalmol Clin Ocul* 91(6):371–386.

Foster, S. 1996. Bilberry: A Long History. *Health Food Business.* August 1996: 40.

Friedrich, V.H. and J. Schönert. 1973. Untersuchungen über einige Inhaltsstoffe der *Blätter* und *Früchte von Vaccinium myrtillus* [Phytochemical investigation of leaves and fruits of *Vaccinium myrtillus*]. *Planta Med* 24(1):90–100.

German Homeopathic Pharmacopoeia (GHP). 1993. Translation of the *Deutsches Homöopathisches Arzneibuch* (HAB 1), 1st ed., 5th suppl. 1991. Stuttgart: Deutscher Apotheker Verlag. 383–384.

Ghiringhelli, C., F. Gregoratti, F. Marastoni. 1978. Attivita capillarotrop di antocianosidi e alto dosaggio nella stasi da flebopatia [Capillarotropic activity of anthocyanosides in high doses in phlebopathic statis]. *Minerva Cardioangiol* 26(4):255–276.

Grieve, M. 1979. *A Modern Herbal.* New York: Dover Publications, Inc.

Hänsel, R., K. Keller, H. Rimpler, G. Schneider (eds.). 1992–1994. *Hagers Handbuch der Pharmazeutischen Praxis,* 5th ed. Vol. 4–6. Berlin-Heidelberg: Springer Verlag.

Jayle, G.E. and L. Aubert. 1964. [Action des glucosides d'anthocyanes sur la vision scotopique et mesopique du sujet normal] [in French]. *Therapie* 19:171.

Jayle, G.E. et al. 1965. [Study concerning the action of anthocyanoside extracts of *Vaccinium Myrtillus* on night vision] [In French]. *Ann Ocul (Paris)* 198(6):556–562.

Lagrue, G. et al. 1979. Pathology of the microcirculation in diabetes and alterations of the biosynthesis of intracellular matrix molecules. *Front Matrix Biol S Karger* 7:324–325.

Leung, A.Y. and S. Foster. 1996. *Encyclopedia of Common Natural Ingredients Used in Food, Drugs, and Cosmetics,* 2nd ed. New York: John Wiley & Sons, Inc. 84–85.

Lietti, A., A. Cristoni, M. Picci. 1976. Studies on *Vaccinium myrtillus* anthocyanosides. I. Vasoprotective and antiinflammatory activity. *Arzneimforsch* 26(5):829–832.

Meyer-Buchtela, E. 1999. *Tee-Rezepturen—Ein Handbuch für Apotheker und Ärzte.* Stuttgart: Deutscher Apotheker Verlag.

Morazzoni, P. and E. Bombardelli. 1996. *Vaccinium myrtillus* L. *Fitoterapia* 67(1):3–29.

Neumann, L. 1971. Therapeutische Versuche mit Anthozyanosiden bei Langzeitbehandlungen in der Augenheilkunde [In German]. *Klin Monatsbl Augenheilkd* 158:592–597.

Österreichisches Arzneibuch, 1st suppl. (ÖAB). 1983. Wien: Verlag der Österreichischen Staatsdruckerei.

Österreichisches Arzneibuch (ÖAB). 1991. Wien: Verlag der Österreichischen Staatsdruckerei.

Pennarola, R. et al. 1980. The therapeutic action of the anthocyanosides in microcirculatory changes due to adhesive-induced polyneuritis. *Gazz Med Ital* 139:485–491.

Perossini, M. et al. 1987. Diabetic and hypertensive retinopathy therapy with *Vaccinium myrtillus* anthocyanosides (Tegens): Double blind placebo controlled clinical trial. *Ann Ottalmol Clin Ocul* 113:1173.

Pharmacopoeia Helvetica, 7th ed. Vol. 1–4. (Ph.Helv.VII). 1987. Bern: Office Central Fédéral des Imprimés et du Matériel.

Pizzorno, J.E. and M.T. Murray. 1992. *A Textbook of Natural Medicine.* Seattle, WA: Bastyr University Publications.

Politzer, M. 1977. [Experiences in the medical treatment of progressive myopia] [In German]. *Klin Monatsbl Augenheilkd* 171(4):616–619.

Regtop, H. 1998. Age related macular degeneration. *Aust J Med Herbalism* 10(2):38–45.

Scharrer, A. and M. Ober. 1981. Anthocyanoside in der Behandlung von Retinopathien [Anthocyanosides in the treatment of retinopathies] [In German]. *Klin Monatsbl Augenheilkd* 178(5):368–389.

Sevin, R. and J.F. Cuendet. 1966. Effets d'une association d'anthocyanosides de myrtille et de beta-carotene sur la resistance capillaire des diabetiques [In French]. *Ophthalmologica* 152:109–117.

Tyler, V.E. 1994. *Herbs of Choice: The Therapeutic Use of Phytomedicinals.* New York: Pharmaceutical Products Press.

Wichtl, M. and N.G. Bisset (eds.). 1994. *Herbal Drugs and Phytopharmaceuticals.* Stuttgart: Medpharm Scientific Publishers. 351–352.

Wichtl, M. 1996. Monographien—Kommentar. In: Braun, R. et al. 1997. *Standardzulassungen für Fertigarzneimittel—Text and Kommentar.* Stuttgart: Deutscher Apotheker Verlag.

Zavarise, G. 1968. Sull'effetto del trattamento prolungato con antocianosidi sul senso luminoso [Effect of prolonged treatment with anthocyanosides on light senstivity]. *Ann Ottalmol Clin Ocul* 94(2):209–214.

Additional Resources

Alexeeff, T. 1998. Circulatory insufficiency: a historical and modern review of three classic herbs. *Aust J Med Herbalism* 10(4):135–140.

Alfieri, R. and P. Sole. 1964. Influence des anthocyanosides administres par voie parenerale sur l'adaptoelectroretinogramme du lapin. *C R Soc Biol* 158:2338.

Benninger, J. 1997. Understanding Bilberry. *Health Supplement Retailer.* March 1997: 54.

Bettini, V. et al. 1984. Interactions between *Vaccinium myrtillus* anthocyanosides and serotonin on splenic artery smooth muscle. *Fitoterapia* 55(4):201–208.

———. 1984. Interactions between *Vaccinium myrtillus* anthocyanosides on vascular smooth muscle. *Fitoterapia* 55(5):265–272.

Bomser, J., D.L. Madhavi, K. Singletary, M.A. Smith. 1996. *In vitro* anti-cancer activity of fruit extracts from Vaccinium species. *Planta Med* 62(3):212–216.

Der Marderosian, A. (ed.). 1999. *The Review of Natural Products.* St. Louis: Facts and Comparisons.

Detre, Z., H. Jellinek, R. Miskulin. 1986. Studies on vascular permeability in hypertension: action of anthocyanosides. *Clin Physiol Biochem* 4(2):143–149.

This material was adapted from *The Complete German Commission E Monographs—Therapeutic Guide to Herbal Medicines.* M. Blumenthal, W.R. Busse, A. Goldberg, J. Gruenwald, T. Hall, C.W. Riggins, R.S. Rister (eds.) S. Klein and R.S. Rister (trans.). 1998. Austin: American Botanical Council; Boston: Integrative Medicine Communications.

1) The Overview section is new information.

2) Description, Chemistry and Pharmacology, Uses, Contraindications, Side Effects, Interactions with Other Drugs, and Dosage sections have been drawn from the original work. Additional information has been added in some or all of these sections, as noted with references.

3) The dosage for equivalent preparations (tea infusion, fluidextract, and tincture) have been provided based on the following example:
   Unless otherwise prescribed: 2 g per day of [powdered, crushed, cut or whole] [plant part]
   Infusion: 2 g in 150 ml of water
   Fluidextract 1:1 (g/ml): 2 ml
   Tincture 1:5 (g/ml): 10 ml

4) The References and Additional Resources sections are new sections. Additional Resources are not cited in the monograph but are included for research purposes.

Mian, E. et al. 1977. Anthocyanosides and microvessel walls: new findings on the mechanism of action of their protective effect in syndromes due to abnormal capillary fragility. *Min Med* 68:3565.

Morazzoni, P. and M.J. Magistretti. 1990. Activity of bilberry, an anthocyanoside complex from *Vaccinium myrtillus* (VMA), on platelet aggregation and adhesiveness. *Fitoterapia* 61(1):13–21.

Orsucci, P.L. et al. 1983. Treatment of diabetic retinopathy with anthocyanosides: a preliminary report. *Clin Oc* 5:377.

Repossi, P., R. Malagola, C. De Cadilhac. 1987. The role of anthocyanosides on vascular permeability in diabetic retinopathy. *Ann Ottalmol Clin Ocul 357.*

Wichtl, M. (ed.). 1989. *Teedrogen,* 2nd ed. Stuttgart: Wissenschaftliche Verlagsgesellschaft.

BLACK COHOSH ROOT

Latin Name:
Cimicifuga racemosa

Pharmacopeial Name:
Cimicifugae racemosae rhizoma

Other Names:
black snakeroot, rattleroot

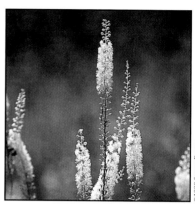

©1999 Steven Foster

Overview

Black cohosh is a plant native to eastern North America. The plant is found in rich, shady woods ranging from Maine to Ontario, and from Wisconsin south to Georgia and Missouri. Native Americans used the rhizome of black cohosh for general malaise, kidney ailments, malaria, rheumatism, sore throat, and for conditions specific to women, such as menstrual irregularities and childbirth. Black cohosh was adopted and used frequently by early settlers and herbal doctors, and in the 1840s by the Eclectic physicians, who used it for many symptoms, especially those associated with rheumatism and rheumatoid pain. Some of the early patent medicines contained high concentrations of black cohosh, and it was the main ingredient in Lydia Pinkham's famous "Vegetable Compound," drunk by women in the early nineteenth century to relieve menstrual stress and nervous tension (Duke, 1985; Felter, 1922; Snow, 1996). Currently, black cohosh has become the largest-selling herbal dietary supplement in the United States for reducing symptoms associated with menopause. Black cohosh influences the endocrine regulatory systems, with effects similar to one of the milder endogenous estrogens, estriol. For a short duration, it binds weakly with estrogen receptors and is thought to exert its effects on the vaginal lining (Murray, 1997). A lack of estrogen-like (hormonal) effect has been demonstrated, in animal experiments (Einer-Jensen et al., 1996; Freudenstein and Bodinet, 1999) and human pharmacological studies (Liske and Wüstenberg, 1999; Liske et al., 1998).

Modern clinical studies have investigated the therapeutic efficacy and safety of black cohosh extracts for indications of the neurovegetative symptoms caused by menopause. These studies used several internationally recognized and validated scales as controls, including Kupperman's Menopause Index for the quantitative determination of menopausal symptoms, the Self-evaluation Depression Scale, the Profile of Mood States, the Hamilton Anxiety Scale, and the Clinical Global Impression scale (CGI), for evaluating the success and the risk-to-benefit assessment of the treatment. Somatic symptoms were determined using vaginal-cytological controls, such as vaginal smears, and measures of gonadotropin secretion (Beuscher, 1995).

Clinical studies using hormone replacement therapy (HRT) and black cohosh have been published based on a particular product called Remifemin® (Shaper & Brümmer, Germany), standardized on the basis of triterpene glycosides; each tablet contains 1 mg of triterpenes, calculated as 27-deoxyacteine and totaling 40 mg of black cohosh extract. In 1996, nearly ten million monthly units of Remifemin were sold in Germany, Australia, and the United States (Murray, 1997). At least eight clinical studies have been published on the therapeutic effects of Remifemin in treating menopausal symptoms (Foster, 1999) although the total in the literature, according to the Napralert database, is 19 (Farnsworth, 1999).

Two studies examined the efficacy of Remifemin in 86 women with climacteric complaints who were at risk with HRT, or who wanted a natural alternative. One open study treated 36 women who either showed contraindications to HRT or wished to be treated with a hormone-free preparation (Daiber, 1983). They were given liquid Remifemin (40 drops twice daily) for a period of 12 weeks. The decrease in values of the Kupperman index was highly significant in the treatment group, as was the improvement in the most frequent climacteric symptoms. Also highly significant was the positive change in the Clinical Global Impression scale. No side effects or incompatibility reactions were observed during the three-month trial. In the other open study, 50 women with menopausal complaints were also treated with 40 drops twice daily of liquid Remifemin for 12 weeks (Vorberg, 1984). Thirty-nine patients had shown contraindications to HRT, and 11 had refused hormone treatment. Improvements in the somatic findings, neurovegetative and psychic symptoms and signs, and the Profile of Mood State and Clinical Global Impression scales were all rated significant to highly significant in the treatment group. No serious side effects were observed, with only mild gastrointestinal disturbances in four patients, and in no case did the treatment need to be discontinued.

Four studies have compared the efficacy of Remifemin with a placebo, conjugated estrogens, diazepam, estriol, and/or an estrogen-gestagen combination. A 1985 study looked at the efficacy of Remifemin with regard to the symptoms of menopause (neurovegetative, psychological, and somatic disorders) in comparison with hormone treatment or therapy with a psychotropic drug (Warnecke, 1985). In this open, controlled study, 60 patients were given Remifemin liquid (40 drops twice daily), conjugated estrogens (0.625 mg daily), or diazepam (Valium, 2 mg daily) for three months. Standard menopausal symptom indexes showed a clear equivalence of the black cohosh extract to both drugs. The effect of Remifemin liquid on relieving the depressive mood and anxiety associated with menopause was far superior to either the conjugated estrogens or diazepam, as demonstrated by the Kupperman index. The author concluded that the results clearly demonstrated the superiority of Remifemin in treatment of menopausal symptoms, especially when safety and side effects were taken into consideration.

In a study designed to test the effectiveness of black cohosh against an estrogenic drug and placebo, 80 patients were treated for 12 weeks (Stoll, 1987). Thirty were given Remifemin tablets (calculated at 8 mg extract daily: 2 tablets twice daily, each tablet containing 2 mg extract), 30 were given conjugated estrogens (0.625 mg daily), and 20 received placebo. Black cohosh extract produced favorable results in the Kupperman index, Hamilton anxiety test, and improvement in the vaginal lining. The number of hot flashes dropped from an average of 5 daily to less than 1 in the black cohosh group, compared to the estrogen group, which dropped from 5 to 3.5 average daily occurrences. Improvements in the vaginal lining were so significant, the author suggests the extract is suited as the drug of first choice to treat menopausal symptoms, particularly if HRT is contraindicated or not desired by the patient. (While the study refers to 8 mg of the preparation, in actuality, the Remifemin was formerly standardized at 2 mg 27-deoxyacteine; the 8 mg is thus presumably the level of this compound at a dosage of 80 mg of the extract per day.)

In another trial, 60 women under the age of 40 whose hysterectomies had left at least one ovary intact were treated with estriol (1 mg daily), conjugated estrogens (1.25 mg daily), estrogen-gestagen therapy (Trisequens®, one tablet daily), or Remifemin (8 mg of black cohosh extract daily). Control was by a modified Kupperman index that assessed the climacteric symptoms associated with menopause, such as hot flashes and nervousness. Serum luteinizing hormone (LH) and follicle stimulating hormone (FSH) levels were also measured. In all groups, the modified Kupperman index became significantly lower, with no significant differences between groups concerning therapy success (Lehmann-Willenbrock and Riedel, 1988).

In one double-blind clinical trial, the efficacy of black cohosh versus placebo in reducing gonadotropin secretion in menopausal women was studied by investigating the effect on the LH and FSH secretions in 110 women (Düker et al., 1991). Half were treated with Remifemin (8 mg of black cohosh extract daily), and half with placebo. The extract was shown to exert improvements in menopausal symptoms and blood hormone measurements. After eight weeks of treatment, levels of LH were reduced in the treatment group compared to placebo. No effect on FSH levels was seen in either group. Analysis of the commercial product suggested the presence of at least three fractions that contribute synergistically to the suppression of LH and bind to estrogen receptors. The authors concluded that Remifemin selectively suppresses LH secretion in menopausal women, pointing to an estrogenic effect, and confirming the estrogenic activity reported in the Stoll study. However, recent experimental and clinical research excludes an estrogen-identical mode of activity (Einer-Jensen et al., 1996; Liske and Wüstenberg, 1999; Liske et al., 1998).

Two further studies examined the efficacy of Remifemin compared to previous treatment with hormones and/or psychoactive drugs, and the practicality of switching from HRT to the black cohosh extract. In a large open study of 629 female patients under the care of 131 doctors, the ability of Remifemin to improve menopausal symptoms was tested, partially in comparison to a preceding therapy with hormones and/or psychoactive drugs (Stolze, 1982). Of the 629 patients, 204 had been previously treated with hormones, 35 with psychotropic agents, 11 with both, 367 had no previous treatment, and in 12 patients premedication could not be evaluated. Remifemin drops (40 drops twice a day) produced clear improvement of menopausal symptoms in over 80% of the patients within six to eight weeks, with relief of both physical and psychological symptoms. In 72% of the cases, physicians observed advantages of the Remifemin therapy in opposition to a preceding hormone treatment, due to a positive response not seen with HRT, or to the safety and tolerability of the extract. The Remifemin was well tolerated, with no discontinuation of therapy, and only 7% of patients reported mild transitory stomach complaints. In 54.3% of the cases, physicians stated advantages of Remifemin compared to previous medication with psychoactive drugs. The author concluded that Remifemin can be an alternative in the treatment of menopausal complaints, especially in those cases where treatment with estrogens or psychotropic agents is not indicated because of the risks and side effects.

In a study to test the practicality of switching from a hormone treatment to black cohosh, 50 patients who had been in hormone treatment because of menopausal complaints were given Remifemin (2 tablets twice a day) for 6 months (Pethö, 1987). Twenty-eight patients required no further hormone injections during the trial, 21 patients needed one injection during this time, and one patient needed two injections. The therapeutic result was evaluated by the gynecologist as very good in 21 patients, good in 20 patients, and of minor effect in nine. No side effects were reported. The author concluded that the therapeutic response was maintained in most cases when changing from HRT to black cohosh, and that Remifemin can be regarded as a valuable enrichment to therapy.

From the evidence cited above there exists considerable documentation of the potential benefit of a proprietary black cohosh for premenstrual and menopausal conditions. Additional well-controlled studies performed in the United States are forthcoming to corroborate the European studies. Several recent reviews have been published on black cohosh (Gruenwald, 1992; Liske and Wüstenberg, 1998; Foster, 1999).

Description

Preparations of black cohosh consist of the fresh or dried rhizome with attached roots of *Cimicifuga racemosa* (L.) Nutt. [Fam. Ranunculaceae] in effective dosage. The preparation contains triterpene glycosides.

Chemistry and Pharmacology

Constituents include oleic, palmitic, and salicylic acids; cimigonite; tannin; and volatile oil (Bruneton, 1995; Leung and Foster, 1996). The tetracyclic triterpenes, which are oxidized and cyclized by ketalization, are derived from cycloartanol (e.g., actein and cimifugoside) (Bruneton, 1995).

Commission E reported estrogen-like action, luteinizing hormone suppression, and binding to estrogen receptors. Recent research on 152 patients suggests no effects of an isopropanolic-aqueous black cohosh extract at two dosages (40 mg and 127 mg) over six months on levels of luteinizing hormone, follicle-stimulating hormone, prolactin and estradiol, demonstrating that this particular black cohosh extract does not have an estrogenic effect (Liske and Wüstenberg, 1998).

Uses

Commission E approved the use of black cohosh root for premenstrual discomfort and dysmenorrhea or climacteric (menopausal) neurovegetative ailments. Acteina, a constituent in black cohosh, has been studied for use in treating peripheral arterial disease (Genazzani and Sorrentino, 1962).

Contraindications

None known.

Side Effects

Occasionally, gastric discomfort.

Use During Pregnancy and Lactation

Not recommended.

Interactions with Other Drugs

None known.

Dosage and Administration

Unless otherwise prescribed: 0.04 g (40 mg) per day of cut rhizome and root or equivalent preparations.
Dried rhizome and root: 40 mg.
Decoction: 0.04 g in 150 ml water.
Fluidextract 1:1 (g/ml), 40–60% alcohol: 0.04 ml.
Tincture 1:10 (g/ml), 40–60% alcohol: 0.4 ml.
Standardized extract (1:1; standardized to 1% 27-deoxyacteine): 8 mg/day.

References

Beuscher, N. 1995. *Cimicifuga racemosa* L.—Black Cohosh. *Z Phytotherapie* 16:301–310.

Bruneton, J. 1995. *Pharmacognosy, Phytochemistry, Medicinal Plants.* Paris: Lavoisier Publishing.

Daiber, W. 1983. Climacteric Complaints: success without using hormones. *Ärztliche Praxis* 35:1946–1947.

Duke, J.A. 1985. *Handbook of Medicinal Herbs.* Boca Raton: CRC Press. 120–121.

Düker E-M, L. Kopanski, H. Jarry, W. Wuttke. 1991. Effects of extracts from *Cimicifuga racemosa* on gonadotropin release in menopausal women and ovariectomized rats. *Planta Med* 57:420–424.

Einer-Jensen, N., J. Zhao, K.P. Andersen, K. Kristoffersen. 1996. Cimicifuga and Melbrosia lack oestrogenic effects in mice and rats. *Maturitas* 25:149–153.

Farnsworth, N.R. 1999. Personal communication to Mark Blumenthal, May 24.

Felter, H.W. 1922. *The Eclectic Materia Medica, Pharmacology and Therapeutics.* Cincinnati, OH: Eclectic Medical Publications.

Foster, S. 1999. Black Cohosh, *Cimicifuga racemosa*—A Literature Review. *HerbalGram* 46:35–50.

Genazzani, E. and L. Sorrentino. 1962. Vascular action of acteina: active constituent of *Actaea racemosa* L. *Nature* 194:544–545.

Gruenwald, J. 1998. Standardized black cohosh (Cimicifuga) extract clinical monograph. *Quarterly Rev Nat Med* Summer:117–125.

Lehmann-Willenbrock, E. and H.-H. Riedel. 1988. Clinical and endocrinologic examinations concerning therapy of climacteric symptoms following hysterectomy with remaining ovaries. *Zentralbl Gynakol* 110:611–618.

Leung, A.Y. and S. Foster. 1996. *Encyclopedia of Common Natural Ingredients Used in Food, Drugs and Cosmetics,* 2nd ed. New York: John Wiley & Sons, Inc.

Liske, E. and P. Wüstenberg. 1999. Efficacy and safety of phytomedicines for gynecologic disorders with particular reference to *Cimicifuga racemosa* and *Hypericum perforatum.* 1st Asian-European Congress on Menopause. Bangkok, Thailand, Jan. 26–31.

———. 1998. Therapy of climacteric complaints with *Cimicifuga racemosa*: herbal medicine with clinically proven evidence. *Menopause* 5(4):250.

Liske, E., P. Wüstenberg, N. Boblitz. 1998. Human-pharmacological investigations during treatment of climacteric complaints with *Cimicifuga racemosa* (Remifemin®): No estrogen-like effects. 5th International ESCOP Symposium, London, Oct. 15–16.

Murray, M. 1997. Remifemin: Answers to some common questions. *Am J Nat Med* 4(3):3–5.

Pethö, A. 1987. Menopausal complaints: Change-over of a hormone treatment to a herbal gynecological remedy practicable? *Ärztl Praxis* 47:1551–1553.

Snow, J.M. 1996. *Cimicifuga racemosa* (L.) Nutt. (Ranunculaceae). *Protocol J Botanical Med* 1(4):17–19.

Stoll, W. 1987. Phytopharmacon influences atrophic vaginal epithelium: Double blind-study—*cimicifuga* vs. estrogenic substances. *Therapeuticum* 1:23–31.

Stolze, H. 1982. An alternative to treat menopausal complaints. *Gyne* 1:14–16.

Vorberg, G. 1984. Treatment of menopause symptoms—Successful hormone-free therapy with Remifemin®. *ZFA* 60:626–629.

Warnecke, G. 1985. Influencing Menopausal Symptoms with a Phytotherapeutic Agent: Successful therapy with *Cimicifuga* mono-extract. *Med Welt* 36:871–874.

British Herbal Pharmacopoeia (BHP). 1983. Keighley: British Herbal Medicine Association.

———. 1990. Exeter, U.K.: British Herbal Medicine Association.

Foster, S. and J.A. Duke. 1990. *A Field Guide to Medicinal Plants: Eastern and Central North America.* Boston: Houghton Mifflin Co.

Jarry, H., G. Harnischfeger, E. Duker. 1985. Untersuchungen zur endokrinen wirksamkeit von inhaltsstoffen aus *Cimicifuga racemosa* 2. In-vitro-bindung von inhaltsstoffen an östrogen-rezeptoren [The endocrine effects of constituents of *Cimicifuga racemosa*. 2. in vitro binding of constituents to estrogen receptors]. *Planta Med* (4):316–319.

Lieberman, S. 1998. A review of the effectiveness of *Cimicifuga racemosa* (black cohosh) for the symptoms of monopause. *J Womens Health* 7(5):525–529.

Liske, E. Therapeutic efficacy and safety of *Cimicifuga racemosa* for gynecological disorders. *Adv Ther* 15(1):45–53.

McGuffin, M., C. Hobbs, R. Upton, A. Goldberg. 1997. American Herbal Product Association's *Botanical Safety Handbook.* Boca Raton: CRC Press.

Resing, K. and A. Fitzgerald. 1978. Crystal data for 15-o-acetylacerinol and two related triterpenes isolated from Japanese Cimicifuga plants. *J Appl Cryst* (11):58.

Wren, R.C. 1988. *Potter's New Cyclopaedia of Botanical Drugs and Preparations.* Essex: The C.W. Daniel Company Ltd.

Additional Resources

Baillie, N. and P. Rasmussen. 1997. Black and blue cohosh in labour. *N Z Med J* 110(1036):20–21.

This material was adapted from *The Complete German Commission E Monographs—Therapeutic Guide to Herbal Medicines.* M. Blumenthal, W.R. Busse, A. Goldberg, J. Gruenwald, T. Hall, C.W. Riggins, R.S. Rister (eds.) S. Klein and R.S. Rister (trans.). 1998. Austin: American Botanical Council; Boston: Integrative Medicine Communications.
1) The Overview section is new information.
2) Description, Chemistry and Pharmacology, Uses, Contraindications, Side Effects, Interactions with Other Drugs, and Dosage sections have been drawn from the original work. Additional information has been added in some or all of these sections, as noted with references.
3) The dosage for equivalent preparations (tea infusion, fluidextract, and tincture) have been provided based on the following example:
   Unless otherwise prescribed: 2 g per day of [powdered, crushed, cut or whole] [plant part]
   Infusion: 2 g in 150 ml of water
   Fluidextract 1:1 (g/ml): 2 ml
   Tincture 1:5 (g/ml): 10 ml
4) The References and Additional Resources sections are new sections. Additional Resources are not cited in the monograph but are included for research purposes.

BLESSED THISTLE HERB

Latin Name:
Cnicus benedictus

Pharmacopeial Name:
Cnici benedicti herba

Other Names:
holy thistle herb

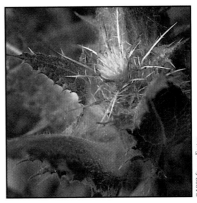

© 1999 Steven Foster

Overview

Blessed thistle is an annual herb native to the Mediterranean region and western Asia, now naturalized throughout Europe and in the eastern United States (Karnick, 1994; Leung and Foster, 1996; Wichtl and Bisset, 1994). The material of commerce in Europe is collected in northern and eastern Europe, Italy, and Spain (BHP, 1996; Wichtl and Bisset, 1994). The material used in Ayurvedic medicine is collected in India from Kashmir to the Khasia Hills, and in Bhutan (Karnick, 1994). It was brought under cultivation in Europe during the early sixteenth century, originally in monastery gardens, and was mentioned as a heal-all in treatises on the Plague from whence the specific epithet *benedictus* was derived (Bown, 1995; Grieve, 1979). Galenical preparations of blessed thistle are used for anorexia, dyspepsia, flatulence, indigestion, and loss of appetite in traditional European herbal medicines, traditional Indian Ayurvedic medicine, and modern naturopathic medicine (Hoffmann, 1990; Karnick, 1994; Leung and Foster, 1996; Lust, 1974; Newall et al., 1996).

The approved modern therapeutic applications for blessed thistle herb are based on its long history of use in well established systems of traditional medicine, *in vitro* and *in vivo* studies in animals, and its documented chemical composition.

In the United States and Germany, blessed thistle herb is used as a component of cholagogic and gastrointestinal remedies in aqueous infusion, alcoholic fluidextract, and tincture form, and in tablets. It is also used as a component of simple bitters, tonic drinks used to stimulate the digestive mucosa (Leung and Foster, 1996; Wichtl and Bisset, 1994).

Pharmacopeial grade blessed thistle herb must have a bitterness value of not less than 800. Assay methods are published for determination of the bitter principle cnicin (Bradley, 1992; DAC, 1986; ÖAB, 1981).

Description

Blessed thistle herb consists of the dried leaves and upper stems, including inflorescence, of *Cnicus benedictus* L. [Fam. Asteraceae], as well as preparations thereof in effective dosage. The herb contains bitter principles, such as cnicin.

Chemistry and Pharmacology

Blessed thistle contains sesquiterpene lactones including cnicin (bitter index = 1:1,800) (0.2–0.7%), tannins (8%), high mineral content (mainly potassium, manganese, magnesium, and calcium), lignan lactones (lignanolides), phytosterols, triterpenoids, volatile oils (0.3%), and small amounts of flavonoids and poly-ynes (polyacetylenes) (Bradley, 1992; Leung and

Foster, 1996; Newall et al., 1996; Wichtl and Bissett, 1994).

The Commission E reported stimulation of the secretion of saliva and gastric juices. The *British Herbal Compendium* reports its actions as bitter, carminative, antidiarrheal, and antimicrobial (Bradley, 1992). Its sesquiterpene lactones constituents are considered to be bitter principles (Wagner et al., 1983). Bitter constituents (mainly cnicin) stimulate the taste buds, causing a reflex increase in the secretion of saliva and gastric juice, thus stimulating the appetite (Bradley, 1992). The whole dried herb, its volatile oil, and the isolated constituent cnicin have all demonstrated antibacterial activity (Newall et al., 1996). Its antimicrobial activity has been attributed to cnicin and to its polyacetylene constituents (Vanhaelen-Fastré, 1968).

Uses

The Commission E approved the internal use of blessed thistle for loss of appetite and dyspepsia. The *British Herbal Compendium* indicates its use for loss of appetite, anorexia, and flatulent dyspepsia (Bradley, 1992). It is used as an aromatic bitter for stimulation of appetite and increasing gastric juice secretion (Wichtl and Bisset, 1994).

Contraindications

Allergies to blessed thistle and other composites.

Side Effects

Allergic reactions are possible.

Use During Pregnancy and Lactation

Not recommended (McGuffin et al., 1997; Bradley, 1992).

Interactions with Other Drugs

None known.

Dosage and Administration

Unless otherwise prescribed: 4–6 g per day of cut herb or dried extract.
Infusion: 1.5–2 g in 150 ml water, three times daily.
Fluidextract 1:1 (g/ml): 1.5–2 ml, three times daily.
Tincture 1:5 (g/ml): 7.5–10 ml, three times daily.

References

Bown, D. 1995. *Encyclopedia of Herbs and Their Uses*. New York: DK Publishing, Inc. 264.
British Herbal Pharmacopoeia (BHP). 1996. Exeter, U.K.: British Herbal Medicine Association. 104–5.
Bradley, P.R. (ed.). 1992. *British Herbal Compendium*, Vol. 1. Bournemouth: British Herbal Medicine Association.
Deutscher Arzneimittel-Codex (DAC). 1986. Stuttgart: Deutscher Apotheker Verlag.
Grieve, M. 1979. *A Modern Herbal*. New York: Dover Publications, Inc.
Hoffmann, D. 1990. *The New Holistic Herbal*. Dorset: Element Books Ltd. 182.
Karnick, C.R. 1994. *Pharmacopoeial Standards of Herbal Plants*, Vols. 1–2. Delhi: Sri Satguru Publications. Vol. 1:98–100; Vol. 2:18.
Leung, A.Y. and S. Foster. 1996. *Encyclopedia of Common Natural Ingredients Used in Food, Drugs and Cosmetics*, 2nd ed. New York: John Wiley & Sons, Inc.
Lust, J.B. 1974. *The Herb Book*. New York: Bantam Books. 343.
McGuffin, M., C. Hobbs, R. Upton, A. Goldberg. 1997. American Herbal Product Association's *Botanical Safety Handbook*. Boca Raton: CRC Press.
Newall, C.A., L.A. Anderson, J.D. Phillipson. 1996. *Herbal Medicines: A Guide for Health-Care Professionals*. London: The Pharmaceutical Press.
Österreichisches Arzneibuch (ÖAB). 1981–1983. Vols. 1–2; 1st suppl.
Vanhaelen-Fastré, R. 1968. *Cnicus benedictus*: Separation of antimicrobial constituents. *Plant Med Phytother* 2:294–299.
Wagner, H., S. Bladt, E.M. Zgainski. 1983. *Plant Drug Analysis*. Berlin-Heidelberg: Springer Verlag.
Wichtl, M. and N.G. Bisset (eds.). 1994. *Herbal Drugs and Phytopharmaceuticals*. Stuttgart: Medpharm Scientific Publishers.

Additional Resources

Harnischfeger, G. and H. Stolze. 1983. *Bewährte Pflanzendrogen in Wissenschaft und Medizin*. Bad Homburg/Melsungen: Notamed Verlag. 74–81.
Schneider, G. and I.A. Lachner. 1987. A contribution to analytics and pharmacology of Cnicin. *Planta Med* 53(3):247–251.

Vanhaelen-Fastré, R. 1973. [Constitution and antibiotical properties of the essential oil of *Cnicus benedictus*] [In French]. *Planta Med* 24(2):165–175.

Vanhaelen-Fastré, R. and M. Vanhaelen. 1976. [Antibiotic and cytotoxic activity of Cnicin and of its hydrolysis products. Chemical structure—biological activity relationship] [In French]. *Planta Med* 29(2):179–189.

This material was adapted from *The Complete German Commission E Monographs—Therapeutic Guide to Herbal Medicines.* M. Blumenthal, W.R. Busse, A. Goldberg, J. Gruenwald, T. Hall, C.W. Riggins, R.S. Rister (eds.) S. Klein and R.S. Rister (trans.). 1998. Austin: American Botanical Council; Boston: Integrative Medicine Communications.

1) The Overview section is new information.
2) Description, Chemistry and Pharmacology, Uses, Contraindications, Side Effects, Interactions with Other Drugs, and Dosage sections have been drawn from the original work. Additional information has been added in some or all of these sections, as noted with references.
3) The dosage for equivalent preparations (tea infusion, fluidextract, and tincture) have been provided based on the following example:
   Unless otherwise prescribed: 2 g per day of [powdered, crushed, cut or whole] [plant part]
   Infusion: 2 g in 150 ml of water
   Fluidextract 1:1 (g/ml): 2 ml
   Tincture 1:5 (g/ml): 10 ml
4) The References and Additional Resources sections are new sections. Additional Resources are not cited in the monograph but are included for research purposes.

BOLDO LEAF

Latin Name:
Peumus boldus

Pharmacopeial Name:
Boldo folium

Other Names:
n/a

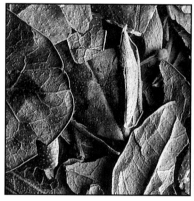

©1999 Steven Foster

Overview

Boldo is an evergreen native to Chile, Ecuador, Argentina, Bolivia, and Peru. Explorers to South America observed natives using leaves as culinary spice, and also as a carminative agent with numerous therapeutic applications, including the treatment of gout and disorders of the liver, bladder, and prostate. In 1875, it was introduced to British and American pharmacists as a treatment for mild stomach, liver, and bladder discomforts, and also as a mild nervine, or sedative (Bastien, 1997).

Recent excavation of Monte Verde, an area in southern Chile, unearthed evidence of the medicinal use of 22 varieties of plants by people thought to have lived there more than 12,500 years ago. Among these plants is boldo, which archeologists found wrapped in seaweed. When chewed by individuals who had been severely injured or who required some kind of surgery, this combination of plants may have provided both painkilling and mind-altering properties (Gore, 1997).

Today, boldo leaves are used to treat gallstones, liver or gall bladder discomfort, cystitis, and rheumatism (Newall et al., 1996), and for heartburn or other mild stomach cramps. Its choleretic actions release bile, and its diuretic actions increase fluid excretion, possibly cleansing sediment or bacteria from the biliary tract itself (Schulz et al., 1998). The constituent boldine stimulates choleretic action (Tyler, 1994), which may provide relief to patients with gallstones for whom surgery is not an option or drugs have not been effective (Schulz et al., 1998). Although herbs that have been used over time to treat biliary tract diseases rely largely on empirical evidence as proof of efficacy, researchers, in a recent study of 12 human volunteers, concluded that a dry boldo extract lengthens intestinal transit time (Gotteland et al., 1995). Most human studies have used herbal combination formulas and not boldo alone (Newall et al., 1996).

Contemporary studies using laboratory animals suggest that boldo may reduce inflammation and fever through prostaglandin biosynthesis inhibition (Backhouse et al., 1994). Recent studies in animals showed that certain components of boldo relax smooth muscle and prolong intestinal transit (Gotteland et al., 1995). Boldo may provide the liver with protection against harmful chemicals, appearing to maintain adequate liver enzyme levels in response to toxic agents (Lanhers et al., 1991). The therapeutic implications of these actions require further study, as do boldo's use in folk medicine as a sedative; mechanisms of action and scope of activity have not been determined in this regard.

As with many herbs that have diuretic action, it is unclear whether boldo's actions are truly diuretic (stimulating both fluid and electrolyte secretion), or whether they are in fact aquaretic (stimulating only fluid excretion), a distinction that hypertensive or edematous patients need to consider (Tyler, 1994).

Boldo's aromatic essential oil contains a toxic constituent, ascaridole, which is contained in some plants used by traditional healers to treat parasitic diseases

(Montoya-Cabrera et al., 1996); Germany's Commission E approves only boldo formulas that do not contain ascaridole.

Description

Boldo leaf consists of the dried leaves of *Peumus boldus* Molina [Fam. Monimiaceae], as well as its preparations in effective dosage. The leaves contain at least 0.1% alkaloids, calculated as boldine, and flavonoids.

Chemistry and Pharmacology

The plant contains 0.25–0.70% alkaloids (Leung and Foster, 1996). Other constituents include 1–3% essential oil composed of monoterpenoids (including volatile oils (limonene, β-pinene, p-cymene), linalol, cineole, camphor, ascaridole (Bruneton, 1995; Newall et al., 1996; Wichtl and Bisset, 1994). Common flavonol glycosides (e.g., rhamnetin, isorhamnetin, and kaempferol derivatives), resin, and tannins can be found in the plant (Bruneton, 1995; Leung and Foster, 1996).

The Commission E reported that boldo increases gastric secretions and has antispasmodic properties. Boldo's alkaloidal constituents are apparently responsible for its confirmed choleretic activity (Newall et al., 1996). *In vitro*, boldine protects against damaging free radicals, as shown in animal studies. Boldine also acts *in vitro* as a smooth muscle relaxant and as a contraction impediment (Bruneton, 1995).

Uses

The Commission E approved boldo as treatment for mild dyspepsia and spastic gastrointestinal complaints. It has been used successfully as treatment for gallstones, liver ailments, cystitis, and rheumatism (Newall et al., 1996).

Contraindications

Obstruction of bile ducts, severe liver diseases. In case of gallstones, to be used only after consultation with a physician.

Side Effects

None known.

Use During Pregnancy and Lactation

No restrictions known.

Interactions with Other Drugs

None known.

Dosage and Administration

Unless otherwise prescribed: 3 g per day of cut herb.
Infusion: 3 g in 150 ml water.
Fluidextract 1:1 (g/ml): 3 ml.
Tincture 1:5 (g/ml): 15 ml.
Note: Because of the ascaridole content, essential oil and distillates of boldo leaf should not be used.

References

Backhouse, N. et al. 1994. Anti-inflammatory and antipyretic effects of boldine. *Agents Actions* 42(3–4):114–117.

Bastien, J.W. 1987. *Healers of the Andes—Kallaway Herbalists and Their Medicinal Plants.* Salt Lake City: University of Utah Press.

Bruneton, J. 1995. *Pharmacognosy, Phytochemistry, Medicinal Plants.* Paris: Lavoisier Publishing.

Gore, R. 1997. The most ancient Americans. *National Geographic* 192(4):98–99.

Gotteland, M., J. Espinoza, B. Cassels, H. Speisky. 1995. [Effect of a dry boldo extract on oro-cecal intestinal transit in healthy volunteers] [In Spanish]. *Rev Med Chil* 123(8):955–960.

Lanhers, M.C. et al. 1991. Hepatoprotective and anti-inflammatory effects of a traditional medicinal plant of Chile, *Peumus boldus. Planta Med* 57(2):110–115.

Leung, A.Y. and S. Foster. 1996. *Encyclopedia of Common Natural Ingredients Used in Food, Drugs, and Cosmetics,* 2nd ed. New York: John Wiley & Sons, Inc.

Montoya-Cabrera, M.A. et al. 1996. Fatal poisoning caused by oil of epazote, *Chenopodium graveolens.* Gac Med Mex 132(4):433–437.

Newall, C.A., L.A. Anderson, J.D. Phillipson. 1996. *Herbal Medicines: A Guide for Health-Care Professionals.* London: The Pharmaceutical Press.

Schulz, V., R. Hänsel, V.E. Tyler. 1998. *Rational Phytotherapy: A Physicians' Guide to Herbal Medicine.* New York: Springer.

Tyler, V.E. 1994. *Herbs of Choice: The Therapeutic Use of Phytomedicinals.* New York: Pharmaceutical Products Press.

Wichtl, M. and N.G. Bisset (eds.). 1994. *Herbal Drugs and Phytopharmaceuticals.* Stuttgart: Medpharm Scientific Publishers.

Additional Resources

British Herbal Pharmacopoeia (BHP). 1983. Keighley, U.K.: British Herbal Medicine Association.

Borgia, M. et al. 1981. Pharmacological activity of a herb extract: A controlled clinical study. *Curr Ther Res* (29):525–536.

Borgia, M. et al. 1985. Studio policentrico doppio-cieco doppio-controllato sull'attivita terapeutica di una nota associazione di erbe medicamentose. *Clin Ter* (114):401–409.

Deutscher Arzneimittel-Codex (DAC). 1986. Stuttgart: Deutscher Apotheker Verlag.

List, P.H. and L. Hörhammer (eds.). 1977. *Hagers Handbuch der Pharmazeutischen Praxis,* 4th ed. Vol. 6A. New York: Springer Verlag.

Pharmacopoeia Helvetica, 7th ed. (Ph.Helv.VII), Vol. 1–4. 1987. Bern: Office Central Fédéral des Imprimés et du Matériel.

Reynolds, J.E.F. (ed.). 1982. *Martindale: The Extra Pharmacopoeia.* London: The Pharmaceutical Press.

Salati R, R. Lugli, E. Tamborino. 1984. Valutazione delle proprieta coleretiche di due preparati contenenti estratti di boldo e cascara [Evaluation of the choleretic property of 2 preparations containing extracts of boldo and cascara]. *Minerva Dietol Gastroenterol* 30(3):269–272.

Wagner, H. and P. Wolff (eds.). 1977. *New Natural Products and Plant Drugs with Pharmacological, Biological, or Therapeutic Activity.* Berlin-Heidelberg: Springer Verlag.

Wren, R.C. 1988. *Potter's New Cyclopaedia of Botanical Drugs and Preparations.* Essex: The C.W. Daniel Company Ltd.

This material was adapted from *The Complete German Commission E Monographs—Therapeutic Guide to Herbal Medicines.* M. Blumenthal, W.R. Busse, A. Goldberg, J. Gruenwald, T. Hall, C.W. Riggins, R.S. Rister (eds.) S. Klein and R.S. Rister (trans.). 1998. Austin: American Botanical Council; Boston: Integrative Medicine Communications.

1) The Overview section is new information.
2) Description, Chemistry and Pharmacology, Uses, Contraindications, Side Effects, Interactions with Other Drugs, and Dosage sections have been drawn from the original work. Additional information has been added in some or all of these sections, as noted with references.
3) The dosage for equivalent preparations (tea infusion, fluidextract, and tincture) have been provided based on the following example:
   Unless otherwise prescribed: 2 g per day of [powdered, crushed, cut or whole] [plant part]
   Infusion: 2 g in 150 ml of water
   Fluidextract 1:1 (g/ml): 2 ml
   Tincture 1:5 (g/ml): 10 ml
4) The References and Additional Resources sections are new sections. Additional Resources are not cited in the monograph but are included for research purposes.

BROMELAIN

Latin Name:
Ananas comosus

Pharmacopeial Name:
Bromelainum

Other Names:
pineapple enzyme

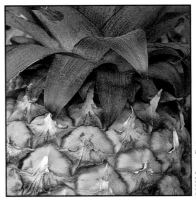

©1999 Steven Foster

Overview

Bromelain is the proteolytic enzyme from juice wastes of pineapple stem and ripe or unripe fruits combined with solvents, such as acetone or methanol, or following filtration (Leung and Foster, 1996; Samuelsson, 1992; Schulz et al., 1998). For the past 25 years, proteolytic enzymes that contain chemically active thiol groups that can tenderize meat have been used by the food industry (Samuelsson, 1992). Other enzymes such as papain, derived from papaya latex (*Carica papaya*), and ficin, from fig latex (*Ficus* species), also contain thiol groups. Other uses of proteolytic enzymes include animal skin preparation, fish oil production, soap manufacture, and cloth shrinkage (Leung and Foster, 1996).

In Europe, a patented tape that contains bromelain is used for debriding escharotic skin (Leung and Foster, 1996). Bromelain is also used to treat traumatic or post-surgical swelling; Commission E approves the use of bromelain to quell surgical swelling, particularly nasal sinus swelling. This approval, however, has been questioned by some scientists, who note that the Commission E's assessment involved five studies, three positive and two negative, leading to an equivocal proof of efficacy (Schulz et al., 1998).

In pharmacological tests, bromelain inhibits platelet aggregation, which explains, at least partially, its anti-inflammatory activity (Taussig and Batkin, 1988). Bromelain may also therapeutically influence fibrinolysis, tumor growth, drug absorption, blood coagulation and the debridement of third-degree burns (Taussig and Batkin, 1988). Another study demonstrated intestinal and antibacterial effects beneficial in the treatment of diarrhea (Mynott et al., 1997).

One obstacle to determining bromelain's therapeutic effects in humans is its bioavailability. Because the proteins contained in bromelain are usually broken down prior to absorption in the gastrointestinal tract, bromelain's active enzymes may not survive digestion. In rats, bromelain absorption rate is about 50%; other animal tests show that some undegraded protein winds up in lymph and the blood-stream (Schulz et al., 1998). Human rates are unknown, but one study using 19 healthy human males suggests that small amounts of undegraded bromelain may pass through the gastrointestinal tract intact (Castell et al., 1997).

The source of commercial bromelain tends to be the pineapple stem (Leung and Foster, 1996; Schulz et al., 1998); ripe fruits are sold as food products. Histori-cally, the juice, fruit, and stem latex were used. In Hawaii, Japan, and Taiwan, folk medicine and contemporary descriptions of fruit latex report its use to cleanse and heal wounds and burns, to relieve digestive disturbances, and to treat some cancers (Taussig and Batkin, 1988).

Description

Bromelain (EC 3.4.22.4) is the genuine mixture of bromelin A and B, the proteolytic enzymes of pineapple fruit, *Ananas comosus* (L.) Merrill [Fam. Bromeliaceae], in effective dosage.

Chemistry and Pharmacology

Bromelain constituents are a mixture of basic glycoproteins similar to papain (Bruneton, 1995). The fruit consists of soluble monosaccharides and disaccharides, organic acids, and vitamins (Bruneton, 1995).

In various animal experiments (egg white-, carrageen-, dextran-, and yeast-induced edemas, traumatic edema, adrenalin-caused edema of the lungs), an edema-inhibiting effect was demonstrated with high dosages of bromelain upon oral and intraperitoneal administration. Upon oral intake, bromelain can prolong prothrombin and bleeding time, as well as inhibit the aggregation of thrombocytes. There is no information available on the absorption of the compound in humans after oral ingestion. Only older data are known regarding acute and chronic toxicity of the compound. The LD_{50} after parenteral application is 85.2 mg/kg for rats, 30–35 mg/kg for mice, and for rabbits greater than 20 mg/kg of body weight. There are no data for mutagenicity and carcinogenicity. With rats and rabbits, there were no indications of embryotoxic or teratogenic effects.

Uses

The Commission E approved the use of bromelain for acute post-operative and post-traumatic conditions of swelling, especially of the nasal and paranasal sinuses. Additionally, bromelain, combined with pancreatic extracts of titrated trypsin, amylase, and lipase enzymes, is suggested as treatment for the symptoms of dyspepsia and exocrine hepatic insufficiency (Bruneton, 1995).

Contraindications

Hypersensitivity to bromelain.

Side Effects

Occasionally gastric disturbances or diarrhea. Sometimes allergic reactions.

Use During Pregnancy and Lactation

No restrictions known.

Interactions with Other Drugs

An increased tendency for bleeding in the case of simultaneous administration of anticoagulants and inhibitors of thrombocytic aggregation may occur. The levels of tetracyclines in plasma and urine are increased by simultaneous intake of bromelain.

Dosage and Administration

Unless otherwise prescribed: 80–320 mg, two to three times daily for oral ingestion for 8 to 10 days. If necessary, administration may be prolonged. Solid dosage forms: 80–320 mg of bromelain (200–800 FIP units) in 2 or 3 doses.

References

Bruneton, J. 1995. *Pharmacognosy, Phytochemistry, Medicinal Plants.* Paris: Lavoisier Publishing.

Castell, J.V., G. Friedrich, C.S. Kuhn, G.E. Poppe. 1997. Intestinal absorption of undegraded proteins in men: presence of bromelain in plasma after oral intake. *Am J Physiol* 273(1 Pt. 1):G139–146.

Leung, A.Y. and S. Foster. 1996. *Encyclopedia of Common Natural Ingredients Used in Food, Drugs and Cosmetics*, 2nd ed. New York: John Wiley & Sons, Inc.

Mynott, T.L., S. Guandalini, F. Raimondi, A. Fasano. 1997. Bromelain prevents secretion caused by *Vibrio cholerae* and *Escherichia coli* enterotoxins in rabbit ileum *in vitro. Gastroenterol* 113(1):175–184.

Samuelsson, G. 1992. *Drugs of Natural Origin: A Textbook of Pharmacognosy.* Stockholm: Sweden Pharmaceutical Press.

Schulz, V., R. Hänsel, V.E. Tyler. 1998. *Rational Phytotherapy: A Physicians' Guide to Herbal Medicine.* New York: Springer.

Taussig, S.J. and S. Batkin. 1988. Bromelain, the enzyme complex of pineapple (*Ananas comosus*) and its clinical application. An update. *J Ethnopharmacol* 22(2):191–203.

Additional Resources

Baur, X. et al. 1979. Allergic reactions, including asthma, to the pineapple protease bromelain following occupational exposure. *Clin Allergy* 9(5):443–450.

Der Marderosian, A. (ed.). 1999. *The Review of Natural Products*. St. Louis: Facts and Comparisons.

Duke, J.A. 1985. *Handbook of Medicinal Herbs*. Boca Raton: CRC Press.

Edenharder, R., K. John, H. Ivo-Boor. 1990. [Antimutagenic activity of vegetable and fruit extracts against in-vitro benzo(a)pyrene] [In German]. *Z Gesamte Hyg* 36(3):144–147.

International Commission on Pharmaceutical Enzymes. 1977. *Farm Tijdschr Belg* 54(85).

Lenarcic, B., A. Ritonja, B. Turk, I. Dolenc, V. Turk. 1992. Characterization and structure of pineapple stem inhibitor of cysteine proteinases. *Biol Chem Hoppe Seyler* 373(7):459–464.

Lotz-Winter, H. 1990. On the pharmacology of bromelain: an update with special regard to animal studies on dose-dependent effects. *Planta Med* 56(3):249–253.

Morton, J.F. 1977. *Major Medicinal Plants*. Springfield: C.C. Thomas.

Reynolds, J.E.F. (ed.). 1989. *Martindale: The Extra Pharmacopoeia,* 29th ed. London: The Pharmaceutical Press.

Rowan, A.D., D.J. Buttle, A.J. Barrett. 1990. The cysteine proteinases of the pineapple plant. *Biochem J* (266):869–875.

Stecher, P.G. et al. 1968. *The Merck Index: An Encyclopedia of Chemicals and Drugs,* 8th ed. Rahway, N.J.: Merck & Co., Inc.

Taussig, S.J., J. Szekerczes, S. Batkin. 1985. Inhibition of tumour growth *in vitro* by bromelain, an extract of the pineapple plant (*Ananas comosus*). *Planta Med* (6):538–539.

Werbach, M. and M. Murray. 1994. *Botanical Influences on Illness: A Sourcebook of Clinical Research*. Tarzana: Third Line Press.

This monograph, published by the Commission E in 1994, was modified based on new scientific research. It contains more extensive pharmacological and therapeutic information taken directly from the Commission E.

This material was adapted from *The Complete German Commission E Monographs—Therapeutic Guide to Herbal Medicines*. M. Blumenthal, W.R. Busse, A. Goldberg, J. Gruenwald, T. Hall, C.W. Riggins, R.S. Rister (eds.) S. Klein and R.S. Rister (trans.). 1998. Austin: American Botanical Council; Boston: Integrative Medicine Communications.

1) The Overview section is new information.
2) Description, Chemistry and Pharmacology, Uses, Contraindications, Side Effects, Interactions with Other Drugs, and Dosage sections have been drawn from the original work. Additional information has been added in some or all of these sections, as noted with references.
3) The dosage for equivalent preparations (tea infusion, fluidextract, and tincture) have been provided based on the following example:
   Unless otherwise prescribed: 2 g per day of [powdered, crushed, cut or whole] [plant part]
   Infusion: 2 g in 150 ml of water
   Fluidextract 1:1 (g/ml): 2 ml
   Tincture 1:5 (g/ml): 10 ml
4) The References and Additional Resources sections are new sections. Additional Resources are not cited in the monograph but are included for research purposes.

BUCKTHORN BARK

Latin Name:
Rhamnus frangula

Pharmacopeial Name:
Frangulae cortex

Other Names:
frangula, alder buckthorn

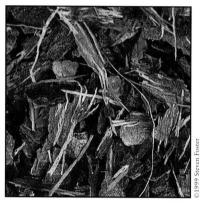

© 1999 Steven Foster

Overview

The source of dried buckthorn bark, the alder buckthorn, is a shrub native to Europe and western parts of Asia (Schulz et al., 1998). Its medicinal use as a purgative laxative dates back to at least 1650, when buckthorn berries first appeared in the *London Pharmacopoeia* (Trease and Evans, 1989). In the United States, buckthorn was included in the *National Formulary* as an official drug from 1820 to 1830 and again from 1880 to 1910 (Boyle, 1991; Tyler, 1994).

Buckthorn bark is an ingredient in laxative teas, extracts, and tablets in Europe. It is also added to sunscreens (Leung and Foster, 1996). In the past, buckthorn was among the botanicals included in Harry Hoxsey's folk cancer remedy, the Hoxsey formula (Hartwell, 1971). Although current adaptations of the Hoxsey formula tend not to include buckthorn bark, tests have demonstrated that the anthraquinone derivatives in buckthorn may have anticancer effects. In particular, emodin, which is sometimes referred to as frangula emodin, frangulic acid, and rheum emodin, has stopped the growth of potato tubers, inhibited Walkers sarcoma *in vitro*, and is cytotoxic to at least three human tumor cell lines. These effects may be due to antiangiogenic actions. The same constituent is also found in many other plant species, including yellow dock and rhubarb (Trease and Evans, 1989; Harborne and Baxter, 1993; Kupchan and Karim, 1976).

Many *Rhamnus* species share anthraquinone derivative constituents and provide characteristic laxative actions. These constituents were isolated by botanists early on in the study of plant chemistry. They are chemically classified as anthraquinone derivatives and give buckthorn heartwood a bright red-yellow color, used for centuries as a dye for textiles (Trease and Evans, 1989).

In the United States, *Rhamnus purshiana*, more commonly known as cascara sagrada, grows throughout northern California and British Columbia. Further down the Pacific coast, *R. californica* grows; this was a source of cathartic remedies used by Spanish priests. *R. frangula* is the European species; its fragile wood tastes extremely bitter and the strong odor it imparts is evidenced by its German common name, *faulbaum*, meaning rotten tree (Schulz et al., 1998). Although European buckthorn has been cultivated in the United States, most commercial European buckthorn is grown in Eastern Europe and Russia and sold in Europe (Trease and Evans, 1989).

Because the anthraquinones in freshly dried buckthorn bark can cause extreme gastrointestinal irritation, including severe intestinal spasm, as well as vomiting, the bark is aged for a year to allow oxidation of the anthrones (Samuelsson, 1992), or it is heated and dried in order to induce artificial aging. Either process makes the effects of buckthorn preparations suitable for treating constipation that occurs in patients with hemorrhoids, anal fissures, or post-surgical pain (Schulz et al., 1998).

Description

Buckthorn bark consists of the dried bark of the trunks and branches of *R. frangula* L. (syn. *Frangula alnus* Miller) [Fam. Rhamnaceae], as well as its preparations in effective dosage. The bark contains anthranoids, mainly of the emodin-physcion and chrysophanol type. These preparations must conform to the currently valid pharmacopeia.

Chemistry and Pharmacology

The main constituents of the dried bark are the anthraquinone glycosides A and B and frangulins A and B, which make up 3–7%, other anthraquinones, glycosides, dianthrones, aglycones, flavonoids, and tannins (Bradley, 1992; ESCOP, 1997; Newall et al., 1996; Wichtl and Bisset, 1994).

1,8-dihydroxy-anthracene derivatives have a laxative effect. These compounds increase the motility of the colon by inhibiting stationary and stimulating propulsive contractions. This results in accelerated intestinal passage and, because of the shortened contraction time, a reduction in liquid absorption through the lumen. In addition, stimulation of active chloride secretion increases the water and electrolyte content of intestinal contents. Systematic studies pertaining to the kinetics of buckthorn bark preparations are not available; however, it must be supposed that the aglycones contained in the drug are already absorbed in the upper small intestine. The β-glycosides are prodrugs which are neither absorbed nor cleaved in the upper gastrointestinal tract. They are degraded in the colon by bacterial enzymes to anthrones. Anthrones are the laxative metabolites. Active metabolites of other anthronoids, such as rhein, infiltrate in small amounts into the milk ducts. A laxative effect on nursing infants has not been observed. The placental permeability for rhein is very small.

Drug preparations (i.e., herbal stimulant laxatives) have a higher general toxicity than the pure glycosides, presumably due to the content of aglycones. Experiments pertaining to the genotoxicity of buckthorn and its preparations are not available. Some positive data were obtained for aloe-emodin, emodin, physcion, and chrysophanol. No data are available for their carcinogenicity.

The fresh bark contains free anthrone and must be stored for one year or artificially aged by heat and aeration. The use of illegally processed buckthorn bark, e.g., fresh bark, will cause severe vomiting, possibly with spasms.

Uses

The Commission E approved the internal use of buckthorn bark for constipation. Other conditions for use include conditions in which soft feces are desirable (hemorrhoids and post rectal-anal operations) (Bradley, 1992; Wichtl and Bisset, 1994).

Contraindications

Intestinal obstruction, acute intestinal inflammation, e.g., Crohn's disease, colitis ulcerosa, appendicitis, abdominal pain of unknown origin. Children under 12 years of age.

Side Effects

In some cases, cramp-like discomforts of the gastrointestinal tract can occur. These incidents require a dosage reduction.

With long-term use/abuse: disturbances of electrolyte balance, especially potassium deficiency, albuminuria, and hematuria. Pigment implantation into the intestinal mucosa (*Pseudomelanosis coli*) is harmless and usually reverses upon discontinuation of the preparation. The potassium deficiency can lead to disorders of heart function and muscular weakness, especially with concurrent use of cardiac glycosides, diuretics, and corticosteroids.

Use During Pregnancy and Lactation

Not recommended.

Interactions with Other Drugs

With chronic use or in cases of abuse of the preparation, a potentiation of cardiac glycosides due to a loss of serum potassium is possible. Also possible is an effect on antiarrhythmic agents. Potassium deficiency can be increased by simultaneous application of thiazide diuretics, corticosteroids, or licorice root.

Dosage and Administration

Unless otherwise prescribed: Cut bark, powder, or dried extracts (corresponding to 20–30 mg hydroxyanthracene derivatives, calculated as glycofrangulin A) for teas, decoction, cold maceration, or elixir. Liquid or solid forms of medication exclusively for oral use. The individually correct dosage is the smallest dosage necessary to maintain a soft stool.

[Note: According to the *Austrian Pharmacopeia*, the average single dose for the decoction dosage form is 1.5 g (Meyer-Buchtela, 1999; ÖAB, 1991).]
Decoction: Boil 0.5–2.5 g (Bradley, 1992) in 150–250 ml water.
Infusion: Steep $1/2$ teaspoon (1.2 g) in 150 ml hot water for 10 to 15 minutes (Braun et al., 1997; Meyer-Buchtela, 1999); Or: Steep 2 g of finely cut bark in 150–250 ml boiled water for 10 minutes. Drink one cup mornings and/or evenings at bedtime (Meyer-Buchtela, 1999; Wichtl and Bisset, 1994).
Cold macerate: Soak 2 g in 150–250 ml cold water for 12 hours at room temperature (Meyer-Buchtela, 1999; Wichtl, 1989; Wichtl and Bisset, 1994). Fluidextract 1:1 (g/ml), 25% ethanol: 0.5–2.5 ml, at bedtime (Bradley, 1992); Or: 2–4 ml, twice daily (Karnick, 1994).
Note: The form of administration should be smaller than the normal daily dose.

References

Boyle, W. 1991. *Official Herbs: Botanical Substances in the United States Pharmacopoeias 1820–1990.* East Palestine, OH: Buckeye Naturopathic Press.

Bradley, P.R. (ed.). 1992. *British Herbal Compendium*, Vol. 1. Bournemouth: British Herbal Medicine Association. 99–101.

Braun, R. et al. 1997. *Standardzulassungen für Fertigarzneimittel—Text und Kommentar.* Stuttgart: Deutscher Apotheker Verlag.

ESCOP. 1997. "Frangulae cortex." *Monographs on the Medicinal Uses of Plant Drugs.* Exeter, U.K.: European Scientific Cooperative on Phytotherapy.

Harborne, J. and H. Baxter. 1993. *Phytochemical Dictionary: A Handbook of Bioactive Compounds from Plants.* Washington, D.C.: Taylor and Francis.

Hartwell, J.L. 1971. Plants used against cancer: a survey. *Lloydia* 34(1):103–160.

Karnick, C.R. 1994. *Pharmacopoeial Standards of Herbal Plants,* Vol. 1. Delhi: Sri Satguru Publications. 142–143.

This monograph, published by the Commission E in 1993, was modified based on new scientific research. It contains more extensive pharmacological and therapeutic information taken directly from the Commission E.

This material was adapted from *The Complete German Commission E Monographs—Therapeutic Guide to Herbal Medicines.* M. Blumenthal, W.R. Busse, A. Goldberg, J. Gruenwald, T. Hall, C.W. Riggins, R.S. Rister (eds.) S. Klein and R.S. Rister (trans.). 1998. Austin: American Botanical Council; Boston: Integrative Medicine Communications.

1) The Overview section is new information.
2) Description, Chemistry and Pharmacology, Uses, Contraindications, Side Effects, Interactions with Other Drugs, and Dosage sections have been drawn from the original work. Additional information has been added in some or all of these sections, as noted with references.
3) The dosage for equivalent preparations (tea infusion, fluidextract, and tincture) have been provided based on the following example:
   Unless otherwise prescribed: 2 g per day of [powdered, crushed, cut or whole] [plant part]
   Infusion: 2 g in 150 ml of water
   Fluidextract 1:1 (g/ml): 2 ml
   Tincture 1:5 (g/ml): 10 ml
4) The References and Additional Resources sections are new sections. Additional Resources are not cited in the monograph but are included for research purposes.

Kupchan, S. and A. Karim. 1976. Tumor inhibitors. 114. Aloe emodin: antileukemic principle isolated from *Rhamnus frangula* L. *Lloydia* 39(4):223–224.

Leung, A.Y. and S. Foster. 1996. *Encyclopedia of Common Natural Ingredients Used in Food, Drugs, and Cosmetics*, 2nd ed. New York: John Wiley & Sons, Inc.

Meyer-Buchtela, E. 1999. *Tee-Rezepturen—Ein Handbuch für Apotheker und Ärzte*. Stuttgart: Deutscher Apotheker Verlag.

Newall, C.A., L.A. Anderson, J.D. Phillipson. 1996. *Herbal Medicines: A Guide for Health-Care Professionals*. London: The Pharmaceutical Press.

Österreichisches Arzneibuch. (ÖAB). 1991. Wien: Verlag der Österreichischen Staatsdruckerei.

Samuelsson, G. 1992. *Drugs of Natural Origin: A Textbook of Pharmacognosy*. Stockholm: Sweden Pharmaceutical Press.

Schulz, V., R. Hänsel, V.E. Tyler. 1998. *Rational Phytotherapy: A Physicians' Guide to Herbal Medicine*. New York: Springer.

Trease, G.E. and W.C. Evans. 1989. *Trease and Evans' Pharmacognosy*, 13th ed. London; Philadelphia: Baillière Tindall.

Tyler, V.E. 1994. *Herbs of Choice: The Therapeutic Use of Phytomedicinals*. New York: Pharmaceutical Products Press.

Wichtl, M. (ed.). 1989. *Teedrogen*, 2nd ed. Stuttgart: Wissenschaftliche Verlagsgesellschaft.

Wichtl, M. and N.G. Bisset (eds.). 1994. *Herbal Drugs and Phytopharmaceuticals*. Stuttgart: Medpharm Scientific Publishers. 208–211.

Additional Resources

Demuth, G., H. Hinz, O. Seligmann, H. Wagner. 1978. Investigations on anthraquinon glycosides of *Rhamnus* species, V Emodin-8-O-beta-gentiobioside, a new O-glycoside from *Rhamnus frangula*. *Planta Med* 33(1):53–56.

BUTCHER'S BROOM

Latin Name:
Ruscus aculeatus

Pharmacopeial Name:
Rusci aculeati rhizoma

Other Names:
box holly

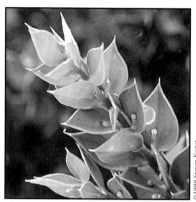

©1999 Steven Foster

Overview

Butcher's broom is an evergreen shrub native to Mediterranean Europe and Africa from the Azores islands, west of Portugal, to Iran in southwestern Asia (Der Marderosian, 1999; Tyler, 1987; Weiss, 1988). It has been used in European medicine for nearly two thousand years as a laxative and diuretic agent to treat urinary, gastrointestinal, and reproductive disorders (Der Marderosian, 1999; Foster and Tyler, 1999). Traditionally, the rootstock was decocted in water or wine as a treatment for abdominal complaints (Weiss, 1988). In the first century C.E., Greek physician Dioscorides reported its laxative effects as well as its use as a treatment for kidney stones (Bown, 1995; Foster and Tyler, 1999). Nicholas Culpepper, the seventeenth century English herbalist, reported that the decoction of the root taken orally, and a poultice of the berries applied topically, assisted in the knitting of fractured bones (Foster and Tyler, 1999; Tyler, 1987).

Today, it is used in Europe for disorders involving the venous system, including venous fragility or varicose veins, and clinical data supports claims that it has positive effects on circulation (Foster and Tyler, 1999). Ruscogenin, a sapogenin first isolated from butcher's broom root in the 1950s by French researchers H. Lapin and C. Sannié, is chemically similar to the steroid saponin diosgenin, which occurs in the Mexican yam root (*Dioscorea* species) (Reynolds, 1989; Tyler, 1987; Weiss, 1988). European preparations standardized to ruscogenin include Ruscorectal® (Endopharm, Germany and Juste, Spain) rectal ointment and suppositories and Hemodren® Simple (Llorens, Spain) indicated for local treatment of hemorrhoids (Reynolds, 1989; Weiss, 1988). In the United States, butcher's broom is not yet widely used, though capsules containing a combination of butcher's broom with rosemary oil have been found in health food stores (Tyler, 1987).

Several clinical studies have been documented. Human studies have investigated its effects on venous insufficiency of the lower limbs when taken in combination with trimethylhesperidine chalcone and ascorbic acid (Weindorf and Schultz-Ehrenburg, 1987), its use to treat lower limb venous disease in patients with chronic phlebopathy when taken in combination with hesperidin and ascorbic acid (Cappelli et al., 1988), its effects on venous tone and capillary sealing when taken in combination with hesperidine methyl chalcone (Rudofsky, 1989), its venoconstrictive action by local application (Berg, 1990), and its effects on retinopathy and lipids in diabetic patients (Archimowicz-Cyrylowska et al., 1996).

A Polish study tested an oral dose of 75 mg of the entire butcher's broom plant extract showing improvement in diabetic retinopathy (Archimowicz-Cyrylowska et al., 1996). The same study showed the extract inactive for hypocholesteremic activity and active in lowering triglycerides. In a double-blind placebo-controlled crossover trial, the effectiveness and tolerability of a venotropic drug (RAES) were evaluated in 40 patients (30 female, 10 male), between the ages of 28 and 74 years, suffering from chronic phlebopathy (venous insufficiency) of the lower limbs. Each RAES capsule dose contained 16.5 mg butcher's broom extract (presumably root) combined with 75 mg hesperidin and 50 mg ascorbic acid. There were two treatment periods of 2 months duration with an interim period of 15 days for wash-out. The daily dosage was 2 capsules, 3 times daily. The authors reported an overall trend toward improvement in the treatment group. Symptoms (e.g., edema, itching, paresthesias, leg heaviness, and cramps) and plethysmographic parameters improved immediately and significantly with the RAES treatment compared to placebo. (A plethysmograph is a device for finding variations in size due to vascular changes.) No side effects were reported (Cappelli et al., 1988).

The approved modern therapeutic applications for butcher's broom are supportable based on its long history of use in well established systems of traditional medicine, phytochemical investigations, *in vitro* studies and pharmacological studies in animals, and several modern clinical studies. Pharmacopeial grade butcher's broom has not been defined at this point.

Description
Butcher's broom is the dried rhizome and root of *Ruscus aculeatus* L. [Fam. Liliaceae], as well as its preparations in effective dosage. The rhizome and root contain the steroid saponins ruscin and ruscoside.

Chemistry and Pharmacology
Butcher's broom contains 4–6% of a mixture of steroidal saponin compounds including approximately 0.12% ruscogenin, neoruscogenin, ruscin and ruscoside (List and Hörhammer, 1979; Nikolov et al., 1976; Der Marderosian, 1999; Pourrat et al., 1983; Reynolds, 1989; Weiss, 1988); fatty acids, mainly tetracosanoic acid; flavonoids; sterols including sitosterol, campesterol, and stigmasterol; benzofuranes, including euparone and ruscodibenzofurane (Bruneton, 1995; ElSohly et al., 1974; ElSohly et al., 1975; Der Marderosian, 1999).

The Commission E reported increase in venous tone, electrolyte-like reaction on the cell wall of capillaries, antiphlogistic and diuretic actions from animal experiments.

Oral absorption may stimulate the post-junctional α-adrenergic receptors of the smooth muscle cells of the vascular wall. Preparations containing high doses of the vasoprotective butcher's broom have been shown to assist with symptoms of venous insufficiency and acute attacks of hemorrhoids. Butcher's broom has also demonstrated antiphlogistic and diuretic activity (Bruneton, 1995).

Uses
The Commission E approved its use as a supportive therapy for discomforts of chronic venous insufficiency, such as pain and heaviness, as well as cramps in the legs, itching, and swelling. It is also approved as a supportive therapy for complaints of hemorrhoids, such as itching and burning.

Contraindications
None known.

Side Effects
In rare cases, gastric disorders or nausea may occur.

Use During Pregnancy and Lactation
No restrictions known.

Interactions with Other Drugs
None known.

Dosage and Administration
Unless otherwise prescribed: Daily dosage: Extracts and their preparations for internal use equivalent to 7–11 mg

total ruscogenin (determined as the sum of neoruscogenin and ruscogenin obtained after fermentation or acid hydrolysis).
Solid dosage forms: Dry native extract containing 7–11 mg total ruscogenin.

References

Archimowicz-Cyrylowska, B. et al. 1996. Clinical effect of buckwheat herb, ruscus extract and troxerutin on retinopathy and lipids in diabetic patients. *Phytother Res* 10(8): 659–662.

Berg, D. 1990. Venenkonstriktion durch lokale Anwendung von Ruscusextrakt. [Venous constriction by local administration of *Ruscus* extract]. *Fortschr Med* 108(24):473–476.

Bown, D. 1995. *Encyclopedia of Herbs and Their Uses.* New York: DK Publishing, Inc. 345.

Bruneton, J. 1995. *Pharmacognosy, Phytochemistry, Medicinal Plants.* Paris: Lavoisier Publishing.

Cappelli, R., M. Nicora, T. Di Perri. 1988. Use of extract of *Ruscus aculeatus* in venous disease in the lower limbs. *Drugs Exp Clin Res* 14(4):277–283.

Der Marderosian, A. (ed.). 1999. *The Review of Natural Products.* St. Louis: Facts and Comparisons.

ElSohly, M.A. et al. 1974. Euparone, a new benzofuran from *Ruscus aculeatus* L. *J Pharm Sci* 63(10):1623–1624.

ElSohly, M.A. et al. 1975. Constituents of *Ruscus aculeatus. Lloydia* 38(2):106–108.

Foster, S. and V. Tyler. 1999. *Tyler's Honest Herbal,* 4th ed. New York: The Haworth Herbal Press.

List, P.H. and L. Hörhammer (eds.). 1979. *Hagers Handbuch der Pharmazeutischen Praxis,* 4th ed. Vol. 6. Berlin-Heidelberg: Springer Verlag. 200–201.

Nikolov, S., M. Joneidi, D. Panova. 1976. Quantitative determination of ruscogenin in *Ruscus* species by densitometric thin-layer chromatography. *Pharmazie* 31(9):611–612.

Pourrat, H., J.L. Lamaison, J.C. Gramain, R. Remuson. 1983. [Isolation and confirmation of the structure by 13C-NMR of the main prosapogenin from *Ruscus aculeatus* L.] [In French]. *Ann Pharm Fr* 40(5):451–458.

Reynolds, J.E.F. (ed.). 1989. *Martindale: The Extra Pharmacopoeia,* 29th ed. London: The Pharmaceutical Press.

Rudofsky, G. 1989. Venentonisierung und Kapillarabdichtung. Die Wirkung der Kombination aus *Ruscus*-Extrakt und Trimethylhesperidin-chalkon bei gesunden Probanden unter Warmebelastung [Improving venous tone and capillary sealing. Effect of a combination of *Ruscus* extract and hesperidine methyl chalcone in healthy probands in heat stress]. *Fortschr Med* 107(19):52, 55–58.

Tyler, V.E. 1987. *The New Honest Herbal.* Philadelphia, PA: George F. Stickley Company. 51–52.

Weindorf, N. and U. Schultz-Ehrenburg. 1987. Kontrollierte Studie zur oralen Venentonisierung der primaren Varikosis mit *Ruscus aculeatus* und Trimethylhesperidinchalkon [Controlled study of increasing venous tone in primary varicose veins by oral administration of *Ruscus aculeatus* and trimethylhespiridinchalcone]. *Z Hautkr* 62(1):28–38.

Weiss, R.F. 1988. *Herbal Medicine.* Beaconsfield, England: Beaconsfield Publishers.

Additional Resources

Bouskela, E., F.Z. Cyrino, G. Marcelon. 1994. Possible mechanisms for the inhibitory effect of *Ruscus* extract on increased microvascular permeability induced by histamine in hamster cheek pouch. *J Cardiovasc Pharmacol* 24(2):281–285.

———. 1993. Effects of *Ruscus* extract on the internal diameter of arterioles and venules of the hamster cheek pouch microcirculation. *J Cardiovasc Pharmacol* 22(2):221–224.

This material was adapted from *The Complete German Commission E Monographs—Therapeutic Guide to Herbal Medicines.* M. Blumenthal, W.R. Busse, A. Goldberg, J. Gruenwald, T. Hall, C.W. Riggins, R.S. Rister (eds.) S. Klein and R.S. Rister (trans.). 1998. Austin: American Botanical Council; Boston: Integrative Medicine Communications.

1) The Overview section is new information.

2) Description, Chemistry and Pharmacology, Uses, Contraindications, Side Effects, Interactions with Other Drugs, and Dosage sections have been drawn from the original work. Additional information has been added in some or all of these sections, as noted with references.

3) The dosage for equivalent preparations (tea infusion, fluidextract, and tincture) have been provided based on the following example:
   Unless otherwise prescribed: 2 g per day of [powdered, crushed, cut or whole] [plant part]
   Infusion: 2 g in 150 ml of water
   Fluidextract 1:1 (g/ml): 2 ml
   Tincture 1:5 (g/ml): 10 ml

4) The References and Additional Resources sections are new sections. Additional Resources are not cited in the monograph but are included for research purposes.

Facino, R.M., M. Carini, R. Stefani, G. Aldini, L. Saibene. 1995. Anti-elastase and anti-hyaluronidase activities of saponins and sapogenins from *Hedera helix*, *Aesculus hippocastanum*, and *Ruscus aculeatus*: factors contributing to their efficacy in the treatment of venous insufficiency. *Arch Pharm (Weinheim)* 328(10):720–724.

Harborne, J.B. and H. Baxter. 1993. *Phytochemical Dictionary: A Handbook of Bioactive Compounds from Plants*. Washington, D.C.: Taylor & Francis.

Marcelon, G., T.J. Verbeuren, H. Lauressergues, P.M. Vanhoutte. 1983. Effect of *Ruscus aculeatus* on isolated canine cutaneous veins. *Gen Pharmacol* 14(1):103–106.

Rubanyi, G., G. Marcelon, P.M. Vanhoutte. 1984. Effect of temperature on the responsiveness of cutaneous veins to the extract of *Ruscus aculeatus*. *Gen Pharmacol* 15(5):431–434.

Salzmann, P. et al. 1977. [*Ruscus aculeatus* L. Butcher's broom, a therapeutic agent in proctology] [In German]. *Fortschr Med* 95(21):1419–1422.

Vanhoutte, P.M. 1986. *Advances in Medicinal Phytochemistry*. New York: John Wiley & Sons, Inc.

Werbach, M.R. and M.T. Murray. 1994. *Botanical Influences on Illness: A Sourcebook of Clinical Research*. Tarzana, CA: Third Line Press.

CALENDULA FLOWER

Latin Name:
Calendula officinalis

Pharmacopeial Name:
Calendulae flos

Other Names:
marigold, poet's marigold,
pot marigold

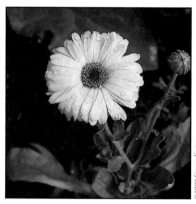

©1999 Steven Foster

Overview

Calendula, or pot marigold, is native to the Mediterranean countries. The name, calendula, refers to the plant's tendency to bloom in accordance with the calendar—every month in some regions, or during the new moon. "Marigold" refers to the Virgin Mary, and marigolds are traditionally used in Catholic events concerning the Virgin Mary. *Calendula officinalis* is sometimes confused with *Tagetes* species of marigolds, more frequently planted in gardens than calendula (Foster, 1993). Used historically as "poor man's saffron," calendula adds both color and flavor to some foods, typically rice and chowders. It was prevalent in European marketplaces during the Middle Ages and was a common soup-starter. Today, petals are sometimes added to salads.

Medicinally, infusions, extracts, and ointments prepared with these petals were used by folk medicine healers in Europe to induce menses, produce sweat during fevers, and to cure jaundice. American Eclectic physicians of the nineteenth century considered calendula helpful in treating stomach ulcers, liver complaints, conjunctivitis, and superficial wounds, sores, and burns (Ellingwood, 1983). Calendula flower preparations were observed to be anti-inflammatory and astringent. In both contemporary and historic times, calendula tinctures, ointments, and washes have been used to notably speed the healing of burns, bruises, cuts, and the minor infections that they cause (Foster, 1993; Tyler, 1994).

While calendula's mechanism of action in stimulating wound healing is poorly understood, effects are localized (Foster, 1993), and the triterpenes clearly demonstrate anti-inflammatory actions, in some cases exceeding the effects of indomethacin (Zitterl-Eglseer et al., 1997). In Europe, ointments used to treat oral lesions or slow-healing cuts and sores rely on the immunostimulating and antibacterial actions of calendula (Foster, 1993). Tests also demonstrate that ointments containing calendula activate tissue regeneration and epithelial tissue development (Klouchek-Popova et al., 1982).

Some clinical studies validate the early treatment of stomach ulcers, although further research is needed (Chakurski et al., 1981; Krivenko et al., 1989). Antiviral and immunostimulating effects have also been reported; calendula's high-molecular weight polysaccharides stimulate immune system activity (Wagner et al., 1985). Calendula has been researched for immune system activity and was initially determined to have some potential therapeutic activity against the human immunodeficiency virus (HIV): extracts significantly inhibited HIV-1 *in vitro*, and reduced HIV-1 reverse transcriptase in a dose- and time-dependent manner (Kalvatchev et al., 1997).

Description

Calendula flower consists of the dried flower heads or the dried ligulate flowers (ray florets) of C. *officinalis* L. [Fam. Asteraceae], as well as its preparations in effective dosage. The preparation contains triterpene glycosides and aglycones, as well as carotenoids and essential oils.

Chemistry and Pharmacology

Constituents include the flavonol glycosides isoquercitrin, narcissin, neohesperidoside, and rutin, terpenoids α- and β-amyr-in, lupeol, longispinogenin, and sterols, volatile oils, arvoside A, carotenoid pigments, calendulin, and polysaccharides (Newall et al., 1996).

The Commission E reported anti-inflammatory, granulatory, and wound healing action with topical application.

Human studies of post-mastectomy lymphedema indicate that external applications of calendula (in conjuction with other plant extracts) possess pain reduction properties (Newall et al., 1996). In vitro research suggests antibacterial activity as well, due to the presence of ethanol (Bruneton, 1995). Other activities include an increase of glycoprotein, nucleoprotein, and collagen metabolism at wound sites; and antibacterial, antifungal, antiviral, and antiparasitic properties (Leung and Foster, 1996).

Uses

The Commission E approved the internal and topical use of calendula flower for inflammation of the oral and pharyngeal mucosa. It was also approved externally for poorly healing wounds. Specifically, herbal infusions, tinctures, and ointments are used to respond to skin and mucous membrane inflammations such as pharyngitis, dermatitis, leg ulcers, bruises, boils, and rashes (Wichtl and Bisset, 1994).

Contraindications

None known.

Side Effects

None known.

Use During Pregnancy and Lactation

No restrictions known.

Interactions with Other Drugs

None known.

Dosage and Administration

Internal: Unless otherwise prescribed: 1–2 g per day whole dried flower.
Infusion: 1–2 g dried herb in 150 ml.
Fluidextract 1:1 (g/ml): 1–2 ml.
Tincture 1:5 (g/ml): 5–10 ml.

References

Bruneton, J. 1995. *Pharmacognosy, Phytochemistry, Medicinal Plants*. Paris: Lavoisier Publishing.

Chakurski I., M. Matev, A. Koichev, I. Angelova, G. Stefanov. 1981. [Treatment of chronic colitis with an herbal combination of *Taraxacum officinale, Hipericum perforatum, Melissa officinalis, Calendula officinalis* and *Foeniculum vulgare*] [In Bulgarian]. *Vutr Boles* 20(6):51–54.

Ellingwood, F. 1983. *American Materia Medica, Therapeutics and Pharmacognosy*. Portland, OR: Eclectic Medical Publications [reprint of 1919 original].

Foster, S. 1993. *101 Medicinal Herbs: An Illustrated Guide*. Loveland: Interweave Press.

Kalvatchev, Z., R. Walder, D. Garzaro. 1997. Anti-HIV activity of extracts from *Calendula officinalis* flowers. *Biomed Pharmacother* 51(4):176–180.

Klouchek-Popova, E. et al. 1982. Influence of the physiological regeneration and epithelialization using fractions isolated from *Calendula officinalis*. *Acta Physiol Pharmacol Bulg* 8(4):63–67.

Krivenko, V.V., G.P. Potebnia, V.V. Loiko. 1989. [Experience in treating digestive organ diseases with medicinal plants] [In Russian]. *Vrach Delo* (3):76–78.

Leung, A.Y. and S. Foster. 1996. *Encyclopedia of Common Natural Ingredients Used in Food, Drugs and Cosmetics*, 2nd ed. New York: John Wiley & Sons, Inc.

Newall, C.A., L.A. Anderson, J.D. Phillipson. 1996. *Herbal Medicines: A Guide for Health-Care Professionals*. London: The Pharmaceutical Press.

Tyler, V.E. 1994. *Herbs of Choice: The Therapeutic Use of Phytomedicinals*. New York: Pharmaceutical Products Press.

Wagner, H. et al. 1985. [Immunostimulating action of polysaccharides (heteroglycans) from higher plants] [In German]. *Arzneimforsch* 35(7):1069–1075.

Wichtl, M. and N.G. Bisset (eds.). 1994. *Herbal Drugs and Phytopharmaceuticals.* Stuttgart: Medpharm Scientific Publishers.

Zitterl-Eglseer, K. et al. 1997. Anti-oedematous activities of the main triterpendiol esters of marigold (*Calendula officinalis* L.). *J Ethnopharmacol* 57(2):139–144.

Additional Resources

Akihisa, T. et al. 1996. Triterpene alcohols from the flowers of compositae and their anti-inflammatory effects. *Phytochemistry* 43(6):1255–1260.

Boucaud-Maitre, Y., O. Algernon, J. Raynaud. 1988. Cytotoxic and antitumoral activity of *Calendula officinalis* extracts. *Pharmazie* 43(3):220–221.

Della Loggia, R. et al. 1994. The role of triterpenoids in the topical anti-inflammatory activity of *Calendula officinalis* flowers. *Planta Med* 60(6):516–520.

Gasiorowska, I., M. Jachimowicz, B. Patalas, A. Mlynarczyk. 1983. [The use of *Calendula officinalis* in the treatment of periodontopathies] [In Polish]. *Czas Stomatol* 36(4):307–311.

This material was adapted from *The Complete German Commission E Monographs—Therapeutic Guide to Herbal Medicines.* M. Blumenthal, W.R. Busse, A. Goldberg, J. Gruenwald, T. Hall, C.W. Riggins, R.S. Rister (eds.) S. Klein and R.S. Rister (trans.). 1998. Austin: American Botanical Council; Boston: Integrative Medicine Communications.

1) The Overview section is new information.
2) Description, Chemistry and Pharmacology, Uses, Contraindications, Side Effects, Interactions with Other Drugs, and Dosage sections have been drawn from the original work. Additional information has been added in some or all of these sections, as noted with references.
3) The dosage for equivalent preparations (tea infusion, fluidextract, and tincture) have been provided based on the following example:
   Unless otherwise prescribed: 2 g per day of [powdered, crushed, cut or whole] [plant part]
   Infusion: 2 g in 150 ml of water
   Fluidextract 1:1 (g/ml): 2 ml
   Tincture 1:5 (g/ml): 10 ml
4) The References and Additional Resources sections are new sections. Additional Resources are not cited in the monograph but are included for research purposes.

Cascara Sagrada Bark

Latin Name:
Rhamnus purshiana

Pharmacopeial Name:
Rhamni purshianae cortex

Other Names:
cascara, chittem bark, sacred bark

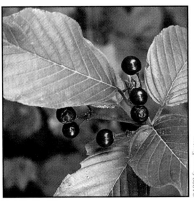

©1999 Steven Foster

Overview

Cascara sagrada is a deciduous tree native to forests of the North American Pacific Coast, ranging from northern California to British Columbia and almost to the Alaska panhandle, in moist areas below 1,500 m elevation. It is also found in the Rockies of Idaho and in Montana (HPUS, 1992; Leung and Foster, 1996; Moore, 1993). The material of commerce comes mainly from Oregon, Washington, and British Columbia in the form of dried quills, flattened and/or curved pieces of dried bark. It is harvested from trees with a trunk diameter of at least 10 cm and it is cured for at least one year before use (BHP, 1996; HPUS, 1992; Leung and Foster, 1996; Wichtl and Bisset, 1994). Because the anthraquinones in freshly dried cascara bark can cause extreme gastrointestinal irritation, including severe intestinal spasms or vomiting, it is either aged for a year to allow oxidation of the anthrones (Samuelsson, 1992), or it is heated and dried to induce artificial aging. Either process makes the laxative effects mild enough so that the relief of constipation is gentle, even when constipation occurs in patients with hemorrhoids, anal fissures, or pain following anorectal surgery (Schulz et al., 1998).

The modern clinical applications for cascara originate from its traditional use in North American aboriginal medicine. Numerous tribes throughout the Northwest have traditionally used cascara bark as a laxative drug in various dosage forms, including aqueous decoction and/or infusion, cold macerate as well as chewing the bark directly. For example, the Flathead, a Salish people of northwest Montana, and the Kutenai people of Montana, Idaho and British Columbia both prepare a cathartic infusion of the bark as a purgative. The Sanpoil, Shuswap, Skagit, and Yurok peoples prepare the bark as a decoction for laxative action (Moerman, 1998). Cascara was not mentioned in the literature until 1805 and it was not brought into western medical use until 1877 (Der Marderosian, 1999; Trease and Evans, 1989), when its traditional use was reported by Eclectic physician Dr. J.H. Bundy in his *"New Preparations."* Parke-Davis & Co. then introduced it as a laxative drug in an alcoholic fluidextract form. Eli Lilly & Co. also introduced their laxative product "Elixir Purgans," a compound elixir containing cascara (*Rhamnus purshiana* DC), wahoo (*Euonymus atropurpureus* Jacq.), senna (*Cassia acutifolia* Delile), blue flag (*Iris versicolor* L.), and hyoscyamus leaves (*Hyoscyamus niger* L.) combined with aromatics (Felter and Lloyd, 1983).

Many *Rhamnus* species share anthraquinone derivative constituents and provide similar laxative actions. These constituents were isolated by botanists early in the study of plant chemistry. They are chemically classified as anthraquinone derivatives. The cascarosides in cascara sagrada provide up to two thirds of the plant's anthraquinone content. They induce peristalsis in the large intestine, with few side effects (Harborne and Baxter, 1993).

Very few modern human studies have been done. Some studies have investigated its use as a colon cleansing method for colonoscopy (Hangartner et al., 1989; Phillip et al., 1990) and its effectiveness as a laxative to treat elderly people suffering from chronic functional constipation (Petticrew et al., 1997).

In Germany, cascara is official in the *German Pharmacopoeia*, approved in the Commission E monographs, and the tea form is official in the German Standard License monographs. It is typically combined with other laxatives in various dosage forms including dry extract, fluidextract, and infusion (Bradley, 1992; Braun et al., 1997; DAB 10, 1994; Wichtl and Bisset, 1994). In the United States, cascara was official in the *United States Pharmacopoeia* from 1890 up through the 22nd revision in 1990, and recognized in the *National Formulary* 14th edition (Boyle, 1991; CFR 21, 1985; Leung and Foster, 1996; NF XIV, 1975; USP XXII, 1990). It is a component of numerous over-the-counter laxative preparations (e.g., Cas-Evac, Parke-Davis; Concentrated Milk of Magnesia-Cascara) (Budavari, 1996; Der Marderosian, 1999; Reynolds, 1989; Tyler, 1994). Aromatic Cascara Fluidextract (USP) is a 1:1 (w/v) aqueous extract of cascara with licorice root, preserved in alcohol 20% (v/v). Cascara Sagrada Extract (USP) is a dry extract containing 11% hydroxyanthracene derivatives (Reynolds, 1989). Cascara sagrada is also classified in the *Homeopathic Pharmacopoeia of the United States* as an OTC Class C drug prepared as a 1:10 (w/v) alcoholic tincture of the bark, in 65% v/v alcohol (HPUS, 1992).

Pharmacopeial grade cascara sagrada bark consists of the dried whole or cut bark of *R. purshiana* D.C. It must contain not less than 8.0% hydroxyanthracene glycosides of which 60% must be cascarosides, both calculated as cascaroside A with reference to the dried drug. Botanical identity must be confirmed by thin-layer chromatography (TLC), macroscopic and microscopic examinations, and organoleptic evaluation. Tests for adulteration with fresh uncured bark and/or other species of *Rhamnus* are carried out (BP, 1980; DAB 10, 1994; Ph.Eur.3, 1997; Wichtl and Bisset, 1994). It should contain not less than 15% water-soluble extractive (Karnick, 1994). The ESCOP monograph requires that the material comply with the *European Pharmacopoeia* (ESCOP, 1997).

Description

Cascara sagrada bark is the dried bark of *R. purshiana* D.C. (syn. *Frangula purshiana* (D.C.) A. Gray ex J.C. Cooper) [Fam. Rhamnaceae], as well as its preparations in effective dosage. The bark contains anthranoids, mainly of the aloe-emodin type, in addition to those of the chrysophanol and physcion type.The commercial product must conform to the currently valid pharmacopeia.

Chemistry and Pharmacology

Cascara contains 8–10% of a complex mixture of hydroxyanthracene derivatives, of which 60–70% are cascarosides A, B, C, D, E, and F, 10–30% are aloins A and B with chrysaloins A and B, and 10–20% are a mixture of anthraquinone O-glycosides and free anthraquinones (e.g., aloe-emodin, frangula-emodin, iso-emodin, chrysophanol, and physcion); resins; tannins; lipids (Bradley, 1992; Budavari, 1996; ESCOP, 1997; Leung and Foster, 1996; Meyer-Buchtela, 1999; Wichtl and Bisset, 1994).

The Commission E reported that 1,8-dihydroxy-anthracene derivatives have a laxative effect, due to the influence of the herb on the motility of the colon, inhibiting stationary and stimulating propulsive contractions. This results in an accelerated intestinal passage and, because of the shortened contact time, a reduction in liquid absorption. In addition, stimulation of chloride secretion increases water and electrolyte content. Systematic studies pertaining to the kinetics of cascara sagrada bark preparations are not available. However, it must be concluded that the aglycones contained in the preparation are already absorbed in the upper small intestine.

The β-glycosides are prodrugs that are neither absorbed nor cleaved in the upper gastrointestinal tract. They are degraded in the colon by bacterial enzymes to anthrones, laxative metabolites. Active metabolites of other anthronoids, such as rhein, infiltrate in small amounts into the milk ducts. A laxative effect on nursing infants has not been observed. The placental permeability for rhein is very small.

Commercial preparations (i.e., herbal stimulant laxatives) have a higher general toxicity than the pure glycosides, presumably due to the content of aglycones. Experiments pertaining to the genotoxicity of cascara sagrada and its preparations are not available. Some positive data were obtained for aloe-emodin, emodin, physcion, and chrysophanol. No data are available for carcinogenicity.

The fresh bark contains free anthrone and must be stored for one year or artificially aged by heat and aeration. The use of illegally processed cascara sagrada bark, e.g., fresh bark, will cause severe vomiting, possibly spasms.

The *British Herbal Pharmacopoeia* and the *British Pharmacopoeia* both reported laxative action (BP, 1980; Bradley, 1992). The Canadian Health Protection Branch Status Manual reported cascara to be an anthraquinone purgative drug with a mild action (HPB, 1992). *The Merck Index* reported its therapeutic category as cathartic (Budavari, 1996).

Uses

The Commission E approved the use of cascara sagrada bark for constipation.

ESCOP reported its therapeutic indications for short term use in cases of occasional constipation based on the U.S. FDA monograph (CFR 21, 1985; ESCOP, 1997). The German Standard License for cascara bark tea indicates its use for constipation; all disorders in which easy bowel evacuation with soft stools is desired, e.g., in cases of anal fissures, hemorrhoids, and after recto-anal operations (Bradley, 1992; Braun et al., 1997; Wichtl and Bisset, 1994).

The *British Herbal Pharmacopoeia* indicates its use for occasional constipation; conditions in which a soft stool is desirable, such as anal fissure or hemorrhoids (Bradley, 1992).

Contraindications

Intestinal obstruction, acute intestinal inflammation, e.g., Crohn's disease, colitis ulcerosa, appendicitis, abdominal pain of unknown origin. Children under 12 years of age.

Side Effects

In single incidents, cramp-like discomforts of the gastrointestinal tract. These cases require a dosage reduction.

Long-time use/abuse: Disturbances of electrolyte balance, especially potassium deficiency, albuminuria, and hematuria. Pigment implantation into the intestinal mucosa (*Pseudomelanosis coli*) is harmless and usually reverses upon discontinuation of the preparation. Potassium deficiency can lead to disorders of heart function and muscular weakness, especially with concurrent use of heart glycosides, diuretics, or corticosteroids.

Use During Pregnancy and Lactation

Because of insufficient toxicological investigation, this drug should not be used during pregnancy and lactation.

Interactions with Other Drugs

With chronic use/abuse, potassium loss may cause an increase in the effectiveness of cardiac glycosides. An effect on antiarrhythmics is possible. Potassium deficiency increases with simultaneous application of thiazide diuretics, corticosteroids, or licorice root.

Dosage and Administration

Unless otherwise prescribed: 1–2 g per day cut or powdered aged bark yielding 20–30 mg hydroxyanthracene derivatives (calculated as cascaroside A) in tea, decoction, cold maceration, elixir, or dry extract. Liquid or solid forms of medication exclusively for oral use. The individually correct dosage is the smallest dosage necessary to maintain a soft stool. Note: The form of administration should be smaller than the normal daily dosage.

Bark: 0.3–1 g in a single daily dose (Bradley, 1992; CFR 21, 1985; ESCOP, 1997).

Infusion: Steep 1–2 g in 150 ml boiled water for 10 to 15 minutes (Braun et al., 1997; ESCOP, 1997; Meyer-Buchtela, 1999; Wichtl and Bisset, 1994).

[Note: Extraction with boiling water prevents some of the losses and chemical changes that occur during cold water extraction (Fairbairn and Simic, 1970; Der Marderosian, 1999).]

Cold macerate: 1–2 g in 150 ml cold water for several hours, then boil and strain. [Note: 90% of the available hydroxyanthracene derivatives are released into cold water after six hours of maceration (Meyer-Buchtela, 1999).]

Elixir: 1–2 ml flavored and sweetened alcoholic fluidextract.

[Note: Cascara Elixir of the *British Pharmacopoeia* contains cascara in combination with licorice, light magnesium oxide, coriander oil, anise oil, ethanol, saccharin sodium, glycerol, and water (BP, 1980).]

Fluidextract 1:1 (g/ml): 1–2 ml.

[Note: Cascara Liquid Extract dosage range in the *British Pharmacopoeia* is 2–5 ml (BP, 1980).]

Tincture 1:5 (g/ml): 2–4 ml.

Dry extract 4.0–5.5:1 (w/w) containing approximately 13% (130 mg/g) hydroxyanthracene derivatives: 0.15–0.23 g (BP, 1980; Bradley, 1992; Braun et al., 1997; CFR 21, 1985; ESCOP, 1997; Meyer-Buchtela, 1999; Wichtl and Bisset, 1994).

Special caution for use: Stimulating laxatives must not be used over an extended period of time (1–2 weeks) without medical advice.

Overdosage: Electrolyte and fluid imbalance.

Special warnings: Use of a stimulating laxative longer than recommended can cause intestinal sluggishness. The prepa-ration should be used only if no effects can be obtained through change of diet or use of bulk-forming products.

References

Boyle, W. 1991. *Official Herbs: Botanical Substances in the U.S. Pharmacopoeias 1820–1990.* East Palestine, OH: Buckeye Naturopathic Press.

Bradley, P.R. (ed.). 1992. *British Herbal Compendium*, Vol. 1. Bournemouth: British Herbal Medicine Association.

Braun, R. et al. 1997. *Standardzulassungen für Fertigarzneimittel—Text und Kommentar.* Stuttgart: Deutscher Apotheker Verlag.

British Herbal Pharmacopoeia (BHP). 1996. Exeter, U.K.: British Herbal Medicine Association. 53

British Pharmacopoeia (BP). 1980. London: Her Majesty's Stationery Office. Vol. I: 83–84; Vol. II: 551, 561–562.

Budavari, S. (ed.). 1996. *The Merck Index: An Encyclopedia of Chemicals, Drugs, and Biologicals*, 12th ed. Whitehouse Station, N.J.: Merck & Co, Inc.

CFR 21. See U.S.A. Dept. of Health and Human Services: Food and Drug Administration.

Der Marderosian, A. (ed.). 1999. *The Review of Natural Products.* St. Louis: Facts and Comparisons.

Deutsches Arzneibuch, 10th ed., 3rd suppl. (DAB 10). 1994. Stuttgart: Deutscher Apotheker Verlag.

ESCOP. 1997. "Rhamni purshianae cortex." *Monographs on the Medicinal Uses of Plant Drugs.* Exeter, U.K.: European Scientific Cooperative on Phytotherapy.

Europäisches Arzneibuch, 3rd ed., 1st suppl. (Ph.Eur.3). 1998. Stuttgart: Deutscher Apotheker Verlag.

Fairbairn, J.W. and S. Simic. 1970. A new dry extract of cascara (*Rhamnus purshiana* D.C. bark). *J Pharm Pharmacol* 22(10):778–780.

Felter, H.W. and J.U. Lloyd. 1983. *King's American Dispensatory*, 18th ed., 3rd rev. Portland, OR: Eclectic Medical Publications [reprint of 1898 original]. 1654-1657.

Grieve, M. 1979. *A Modern Herbal.* New York: Dover Publications, Inc.

Hangartner, P.J., R. Munch, J. Meier, R. Ammann, H. Buhler. 1989. Comparison of three colon cleansing methods: evaluation of a randomized clinical trial with 300 ambulatory patients. *Endoscopy* 21(6):272–275.

Harborne, J. and H. Baxter. 1993. *Phytochemical Dictionary. A Handbook of Bioactive Compounds from Plants.* Washington, D.C.: Taylor & Francis.

Health Protection Branch (HPB) Status Manual. 1992. Ottawa: Health Protection Branch.

The Homeopathic Pharmacopoeia of the United States (HPUS). 1992. Revision Service Official Compendium. Fairfax, VA: Pharmacopoeia Convention of the American Institute of Homeopathy.

Karnick, C.R. 1994. *Pharmacopoeial Standards of Herbal Plants*. Vol. 1:315–316.

Leung, A.Y. and S. Foster. 1996. *Encyclopedia of Common Natural Ingredients Used in Food, Drugs, and Cosmetics*, 2nd ed. New York: John Wiley & Sons, Inc.

Meyer-Buchtela, E. 1999. *Tee-Rezepturen—Ein Handbuch für Apotheker und Ärzte*. Stuttgart: Deutscher Apotheker Verlag.

Moerman, D.E. 1998. *Native American Ethnobotany*. Portland, OR: Timber Press. 237.

Moore, M. 1993. *Medicinal Plants of the Pacific West*. Santa Fe, NM: Red Crane Books. 304.

National Formulary, 14th ed. (NF XIV).1975. Washington, D.C.: American Pharmaceutical Association.

Petticrew, M., I. Watt, T. Sheldon. 1997. Systematic review of the effectiveness of laxatives in the elderly. *Health Technol Assess* 1(13):i–iv, 1–52.

Ph.Eur.3. See *Europäisches Arzneibuch*.

Phillip J., G.E. Schubert, A. Thiel, U. Wolters. 1990. Vorbereitung zur Koloskopie mit "Golytely" eine sichere Methode? Vergleichende histologische und klinische Untersuchung zwischen Lavage und salinischem Laxans [Preparation for colonoscopy using Golytely—a sure method? Comparative histological and clinical study between lavage and saline laxatives]. *Med Klin* 85(7):415–420.

Reynolds, J.E.F. (ed.). 1989. *Martindale: The Extra Pharmacopoeia*, 29th ed. London: The Pharmaceutical Press.

Samuelsson, G. 1992. *Drugs of Natural Origin: A Textbook of Pharmacognosy*. Stockholm: Sweden Pharmaceutical Press.

Schulz, V., R. Hänsel, V.E. Tyler. 1998. *Rational Phytotherapy: A Physicians' Guide to Herbal Medicine*. New York: Springer.

Trease, G.E. and W.C. Evans. 1989. *Trease and Evans' Pharmacognosy*, 13th ed. London; Philadelphia: Baillière Tindall.

Tyler, V.E. 1994. *Herbs of Choice: The Therapeutic Use of Phytomedicinals*. New York: Pharmaceutical Products Press.

The *United States Pharmacopeia*, 22nd rev. (USP XXII). 1990. Rockville, MD: U.S. Pharmacopoeial Convention.

U.S.A. Dept. of Health and Human Services: Food and Drug Administration. 1985. *Code of Federal Regulations 21* (CFR 21). Part 334. Tentative final monograph. Washington, D.C.: Office of the Federal Register National Archives and Records Administration. 50(10):2124–2156.

Wichtl, M. and N.G. Bisset (eds.). 1994. *Herbal Drugs and Phytopharmaceuticals*. Stuttgart: Medpharm Scientific Publishers.

Additional Resources

Bruneton, J. 1995. *Pharmacognosy, Phytochemistry, Medicinal Plants*. Paris: Lavoisier Publishing.

Giavina-Bianchi, P.F. Jr., F.F. Castro, M.L. Machado, A.J. Duarte. 1997. Occupational respiratory allergic disease induced by *Passiflora alata* and *Rhamnus purshiana*. *Ann Allergy Asthma Immunol* 79(5):449–454.

Hutchens, A.R. 1991. *Indian Herbology of North America*. Boston: Shambala.

Kinget, R. 1967. [Studies of the drugs of anthraquinone principles. XVI. Determination of the structure of anthracene derivatives reduced from the bark of *Rhamnus purshiana* DC] [In French]. *Planta Med* 15(3):233–239.

Muller-Lissner, S. 1993. Adverse effects of laxatives: fact and fiction. *Pharmacology* 47(suppl. 1):138–145.

Newall, C.A., L.A. Anderson, J.D. Phillipson. 1996. *Herbal Medicines: A Guide for Health-Care Professionals*. London: The Pharmaceutical Press.

Reynolds, J.E.F. (ed.). 1996. *Martindale: The Extra Pharmacopoeia*, 31st ed. London: The Pharmaceutical Press.

Steinegger, E. and R. Hänsel. 1992. *Pharmakognosie*, 5th ed. Berlin-Heidelberg: Springer Verlag.

This monograph, published by the Commission E in 1993, was modified based on new scientific research. It contains more extensive pharmacological and therapeutic information taken directly from the Commission E.

This material was adapted from *The Complete German Commission E Monographs—Therapeutic Guide to Herbal Medicines*. M. Blumenthal, W.R. Busse, A. Goldberg, J. Gruenwald, T. Hall, C.W. Riggins, R.S. Rister (eds.). S. Klein and R.S. Rister (trans.). 1998. Austin: American Botanical Council; Boston: Integrative Medicine Communications.

1) The Overview section is new information.
2) Description, Chemistry and Pharmacology, Uses, Contraindications, Side Effects, Interactions with Other Drugs, and Dosage sections have been drawn from the original work. Additional information has been added in some or all of these sections, as noted with references.
3) The dosage for equivalent preparations (tea infusion, fluidextract, and tincture) have been provided based on the following example:
   Unless otherwise prescribed: 2 g per day of [powdered, crushed, cut or whole] [plant part]
   Infusion: 2 g in 150 ml of water
   Fluidextract 1:1 (g/ml): 2 ml
   Tincture 1:5 (g/ml): 10 ml
4) The References and Additional Resources sections are new sections. Additional Resources are not cited in the monograph but are included for research purposes.

CAYENNE PEPPER

Latin Name:
Capsicum species

Pharmacopeial Names:
capsici fructus, capsici fructus acer

Other Names:
Capsicum annuum L. var. *annuum*:
bell pepper, chili pepper, red pepper,
sweet pepper, paprika; *Capsicum
annuum* var. *conoides* Irish: Mexican chili, pimiento; *Capsicum
annuum* var. *glabriusculum* (Dunal) Heiser & Pickersgill: bird pepper;
Capsicum annuum var. *longum* Sendtner: Louisiana long pepper or
hybridized to the Louisiana sport pepper;
Capsicum frutescens L.s.l.: Tabasco pepper, African capsicum, African
chili, capsicum, chili pepper, hot pepper.

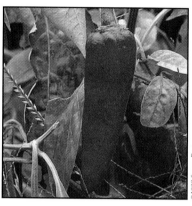

© 1999 Steven Foster

[Note: This herb was published under the monograph heading "Paprika
(Cayenne)" in the original book of Commission E monographs.]

Overview

Capsicum annuum is an annual or biennial plant (Iwu, 1990), while *C. frutescens* is
a perennial shrub. Both species are native to tropical America, now cultivated
worldwide in tropical and subtropical zones (Leung and Foster, 1996; Whistler,
1992). The degree of pungency, calculated in heat units, of dried *Capsicum* and/or
the oleoresin extractive, is what determines its value and end use (Wood, 1987).
The material of commerce comes mainly from tropical Africa, China, and India
(BHP, 1996).

Chili is the Aztec name for cayenne pepper. It has been used by Native Americans
as food and medicine for at least nine thousand years. Based on archeological evidence, its cultivation in Mexico is believed to have begun around seven thousand
years ago. It was first introduced to Europe by Dr. Diego Alvarez Chanca, who
accompanied explorer Cristoforo Colombo (ca. 1451–1506 C.E.) to the West Indies
(Lembeck, 1987; Palevitch and Craker, 1995). From Europe, it was then transported to most tropical, subtropical, and temperate zones around the world (Palevitch and Craker, 1995).

Cayenne was introduced into traditional Indian Ayurvedic medicine as well as
traditional Chinese, Japanese, and Korean medicines, respectively. In Ayurvedic
medicine, a combination of cayenne, garlic, and liquid amber are used externally in
paste or plaster form as a rubefacient (agent which reddens the skin) and local
stimulant. It is also combined with mustard seed in a paste form used as a counterirritant (Kapoor, 1990; Nadkarni, 1976). The dried fruit and/or tincture are also
used internally to treat flatulent dyspepsia and atony of digestive organs (Karnick,
1994; Nadkarni, 1976). In Chinese medicine, cayenne is considered to have digestive stimulant action and is sometimes used to cause diaphoresis (Shih-Chen et al.,
1973). Topically, it is used in China in an ointment form to treat myalgia and frostbite. In Japan, the tincture form is used topically to treat the same conditions (But
et al., 1997).

In Germany, cayenne pepper is official in the *German Pharmacopeia* and approved in the Commission E monographs as a topical ointment for the relief of painful muscle spasms in the upper torso (DAB, 1997). In the United States, capsicum tincture and oleoresin were formerly official in the *United States Pharmacopeia* and *National Formulary*. *Capsicum* USP was used as a carminative, stimulant, and rubefacient (Leung and Foster, 1996; Taber, 1962). Capsaicin, isolated from *Capsicum*, is recognized by the U.S. FDA as a counterirritant for use in OTC topical analgesic drug products (Palevitch and Craker, 1995). It is used as a component in various counterirritant preparations (Leung and Foster, 1996), including ArthriCare® (Del Pharmaceuticals, Inc.) arthritis pain relieving rub, which contains *Capsicum* oleoresin (0.025% capsaicin) in combination with menthol USP and *Aloe vera* gel (Arky et al., 1999). *Capsicum* ointments, such as Zostrix® cream (GenDerm Corp.), containing 0.025% or 0.075% capsaicin, are used topically to treat shingles (herpes zoster) and post-herpetic neuralgia (Bernstein et al., 1987; Der Marderosian, 1999; Palevitch and Craker, 1995).

Cayenne preparations have demonstrated significant efficacy in the treatment of shingles, trigeminal neuralgia, and reduction of pain following surgical amputation (Tyler, 1993). For topical arthritis relief, capsaicin interferes with the pain of inflammatory joint disease. It may block pain fibers by destroying substance P, which normally would mediate pain signals to the brain (Garrett et al., 1997; Tyler, 1993). It may also interfere with oxygen radical transfers that are intrinsic to pain-producing prostaglandin pathways (Leung and Foster, 1996). While its exact mechanisms are not fully understood, capsaicin is regarded as a neuropathic pain reliever, and has recently been the subject of a phase 3 trial that demonstrated significant reductions in the long-term, postsurgical pain of cancer survivors (Ellison et al., 1997).

Numerous studies on topical preparations containing isolated capsaicin have been documented. Human trials have investigated its use as a treatment for chronic post-herpetic neuralgia (Bernstein et al., 1987; Bernstein et al., 1989; Menke and Heins, 1999; Peikert et al., 1991; Watson et al., 1988; Watson et al., 1993), its effects on normal skin and affected dermatomes in herpes zoster (Westerman et al., 1988), the somesthetic and electrophysiologic effects of topical capsaicin (Walker and Lewis, 1990), its use in the treatment of painful diabetic neuropathy (Basha and Whitehouse, 1991; Tandan et al., 1992), the effect of local capsaicin treatment for chronic rhinopathy (Eberle and Gluck, 1994), its use in the management of surgical neuropathic pain in cancer patients (Ellison et al., 1997), and the effect of topical capsaicin on substance P immunoreactivity (Munn et al., 1997). Additionally, a meta-analysis of trials of topical capsaicin for the treatment of diabetic neuropathy, osteoarthritis, post-herpetic neuralgia, and psoriasis has been published (Zhang and Li Wan Po, 1994).

Other studies on the anti-inflammatory action of capsaicin analogs suggest that the antioxidant nature of the methoxyphenol ring of capsaicin may interfere with the oxygen radical transfer mechanism common to lipoxygenase and cyclo-oxygenase. Cayenne is thought to cause a dose-related (1–100 nM) hemolysis of human red blood cells, and is associated with significant changes in erythrocyte membrane lipid components (decreasing phospholipid and cholesterol content), as well as an acetylcholinesterase activity. There are reported alterations in membranes including calcium homeostasis, lysosomal leakage, and alterations in antioxidant enzyme defense systems (Leung and Foster, 1996).

German pharmacopeial grade cayenne pepper consists of dried, ripe fruit of C. *frutescens* L. sensu latiore., usually removed from the calyx. It must contain not less than 0.4% capsaicinoids with reference to the dried drug. Determination of total capsaicinoids is carried out with liquid chromatography. Botanical identification must be confirmed by thin-layer chromatography (TLC), macroscopic and microscopic examinations, and organoleptic evaluation. Fruit from C. *annuum* L.

var. *longum* (de Candolle) Sendtner may not be present (DAB, 1997). The *German Homeopathic Pharmacopoeia*, however, requires the dried ripe fruits of *C. annuum* L. and considers the fruits of *C. frutescens* L. to be foreign constituents (GHP, 1993).

Japanese pharmacopeial grade cayenne pepper consists of the fruit of *C. annuum* L. or its varieties. Identity is confirmed by TLC plus macroscopic and organoleptic evaluations. It must contain not less than 9.0% ether-soluble extractive (JSHM, 1993).

Description

Cayenne consists of the dried fruits of various capsaicin-rich *Capsicum* species [Fam. Solanaceae] and its preparations in effective dosage. Cayenne pepper consists of the dried, ripe, usually removed from the calyx, fruits of *C. frutescens* L., and its preparations in effective dosage. The preparations contain capsaicinoids.

Chemistry and Pharmacology

Cayenne pepper contains up to 1.5% capsaicinoids (pungent principles) including 0.1–1% capsaicin, 6,7-dihydrocapsaicin, nordihydrocapsaicin, homodihydrocapsaicin, and homocapsaicin; fixed oils (Budavari, 1996; Leung and Foster, 1996; Wood, 1987); carotenoid pigments including capsanthin, capsorubin, alpha- and beta-carotene (Budavari, 1996; But et al., 1997; Leung and Foster, 1996); steroid glycosides, including capsicosides A, B, C, and D (But et al., 1997); 9–17% fats; 12–15% proteins; vitamins A and C; trace of volatile oil (Leung and Foster, 1996; Newall et al., 1996).

The Commission E reported local hyperemic and local nerve-damaging activity.

The *British Herbal Pharmacopoeia* reported rubefacient and vasostimulant actions (BHP, 1996). *The Merck Index* reported the therapeutic category of capsaicin, a pungent principle isolated from cayenne or paprika, as topical analgesic (Budavari, 1996). Cayenne has been shown to have counterirritant, antiseptic, diaphoretic, rubefacient, and gastric stimulating properties (Newall et al., 1996; Stecher, 1968).

Uses

The Commission E approved cayenne for painful muscle spasms in areas of shoulder, arm, and spine of adults and children. Preparations are used to treat arthritis, rheumatism, neuralgia, lumbago, and chilblains. It is also used as a deterrent for thumb sucking or nail biting in children (Leung and Foster, 1996). Human studies on cayenne have found different results in duodenal ulcer patients. One study administered 10 g of red chilies in wheatmeal to the control group and duodenal ulcer sufferers and found no significant effect on acid or pepsin secretion, or on sodium, potassium, and chloride concentrations in the gastric aspirate (Pimparkar et al., 1972). In contrast, a study on capsicum showed that it increased acid concentration and DNA content of gastric aspirates in control subjects as well as in patients with duodenal ulcers (Locock, 1985).

Contraindications

Application on injured skin, allergies to cayenne preparations.

Side Effects

In rare cases hypersensitivity reaction may occur (urticaria).

Use During Pregnancy and Lactation

No restrictions known.

Interactions with Other Drugs

None known.

Note: No additional heat application.

Dosage and Administration

Unless otherwise prescribed: Preparations of cayenne exclusively for external uses.

Liniment: Hot oil emulsion containing dried cayenne powder or alcoholic tincture, applied locally by friction method.

Ointment or cream: Semi-liquid preparation containing 0.02–0.05% capsaicinoids in an emulsion base, applied to affected area.

Poultice: Semi-solid paste or plaster containing 10–40 g capsaicinoids per cm², applied locally.

Tincture 1:10 (g/ml), 90% ethanol: Aqueous-alcoholic preparation containing 0.005–0.01% capsaicinoids, applied locally.

Duration of administration: Not longer than two days; 14 days must pass before a new application can be used in the same location. Longer use on the same area may cause damage to sensitive nerves.

Warning: Cayenne preparations irritate the mucous membranes even in very low concentrations and cause a painful burning sensation. Avoid contact of cayenne preparations with mucous membranes, especially the eyes.

References

Arky, R. et al., 1999. *Physicians' Desk Reference for Nonprescription Drugs and Dietary Supplements.* Montvale, NJ: Medical Economics Company, Inc. 642.

Basha, K.M. and F.W. Whitehouse. 1991. Capsaicin: a therapeutic option for painful diabetic neuropathy. *Henry Ford Hosp Med J* 39(2):138–140.

Bernstein J.E., D.R. Bickers, M.V. Dahl, J.Y. Roshal. 1987. Treatment of chronic postherpetic neuralgia with topical capsaicin. A preliminary study. *J Am Acad Dermatol* 17(1):93–96.

Bernstein J.E., N.J. Korman, D.R. Bickers, M.V. Dahl, L.E. Millikan. 1989. Topical capsaicin treatment of chronic postherpetic neuralgia. *J Am Acad Dermatol* 21(2 Pt 1):265–270.

British Herbal Pharmacopoeia (BHP). 1996. Exeter, U.K.: British Herbal Medicine Association. 55–56.

Budavari, S. (ed.). 1996. *The Merck Index: An Encyclopedia of Chemicals, Drugs, and Biologicals,* 12th ed. Whitehouse Station, N.J.: Merck & Co, Inc. 287–289.

But, P.P.H. et al. (eds.). 1997. *International Collation of Traditional and Folk Medicine.* Singapore: World Scientific. 138–139.

Der Marderosian, A. (ed.). 1999. *The Review of Natural Products.* St. Louis: Facts and Comparisons.

Deutsches Arzneibuch (DAB 1997). 1997. Stuttgart: Deutscher Apotheker Verlag.

Eberle L. and U. Gluck. 1994. Klinische Erfahrungen mit lokaler Capsaicinbehandlung bei chronischer Rhinopathie [Clinical experiences with local capsaicin treatment of chronic rhinopathy]. *HNO* 42(11):665-669.

Ellison, N. et al. 1997. Phase III placebo-controlled trial of capsaicin cream in the management of surgical neuropathic pain in cancer patients. *J Clin Oncol* 15(8):2974–2980.

Garrett, N.E., S.C. Cruwys, B.L. Kidd, D.R. Tomlinson. 1997. Effect of capsaicin on substance P and nerve growth factor in adjuvant arthritic rats. *Neurosci Lett* 230(1):5–8.

The *German Homeopathic Pharmacopoeia* (GHP). 1993. Translation of *Homöopathisches Arzneibuch* (HAB 1), 5th suppl. 1991 to the first edition 1978. Stuttgart: Deutscher Apotheker Verlag. 275–277.

Iwu, M.M. 1990. *Handbook of African Medicinal Plants.* Boca Raton: CRC Press. 139–140.

The *Japanese Standards for Herbal Medicines* (JSHM). 1993. Tokyo: Yakuji Nippo, Ltd. 59–60.

Kapoor, L.D. 1990. *Handbook of Ayurvedic Medicinal Plants.* Boca Raton: CRC Press. 98.

Karnick, C.R. 1994. *Pharmacopoeial Standards of Herbal Plants,* Vol. 1. Delhi: Sri Satguru Publications. 79–80.

Lembeck, F. 1987. Columbus, *Capsicum* and capsaicin: past, present and future. *Acta Physiol Hung* 69(3–4):265-273.

Leung, A.Y. and S. Foster. 1996. *Encyclopedia of Common Natural Ingredients Used in Food, Drugs and Cosmetics,* 2nd ed. New York: John Wiley & Sons, Inc.

Locock, R.A. 1985. *Capsicum. Can Pharm J* 118:517–519.

Menke, J.J. and J.R. Heins. 1999. Treatment of postherpetic neuralgia. *J Am Pharm Assoc (Wash)* 39(2):217–221.

Munn, S.E. et al. 1997. The effect of topical capsaicin on substance P immunoreactivity: a clinical trial and immunohistochemical analysis [letter]. *Acta Derm Venereol (Stockh)* 77(2):158–159.

Nadkarni, K.M. 1976. *Indian Materia Medica.* Bombay: Popular Prakashan. 268–271.

Newall, C.A., L.A. Anderson, J.D. Phillipson. 1996. *Herbal Medicines: A Guide for Health-Care Professionals.* London: The Pharmaceutical Press.

Palevitch, D. and L.E. Craker. 1995. Nutritional and medical importance of red pepper (*Capsicum* spp.). *J Herbs Spices Med Plants* 3(2):55–83.

Peikert A., M. Hentrich, G. Ochs. 1991. Topical 0.025% capsaicin in chronic post-herpetic neuralgia: efficacy, predictors of response and long-term course. *J Neurol* 238(8):452–456.

Pimparkar, B.N.D. et al. 1972. Effects of commonly used spices on human gastric secretion. *J Assoc Physicians India* 20:901–910.

Shih-Chen, L., F.P. Smith, G.A. Stuart. 1973. *Chinese Medicinal Herbs*. San Francisco, CA: Georgetown Press.

Stecher, P.G. et al. 1968. *The Merck Index: An Encyclopedia of Chemicals and Drugs*, 8th ed. Rahway, N.J.: Merck & Co., Inc.

Taber, C.W. 1962. *Taber's Cyclopedic Medical Dictionary*, 9th ed. Philadelphia: F.A. Davis Company. C-11.

Tandan, R., G.A. Lewis, P.B. Krusinski, G.B. Badger, T.J. Fries. 1992. Topical capsaicin in painful diabetic neuropathy. Controlled study with long-term follow-up. *Diabetes Care* 15(1):8–14.

Tyler, V. 1993. *The Honest Herbal*, 3rd ed. New York: Pharmaceutical Products Press.

Walker, F.O. and S.F. Lewis. 1990. Somesthetic and electrophysiologic effects of topical 0.025% capsaicin in man. *Reg Anesth* 15(2):61–66.

Watson, C.P., R.J. Evans, V.R. Watt. 1988. Post-herpetic neuralgia and topical capsaicin. *Pain* 33(3):333–340.

Watson C.P. et al. 1993. A randomized vehicle-controlled trial of topical capsaicin in the treatment of postherpetic neuralgia. *Clin Ther* 15(3):510–526.

Westerman, R.A. et al. 1988. Effects of topical capsaicin on normal skin and affected dermatomes in herpes zoster. *Clin Exp Neurol* 25:71–84.

Whistler, W.A. 1992. *Polynesian Herbal Medicine*. Lawai, Kauai, Hawaii: National Tropical Botanical Garden. 237.

Wood, A.B. 1987. Determination of the pungent principles of chilies and ginger by reversed-phase high-performance liquid chromatography with use of a single standard substance. *Flavour Fragrance J* 2:1–12.

Zhang, W.Y. and A. Li Wan Po. 1994. The effectiveness of topically applied capsaicin. A meta-analysis. *Eur J Clin Pharmacol* 46(6):517–522.

Additional Resources

British Herbal Pharmacopoeia (BHP). 1983. Keighley, U.K.: British Herbal Medicine Association.

Bruneton, J. 1995. *Pharmacognosy, Phytochemistry, Medicinal Plants*. Paris: Lavoisier Publishing.

Deutsches Arzneibuch, 10th ed. (DAB 10). 1991. (With subsequent supplements through 1996.) Stuttgart: Deutscher Apotheker Verlag.

Grieve, M. 1979. *A Modern Herbal*. New York: Dover Publications, Inc.

Wren, R.C. 1988. *Potter's New Cyclopaedia of Botanical Drugs and Preparations*. Essex: The C.W. Daniel Company Ltd.

This material was adapted from *The Complete German Commission E Monographs—Therapeutic Guide to Herbal Medicines*. M. Blumenthal, W.R. Busse, A. Goldberg, J. Gruenwald, T. Hall, C.W. Riggins, R.S. Rister (eds.) S. Klein and R.S. Rister (trans.). 1998. Austin: American Botanical Council; Boston: Integrative Medicine Communications.

1) The Overview section is new information.

2) Description, Chemistry and Pharmacology, Uses, Contraindications, Side Effects, Interactions with Other Drugs, and Dosage sections have been drawn from the original work. Additional information has been added in some or all of these sections, as noted with references.

3) The dosage for equivalent preparations (tea infusion, fluidextract, and tincture) have been provided based on the following example:
Unless otherwise prescribed: 2 g per day of [powdered, crushed, cut or whole] [plant part]
Infusion: 2 g in 150 ml of water
Fluidextract 1:1 (g/ml): 2 ml
Tincture 1:5 (g/ml): 10 ml

4) The References and Additional Resources sections are new sections. Additional Resources are not cited in the monograph but are included for research purposes.

CHAMOMILE FLOWER, GERMAN

Latin Name:
Matricaria recutita (syn. *Chamomilla recutita)*

Pharmacopeial Name:
Matricariae flos

Other Names:
Hungarian chamomile, wild chamomile

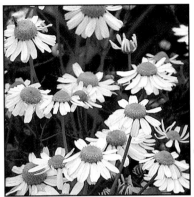

©1999 Steven Foster

Overview

German chamomile is a low-growing, annual herbaceous plant native to southern and eastern Europe and northern and western Asia, now common in wastelands and neglected fields as well as cultivated ground throughout Europe, extending to northern Asia and India. It is particularly abundant in Hungary and Croatia and northern and eastern Africa; it is also naturalized in Australia and the United States (Bruneton, 1995; Felter and Lloyd, 1983; Foster, 1990; HPUS, 1992; Iwu, 1990; Leung and Foster, 1996; Wichtl and Bisset, 1994). The material of commerce, however, comes from cultivated plants from Argentina, Egypt, Bulgaria, and Hungary, and to a lesser extent from Spain, the Czech Republic, and Germany (BHP, 1996; Wichtl and Bisset, 1994). In Germany, chamomile is one of the most important medicinal plants obtained from cultivation. It is cultivated on "set-aside areas" in accordance with EEC regulations (Lange and Schippmann, 1997). The material used in Indian Ayurvedic medicine grows in the Punjab and Upper Gangetic plains (Karnick, 1994; Nadkarni, 1976). The material used in African medicine grows in north Africa and cooler regions of south and eastern Africa (Iwu, 1990).

Chamomile has been described in medical writings since ancient times and was an important drug in ancient Egyptian, Greek, and Roman medicines. Its name is derived from the Greek *chamos* (ground) and *melos* (apple), referring to its low-growing habit and the apple scent of its fresh blooms. Descriptions of the plant are found in the writings of Hippocrates, Dioscorides, and Galen. Over the past 30 years, extensive scientific investigations have confirmed its traditional uses (Foster, 1990; Salaman, 1992). In the United States, chamomile was first cultivated by German settlers and was formerly official in the *United States Pharmacopoeia* and the National Formulary. During the nineteenth century it became an important drug prescribed by American Eclectic physicians, particularly in diseases of young children (Felter and Lloyd, 1983; Leung and Foster, 1996). Today, it is official in many national pharmacopeias, including those of Austria, Egypt, France, Germany, Hungary, Italy, the Netherlands, Switzerland, and Russia (Bradley, 1992; Newall et al., 1996).

In Germany, chamomile flower is licensed as a standard medicinal tea (infusion) for oral ingestion, for topical application as a rinse or gargle, cream, or ointment, as a vapor inhalant, and as an additive for sitz baths or vapor baths. It is official in the *German Pharmacopoeia* and is an approved herb in the Commission E monographs. Aqueous infusions, hydroalcoholic dry extracts, fluidextracts, and tinctures, and the volatile oil are all used as monopreparations and as active components of more than 90 licensed prepared medicines (ABDA, 1982; BAnz, 1998; Bradley, 1992; Braun et al., 1997; DAB 10, 1991; Meyer-Buchtela, 1999; Schilcher, 1997;

Wichtl and Bisset, 1994). In German pediatric medicine, chamomile preparations are the first choice in caring for the sensitive skin of infants and young children, especially for inflammatory skin conditions such as nappy rash and milk crust (Schilcher, 1997). In the United States, it is now one of the most widely used herbal tea ingredients. It is used singly or as a primary component in a wide range of dietary supplement and health food products for oral ingestion, and in skin care for topical application (Foster, 1990; Leung and Foster, 1996). German chamomile is also classified in the *Homeopathic Pharmacopoeia of the United States* as an OTC Class C drug prepared as a 1:10 (w/v) alcoholic tincture of the whole flowering plant, in 45% v/v alcohol (HPUS, 1992).

Modern human studies have investigated its anti-inflammatory, antipeptic, antiphlogistic, antispasmodic, antibacterial, and sedative actions (Bradley, 1992; Leung and Foster, 1996; Mann and Staba, 1986; Szabo-Szalontai and Verzar-Petri, 1977; Newall et al., 1996). One *in vivo* skin penetration study of chamomile flavones was carried out with nine healthy female volunteers. The study concluded that the flavonoids are not only absorbed at the skin surface, but penetrate into deeper skin layers, which is important for their topical use as antiphlogistic agents (Merfort et al., 1994).

In another controlled bilateral comparative study, the efficacy of a chamomile ointment (Kamillosan®) vs. 0.25% hydrocortisone, 0.75% fluocortin butyl ester, and 5% bufexamac was studied as dermatologic agents in maintenance therapy of eczematous diseases. Over a period of three to four weeks, maintenance therapy was carried out on 161 patients suffering from inflammatory dermatoses on hands, forearms, and lower legs who had been initially treated with 0.2% difluorcortolone valerate. The chamomile preparation showed more or less equally effective therapeutic results as the hydrocortisone. It proved superior, however, to the non-steroidal anti-inflammatory agent 5% bufexamac as well as to the 0.75% fluocortin butyl ester. The authors concluded that for treatment of neurodermitis, chamomile ointment is therapeutically comparable to hydrocortisone and superior to the other tested products (Aertgeerts et al., 1985).

In a prospective, double-blind, randomized, multicenter, parallel group study, 79 children (6 months to 5.5 years of age) with acute, non-complicated diarrhea received either an apple pectin-chamomile extract preparation or placebo in addition to the usual rehydration and alimentation diet. After three days of treatment, the diarrhea had ended significantly more in the experimental group than in the placebo group. The pectin-chamomile preparation reduced the duration of diarrhea significantly (p <0.05) by at least 5.2 hours. The parents documented the well-being in a diary twice daily and, in contrast to placebo, a trend of continuous improvement was observed in the pectin-chamomile group (de la Motte et al., 1997).

In a clinical double-blind study the therapeutic efficacy of a chamomile extract on wound healing was investigated on 14 patients after receiving tattoos. Objective parameters were used to evaluate the epithelial and drying effect of the chamomile preparation topically applied to the weeping wound area after dermabrasion from tattoos. The authors reported the decrease of weeping wound area as well as the drying tendency to be statistically significant (Glowania et al., 1987).

Despite popular use of chamomile teas as mild sedatives and sleep aids in Germany and elsewhere, Commission E did not grant approval for such use due to the lack of published research in this area. However, a study indicated that apigenin, a watersoluble component of chamomile, binds at benzodiazepine receptor sites, thus providing a molecular basis for a possible weak central nervous system-depressing activity (Viola et al., 1995).

Pharmacopeial grade German chamomile must be composed of the dried flowerheads (capitulums) containing not less than 0.4% (v/m) blue volatile oil (Ph.Eur.3 method 2.8.12). Additionally, not more than 25% flower fragments, able to pass through a 710 sieve, are allowed. Botanical identity must be confirmed by thin-layer chromatography (TLC) as well as macroscopic and microscopic examinations (Bruneton, 1995; Ph.Eur.3, 1997; Ph.Fr.X, 1990; Wichtl and Bisset, 1994). Both the *British Herbal Pharmacopoeia* and ESCOP monographs require that the material comply with the *European Pharmacopoeia* (BHP, 1996; ESCOP, 1997; Schilcher, 1997).

Description

Chamomile, consisting of fresh or dried flowerheads of *Matricaria recutita* L. (syn. *Chamomilla recutita* (L.) Rauschert) [Fam. Asteraceae] and its preparations in effective dosage. The flowers contain at least 0.4% (v/w) essential oil. Main ingredients of the essential oil are x-bisabolol or bisabolol oxide A and B. The flowers also contain matricin and flavone derivatives such as apigenin and apigenin-7-glucoside.

Chemistry and Pharmacology

Chamomile contains flavonoids (up to 8%), including apigenin and luteolin, volatile oils (0.4–2.0%) composed of x-bisabolol (up to 50%) and chamazulene (1–15%), sesquiterpene lactones (matricin and matricarin), mucilage (10%) composed of polysaccharides, amino acids, fatty acids, phenolic acids, choline (up to 0.3%), and coumarins (0.1%) (Bradley, 1992; Bruneton, 1995; Leung and Foster, 1996; Newall et al., 1996; Wichtl and Bisset, 1994).

The Commission E reported antiphlogistic, musculotropic, antispasmodic, wound-healing promotional, deodorant, antibacterial, bacteriostatic, and skin metabolism stimulant activities.

Chamomile exhibited anti-inflammatory, antipeptic, and antispasmodic activities on the human stomach and duodenum. Oral administration of chamomile extract induced a deep sleep in 10 of 12 patients undergoing cardiac catheterization (Mann and Staba, 1986). Chamomile tea has a marked hypnotic effect (Reynolds, 1989). A hydroalcoholic extract of chamomile flower heads had spasmolytic action on guinea pig ileum (Bruneton, 1995;

Newall et al., 1996). The flavones, especially apigenin, as well as α-bisabolol and other volatile oil constituents, are responsible for its spasmolytic actions (Bradley, 1992). *In vitro*, chamomile has demonstrated antistaphylococcal properties (Molochko et al., 1990).

Uses

The Commission E approved the internal use of chamomile for gastrointestinal spasms and inflammatory diseases of the gastrointestinal tract and approved its external use for skin and mucous membrane inflammations, as well as bacterial skin diseases, including those of the oral cavity and gums. It is also approved for inflammations and irritations of the respiratory tract (inhalations) and ano-genital inflammation (baths and irrigation). The *British Herbal Compendium* lists chamomile internally for spasms or inflammatory conditions of the gastrointestinal tract, peptic ulcer, and mild sleep disorders, and its external use for inflammations and irritations of skin and mucosa in any part of the body and for eczema (Bradley, 1992). The German Standard License for chamomile tea indicates its use for gastrointestinal complaints and irritation of the mucous membranes of the mouth and throat and of the upper respiratory tract (Wichtl and Bisset, 1994).

Contraindications

None known.

Side Effects

None known.

Use During Pregnancy and Lactation

No restrictions known.

Interactions with Other Drugs

None known.

Dosage and Administration

Unless otherwise prescribed: 3 g of whole flower head three to four times daily between meals.

Internal: Infusion: 3 g in 150 ml water, three or four times daily for gastrointestinal complaints. Use the tea infusion as a wash or gargle for inflammation of the mucous membranes of the mouth and throat.

Fluidextract 1:1 (g/ml): 3 ml, three or four times daily.

Tincture 1:5 (g/ml): 15 ml, three or four times daily.

External: Bath additive: 50 g per 10 liters (approximately $2^1/_2$ gallons) of hot water.

Inhalation: Inhale steam vapor of hot aqueous infusion for inflammation of the upper respiratory tract.

Poultice: Semi-solid paste or plaster containing 3–10% m/m of flower head.

Rinse: Hot aqueous rinse containing 3–10% infusion.

References

ABDA (ed.). 1982. *Pharmazeutische Stoffliste*, 4th ed., with supplements. Frankfurt am Main: Arzneibüro der ABDA.

Aertgeerts, P. et al. 1985. [Comparative testing of Kamillosan cream and steroidal (0.25% hydrocortisone, 0.75% fluocortin butyl ester) and non-steroidal (5% bufexamac) dermatologic agents in maintenance therapy of eczematous diseases] [In German]. *Z Hautkr* 60(3):270–277.

BAnz. See *Bundesanzeiger*.

Bradley, P.R. (ed.). 1992. *British Herbal Compendium*, Vol. 1. Bournemouth: British Herbal Medicine Association.

Braun, R. et al. 1997. *Standardzulassungen für Fertigarzneimittel—Text und Kommentar*. Stuttgart: Deutscher Apotheker Verlag.

British Herbal Pharmacopoeia (BHP). 1996. Exeter, U.K.: British Herbal Medicine Association. 131.

Bruneton, J. 1995. *Pharmacognosy, Phytochemistry, Medicinal Plants*. Paris: Lavoisier Publishing.

Bundesanzeiger (BAnz). 1998. Monographien der Kommission E (Zulassungs- und Aufbereitungskommission am BGA für den humanmed. Bereich, phytotherapeutische Therapierichtung und Stoffgruppe). Köln: Bundesgesundheitsamt (BGA).

de la Motte, S., S. Bose-O'Reilly, M. Heinisch, F. Harrison. 1997. Doppelblind-vergleich zwischen einem apfelpektin/kamillenextrakt-präparat und plazebo bei kindern mit diarrhoe [Double-blind comparison of an apple pectin-chamomile extract preparation with placebo in children with diarrhea]. *Arzneimforsch* 47(11):1247–1249.

Deutsches Arzneibuch, 10th ed. (DAB 10). 1991. (With subsequent supplements through 1996.) Stuttgart: Deutscher Apotheker Verlag.

ESCOP. 1997. "Matricariae flos." *Monographs on the Medicinal Uses of Plant Drugs*. Exeter, U.K.: European Scientific Cooperative on Phytotherapy.

Europäisches Arzneibuch, 3rd ed. (Ph.Eur.3). 1997. Stuttgart: Deutscher Apotheker Verlag. 1161–1162.

Felter, H.W. and J.U. Lloyd. 1983. *King's American Dispensatory*, 18th ed., 3rd rev. Portland, OR: Eclectic Medical Publications [reprint of 1898 original]. 1246–1247.

Foster, S. 1990. Chamomile. *Botanical Booklet Series*, No. 307. Austin: American Botanical Council.

Glowania, H.J., C. Raulin, M. Swoboda. 1987. [Effect of chamomile on wound healing—a clinical double-blind study] [In German]. *Z Hautkr* 62(17):1262, 1267–1271.

The Homeopathic Pharmacopoeia of the United States (HPUS). 1992. Arlington, VA: Pharmacopoeia Convention of the American Institute of Homeopathy.

Iwu, M.M. 1990. *Handbook of African Medicinal Plants*. Boca Raton: CRC Press. 203–204.

Karnick, C.R. 1994. *Pharmacopoeial Standards of Herbal Plants*. Delhi: Sri Satguru Publications. 251–252.

Lange, D. and U. Schippmann. 1997. *Trade Survey of Medicinal Plants in Germany—A Contribution to International Plant Species Conservation*. Bonn: Bundesamt für Naturschutz. 29–35

Leung, A.Y. and S. Foster. 1996. *Encyclopedia of Common Natural Ingredients Used in Food, Drugs, and Cosmetics*, 2nd ed. New York: John Wiley & Sons, Inc.

Mann, C. and E.J. Staba. 1986. In: Craker, L.E. and J.E. Simon (eds.). *Herbs, Spices, and Medicinal Plants—Recent Advances in Botany, Horticulture, and Pharmacology*. Phoenix: Oryx Press. 235–280.

Merfort, I., J. Heilmann, U. Hagedorn-Leweke, B.C. Lippold. 1994. *In vivo* skin penetration studies of camomile flavones. *Pharmazie* 49(7):509–511.

Meyer-Buchtela, E. 1999. *Tee-Rezepturen—Ein Handbuch für Apotheker und Ärzte*. Stuttgart: Deutscher Apotheker Verlag.

Molochko, V.A., T.M. Lastochkina, I.A. Krylov, K.A. Brangulis. 1990. [The antistaphylococcal properties of plant extracts in relation to their prospective use as therapeutic and prophylactic formulations for the skin] [In Russian]. *Vestn Dermatol Venerol* (8):54–56.

Nadkarni, K.M. 1976. *Indian Materia Medica.* Bombay: Popular Prakashan. 772–773.

Newall, C.A., L.A. Anderson, J.D. Phillipson. 1996. *Herbal Medicines: A Guide for Health-Care Professionals.* London: The Pharmaceutical Press.

Ph.Eur.3. See *Europäisches Arzneibuch.*

Pharmacopée Française Xe Édition (Ph.Fr.X.). 1983–1990. Moulins-les-Metz: Maisonneuve S.A.

Reynolds, J.E.F. (ed.). 1989. *Martindale: The Extra Pharmacopoeia*, 29th ed. London: The Pharmaceutical Press.

Salaman, I. 1992. Chamomile: A Medicinal Plant. *Herb Spice Med Plant Digest* 10(1):1–4.

Schilcher, H. 1997. *Phytotherapy in Paediatrics: Handbook for Physicians and Pharmacists.* Stuttgart: Medpharm Scientific Publishers. 19–26, 123–124, 157–158.

Szabo-Szalontai, M. and G. Verzar-Petri. 1977. The antibacterial effect of chamomile oil and its isolated compounds. May *Parfumerie und Kosmetik.*

Viola, H. et al. 1995. Apigenin, a component of *Matricaria recutita* flowers, is a central benzodiazepine receptors-ligand with anxiolytic effects. *Planta Med* 61(3):213–216.

Wichtl, M. and N.G. Bisset (eds.). 1994. *Herbal Drugs and Phytopharmaceuticals.* Stuttgart: Medpharm Scientific Publishers.

Additional Resources

Achterrath-Tuckermann, U., R. Kunde, E. Flaskamp, O. Isaac, K. Thiemer. 1980. [Pharmacological investigations with compounds of chamomile. V. Investigations on the spasmolytic effect of compounds of chamomile and Kamillosan on the isolated guinea pig ileum] [In German]. *Planta Med* 39(1):38–50.

Carle, R. and O. Isaac. 1987. Die Kamille—Wirkung und Wirksamkeit. Ein Kommentar zur Monographie Matricariae flos (Kamillenblüten). *Z Phytotherapie* 8:67–77.

Della Loggia, R. 1985. Lokale antiphlogistische Wirkung der Kamillen-Flavone. *Dtsch Apoth Ztg* 125:9–11(43, suppl. 1).

Grieve, M. 1967. *A Modern Herbal*, Vol. 2. New York; London: Hafner Publishing Co.

Isaac, O. 1980. Therapy with chamomile—experiences and verifications. *Dtsh Apoth Ztg* 120:567–570.

List, P.H. and L. Hörhammer (eds.). 1973–1979. *Hagers Handbuch der Pharmazeutischen Praxis,* Vols. 1–7. New York: Springer Verlag.

McGuffin, M., C. Hobbs, R. Upton, A. Goldberg. 1997. American Herbal Product Association's *Botanical Safety Handbook.* Boca Raton: CRC Press.

Stuppner, H., M. Huber, R. Bauer. 1993. Zur Analytik des ätherischen Öles in Kamillenpräparaten - Headspace-Gaschromatographie. *Pharm Ztg Wiss* 138(2–6):46–49.

This material was adapted from *The Complete German Commission E Monographs—Therapeutic Guide to Herbal Medicines.* M. Blumenthal, W.R. Busse, A. Goldberg, J. Gruenwald, T. Hall, C.W. Riggins, R.S. Rister (eds.) S. Klein and R.S. Rister (trans.). 1998. Austin: American Botanical Council; Boston: Integrative Medicine Communications.

1) The Overview section is new information.

2) Description, Chemistry and Pharmacology, Uses, Contraindications, Side Effects, Interactions with Other Drugs, and Dosage sections have been drawn from the original work. Additional information has been added in some or all of these sections, as noted with references.

3) The dosage for equivalent preparations (tea infusion, fluidextract, and tincture) have been provided based on the following example:
   Unless otherwise prescribed: 2 g per day of [powdered, crushed, cut or whole] [plant part]
   Infusion: 2 g in 150 ml of water
   Fluidextract 1:1 (g/ml): 2 ml
   Tincture 1:5 (g/ml): 10 ml

4) The References and Additional Resources sections are new sections. Additional Resources are not cited in the monograph but are included for research purposes.

CHASTE TREE FRUIT

Latin Name:
Vitex agnus castus

Pharmacopeial Name:
Agni casti fructus

Other Names:
chaste berry, vitex, monk's pepper

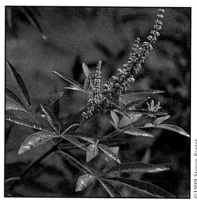

©1999 Steven Foster

Overview

Chaste tree is a small shrub native to Greece and Italy and naturalized to warm climates in the United States. Its peppery fruit has been used medicinally for at least two thousand years. It is mentioned by the Greek physician, Dioscorides, as a beverage taken to lower libido (Schulz et al., 1998). According to the Greek historian, Pliny (first century C.E.), chaste berry strewn on the beds of soldiers' wives was a testimony of the wives' faithfulness while their husbands were at battle (Hobbs, 1996). Despite historical and folk use, there is no scientific evidence to suggest that chaste berry actually reduces libido.

Chaste berry has historically been used to treat hangovers, flatulence, fevers, and constipation (Hobbs, 1996). It was also recognized to bring on menstruation and to relieve uterine cramps (Mills, 1985). American Eclectic physicians of the nineteenth century recommended chaste berry not only as an emmenagogue but also to stimulate lactation (Felter and Lloyd, 1985). Today, chaste berry is used primarily for conditions of the female reproductive system that may stem from latent hyperprolactinemia or corpus luteum insufficiency (luteal phase defect).

In latent hyperprolactinemia, excessive secretion of prolactin may cause breast swelling and breast pain (Schneider and Bohnet, 1981). Studies have determined that chaste berry may help to correct prolactin levels through effects on dopamine receptors (Jarry et al., 1991; Jarry et al., 1994). Chaste berry also affects beneficially "luteal phase defect," a condition marked by short menstrual cycles, thought to be caused by insufficient progesterone secretion consequent to deficits in the corpus luteum (Mühlenstedt et al., 1978). Drugs that lower prolactin secretion have been shown to prolong the luteal phase of the menstrual cycle, as chaste berry has also been shown to do (Schulz et al., 1998; Milewicz et al., 1993).

Both hyperprolactinemia and luteal phase defect have been pointed to as causal to premenstrual syndrome (PMS) and cyclic mastalgia. In clinical trials, chaste berry was shown to relieve both PMS, and, especially, breast swelling and pain (Wuttke et al., 1995). Compared to vitamin B_6, chaste berry was superior in reducing mastalgia, premenstrual fluid retention, headache, and fatigue (Lauritzen et al., 1997).

From 1943 to 1997, approximately 32 clinical studies were conducted on a proprietary chaste berry product (Angolyt®, Madaus, Germany). Seven studies evaluated its effectiveness in treating PMS, four on mastitis and fibrocystic disease, three on menopausal symptons, three on increasing lactation, four on hyperprolactinemia, seven on uterine bleeding diorders, three on acne, and four on miscellaneous menstrual irregularities (Hobbs and Blumenthal, 1999). Commercial chaste berry is administered in capsules and extract forms standardized to the iridoid constituent content, agnuside. Agnuside reduces pain in laboratory mice (Okuyama et al., 1998).

Description

Chaste tree fruit is the ripe, dried fruits of *Vitex agnus castus* L. [Fam. Verbenaceae], as well as their preparations in effective dosage.

Chemistry and Pharmacology

Constituents include the flavonoids casticin, penduletin, and chrysophanol D; alkaloids (viticin); iridoids acucbin and agnuside, volatile oil (0.5%), and essential oil containing *α*-pinene and *β*-pinene (Leung and Foster, 1996; Newall et al., 1996). Vitexin and isovitexin are the primary water-soluble flavones (Hobbs and Blumenthal, 1999).

According to the Commission E, there is evidence that aqueous-alcoholic extracts of chaste tree fruit inhibit secretion of prolactin *in vitro*. In human pharmacology there are no data about the lowering of prolactin levels. There is no knowledge regarding pharmacokinetics and systematic toxicological studies have not been conducted.

Uses

The Commission E approved the use of chaste tree fruit for irregularities of the menstrual cycle, premenstrual complaints, and mastodynia. The herb has been studied for use in cases of insufficient lactation (Bruckner, 1989).
Note: If tension, swelling of the breasts, and disturbances of menstruation occur, a physician should be consulted.

Contraindications

None known.

Side Effects

Occasional itching, urticarial exanthemas.

Use During Pregnancy and Lactation

Not recommended.

Interactions with Other Drugs

In animal experiments, there is evidence of a dopaminergic effect; therefore, ingestion of dopamine-receptor antagonists may weaken the effect.

Dosage and Administration

Unless otherwise prescribed: 30–40 mg (0.03–0.04 g) per day of crushed fruit for aqueous-alcoholic extracts in dry or fluid form.
Fluidextract 1:1 (g/ml), 50–70% alcohol (v/v): 0.03–0.04 ml.
Tincture 1:5 (g/ml), 50–70% alcohol (v/v): 0.15–0.2 ml.
Dry native extract 9.5–11.5:1 (w/w): 2.6–4.2 mg.

References

Bruckner, C. 1989. In mitteleuropa genutzte heilpflanzen mit milchsekretionsfoerdernder wirkung (galactagoga). *Gleditschia* 17:189–201.

Felter, H.W. and J.U. Lloyd. 1985. *King's American Dispensatory*, Vols. 1–2. Portland, OR: Eclectic Medical Publications [reprint of 1898 original].

Hobbs, C. 1996. *Vitex, The Women's Herb*. Santa Cruz: Botanica Press.

Hobbs, C. and M. Blumenthal. 1999. *Vitex agnus-castus*: A Literature Review. *HerbalGram* 47 (in press).

Jarry, H., S. Leonhardt, C. Gorkow, W. Wuttke. 1994. In vitro prolactin but not LH and FSH release is inhibited by compounds in extracts of Agnus castus: direct evidence for a dopaminergic principle by the dopamine receptor assay. *Exp Clin Endocrinol* 102(6):448–454.

Jarry, H. et al. 1991. *Agnus castus* as a dopaminergic active constituent in Mastodynon®N. *Z Phytother* 12:77–82.

Lauritzen, C. et al. 1997. Treatment of premenstrual tension syndrome with vitex agnus castus. Controlled, double-blind study versus pyridoxine. *Phytomedicine* 4:183–189.

Leung, A.Y. and S. Foster. 1996. *Encyclopedia of Common Natural Ingredients Used in Food, Drugs, and Cosmetics*, 2nd ed. New York: John Wiley & Sons, Inc.

Milewicz, A. et al. 1993. *Vitex agnus castus* extract in the treatment of luteal phase defects due to latent hyperprolactinemia. Results of a randomized placebo-controlled double-blind study. *Arzneimforsch* 43(7):752–756.

Mills, S.Y. 1985. *The Dictionary of Modern Herbalism*. Wellingborough: Thorsons.

Mühlenstedt, D., H.G. Bohnet, J.P. Hanker, H.P. Schneider. 1978. Short luteal phase and prolactin. *Int J Fertil* 23(3):213–218.

Newall, C.A., L.A. Anderson, J.D. Phillipson. 1996. *Herbal Medicines: A Guide for Health-Care Professionals.* London: The Pharmaceutical Press.

Okuyama E., S. Fujimori, M.Yamazaki et al. 1998. Pharmacologically active components of viticis fructus (*Vitex rotundifolia*). II. The components having analgesic effects. *Chem Pharm Bull* 46(4):655–662.

Schneider, H.P., H.G. Bohnet. 1981. [Hyperpro-lactinemic ovarian insufficiency] [In German]. *Gynakologe* 14(2):104–118.

Schulz, V., R. Hänsel, V.E. Tyler. 1998. *Rational Phytotherapy: A Physicians' Guide to Herbal Medicine.* New York: Springer.

Wuttke, W., Gorkow, J. Jarry. 1995. Dopaminergic compounds in *Vitex agnus castus*. In: Loew D. and N. Rietbrock. (eds.). *Phytopharmaka in Forschung and klinischer Anwendung.* Darm-stadt: Steinkopff Verlag. 81–91.

Additional Resources

Bruneton, J. 1995. *Pharmacognosy, Phytochem-istry, Medicinal Plants.* Paris: Lavoisier Publish-ing.

Halaska, M. et al. 1998. [Treatment of cyclical mastodynia using an extract of *Vitex agnus cas-tus*: results of a double-blind comparison with a placebo] [In Czech]. *Ceska Gynekol* 63(5):388–392.

Leow, D. and N. Rietbrock. (eds.). 1995. *Phy-topharmaka in forschung und klinischer Anwen-dung* Steinkopff Verlag, Darmstadt.

McGuffin, M., C. Hobbs, R. Upton, A. Goldberg. 1997. American Herbal Product Association's *Botanical Safety Handbook.* Boca Raton: CRC Press.

Turner, S. and S. Mills. 1993. A double blind clini-cal trial on a herbal remedy for premenstrual syndrome; a case study. *Complementary Thera-pies in Medicine* (1):73–77.

This monograph, published by the Commission E in 1992, was modified based on new scientific research. It contains more extensive pharmacological and therapeutic information taken directly from the Commission E.

This material was adapted from *The Complete German Commission E Monographs—Therapeutic Guide to Herbal Medicines.* M. Blumenthal, W.R. Busse, A. Goldberg, J. Gruenwald, T. Hall, C.W. Riggins, R.S. Ris-ter (eds.). S. Klein and R.S. Rister (trans.). 1998. Austin: American Botanical Council; Boston: Integrative Medicine Communications.

1) The Overview section is new information.
2) Description, Chemistry and Pharmacology, Uses, Contraindications, Side Effects, Interactions with Other Drugs, and Dosage sections have been drawn from the original work. Additional information has been added in some or all of these sections, as noted with references.
3) The dosage for equivalent preparations (tea infusion, fluidextract, and tincture) have been provided based on the following example:
   Unless otherwise prescribed: 2 g per day of [powdered, crushed, cut or whole] [plant part]
   Infusion: 2 g in 150 ml of water
   Fluidextract 1:1 (g/ml): 2 ml
   Tincture 1:5 (g/ml): 10 ml
4) The References and Additional Resources sections are new sections. Additional Resources are not cited in the monograph but are included for research purposes.

CINNAMON BARK

Latin Name:
Cinnamomum verum

Pharmacopeial Name:
Cinnamomi ceylanici cortex

Other Names:
Ceylon cinnamon, true cinnamon

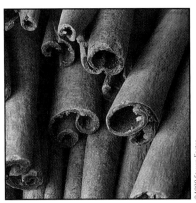

©1999 Steven Foster

Overview

Cinnamon is a small evergreen tree native to tropical southern India and Sri Lanka, growing from sea level to nine hundred meters. It was later introduced throughout the islands of the Indian Ocean and southeast Asia, and is now cultivated extensively in Sri Lanka and the coastal regions of India (Bruneton, 1995; HPUS, 1990; Karnick, 1994; Der Marderosian, 1999; Wichtl and Bisset, 1994). It was not brought into cultivation until 1776 (Grieve, 1979). Sri Lanka is the main producing country, though the material of commerce also comes from India, Malaysia, Madagascar, and the Seychelles (BHP, 1996; Karnick, 1994; Wichtl and Bisset, 1994). Cinnamon bark has been used for several thousand years in traditional Eastern and Western medicines (Leung and Foster, 1996). Galenical preparations of cinnamon bark are used to treat anorexia, bloating, dyspepsia with nausea, flatulent colic, and spastic conditions of the gastrointestinal tract as a component of compounds used in traditional Greco-European medicines and traditional Indian Ayurvedic medicine (Bruneton, 1995; Karnick, 1994; Newall et al., 1996; Wichtl and Bisset, 1994).

The approved modern therapeutic applications for cinnamon are supportable based on a combination of factors including its long history of traditional use in well established systems of traditional medicine, *in vitro* studies, experimental studies in animals, and phytochemical investigations.

In the United States and Germany cinnamon is used as a carminative and stomachic component of herbal compounds in dosage forms including aqueous infusion or decoction, alcoholic fluidextract or tincture, and essential oil. It also appears in both countries as a component of multi-herb cough, cold, and fever formulas.

Pharmacopeial grade cinnamon bark must contain not less than 1.2% volatile oil (Ph.Eur.3, 1997; Wichtl and Bisset, 1994).

Description

Cinnamon consists of the dried bark, separated from cork and the underlying parenchyma, of young branches and shoots of *Cinnamomum verum* J.S. Presl (syn. *C. zeylanicum* Blume) [Fam. Lauraceae], and its preparations in effective dosage. The bark contains essential oil.

Chemistry and Pharmacology

Cinnamon contains volatile oils (1–4%) of cinnamaldehyde (60–80%), eugenol (up to 10%) and *trans*-cinnamic acid (5–10%); phenolic compounds (4–10%), condensed tannins, catechins, and proanthocyanidins; monoterpenes and sesquiterpenes (pinene); calcium-monoterpenes oxalate; gum; mucilage; resin, starch, sugars, and traces of coumarin (Bruneton, 1995; Leung and Foster, 1996; List and Hörhammer,

1973; Hänsel et al., 1992; Newall et al., 1996; Wichtl and Bisset, 1994).

The Commission E reported antibacterial and fungistatic properties in cinnamon as well as the promotion of intestinal motility. The *British Herbal Pharmacopoeia* reported its action as bitter (BHP, 1996). Its essential oil has demonstrated strong antibacterial and antifungal activities *in vitro* (Bruneton, 1995). Antifungal, antiviral, bactericidal, and larvicidal actions have been reported for the volatile oil. Its constituents eugenol, eugenol acetate, and methyl eugenol have been reported to enhance trypsin activity *in vitro*. Cinnamon bark has also shown strong lipolytic (ability to hydrolyze fats) action (Leung and Foster, 1996).

Uses

The Commission E approved the internal use of cinnamon for loss of appetite, dyspeptic complaints such as mild, spastic condition of the gastrointestinal tract, bloating, and flatulence. The German Standard License for cinnamon bark tea infusion lists it for complaints such as a feeling of distension, flatulence, and mild cramp-like gastrointestinal disorders due to reduced production of gastric juice (Braun et al., 1997). In France, cinnamon bark is traditionally used to treat symptoms of digestive disorders, functional asthenias, and also to facilitate weight gain (Bruneton, 1995).

Contraindications

Allergy to cinnamon and Peruvian balsam.

Side Effects

Frequently, allergic reactions of skin and mucosa.

Use During Pregnancy and Lactation

Not recommended (McGuffin et al., 1997).

Interactions with Other Drugs

None known.

Dosage and Administration

Internal: Unless otherwise prescribed: 2–4 g per day of cut or ground bark. Infusion or decoction: 0.7–1.3 g in 150 ml water, three times daily.
Fluidextract 1:1 (g/ml): 0.7–1.3 ml, three times daily.
Tincture 1:5 (g/ml): 3.3–6.7 ml, three times daily.
Essential oil: 0.05–0.2 ml.

References

Braun, R. et al. 1997. *Standardzulassungen für Fertigarzneimittel—Text and Kommentar.* Stuttgart: Deutscher Apotheker Verlag.

British Herbal Pharmacopoeia (BHP). 1996. Exeter, U.K.: British Herbal Medicine Association.

Bruneton, J. 1995. *Pharmacognosy, Phytochemistry, Medicinal Plants.* Paris: Lavoisier Publishing.

Der Marderosian, A. (ed.). 1999. *The Review of Natural Products.* St. Louis: Facts and Comparisons.

Europäisches Arzneibuch, 3rd ed. (Ph.Eur.3). 1997. Stuttgart: Deutscher Apotheker Verlag.

Grieve, M. 1979. *A Modern Herbal.* New York: Dover Publications, Inc.

The Homeopathic Pharmacopoeia of the United States (HPUS). 1992. Revision Service Official Compendium. Boston: Pharmacopoeia Convention of the American Institute of Homeopathy.

Karnick, C.R. 1994. *Pharmacopoeial Standards of Herbal Plants,* Vol. 1. Delhi: Sri Satguru Publications. 94–95.

Leung, A.Y. and S. Foster. 1996. *Encyclopedia of Common Natural Ingredients Used in Food, Drugs, and Cosmetics*, 2nd ed. New York: John Wiley & Sons, Inc.

List, P.H. and L. Hörhammer (eds.). 1973. *Hagers Handbuch der Pharmazeutischen Praxis*, 4th ed. Vol. 4. New York: Springer Verlag. 54, 884.

Hänsel, R., K. Keller, H. Rimpler, G. Schneider (eds.). 1992. *Hagers Handbuch der Pharmazeutischen Praxis*, 5th ed. Vol. 4. Berlin-Heidelberg: Springer Verlag. 884.

McGuffin, M., C. Hobbs, R. Upton, A. Goldberg. 1997. American Herbal Product Association's *Botanical Safety Handbook.* Boca Raton. CRC Press.

Newall, C.A., L.A. Anderson, J.D. Phillipson. 1996. *Herbal Medicines: A Guide for Health-Care Professionals.* London: The Pharmaceutical Press.

Ph.Eur.3. See *Europäisches Arzneibuch.*

Wichtl, M. and N.G. Bisset (eds.). 1994. *Herbal Drugs and Phytopharmaceuticals.* Stuttgart: Medpharm Scientific Publishers.

Additional Resources

Angmor, J.E., D.M. Dicks, W.C. Evans, D.K. Santra. 1972. Studies on Cinnamomum *zeylanicum*. *Planta Med* 21(4):416–420.

Angmor, J.E., P.M. Dewick, W.C. Evans. 1975. Proceedings: Chemical changes in cinnamon oil during its preparation. *J Pharm Pharmacol* 27(suppl. 2):89P.

British Herbal Pharmacopoeia (BHP). 1983. Keighley, U.K.: British Herbal Medicine Association.

British Pharmaceutical Codex (BPC). 1949. London: The Pharmaceutical Press.

———. 1973. London: The Pharmaceutical Press.

Formácek, V. and K.H. Kubeczka. 1982. *Essential oil analysis by capillary gas chromatography and carbon-13 NMR spectroscopy*. New York: John Wiley & Sons, Inc.

Deutsches Arzneibuch, 10th ed. Vol. 1–6. (DAB 10). 1991. Kommentar. Stuttgart: Wissenschaftliche Verlagsgesellschaft.

Lima, E.O., O.F. Gompertz, A.M. Giesbrecht, M.Q. Paulo. 1993. *In vitro* antifungal activity of essential oils obtained from officinal plants against dermatophytes. *Mycoses* 36(9–10):333–336.

Masada, Y. 1976. *Analysis of Essential Oils by Gas Chromatography and Mass Spectrometry*. New York: Halsted (Wiley).

Morozumi, S. 1978. Isolation, purification, and antibiotic activity of o-methoxycinnamaldehyde from cinnamon. *Appl Environ Microbiol* 36(4):577–583.

Quale, J.M., D. Landman, M.M. Zaman, S. Burney, S.S. Sathe. 1996. In vitro activity of Cinnamomum *zeylanicum* against azole resistant and sensitive *Candida* species and a pilot study of cinnamon for oral candidiasis. *Am J Chin Med* 24(2):103–109.

Raharivelomanana, P.J., G.P. Terrom, J.P. Bianchini, P. Coulanges. 1989. [Study of the antimicrobial action of various essential oils extracted from Malagasy plants. II: Lauraceae] [In French]. *Arch Inst Pasteur Madagascar* 56(1):261–271.

Reynolds, J.E.F. (ed.). 1993. *Martindale: The Extra Pharmacopoeia,* 30th ed. London: The Pharmaceutical Press.

Singh, H.B., M. Srivastava, A.B. Singh, A.K. Srivastava. 1995. Cinnamon bark oil, a potent fungitoxicant against fungi causing respiratory tract mycoses. *Allergy* 50(12):995–999.

Trease, G.E. and W.C. Evans. 1989. *Trease and Evans' Pharmacognosy*, 13th ed. London; Philadelphia: Baillière Tindall. 453.

This material was adapted from *The Complete German Commission E Monographs—Therapeutic Guide to Herbal Medicines*. M. Blumenthal, W.R. Busse, A. Goldberg, J. Gruenwald, T. Hall, C.W. Riggins, R.S. Rister (eds.) S. Klein and R.S. Rister (trans.). 1998. Austin: American Botanical Council; Boston: Integrative Medicine Communications.

1) The Overview section is new information.

2) Description, Chemistry and Pharmacology, Uses, Contraindications, Side Effects, Interactions with Other Drugs, and Dosage sections have been drawn from the original work. Additional information has been added in some or all of these sections, as noted with references.

3) The dosage for equivalent preparations (tea infusion, fluidextract, and tincture) have been provided based on the following example:
   Unless otherwise prescribed: 2 g per day of [powdered, crushed, cut or whole] [plant part]
   Infusion: 2 g in 150 ml of water
   Fluidextract 1:1 (g/ml): 2 ml
   Tincture 1:5 (g/ml): 10 ml

4) The References and Additional Resources sections are new sections. Additional Resources are not cited in the monograph but are included for research purposes.

CINNAMON BARK, CHINESE

Latin Name:
Cinnamomum aromaticum

Pharmacopeial Name:
Cinnamomi cassiae cortex

Other Names:
cassia, cassia cinnamon

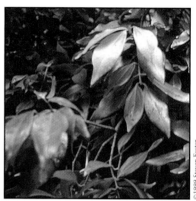

©1999 Steven Foster

Overview

Chinese cinnamon is a medium-sized evergreen tree native to China and Vietnam, now cultivated in southwestern China, Cambodia, India, Japan, Java, Sri Lanka, Sumatra, and Vietnam (Bruneton, 1995; Grieve, 1979; Tyler et al., 1988; Yen, 1992). The cultivated trees are kept as coppices, and prevented from growing higher than 10 feet (Grieve, 1979; Leung and Foster, 1996). The material of commerce used in Chinese medicine is produced in Guangdong, Guangxi, and Yunnan provinces, Cambodia, and Vietnam (Yen, 1992). The genus name *Cinnamomum* may be from Arabic, Hebrew, or Malay language origins and its species name, *cassia*, is from the Greek *kassia*, meaning to strip off the bark. Its medical use is recorded in Chinese formularies around 2700 B.C.E. and somewhat later in ancient Greek and Latin texts (Leung and Foster, 1996; Tyler et al., 1988). According to the energetics theory in traditional Chinese medicine (TMC), it acts to supplement body "fire," to "warm" and tone the "spleen" and "kidney," thus making it effective for precordial and abdominal pain with "cold" sensation, diarrhea due to asthenia and pathogenic "cold," and hypofunction of the kidney (Chang and But, 1986; Tu, 1992). Galenical preparations of Chinese cinnamon bark are used as a carminative, digestive, or stomachic component of compounds in traditional TCM, traditional Greco-European medicines, and traditional Indian Ayurvedic and Unani medicine (Bruneton, 1995; Grieve, 1979; Nadkarni, 1976; Tu, 1992).

Modern clinical studies have investigated its use to treat abdominal pain, diarrhea, gastrointestinal disturbances, bronchial asthma, and asthenia of blood and vital energy. (Chang and But, 1986). Its clinical use is usually as a component in polypharmacy and only rarely as a monopreparation.

One clinical study reported the stimulation of blood circulation and improved digestive function with two different herbal formulas containing Chinese cinnamon, prescribed in TCM in an aqueous decoction, to supplement "vital energy and blood" (Chang and But, 1986; ZMC, 1975). Another study reported improvement in 21 cases treated for bronchial asthma using an alcoholic fluidextract (0.15–0.3 ml) combined with procaine hydrochloride to make a 2 ml dose. The drug was injected into the bilateral "Feishu" acupoints. Asthmatic attacks were controlled in 20 cases and improvement reported in all 21 cases (Chang and But, 1986). Because the cinnamon was combined with other therapeutic agents, either an herbal or a conventional drug, it is not clear what conclusions can be attributed to the action of cinnamon alone.

The modern therapeutic applications for Chinese cinnamon are supportable based on thousands of years of use in well established systems of traditional medicine, *in vitro* studies, *in vivo* studies in animals, phytochemical investigations, and some modern clinical studies. Its composition is similar to that of Ceylon cinnamon and the two herbs are often used interchangeably.

In both the United States and Germany, Chinese cinnamon is used as a digestive or stomachic component of herbal compounds, in aqueous infusion or decoction, alcoholic fluidextract and/or tincture, dry powder in capsules and tablets, and essential oil. It also appears in both countries as one herb among many in cough, cold, and fever formulas.

Pharmacopeial grade Chinese cinnamon bark contains 1–2% volatile oils composed mainly of cinnamaldehyde and cinnamic acid (Chang and But, 1986).

Description

Chinese cinnamon consists of the dried branch bark and occasionally stem bark, separated from the cork, of *Cinnamomum aromaticum* Nees (syn. *C. cassia* Blume) [Fam. Lauraceae] and preparations thereof in effective dosage. The bark contains essential oil.

Chemistry and Pharmacology

Chinese cinnamon contains volatile oils (1–2%) mainly composed of cinnamaldehyde (75–90%); phenolic compounds (condensed tannins), flavonoid derivatives (proanthocyanidins and oligomers or cinnamtannins); mucilage; calcium oxalate, resins, sugars, and coumarins (Bruneton, 1995; Leung and Foster, 1996; Hänsel et al., 1992; List and Hörhammer, 1973; Newall et al., 1996).

The Commission E reported antibacterial, fungistatic, and motility-promotion effects. Antifungal, antiviral, bactericidal, and larvicidal actions have been reported for the volatile oil (Leung and Foster, 1996). Due to autooxidation and evaporation during decoction, it is doubtful that cinnamaldehyde contributes much to the overall therapeutic efficacy of Chinese cinnamon (Hikino, 1985). An aqueous extract demonstrated anti-ulcerogenic activities in rats as effectively as cimetidine (Akira et al., 1986). Chinese cinnamon has shown *in vivo* inhibitory activity against complement formation due to its diterpenoid and condensed tannin content (Hikino, 1985). The aqueous decoction of Chinese cinnamon bark had an inhibitory action against fungi *in vitro* (Chang and But, 1986). A hydroalcoholic extractive of cinnamon bark was found to inhibit bacterial endotoxins (Azumi et al., 1997).

Uses

The Commission E approved the internal use of cinnamon for loss of appetite, and dyspeptic complaints such as mild spasms of the gastrointestinal tract, bloating, and flatulence. The *British Herbal Pharmacopoeia* indicates its use for flatulent dyspepsia, flatulent colic, and diarrhea, specifically colic or dyspepsia with flatulent distension and nausea (BHP, 1983; Newall et al., 1996). The German Standard License for cinnamon bark tea infusion recommends it for a feeling of distension, flatulence, and mild cramp-like gastrointestinal disorders due to reduced production of gastric juice (Braun et al., 1997). The French Herbal Remedies, Notice to Applicants for Marketing Authorization of 1990 allows the same indications for use for Chinese cinnamon as for Ceylon cinnamon (Bruneton, 1995).

Contraindications

Allergy to cinnamon or Peruvian balsam.

Side Effects

Frequently, allergic reaction of the skin and mucosa.

Use During Pregnancy and Lactation

Not recommended (McGuffin et al., 1997).

Interactions with Other Drugs
None known.

Dosage and Administration
Unless otherwise prescribed: 2–4 g per day of ground bark.
Infusion or decoction: 0.7–1.3 g in 150 ml water, three times daily.
Fluidextract 1:1 (g/ml): 0.7–1.3 ml, three times daily.
Tincture 1:5 (g/ml): 3.3–6.7 ml, three times daily.
Essential oil: 0.05–0.2 ml.

References
Akira, T., S. Tanaka, M. Tabata. 1986. Pharmacological studies on the antiulcerogenic activity of Chinese cinnamon. *Planta Med* 52(6):440–443.

Azumi, S., A. Tanimura, K. Tanamoto. 1997. A novel inhibitor of bacterial endotoxin derived from cinnamon bark. *Biochem Biophys Res Commun* 234(2):506–510.

Braun, R. et al. 1997. *Standardzulassungen für Fertigarzneimittel—Text and Kommentar.* Stuttgart: Deutscher Apotheker Verlag.

British Herbal Pharmacopoeia (BHP). 1983. Keighley, U.K.: British Herbal Medicine Association.

Bruneton, J. 1995. *Pharmacognosy, Phytochemistry, Medicinal Plants.* Paris: Lavoisier Publishing.

Chang, H.M. and P.P.H. But (eds.) 1986. *Pharmacology and Applications of Chinese Materia Medica.* Philadelphia: World Scientific. 510–514.

Grieve, M. 1979. *A Modern Herbal.* New York: Dover Publications, Inc.

Hänsel, R., K. Keller, H. Rimpler, G. Schneider (eds.). 1992. *Hagers Handbuch der Pharmazeutischen Praxis,* 5th ed. Vol. 4. Berlin-Heidelberg: Springer Verlag.

Hikino, H. 1985. Oriental Medicinal Plants. In: Wagner, H., H. Hikino, N.R. Farnsworth. 1985. *Economic and Medicinal Plant Research,* Vol. 1. London: Academic Press. 69–70.

Leung, A.Y. and S. Foster. 1996. *Encyclopedia of Common Natural Ingredients Used in Food, Drugs, and Cosmetics,* 2nd ed. New York: John Wiley & Sons, Inc.

List, P.H. and L. Hörhammer (eds.). 1973. *Hagers Handbuch der Pharmazeutischen Praxis,* Vol. 4. New York: Springer Verlag. 54, 884.

McGuffin, M., C. Hobbs, R. Upton, A. Goldberg. 1997. *American Herbal Product Association's Botanical Safety Handbook.* Boca Raton: CRC Press.

Nadkarni, K.M. 1976. *Indian Materia Medica.* Bombay: Popular Prakashan. 328–330.

Newall, C.A., L.A. Anderson, J.D. Phillipson. 1996. *Herbal Medicines: A Guide for Health-Care Professionals.* London: The Pharmaceutical Press.

Tu, G. (ed.). 1992. *Pharmacopoeia of the People's Republic of China* (English Edition 1992). Beijing: Guangdong Science and Technology Press. 31.

Tyler, V.E., L.R. Brady, J.E. Robbers. 1988. *Pharmacognosy,* 9th ed. Philadelphia: Lea & Febiger. 119–122.

Yen, K.Y. 1992. *The Illustrated Chinese Materia Medica—Crude and Prepared.* Taipei: SMC Publishing, Inc.

Zhongshan Medical College Editorial Group (ZMC). 1975. *Clinical Application of Chinese Traditional Drugs,* 1st ed. Guangdong: Guangdong People's Publishing House. 8, 201.

Additional Resources
British Herbal Pharmacopoeia (BHP). 1996. Exeter, U.K.: British Herbal Medicine Association.

Der Marderosian, A. (ed.). 1999. *The Review of Natural Products.* St. Louis: Facts and Comparisons.

Hili, P., C.S. Evans, R.G. Veness. 1997. Antimicrobial action of essential oils: the effect of dimethylsulphoxide on the activity of cinnamon oil. *Lett Appl Microbiol* 24(4):269–275.

This material was adapted from *The Complete German Commission E Monographs—Therapeutic Guide to Herbal Medicines.* M. Blumenthal, W.R. Busse, A. Goldberg, J. Gruenwald, T. Hall, C.W. Riggins, R.S. Rister (eds.) S. Klein and R.S. Rister (trans.). 1998. Austin: American Botanical Council; Boston: Integrative Medicine Communications.

1) The Overview section is new information.

2) Description, Chemistry and Pharmacology, Uses, Contraindications, Side Effects, Interactions with Other Drugs, and Dosage sections have been drawn from the original work. Additional information has been added in some or all of these sections, as noted with references.

3) The dosage for equivalent preparations (tea infusion, fluidextract, and tincture) have been provided based on the following example:
   Unless otherwise prescribed: 2 g per day of [powdered, crushed, cut or whole] [plant part]
   Infusion: 2 g in 150 ml of water
   Fluidextract 1:1 (g/ml): 2 ml
   Tincture 1:5 (g/ml): 10 ml

4) The References and Additional Resources sections are new sections. Additional Resources are not cited in the monograph but are included for research purposes.

Koh, W.S. et al. 1998. Cinnamaldehyde inhibits lymphocyte proliferation and modulates T-cell differentiation. *Int J Immunopharmacol* 20(11):643–660.

Nagai, H. et al. 1982. Immunopharmacological studies of the aqueous extract of *Cinnamomum cassia* (CCAq). II. Effect of CCAq on experimental glomerulonephritis. *Jpn J Pharmacol* 32(5):823–831.

Nagai, H., T. Shimazawa, N. Matsuura, A. Koda. 1982. Immunopharmacological studies of the aqueous extract of *Cinnamomum cassia* (CCAq). I. Anti-allergic action. *Jpn J Pharmacol* 32(5):813–822.

Tanaka, S. et al. 1989. Antiulcerogenic compounds isolated from Chinese Cinnamon. *Planta Med* 55(3):245–248.

Trease, G.E. and W.C. Evans. 1989. *Trease and Evans' Pharmacognosy*, 13th ed. London; Philadelphia: Baillière Tindall. 453.

Wichtl, M. and N.G. Bisset (eds.). 1994. *Herbal Drugs and Phytopharmaceuticals*. Stuttgart: Medpharm Scientific Publishers.

Zhu, Z.P., M.F. Zhang, Y.Q. Shen, G.J. Chen. 1993. [Pharmacological study on spleen-stomach warming and analgesic action of *Cinnamomum cassia* Presl] [In Chinese]. *Chung Kuo Chung Yao Tsa Chih* 18(9): 513–515, 553–557.

COLA NUT

Latin Name:
Cola nitida

Pharmacopeial Name:
Colae semen

Other Names:
kola nut, bissy nut, guru nut

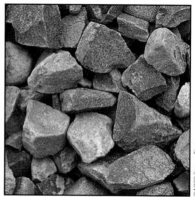

© 1999 Steven Foster

Overview

The cola nut tree is native to West Africa. It has been naturalized to South America, Central America, the West Indies, Sri Lanka, and Malaysia. Related to cocoa, cola nut is the source of a stimulant, and contains the methylxanthine alkaloids that occur also in coffee, cocoa, tea, maté, and guarana. Of the 40 known species, *Cola acuminata* and C. *nitida* bear the nuts most readily available in the United States and Europe; other species frequently used in commerce include C. *verticillata* and C. *anomala* (Trindall, 1997).

West Africans have been chewing cola nuts for thousands of years. Its stimulant effects are its predominant application in the United States and Europe. Commission E approves cola nut during conditions of mental and physical fatigue. In Africa, however, cola nuts have been used as an appetite and thirst suppressant, enabling soldiers who chewed them to travel long distances without much food. Cola twigs, with an extremely bitter taste, are used to clean the teeth and gums (Trindall, 1997).

Cola maintains strong cultural significance in West Africa, partly due to the fact that cola is a valuable commodity. It has been traded to other countries since at least the fourteenth century and it is used particularly by Islamic people, who, according to their religion, cannot drink alcohol, but desire a "social lubricant" (Trindall, 1997). Today, cola nut is exported worldwide. It is used in the manufacture of methylxanthine-based pharmaceuticals. Methylxanthines (caffeine, theophylline, and theobromine) are used to treat pre-term infant apnea, chronic obstructive pulmonary disease, and especially asthma. Pharmacologically, these alkaloids relax bronchial smooth muscle, stimulate the central nervous system and cardiac muscle, and are diuretic (Goodman et al., 1990). However, the most active alkaloid in regard to asthma is theophylline, not present in cola nut (Schulz et al., 1998). Caffeine is sometimes given in conjunction with other analgesics to produce stronger and quicker pain-killing actions (Goodman et al., 1990). These alkaloids have adverse side effects; it is not advisable for an asthmatic to drink copious amounts of any beverage containing significant amounts of methylxanthines: 3–10 g of caffeine can be lethal (Schulz et al., 1998).

Cola nut is also used in non-pharmaceutical preparations, including (at least formerly) cola-based beverages such as Coca Cola®. It is on the GRAS (generally recognized as safe) list for food additives in the United States (Leung and Foster, 1996).

Description

Cola nut consists of the endosperm freed from the testa of various *Cola* species Schott et Endlicher, particularly *C. nitida* (Ventenat) Schott et Endlicher [Fam. Sterculiaceae], and its preparations in effective dosage. The preparation contains at least 1.5% methylxanthine (caffeine, theobromine).

Chemistry and Pharmacology

Constituents include caffeine (1.5–2.5%), alkaloids (xanthines), and tannins (catechins) (Bradley, 1992; Newall et al., 1996). Other constituents include betaine, cellulose, enzyme, fats, a glucoside, protein, red pigments, and sugars (Newall et al., 1996). Caffeine, which stimulates the central nervous system, accounts for the pharmacological activity of the cola nut (Steinegger and Hänsel, 1992). In addition to being a central nervous system stimulant, thymoleptic, antidepressant, diuretic, and antidiarrheal effects have been observed with its use. Peripheral actions on the heart, circulatory system, skeletal muscle, and autonomic functions are attributed to the caffeine content (Bradley, 1992).

The Commission E reported, from animal experiments, analeptic and lipolytic activity, as well as stimulation of the production of gastric acid and an increase in motility. In humans the herb can be compared to methylxanthine, however caffeine is a weaker diuretic and positively chronotropic.

Uses

The Commission E approved the use of cola nut for mental and physical fatigue. It is also indicated as a supportive treatment for depressive states (Bradley, 1992).

Contraindications

Gastric and duodenal ulcers.

Side Effects

Sleep disorders, over-excitability, nervous restlessness, and gastric irritations may occur.

Use During Pregnancy and Lactation

No restrictions known.

Interactions with Other Drugs

Strengthening of the action of psychoanaleptic drugs and caffeine-containing beverages.

Dosage and Administration

Unless otherwise prescribed: 2–6 g per day of powdered cotyledon and other galenical preparations for internal use.
Dried powder: 1–3 g, two to three times daily.
Decoction: 1–3 g in 150 ml water, two to three times daily.
Dry extract: 0.25–0.75 g (Erg.B.6).
Fluidextract: 2.5–7.5 ml (Erg.B.6).
Tincture: 10–30 ml (Erg.B.6).
Cola wine: 60–180 ml (Erg.B.6).

References

Bradley, P.R. (ed.). 1992. *British Herbal Compendium*, Vol. 1. Bournemouth: British Herbal Medicine Association.

Goodman, L.S., A. Gilman, A.G. Gilman. 1990. *The Pharmacological Basis of Therapeutics*, 8th ed. New York: Pergamon Press.

Leung, A.Y. and S. Foster. 1996. *Encyclopedia of Common Natural Ingredients Used in Food, Drugs, and Cosmetics*, 2nd ed. New York: John Wiley & Sons, Inc.

Newall, C.A., L.A. Anderson, J.D. Phillipson. 1996. *Herbal Medicines: A Guide for Health-Care Professionals*. London: The Pharmaceutical Press.

Schulz, V., R. Hänsel, V.E. Tyler. 1998. *Rational Phytotherapy: A Physicians' Guide to Herbal Medicine*. New York: Springer.

Steinegger, E. and R. Hänsel. 1992. *Pharmakognosie*, 5th ed. Berlin-Heidelberg: Springer Verlag.

Trindall, R. 1997. *Ethnobotanical Leaflets: The Culture of Cola: Social and Economic Aspects of a West African Domesticate*. Carbondale: Southern Illinois University Herbarium.

Additional Resources

Maillard C., A. Babadjamian, G. Balansard, B. Ollivier, D. Bamba. 1985. Study of caffein-catechin association in lyophilized fresh seeds and in stabilized extract of *Cola nitida*. *Planta Med* (51):515–517.

List, P.H. and L. Hörhammer (eds.). 1973–1979. *Hagers Handbuch der Pharmazeutischen Praxis,* Vols. 1–7. New York: Springer Verlag.

Ibu, J.O. et al. 1986. The effect of cola acuminata and *cola nitida* on gastric acid secretion. *Scand J Gastroenterol Suppl* 124:39–45.

Morton, J.F. 1992. Widespread tannin intake via stimulants and masticatories, especially guarana, kola nut, betel vine, and accessories. *Basic Life Sci* (59):739–765.

Wren, R.C. 1988. *Potter's New Cyclopedia of Botanical Drugs and Preparations.* Essex: The C.W. Daniel Company Ltd.

This material was adapted from *The Complete German Commission E Monographs—Therapeutic Guide to Herbal Medicines.* M. Blumenthal, W.R. Busse, A. Goldberg, J. Gruenwald, T. Hall, C.W. Riggins, R.S. Rister (eds.) S. Klein and R.S. Rister (trans.). 1998. Austin: American Botanical Council; Boston: Integrative Medicine Communications.

1) The Overview section is new information.

2) Description, Chemistry and Pharmacology, Uses, Contraindications, Side Effects, Interactions with Other Drugs, and Dosage sections have been drawn from the original work. Additional information has been added in some or all of these sections, as noted with references.

3) The dosage for equivalent preparations (tea infusion, fluidextract, and tincture) have been provided based on the following example:
Unless otherwise prescribed: 2 g per day of [powdered, crushed, cut or whole] [plant part]
Infusion: 2 g in 150 ml of water
Fluidextract 1:1 (g/ml): 2 ml
Tincture 1:5 (g/ml): 10 ml

4) The References and Additional Resources sections are new sections. Additional Resources are not cited in the monograph but are included for research purposes.

CORIANDER SEED

Latin Name:
Coriandrum sativum

Pharmacopeial Name:
Coriandri fructus

Other Names:
coriander fruit

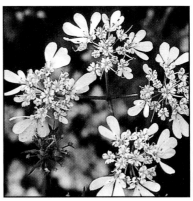

©1999 Steven Foster

Overview

Coriander is an annual herb native to Mediterranean Europe and western Asia, naturalized in North America, now extensively cultivated in many temperate countries (BHP, 1996; Leung and Foster, 1996; Wichtl and Bisset, 1994). The material of commerce comes mostly from Morocco, Bulgaria, Romania, Turkey, India, and the former U.S.S.R. (BHP, 1996; Kapoor, 1990; Wichtl and Bisset, 1994). Coriander is also cultivated on a small scale in some German states (Lange and Schippmann, 1997). Coriander was used in traditional Greek medicine by Hippocrates (ca. 460–377 B.C.E.) and other Greek physicians. Roman naturalist Pliny the Elder (ca. 23–79 B.C.E.) first used the genus name *Coriandrum*, derived from *koros*, in reference to the fetid smell of the leaves. It was later introduced to Great Britain by the Romans (Grieve, 1979). It was first introduced into Chinese medicine around 600 C.E. (Bown, 1995). Galenical preparations of coriander seed have similar uses as a carminative, digestive, or stomachic in traditional Chinese, Indian, and Greco-European medicines. In Ayurvedic medicine it is usually combined with caraway and cardamom seeds, among others, while in European medicine it is usually combined with caraway, fennel, and anise (Kapoor, 1990; Leung and Foster, 1996; Nadkarni, 1976; Wichtl and Bisset, 1994).

Very few, if any, modern clinical studies have been conducted on coriander. The approved modern therapeutic applications for coriander seed are supportable based on its long history of use in well established systems of traditional medicine, pharmacological studies in animals, nutrient composition and dietary value studies, and phytochemical investigations.

In Germany, coriander is used as a medicinal tea and a component of carminative and laxative remedies, in alcoholic distillate and drops dosage forms, often combined with anise, caraway, or fennel (Wichtl and Bisset, 1994). In the United States, coriander is used as a carminative or digestive component of compounds in confection, infusion, syrup, and tincture dosage forms. It is sometimes used in laxative compound preparations (e.g., Confectio Sennae) in order to counteract or modify their harsh stomach-upsetting effects (Duke, 1997; Grieve, 1979; Leung and Foster, 1996; NF V, 1926).

German pharmacopeial grade coriander seed must contain not less than 0.6% (v/m) volatile oil (DAB 1997). The *Austrian Pharmacopoeia* requirement is not less than 0.5% (ÖAB, 1981; Wichtl and Bisset, 1994).

Description

Coriander consists of the ripe, dried, spherical fruit of *Coriandrum sativum* L. var. *vulgare* (synonym var. *macrocarpum*) Alefeld and *C. sativum* L. var. *microcarpum* de Candolle [Fam. Apiaceae], as well as its preparations in effective dosage. The preparation contains at least 0.5% (v/w) essential oil.

Chemistry and Pharmacology

Coriander contains about 1% volatile oil, of which 55–74% is linalool; 20% are monoterpene hydrocarbons (α- and β-pinene and limonene), anethole, and camphor; up to 26% oleic, petroselinic, and linolenic fatty acids; flavonoid glycosides (quercetin, isoquercitrin, and rutin); chlorogenic and caffeic acids; tannins; sugars (approx. 20%); proteins (11–17%); coumarins; mucilage; starch (1%) (Budavari, 1996; Hänsel et al., 1992; Leung and Foster, 1996; List and Hörhammer, 1973; Wichtl and Bisset, 1994).

The Commission E did not report pharmacological actions for coriander fruit. The *British Herbal Pharmacopoeia* reported its actions as carminative and stimulant (BHP, 1996). *The Merck Index* reported its therapeutic categories as carminative and aromatic (Budavari, 1996). It acts as a stomachic, spasmolytic, and carminative due to its essential oil content (Wichtl and Bisset, 1994). Coriander has been reported to have strong lipolytic activity (Leung and Foster, 1996).

Uses

The Commission E approved the internal use of coriander seed for dyspeptic complaints and loss of appetite. The German Standard License for infusion of coriander fruit recommends it as supportive treatment for complaints of the upper abdomen, such as a feeling of distension, flatulence, and mild cramp-like gastrointestinal upsets (Wichtl and Bisset, 1994). Annex II of the French advice to manufacturers of plant based medications, or *avis aux fabricants*, of 1990 allows coriander fruit the same indications for use as aniseed and fennel fruits (Bruneton, 1995).

Contraindications

None known.

Side Effects

None known.

Use During Pregnancy and Lactation

No restrictions known.

Interactions with Other Drugs

None known.

Dosage and Administration

Unless otherwise prescribed: 3 g per day of crushed or powdered fruit or dry extract.
Infusion: 3 g in 150 ml water.
Fluidextract 1:1 (g/ml): 3 ml.
Tincture 1:5 (g/ml): 15 ml.

References

Bown, D. 1995. *Encyclopedia of Herbs and Their Uses*. New York: DK Publishing, Inc. 267.

British Herbal Pharmacopoeia (BHP). 1996. Exeter, U.K.: British Herbal Medicine Association.

British Pharmacopoeia (BP). 1993. London: Her Majesty's Stationery Office.

Bruneton, J. 1995. *Pharmacognosy, Phytochemistry, Medicinal Plants*. Paris: Lavoisier Publishing.

Budavari, S. (ed.). 1996. *The Merck Index: An Encyclopedia of Chemicals, Drugs, and Biologicals*, 12th ed. Whitehouse Station, N.J.: Merck & Co, Inc.

Deutsches Arzneibuch (DAB 1997). 1997. Stuttgart: Deutscher Apotheker Verlag.

Duke, J.A. 1997. *The Green Pharmacy*. Emmaus, PA: Rodale Press. 276–277.

Grieve, M. 1979. *A Modern Herbal*. New York: Dover Publications, Inc.

Hänsel, R., K. Keller, H. Rimpler, G. Schneider (eds.). 1992. *Hagers Handbuch der Pharmazeutischen Praxis*, 5th ed. Vol. 4. Berlin-Heidelberg: Springer Verlag. 996.

Kapoor, L.D. 1990. *Handbook of Ayurvedic Medicinal Plants*. Boca Raton: CRC Press. 137.

Lange, D. and U. Schippmann. 1997. *Trade Survey of Medicinal Plants in Germany—A Contribution to International Plant Species Conservation.* Bonn: Bundesamt für Naturschutz. 32–33.

Leung, A.Y. and S. Foster. 1996. *Encyclopedia of Common Natural Ingredients Used in Food, Drugs, and Cosmetics,* 2nd ed. New York: John Wiley & Sons, Inc.

List, P.H. and L. Hörhammer (eds.). 1973. *Hagers Handbuch der Pharmazeutischen Praxis,* Vol. 1. New York: Springer Verlag. 300.

Nadkarni, K.M. 1976. *Indian Materia Medica.* Bombay: Popular Prakashan. 381–383.

National Formulary, 5th ed. (NF V). 1926. Washington, D.C.: American Pharmaceutical Association. 13.

Österreichisches Arzneibuch, Vols. 1–2, 1st suppl. (ÖAB). 1981–1983. Wien: Verlag der Österreichischen Staatsdruckerei.

Wichtl, M. and N.G. Bisset (eds.). 1994. *Herbal Drugs and Phytopharmaceuticals.* Stuttgart: Medpharm Scientific Publishers.

Additional Resources

Chithra, V. and S. Leelamma. 1997. Hypolipidemic effect of coriander seeds (*Coriandrum sativum*): mechanism of action. *Plant Foods Hum Nutr* 51(2):167–172.

Duke, J. 1997. *Handbook of Phytochemical Constituents of GRAS Herbs and Other Economic Plants.* Boca Raton: CRC Press. 197–199.

Formacék, V. and K.H. Kubeczka. 1982. *Essential oils analysis by capillary chromatography and carbon-13 NMR spectroscopy.* New York: John Wiley & Sons, Inc.

Karlsen, J. et al. 1971. Studies on the essential oil of the fruits of *Coriandrum sativum* L. by means of gas liquid chromatography. Studies on terpenes and related compounds. XI. *Pharm Weekbl* 106(12):293–300.

Kunzemann J. and K. Herrmann. 1977. Isolierung und Identifizierung der Flavon(o1)-0-glykoside in Kummel (*Carum carvi* L.), Fenchel (*Foeniculum vulgare* Mill.), Anis (*Pimpinella anisum* L.), und Koriander (*Coriandrum sativum* L.) und von Flavon-C-glykosiden in Anis. I. Gewurzphenole [Isolation and identification of flavon(ol)-O-glycosides in caraway (*Carum carvi* L.), fennel (*Foeniculum vulgare* Mill.), anise (*Pimpinella anisum* L.), and coriander (*Coriandrum sativum* L.), and of flavon-C-glycosides in anise. I. Phenolics of spices]. *Z Lebensm Unters Forsch* 164(3):194–200.

McGuffin, M., C. Hobbs, R. Upton, A. Goldberg. 1997. *American Herbal Product Association's Botanical Safety Handbook.* Boca Raton: CRC Press.

Mironova, A.N. et al. 1991. [Chemical and biological properties of coriander fatty oil] [In Russian]. *Vopr Pitan* (1):59–62.

Murphy, E.W., A.C. Marsh, B.W. Willis. 1978. Nutrient content of spices and herbs. *J Am Diet Assoc* 72(2):174–176.

National Formulary (NF), 16th ed. 1985. Washington, D.C.: American Pharmaceutical Association.

Reus, W.A. 1996. [Birth representation with reference to the magical coriander prescription of Codex Vindobonensis 93, fol. 102r, of the Austrian National Library] [In German]. *Gynakol Geburtshilfliche Rundsch* 36(2):92–100.

Salzer, U.J. 1977. The analysis of essential oils and extracts (oleoresins) from seasonings—a critical review. *CRC Crit Rev Food Sci Nutr* 9(4):345–373.

Swanston-Flatt, S.K., C. Day, C.J. Bailey, P.R. Flatt. 1990. Traditional plant treatments for diabetes. Studies in normal and streptozotocin diabetic micc. *Diabetologia* 33(8):462–464.

Uma Pradeep, K., P. Geervani, B.O. Eggum. 1993. Common Indian spices: nutrient composition, consumption and contribution to dietary value. *Plant Foods Hum Nutr* 44(2):137–148.

Watt, J.M. and A.L. Merrill. 1975. *Composition of Foods, Raw, Processed, Prepared.* Agriculture Handbook No. 8. Washington, D.C.: Agricultural Research Service, U.S. Department of Agriculture.

This material was adapted from *The Complete German Commission E Monographs—Therapeutic Guide to Herbal Medicines.* M. Blumenthal, W.R. Busse, A. Goldberg, J. Gruenwald, T. Hall, C.W. Riggins, R.S. Rister (eds.) S. Klein and R.S. Rister (trans.). 1998. Austin: American Botanical Council; Boston: Integrative Medicine Communications.

1) The Overview section is new information.

2) Description, Chemistry and Pharmacology, Uses, Contraindications, Side Effects, Interactions with Other Drugs, and Dosage sections have been drawn from the original work. Additional information has been added in some or all of these sections, as noted with references.

3) The dosage for equivalent preparations (tea infusion, fluidextract, and tincture) have been provided based on the following example:
   Unless otherwise prescribed: 2 g per day of [powdered, crushed, cut or whole] [plant part]
   Infusion: 2 g in 150 ml of water
   Fluidextract 1:1 (g/ml): 2 ml
   Tincture 1:5 (g/ml): 10 ml

4) The References and Additional Resources sections are new sections. Additional Resources are not cited in the monograph but are included for research purposes.

DANDELION:

DANDELION HERB
(PAGE 79)

DANDELION ROOT WITH HERB
(PAGE 81)

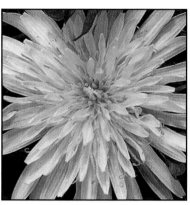

©1999 Steven Foster

Overview

Dandelion is a perennial herb native throughout the northern hemisphere with many varieties and microspecies, found growing wild in meadows, pastures and waste ground in temperate zones (Grieve, 1979; Leung and Foster, 1996; Wichtl and Bisset, 1994). The material of commerce comes from both wild and cultivated plants, mainly from Bulgaria, Hungary, Poland, Romania, the former Yugoslavia, and the United Kingdom (BHP, 1996; Wichtl and Bisset, 1994). The material used in Indian Ayurvedic and Unani medicines grows in the temperate Himalayas from five to twelve thousand feet and in Tibet, though it is also imported (Kapoor, 1990; Karnick, 1994; Nadkarni, 1976).

Dandelion has a long history of traditional use in many systems of medicine in the treatment of hepatobiliary problems. The root is traditionally used to treat liver and spleen ailments (Bradley, 1992; Leung and Foster, 1996). The genus name *Taraxacum* is derived from the Greek *taraxos* (disorder), and *akos* (remedy). The name *dandelion* is derived from its original Greek genus name *leontodon*, meaning lion's teeth. Its use in traditional Arabian medicine is first mentioned in the tenth century C.E. (Grieve, 1979). Dandelion root was formerly official in the United States *National Formulary* (Leung and Foster, 1996). It is official in the national pharmacopeias of Austria and the Czech Republic, and also in the *Ayurvedic Pharmacopoeia*, the *British Herbal Pharmacopoeia*, the *British Herbal Compendium*, the *German Pharmacopoeial Codex*, the German Standard License, and the Commission E (BAnz, 1998; BHP, 1996; Bradley, 1992; Braun, 1991; DAC, 1986; Karnick, 1994; Meyer-Buchtela, 1999; Newall et al., 1996; ÖAB, 1981; Wichtl and Bisset, 1994). ESCOP has also published monographs on the leaf and root (ESCOP, 1997).

Its uses in North American aboriginal medicines are well documented. The Iroquois people prepared infusions and decoctions of the root and herb to treat kidney disease, dropsy, and dermatological problems (Herrick, 1977). The Ojibwe people of Wisconsin prepared an infusion of the root to treat heartburn (Smith, 1932). The Rappahannock people of the eastern United States prepared an infusion of the root as a blood tonic and to treat dyspepsia (Speck et al., 1942). The Bella Coola people of British Columbia prepared a decoction of the roots as an analgesic and to treat stomach pain (Smith, 1929).

In Germany, dandelion root with herb is licensed as a standard medicinal tea to treat biliary disorders, digestive and gastrointestinal complaints, and to stimulate diuresis. Dandelion herb and dandelion root with herb are also approved in the Commission E monographs. Dosage forms, including aqueous decoction and infusion, expressed juice of fresh plant, and hydroalcoholic tincture are used as monopreparations and integral components of about fifty prepared cholagogue, biliary, gastrointestinal, and urological remedies (BAnz, 1998; Bradley, 1992; Braun, 1991; Meyer-Buchtela, 1999; Schilcher, 1997; Wichtl and Bisset, 1994). In the United States, dandelion root and leaf preparations are used as choleretic, diuretic, and tonic components in a wide range of compound dietary supplement and health food products.

The approved modern therapeutic applications for dandelion are supportable based on its long history of use in well established systems of traditional medicine, phytochemical investigations, and pharmacological studies in animals. For a comprehensive review, see Hobbs (1985).

Pharmacopeial grade dandelion leaf must be composed of the dried leaves collected before flowering. It must contain not less than 20% water-soluble extractive, among other quantitative standards. Botanical identity must be confirmed by thinlayer chromatography (TLC) as well as by macroscopic and microscopic examinations (BHP, 1996; Wichtl and Bisset, 1994). The ESCOP monograph requires the material to comply with the *British Herbal Pharmacopoeia* (ESCOP, 1997).

Pharmacopeial grade dandelion root must be composed of the dried root and rhizome collected in the autumn when its inulin content is the highest. Histochemical detection of inulin is carried out. The root must contain not less than 40% water-soluble extractive with reference to the oven-dried material, among other quantitative standards. Botanical identity must be confirmed by TLC as well as by macroscopic and microscopic examinations (BHP, 1996; DAC, 1986; Karnick, 1994; Wichtl and Bisset, 1994). The *Austrian Pharmacopoeia* additionally requires a bitterness value of not less than 100 (ÖAB, 1981; Wichtl and Bisset, 1994). The ESCOP monograph requires the material to comply with both the *Austrian Pharmacopoeia* and the *British Herbal Pharmacopoeia* (ESCOP, 1997).

DANDELION HERB

Latin Name:
Taraxacum officinale

Pharmacopeial Name:
Taraxaci herba

Other Names:
common dandelion, lion's tooth

Description
Dandelion herb, consisting of the fresh or dried aboveground parts of *Taraxacum officinale* G. H. Weber ex Wiggers s.l. [Fam. Asteraceae] and their preparations in effective dosage. The leaf contains bitter principles.

Chemistry and Pharmacology
Dandelion herb contains sesquiterpene lactones (eudesmanolides); triterpenes (β-amyrin, taraxol, and taraxerol); carotenoids (lutein); fatty acids (myristic); flavonoids (apigenin and luteolin); minerals (potassium up to 4.5%); phenolic acids (caffeic acid and chlorogenic acid); phytosterols (sitosterol, stigmasterol, and taraxasterol); sugars (fructose, glucose, and sucrose); vitamins (vitamin A up to 14,000 iu/100g); and inulin (ESCOP, 1997; Leung and Foster, 1996; List and Höerhammer, 1979; Newall et al., 1996; Wichtl and Bisset, 1994).

The Commission E reported that as of the 1992 publication of the monograph, the pharmacological activity of dandelion herb was unknown. In recent rodent experiments, the diuretic and saluretic indices of dandelion herb fluid extract were greater than that of dandelion root and comparable to those of furosemide (ESCOP, 1997; Leung and Foster, 1996; Newall et al., 1996; Wichtl and Bisset, 1994). Intravenous injection of dandelion fresh leaf decoction doubled the volume of bile secreted in dogs (ESCOP, 1997). The high potassium content of dandelion leaf replaces potassium eliminated in urine (ESCOP, 1997; Leung and Foster, 1996). Unusually high potassium content and its bitter substances (sesquiterpene lactones) may play a part in the diuretic effect. Indications of its cholagogic and diuretic actions are found in older clinical studies (Wichtl and Bisset, 1994).

Uses

The Commission E approved the internal use of dandelion herb for loss of appetite and dyspepsia, such as feelings of fullness and flatulence. ESCOP indicates its use as an adjunct to treatments where enhanced urinary output is desirable, as in rheumatism and the prevention of renal gravel (ESCOP, 1997). Dandelion is used for atonic dyspepsia with constipation and specifically for cholecystitis and dyspepsia (Bradley, 1992; Newall et al., 1996).

Contraindications

Obstruction of the bile ducts, gall bladder empyema, ileus. In case of gallstones, first consult a physician. Contact allergies caused by sesquiterpene lactones in the latex have been only rarely observed. Experiments and observations concerning preparations are not available.

Side Effects

None known.

Use During Pregnancy and Lactation

No restrictions known.

Interactions with Other Drugs

None known.

Dosage and Administration

Unless otherwise prescribed: 4–10 g of cut herb three times daily for infusions, as well as for liquid preparations for internal use.
Infusion: 4–10 g in 150–250 ml water, three times daily (Commission E; ESCOP, 1997).
Fluidextract 1:1 (g/ml, ethanol 25% v/v): 4–10 ml, three times daily (Commission E).
Tincture 1:5 (g/ml, ethanol 25% v/v): 2–5 ml, three times daily (Bradley, 1992; ESCOP, 1997).
Succus: 5–10 ml pressed sap from fresh plant, twice daily (Bradley, 1992; ESCOP, 1997).

DANDELION ROOT WITH HERB

Latin Name:
Taraxacum officinale

Pharmacopeial Name:
Taraxaci radix cum herba

Other Names:
common dandelion, lion's tooth

Description

Dandelion root with herb consists of the entire plant *Taraxacum officinale* G. H. Weber ex Wiggers s.l. [Fam. Asteraceae], gathered while flowering, and its preparations in effective dosage. Ingredients include the bitter principles lactucopicrin (taraxacin), triterpenoids, and phytosterol.

Chemistry and Pharmacology

Dandelion root contains sesquiterpene lactones (eudesmanolides and germacranolides); triterpenes (β-amyrin, taraxol, and taraxerol); carbohydrates (inulin 2% in spring and up to 40% in autumn); carotenoids (lutein); fatty acids (myristic); flavonoids (apigenin and luteolin); minerals (potassium 1.8–4.5%); phenolic acids (caffeic acid and chlorogenic acid); phytosterols (sitosterol, stigmasterol, and taraxasterol); sugars (fructose approx. 18% in spring); vitamins (vitamin A up to 14,000 iu/100g); choline; mucilage (approx. 1.1%); and pectin (Bradley, 1992; Budavari, 1996; ESCOP, 1997; Leung and Foster, 1996; List and Hörhammer, 1979; Newall et al., 1996; Wichtl and Bisset, 1994).

The Commission E reported choleretic, diuretic, and appetite-stimulating activities. The *British Herbal Compendium* reported bitter, cholagogue, and mild laxative actions (Bradley, 1992). The *British Herbal Pharmacopoeia* reports its action as hepatic (BHP, 1996). The root contains sesquiterpene lactones beneficial to the digestion process and with a mild purgative effect (Bradley, 1992). Oral administration of dandelion extracts had a diuretic effect in rats and mice (Newall et al., 1996). Intravenous injection of fresh dandelion root decoction doubled the volume of bile secretion in dogs (ESCOP, 1997). The choleretic effect of dandelion root has been confirmed (Bradley, 1992).

Uses

The Commission E approved the internal use of dandelion root with herb for disturbances in bile flow, stimulation of diuresis, loss of appetite, and dyspepsia. The *British Herbal Compendium* indicates its use for hepato-biliary disorders, dyspepsia, lack of appetite, and rheumatic conditions (Bradley, 1992). ESCOP indicates its use for restoration of hepatic and biliary function, dyspepsia, and loss of appetite (ESCOP, 1997). The German Standard License for dandelion decoction indicates its use for biliary disorders, gastrointestinal complaints such as a feeling of distension and flatulence, digestive complaints, and to stimulate diuresis (Wichtl and Bisset, 1996).

Contraindications

Obstruction of bile ducts, gallbladder empyema, ileus. In case of gallstones, use only after consultation with a physician.

Side Effects

As with all drugs containing bitter substances, discomfort due to gastric hyperacidity may occur.

Use During Pregnancy and Lactation

No restrictions known.

Interactions with Other Drugs

None known.

Dosage and Administration

Unless otherwise prescribed: 3–4 g of cut or powdered root and herb three times daily.

Decoction: Boil 3–4 g cut or powdered root and herb in 150 ml water. [Ed. Note: The decoction instructions in the German Standard License monograph are as follows: Boil 1–2 teaspoonfuls (2.4–4.4 g) and strain after 15 minutes, twice daily in the morning and evening.]

Infusion: Steep 1 tablespoon cut root and herb in 150 ml water.

Dry native extract 4:1 (w/w): 0.75–1 g.

Fluidextract 1:1 (g/ml): 3–4 ml.

Tincture: 10–15 drops, three times daily. [Ed. Note: The Commission E-recommended tincture dosage of 10–15 drops, three times daily, does not correlate closely with the Commission E daily dosage of 3–4 g dried root and herb. No justification can be found in the literature for such a low tincture dosage, in drops as opposed to milliliters. Most herbal references recommend 5–10 ml, three times daily, which relates to the Commission E daily dosage of 3–4 g dried root.]

Succus: 5–10 ml pressed sap from fresh plant.

References

BAnz. See *Bundesanzeiger.*

Bradley, P.R. (ed.). 1992. *British Herbal Compendium,* Vol. 1. Bournemouth: British Herbal Medicine Association. 73–75.

Braun, R. (ed.). 1991. *Standardzulassungen für Fertigarzneimittel— mit 7. Ergänzung.* Stuttgart: Deutscher Apotheker Verlag.

British Herbal Pharmacopoeia (BHP). 1996. Exeter, U.K.: British Herbal Medicine Association.

Budavari, S. (ed.). 1996. *The Merck Index: An Encyclopedia of Chemicals, Drugs, and Biologicals,* 12th ed. Whitehouse Station, N.J.: Merck & Co, Inc.

Bundesanzeiger (BAnz). 1998. Monographien der Kommission E (Zulassungs- und Aufbereitungskommission am BGA für den humanmed. Bereich, phytotherapeutische Therapierichtung und Stoffgruppe). Köln: Bundesgesundheitsamt (BGA).

Deutscher Arzneimittel-Codex (DAC). 1986. 3rd suppl. Stuttgart: Deutscher Apotheker Verlag.

ESCOP. 1997. "Taraxaci herba" and "Taraxaci radix." *Monographs on the Medicinal Uses of Plant Drugs.* Exeter, U.K.: European Scientific Cooperative on Phytotherapy.

Grieve, M. 1979. *A Modern Herbal.* New York: Dover Publications, Inc.

Herrick, J.W. 1977. *Iroquois Medical Botany.* Ann Arbor, MI: University Microfilms International. 476–478.

Hobbs, C. 1985. *Dandelion: A Monograph.* Portland, OR: Eclectic Medical Publications.

Kapoor, L.D. 1990. *Handbook of Ayurvedic Medicinal Plants.* Boca Raton: CRC Press. 316.

Karnick, C.R. 1994. *Pharmacopoeial Standards of Herbal Plants,* Vols. 1–2. Delhi: Sri Satguru Publications. Vol. 1:335–336; Vol. 2:47.

Leung, A.Y. and S. Foster. 1996. *Encyclopedia of Common Natural Ingredients Used in Food, Drugs, and Cosmetics,* 2nd ed. New York: John Wiley & Sons, Inc.

List, P.H. and L. Hörhammer (eds.). 1979. *Hagers Handbuch der Pharmazeutischen Praxis,* Vol. 6. Berlin-Heidelberg: Springer Verlag. 16–21.

Meyer-Buchtela, E. 1999. *Tee-Rezepturen—Ein Handbuch für Apotheker und Ärzte.* Stuttgart: Deutscher Apotheker Verlag.

Nadkarni, K.M. 1976. *Indian Materia Medica.* Bombay: Popular Prakashan. 786.

Newall, C.A., L.A. Anderson, J.D. Phillipson. 1996. *Herbal Medicines: A Guide for Health-Care Professionals.* London: The Pharmaceutical Press.

Österreichisches Arzneibuch, Vols. 1–2, 1st suppl. (ÖAB). 1981–1983. Wien: Verlag der Österreichischen Staatsdruckerei.

Schilcher, H. 1997. *Phytotherapy in Paediatrics: Handbook for Physicians and Pharmacists.* Stuttgart: Medpharm Scientific Publishers. 139, 164–165.

Smith, H.H. 1932. Ethnobotany of the Ojibwe Indians. *Bulletin of the Public Museum of Milwaukee* 4:327–525.

Smith, H.I. 1929. *Materia Medica of the Bella Coola and Neigh Tribes of British Columbia.* BC: National Museum of Canada Bulletin. 56:47–68.

Speck, F.G., R.B. Hassrick, E.S. Carpenter. 1942. Rappahannock Herbals, Folk-lore and Science of Cures. *Proc Del County Inst Sci* 10:7–55.

Wichtl, M. and N.G. Bisset (eds.). 1994. *Herbal Drugs and Phytopharmaceuticals.* Stuttgart: Medpharm Scientific Publishers.

Additional Resources

Baba, K., S. Abe, D. Mizuno. 1981. [Antitumor activity of hot water extract of dandelion, *Taraxacum officinale*—correlation between antitumor activity and timing of administration] [In Japanese]. *Yakugaku Zasshi* 101(6):538–543.

British Pharmaceutical Codex (BPC). 1949. London: The Pharmaceutical Press.

Broda, B. and E. Andrzejewska. 1966. Choline content in some medicinal plants. *Farm Polska* 22(3):181–184.

Burrows, S. and J.C.E. Simpson. 1938. The Triterpene Group. Part IV. The triterpene alcohols of *Taraxacum* root. *J Chem Soc* 2042–2047.

Chabrol, E. et al. 1931. L'action cholérétique des Composée. *CR Soc Biol* 108:1100–1102.

Czygan, F.C. 1990. *Taraxacum officinale* Wiggers—Der Löwenzahn. *Z Phytothe* 11:99–102.

Deutsches Arzneibuch, 9th ed. (DAB 9). 1986. Stuttgart: Deutscher Apotheker Verlag.

Faber, K. 1958. Der Löwenzahn—*Taraxacum officinale* Weber. *Pharmazie* 13:423–436.

Hänsel, R., M. Kartarahardja, J.T. Huang, F. Bohlmann. 1980. Sesquiterpenlacton-β-D-glucopyranoside sowie ein neues Eudesmanolid aus *Taraxacum officinale*. *Phytochem* 19:857–861.

Harnischfeger, G. and H. Stolze. 1983. *Bewährte Pflanzendrogen in Wissenschaft und Medizin*. Bad Homburg/Melsungen: Notamed Verlag. 242–249.

Hook, I., A. McGee, M. Henman. 1993. Evaluation of Dandelion for diuretic activity and variation in potassium content. *Int J Pharmacog* 31:29–34.

Kuusi, T., H. Pyysalo, K. Autio. 1985. The bitterness properties of dandelion II. Chemical investigations. *Lebensm Wiss Technol* 18:347–349.

McGuffin, M. (ed.). 1998. *Herbs of Commerce*, 2nd ed. [Draft 3.3]. Bethesda: American Herbal Products Association.

Nadkarni, K.M. 1993. *Indian Materia Medica*. Bombay: Popular Prakashan. 1195–1196.

Pirtkien, R., E. Surke, G. Seybold. 1960. Comparative studies on the choleretic action of various drugs in the rat. *Med Welt* 1417–1422.

Popov, A.I. and K.G. Gromov. 1993. Mineral components of dandelion leaves. *Vopr Pitan* (3):57–58.

Rácz-Kotilla, E., G. Rácz, A. Solomon. 1974. The action of *Taraxacum officinale* extracts on the body weight and diuresis of laboratory animals. *Planta Med* 26(3):212–217.

Rácz-Kotilla, E., J. Bodon, Tölgyesi. 1978. Determination of the mineral content of 41 medicinal plant species by chemotaxonomical and biochemical observations. *Herba Hung* 17:43–54.

Reynolds, J.E.F. (ed.). 1993. *Martindale: The Extra Pharmacopoeia*, 30th ed. London: The Pharmaceutical Press.

Rudenskaya, G.N. et al. 1998. Taraxalisin—a serine proteinase from dandelion *Taraxacum officinale* Webb. s.l. *FEBS Lett* 437(3):237–240.

Rutherford, P.P. and A.C. Deacon. 1972. Fructofuranosidases from roots of dandelion (*Taraxacum officinale* Weber). *Biochem J* 126(3):569–573.

———. 1972. The mode of action of dandelion root-fructofuranosidases on inulin. *Biochem J* 129(2):511–512.

Smith, G.W. 1973. Arctic Pharmacognosia. *Arctic* 26:324–333.

Vogel, H.H. and R. Schaette. 1977. Phytotherapeutische Reflexionen. Betrachtungen über *Silybum marianum* (Carduus marianus), *Taraxacum officinale*, *Cichorium intybus*, *Bryonia alba et dioica*, *Viscum album* und ihre Beziehungen zur Leber. *Erfahrungsheilkunde* 26:347–355.

Weiss, R.F. 1991. *Lehrbuch der Phytotherapie*, 7th ed. Stuttgart: Hippokrates Verlag. 162–163.

Williams, C.A., F. Goldstone, J. Greenham. 1996. Flavonoids, cinnamic acids and coumarins from the different tissues and medicinal preparations of *Taraxacum officinale*. *Phytochemistry* 42(1):121–127.

The dandelion herb monograph, published by the Commission E in 1992, were modified based on new scientific research. They contain more extensive pharmacological and therapeutic information taken directly from the Commission E.

This material was adapted from *The Complete German Commission E Monographs—Therapeutic Guide to Herbal Medicines*. M. Blumenthal, W.R. Busse, A. Goldberg, J. Gruenwald, T. Hall, C.W. Riggins, R.S. Rister (eds.) S. Klein and R.S. Rister (trans.). 1998. Austin: American Botanical Council; Boston: Integrative Medicine Communications.

1) The Overview section is new information.

2) Description, Chemistry and Pharmacology, Uses, Contraindications, Side Effects, Interactions with Other Drugs, and Dosage sections have been drawn from the original work. Additional information has been added in some or all of these sections, as noted with references.

3) The dosage for equivalent preparations (tea infusion, fluidextract, and tincture) have been provided based on the following example:
   Unless otherwise prescribed: 2 g per day of [powdered, crushed, cut or whole] [plant part]
   Infusion: 2 g in 150 ml of water
   Fluidextract 1:1 (g/ml): 2 ml
   Tincture 1:5 (g/ml): 10 ml

4) The References and Additional Resources sections are new sections. Additional Resources are not cited in the monograph but are included for research purposes.

Devil's Claw Root

Latin Name:
Harpagophytum procumbens

Pharmacopeial Name:
Harpagophyti radix

Other Names:
grapple plant, wood spider

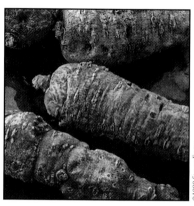

©1999 Steven Foster

Overview

Native to the Kalahari desert, Namibian steppes, Madagascar, and other parts of southern Africa, devil's claw is named for the hooks that cover its fruit. Medicinal preparations made from the secondary storage tubers of the tree have been used in the folk medicine traditions of tribal Africa for the bitter, analgesic, and antipyretic actions of devil's claw root (Schulz et al., 1998). Europeans and Canadians use it, mostly for relief of arthritic symptoms (Der Marderosian, 1999). Apart from its applications as a bitter and fever-reducing agent, devil's claw administered externally to the skin is said to heal sores, boils, and other skin lesions. The conditions that benefit from use of devil's claw include dyspepsia, blood disease, headache, allergy, gout, neuralgia, arthritis, rheumatism, and lower back pain (Leung and Foster, 1996).

Today devil's claw is used as an anti-inflammatory agent for rheumatic or arthitic conditions, and is approved by Commission E to restore appetite and relieve heartburn. Tests demonstrate both anti-inflammatory and anti-exudative activity (Schulz et al., 1998). The constituents most likely responsible for devil's claw root's anti-inflammatory effects are its iridoids, particularly harpagoside (Newall et al., 1996). In animal models, harpagoside is not only anti-inflammatory, but it also lowers blood pressure and heart rate (Der Marderosian, 1999).

Both *in vitro* and *in vivo* tests have resulted in conflicting evidence of devil's claw root's therapeutic activity. Pain-reducing and anti-inflammatory properties were observed in guinea pigs, particularly in chronic pain conditions, but when devil's claw root's effects on rats were compared to those of aspirin and indomethacin, significant efficacy was not found (Newall et al., 1996). When iridoids were isolated and tested, these, too, produced conflicting results. In humans, oral doses of extract of devil's claw root were ineffective compared to indomethacin, according to reports from 13 participants followed in a six week study (Newall et al., 1996). On the other hand, intraperitoneal administration of 100 mg devil's claw root extract/kg was equal to 2.5 mg/kg indomethacin in anti-inflammatory effects (Leung and Foster, 1996). A German study in 1976 found devil's claw root's effects to be comparable to the anti-arthritic drug phenylbutazone (Tyler, 1993).

Most clinical studies of devil's claw root have not been double-blinded and placebo-controlled in design. One that was, however, showed that for a significant number of the study's participants, powdered devil's claw root reduced arthritis pain (Schulz et al., 1998). In another, patients with lower back pain felt significant relief following four weeks of devil's claw root treatment (two 400 mg tablets of extract, three times daily, total of 2400 mg per day), demonstrated by reduction of use of analgesics (Chrubasik et al., 1996).

Description
Devil's claw root is the dried, secondary tubers of *Harpagophytum procumbens* (Burchell) de Candolle [Fam. Pedaliaceae] and their preparations in effective dosage. The commercial product contains bitter substances.

Chemistry and Pharmacology
Constituents include the iridoid glucosides (0.5–3%) harpagoside, harpagide, and procumbide; stachyose and simple sugars; free and glycosylated phytosterols, including β-sitosterol; oleanolic acid; flavonoids kaempferol and luteolin; phenolic acids; and the glycosidic phenylpropanoic esters verbascoside and isoacteoside (Bradley, 1992; Bruneton, 1995). The iridoids are thought to be responsible for the anti-inflammatory activity (Bruneton, 1995; Newall et al., 1996).

The Commission E reported appetite-stimulating, choleretic, antiphlogistic, and mild analgesic properties. Infusions and decoctions of the herb have been used for benign rheumatic disorders (Bruneton, 1995). *In vitro* experiments have shown a significant, dose-dependent, protective action against arrhythmias induced by calcium chloride and epinephrine-chloroform on isolated rabbit heart (ESCOP, 1997). *In vivo* experiments with devil's claw root have determined that anti-inflammatory properties differ by dosage method (ESCOP, 1997). Intraperitoneal and intraduodenal administration reduced carrageenan-induced edema. Oral administration had no effect, regardless of the dose used (ESCOP, 1997).

Uses
The Commission E approved the use of devil's claw root for loss of appetite, dyspepsia, and degenerative disorders of the locomotor system. Devil's claw root has been used to treat painful arthroses, tendonitis, indigestion, blood diseases, headache, allergies, rheumatism, arthritis, lumbago, neuralgia, and fever, and externally for sores, ulcer, boils, and skin lesions (Bradley, 1992;

Leung and Foster, 1996). It has also been used as an anti-inflammatory and analgesic (Bradley, 1992; Wichtl and Bisset, 1994).

Devil's claw root, when administered in aqueous extract containing 2.5% iridoid glucosides at a daily dosage of 3–9 g, divided into three doses, improved the states of 42% to 85% of the 630 patients suffering from arthrosis. A double-blind study of 89 ambulant volunteers established that a dosage of 335 mg (2 capsules three times daily for two months) of powdered devil's claw root with an iridoid glucoside content of 3% decreased the intensity of pain in a significant number of patients (ESCOP, 1997).

Contraindications
Gastric and duodenal ulcers. With gallstones, consult a physician before use.

Side Effects
None known.

Use During Pregnancy and Lactation
No restrictions known.

Interactions with Other Drugs
None known.

Dosage and Administration
Unless otherwise prescribed: For loss of appetite: 1.5 g per day of cut tuber or preparations of equivalent bitter value for teas and other preparations for internal use. Otherwise: 4.5 g per day of cut tuber; equivalent preparations.
For loss of appetite:
Decoction: 0.5 g in 150 ml water, three times daily.
Fluidextract 1:1 (g/ml): 0.5 ml, three times daily.
Other conditions:
Infusion: 4.5 g in 300 ml boiled water, steep at room temperature for 8 hours, strain and drink in three portions daily.

Decoction: 1.5 g in 150 ml water, three times daily.
Fluidextract 1:1 (g/ml): 1.5 ml, three times daily.

References

Bradley, P.R. (ed.). 1992. *British Herbal Compendium*, Vol. 1. Bournemouth: British Herbal Medicine Association.

Bruneton, J. 1995. *Pharmacognosy, Phytochemistry, Medicinal Plants*. Paris: Lavoisier Publishing.

Chrubasik, S. et al. 1996. Effectiveness of *Harpagophytum procumbens* in treatment of acute low back pain. *Phytomedicine* 3(1):1–10.

Der Marderosian, A. (ed.). 1999. *The Review of Natural Products*. St. Louis: Facts and Comparisons.

ESCOP. 1997. "Harpagophyti radix." *Monographs on the Medicinal Uses of Plant Drugs*. Exeter, U.K.: European Scientific Cooperative on Phytotherapy.

Leung, A.Y. and S. Foster. 1996. *Encyclopedia of Common Natural Ingredients Used in Food, Drugs, and Cosmetics*, 2nd ed. New York: John Wiley & Sons, Inc.

Newall, C.A., L.A. Anderson, J.D. Phillipson. 1996. *Herbal Medicines: A Guide for Health-Care Professionals*. London: The Pharmaceutical Press.

Schulz, V., R. Hänsel, V.E. Tyler. 1998. *Rational Phytotherapy: A Physicians' Guide to Herbal Medicine*. New York: Springer.

Tyler, V.E. 1993. *The Honest Herbal: A Sensible Guide to the Use of Herbs and Related Remedies*, 3rd ed. New York: Pharmaceutical Products Press.

Wichtl, M. and N.G. Bisset (eds.). 1994. *Herbal Drugs and Phytopharmaceuticals*. Stuttgart: Medpharm Scientific Publishers.

Additional Resources

Baghdikian, B. et al. 1997. An analytical study, anti-inflammatory and analgesic effects of *Harpagophytum procumbens* and Harpagophytum zeyheri. *Planta Med* 63(2):171–176.

Circost, C. et al. 1984. A drug used in traditional medicine: *Harpagophytum procumbens* DC. II. Cardiovascular activity. *J Ethnopharmacol* 11(3):259–274.

Costa de Pasquale, R. et al. 1985. A drug used in traditional medicine: *Harpagophytum procumbens* DC. III. Effects on hyperkinetic ventricular arrhythmias by reperfusion. *J Ethnopharmacol* 13(2):193–199.

Erdos, A., R. Fontaine, H. Friehe, R. Durand, T. Poppinghaus. 1978. [Contribution to the pharmacology and toxicology of different extracts as well as the harpagoside from *Harpagophytum procumbens* DC] [In German]. *Planta Med* 34(1):97–108.

Grahame, R. and B.V. Robinson. 1981. Devil's claw (*Harpagophytum procumbens*): pharmacological and clinical studies. *Ann Rheum Dis* 40(6):632.

Lanhers, M.C., J. Fleurentin, F. Mortier, A. Vinche, C. Younos. 1992. Anti-inflammatory and analgesic effects of an aqueous extract of *Harpagophytum procumbens*. *Planta Med* 58(2):117–123.

Mestdagh, O. and M. Torck. 1995. [Quality evaluation of Harpagophyton capsules] [In French]. *Ann Pharm Fr* 53(3):135–137.

Moussard, C., D. Alber, M.M. Toubin, N. Thevenon, J.C. Henry. 1992. A drug used in traditional medicine, *Harpagophytum procumbens*: no evidence for NSAID-like effect on whole blood eicosanoid production in human. *Prostaglandins Leukot Essent Fatty Acids* 46(4):283–286.

Occhiuto, F., C. Circosta, S. Ragusa, P. Ficarra, R. Costa de Pasquale. 1985. A drug used in traditional medicine: *Harpagophytum procumbens* DC. IV. Effects on some isolated muscle preparations. *J Ethnopharmacol* 13(2):201–208.

This material was adapted from *The Complete German Commission E Monographs—Therapeutic Guide to Herbal Medicines*. M. Blumenthal, W.R. Busse, A. Goldberg, J. Gruenwald, T. Hall, C.W. Riggins, R.S. Rister (eds.) S. Klein and R.S. Rister (trans.). 1998. Austin: American Botanical Council; Boston: Integrative Medicine Communications.

1) The Overview section is new information.

2) Description, Chemistry and Pharmacology, Uses, Contraindications, Side Effects, Interactions with Other Drugs, and Dosage sections have been drawn from the original work. Additional information has been added in some or all of these sections, as noted with references.

3) The dosage for equivalent preparations (tea infusion, fluidextract, and tincture) have been provided based on the following example:
   Unless otherwise prescribed: 2 g per day of [powdered, crushed, cut or whole] [plant part]
   Infusion: 2 g in 150 ml of water
   Fluidextract 1:1 (g/ml): 2 ml
   Tincture 1:5 (g/ml): 10 ml

4) The References and Additional Resources sections are new sections. Additional Resources are not cited in the monograph but are included for research purposes.

Soulimani, R., C. Younos, F. Mortier, C. Derrieu. 1994. The role of stomachal digestion on the pharmacological activity of plant extracts, using as an example extracts of *Harpagophytum procumbens*. *Can J Physiol Pharmacol* 72(12):1532–1536.

Whitehouse, L.W., M. Znamirowska, C.J. Paul. 1983. Devil's Claw (*Harpagophytum procumbens*): no evidence for anti-inflammatory activity in the treatment of arthritic disease. *Can Med Assoc J* 129(3):249–251.

ECHINACEA:

ECHINACEA ANGUSTIFOLIA HERB AND ROOT/PALLIDA HERB
(page 93)

ECHINACEA PALLIDA ROOT
(page 95)

ECHINACEA PURPUREA HERB
(page 96)

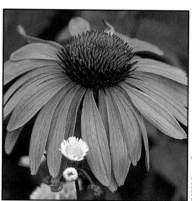

© 1999 Steven Foster

ECHINACEA PURPUREA ROOT
(page 98)

Overview

One of the most popular herbs in the United States marketplace is the native American medicinal plant echinacea. The term refers to several plants in the genus *Echinacea*, derived from the aboveground parts and roots of *Echinacea purpurea* (L.) Moench, *E. angustifolia* D.C., and *E. pallida* (Nutt.) Nutt. [Fam. Asteraceae]. Herbalists and pharmacognosists point out the irony that almost all of the scientific research on this medicinal plant has been conducted not in the United States but in Germany. Echinacea preparations have become increasingly popular in Germany since the early 1900s. The herb was first analyzed and tested for homeopathic purposes in Germany and its medical use was later investigated by Dr. Gerhard Madaus in 1938. Echinacea was formerly used in the United States by native Americans and by Eclectic physicians in the late 1800s and early 1900s. Preparations made from various plants and plant parts of the genus *Echinacea* constituted the top-selling herbal medicine in health food stores in the United States from 1995 to 1998, with an estimated 9.6% of the total health-food dollar spent on herbs, according to a survey of about two hundred independent stores in 1996 (Richman and Witkowski, 1996, 1997, 1998).

Echinacea is used for preventing and treating the common cold, flu, and upper respiratory tract infections (URIs). It is also used to increase general immune system function and to treat vaginal candidiasis. The clinical literature tends to support the *treatment* for symptoms of colds, the flus, and URIs. Recent studies do not support its use to *prevent* URI.

Of the four echinacea monographs published by Commission E, two are positive (i.e., approved) (*E. pallida* root and *E. purpurea* herb) and two are negative (i.e., unapproved) (*E. purpurea* root and *E. angustifolia* root). The latter were given negative assessments due to lack of clinical trials for the specific plant parts. Work on the chemistry of vouchered *Echinacea* species from 1988 onward by Rudolf Bauer and Hildebert Wagner at the Institute for Pharmaceutical Biology in Munich revealed clear chemical profiles for *E. angustifolia* and *E. pallida* (Bauer and Wagner, 1991). It became obvious that earlier pharmacological studies of *E. angustifolia* actually involved *E. pallida*. Historically, *E. pallida* and *E. angustifolia* have been offered to the trade in mixed lots as "Kansas snake root." Therefore, lack of current pharmacological and clinical studies on *E. angustifolia* root and *E. angustifolia/E. pallida* aerial parts resulted in the issuance of a negative monograph until further supporting scientific information becomes available (Leung and Foster, 1996).

However, despite previous problems concerning the botanical identity of *Echinacea* species in commercial preparations and research materials, another reason for the disparity in approvals by Commission E is based on the availability of the research on the respective species. According to Prof. Heinz Schilcher, vice president of Commission E, at the time the monographs were being considered for publication, experimental and clinical studies were available only on the flowering tops and roots of *E. purpurea*, roots of *E. pallida*, and roots of *E. angustifolia*. The Commission decided that only the results from the research conducted on the fresh plant juice from the flowering herb of *E. purpurea* and from the water-alcohol extract of *E. pallida* roots were adequate for a positive monograph. In the meantime, there have been additional studies based on the alcoholic extract of the roots of *E. purpurea* that in Schilcher's opinion should support a positive monograph (Schilcher, 1997). A clinical trial was carried out in 1992 on an extract of the root of *E. purpurea*, suggesting therapeutic benefits in patients with colds and flu (Bräunig et al., 1992). The same year Commission E published a monograph on *E. purpurea* root as an Unapproved Component Characteristic, based on the lack of research of this species and part, although not all members of the Commission supported this decision (Schilcher, 1997).

Since there is a variety of echinacea preparations derived from either one plant or plant part or a variety of plant parts (root, leaf, flower, seed) from various species (*E. purpurea*, *E. pallida*, *E. angustifolia*), it is necessary to clarify which plants and plant parts were used in each clinical trial. Professor R. Bauer of the Institute for Pharmaceutical Biology at Heinrich-Heine University in Düsseldorf, Germany, has evaluated echinacea preparations and determined that they should be grouped according to the species, the part of the plant, and the mode of processing. Based on a review of 23 clinical and pharmacological studies, he determined that significant pharmacological effects have been found *in vitro* and *in vivo* for the expressed juice of the aboveground parts of *E. purpurea* (i.e., Echinacin®) and for alcoholic extracts of the roots of *E. pallida*, *E. angustifolia*, and *E. purpurea* (Bauer, 1996). The effects act mainly on the nonspecific cellular immune system. He reports several active constituent groups: polysaccharides, glycoproteins, caffeic acid derivatives (cichoric acid), and alkamides.

A review of 26 controlled clinical studies (18 randomized, 11 double-blind) that investigated the immunomodulatory activity of preparations containing echinacea extracts (Melchart et al., 1994). Six of the trials used echinacea alone, and 20 tested echinacea in combination with other ingredients. The methodological quality of the trials was assessed and deemed low. However, the authors concluded that existing controlled clinical trials indicated that preparations containing the juice or extracts of echinacea can be efficacious immunomodulators. Further methodologically sound, randomized clinical trials were recommended. Commenting on this study, Professor H. Wagner, a leading figure in European pharmacognosy, commented, "Of the investigated criteria the most striking effects were the reduction in susceptibility to infection and in the incidence of catarrh and pharyngeal inflammation" (Wagner, 1997). In reviewing clinical studies on echinacea, he has written, "The conclusion that can be drawn … is that remedies containing echinacea can effect an improvement in immune defense systems where those systems are temporarily weakened." He pointed out that there is not yet sufficient evidence to give "clear therapeutic recommendations as to which preparation in which dosage and type of application has the optimal effect" (Wagner, 1997).

Many clinical studies on echinacea used fresh stabilized *E. purpurea* juice, in the injectable form, and others have been conducted with oral applications or an externally applied salve (Hobbs, 1994). The *E. purpurea* aerial parts preparations are usually a proprietary fresh-pressed leaf juice (22% ethanol by volume as a preservative), marketed as Echinacin® (manufactured by Madaus AG of Cologne, Germany). Echinacea is often used in combination products such as Esberitox® (Schaper and Brümmer, Germany), which also contains extracts of *Baptisia tinctoria* (wild indigo) and *Thuja occidentalis* (arbor vitae). Clinical studies conducted with this combination product are not reviewed here due to the presence of these presumably active additional ingredients.

In the most recent literature review of clinical trials conducted on various echinacea preparations for prevention or treatment of URIs, focusing on 9 trials designed for treatment and 4 trials for prevention, the authors found that 8 of the 9 treatment trials reported generally positive results, while 3 of the prevention trials reported "marginal benefit" (Barrett et al., 1999). The authors assessed the methodological quality of the trials as "modest." They concluded that various types of preparations from various species of *Echinacea* may be beneficial for the early treatment of URIs, but that there was little evidence to support the extended use of echinacea for prevention of URI. They found it difficult to make specific dosage recommendations due to the variation in composition of commercial preparations. The authors emphasized that the highest quality trials suggest that early dosing of sufficient doses is important.

Another recent review of echinacea (Melchart and Linde, 1999) has found seven placebo-controlled, double-blind, randomized clinical trials testing the efficacy of two different echinacea monopreparations and three combination products in the treatment of non-specific URIs. Combination products are not reviewed in this monograph.

Several studies have examined echinacea's usefulness in the prevention and treatment of colds. A double-blind, placebo-controlled study was conducted with 108 volunteers who had chronic URIs (more than three occurrences in a half year) (Schöneberger, 1992). Half of the patients received a dose of 8 ml/day of fresh-pressed juice of *E. purpurea* (Echinacin®) for eight weeks, with the other half receiving placebo. Compared to the placebo group, in the echinacea group there was a tendancy for more patients (36%) to suffer no infections, or the time between infections increased, the duration of illness shortened, and severity of symptoms lessened. The echinacea preparation was well tolerated, and patients with diminished immune response (expressed by a low T4/T8 cell ratio) seemed to benefit most from the treatment. This same study was recently re-interpreted and re-published with a less positive assessment given by the authors (Grimm and Müller, 1999).

In a more recent randomized, double-blind, placebo-controlled study on this fresh juice preparation (Hoheisel et al., 1997), the clinical efficacy of the proprietary *E. purpurea* expressed juice preparation (Echinagard®, Echinacin's trade name in the United States) was tested on 120 patients with initial symptoms of common cold. The preparation was effective in that significantly fewer patients developed full disease symptoms (40% versus 60%); recovery was much quicker with the echinacea preparation than with placebo (four days versus eight days).

A third study highlighted the importance of dosage in the expected effectiveness of echinacea preparations (Bräunig et al., 1992). This double-blind, placebo-controlled trial examined the effectiveness of an ethanolic extract made from the root of *E. purpurea* (1:5, 55% ethanol) in relieving the symptoms and duration of flu-like infections in 180 volunteers. Subjects were divided into three groups of 60 each and administered the echinacea at 450 mg/dose, 900 mg/dose, or placebo. Those who received only 450 mg/dose showed improvement only comparable to the placebo. Those receiving 900 mg/dose showed a statistically significant improvement. An effect from the higher dose was seen after three to four days, but the full effect was not seen for 8 to 10 days. It is possible that the availability of this study to the Commission E at the time the *E. purpurea* root monograph was given a negative assessment (published in August, 1992) may have influenced a positive (approved) assessment.

In a recent Swedish placebo-controlled double-blind study conducted over eight days with tablets (daily dose, 3x2) made from a proprietary water-alcohol extract of the fresh herb (95%) and roots (5%) of *E. purpurea* (extract ratio 5.9:1; Echinaforce®, Bioforce, Switzerland), 55 patients were given the herbal preparation and 64 received placebo. Thirteen of the echinacea group were allowed to use additional approved medication, such as nose drops and the fever-reducing drug paracetamol. The examining physician concluded that the echinacea preparation was effective in 68% of the patients in reducing several of 12 symptoms (nasal catarrh and/or stuffy nose, sore throat, headache/dizziness, muscle pain, fever, cough, etc.); patients self-assessed the efficacy of the echinacea at 78% of the cases (Brinkeborn et al., 1998). The preparation evoked little concern about safety.

A critical summary of studies on the immunomodulatory activity of preparations of echinacea reported on five randomized trials conducted between 1984 and 1992 (Melchart et al., 1995). A total of 134 healthy, mostly male, volunteers between the ages of 18 and 40 were studied in Germany, using five different echinacea preparations. The results were mixed; not only were different preparations administered, but methods for analyzing the activity of targeted immune cells varied as well, making interpretation difficult. Two of the five studies showed activity of the measured immune cells to be significantly stimulated, while three did not.

In a highly publicized study, researchers ran a clinical study on 302 healthy people (revised to a total of 289 after dropouts) who were divided into three groups. Each group received either an alcoholic extract of *E. purpurea* root, *E. angustifolia* root, or a placebo. Neither echinacea preparation helped prevent the onset of the common cold; cold symptoms appeared within 69 days in the *E. purpurea* group (29.3% with infection), 66 days for the *E. angustifolia* group (32.0%), and 65 days for the placebo group (36.7%). The participants were instructed to take 50 drops (about 20 microliters per drop) twice per day from Monday through Friday for 12 weeks. The two ethanolic echinacea root extracts were prepared at a 1:11 ratio and were dissolved in 30% ethanol. The conclusion was that the study could not show that echinacea helps to prevent the common cold. The study states, "Based on the results of this and two other studies, one could speculate that there might be an effect of echinacea products in the order of magnitude of 10% to 20% relative risk reduction" (Melchart et al., 1998). The conclusion to be drawn from this research is that the study could not show preventive activity with the specific preparation according to the particular study design; the authors acknowledged the need for a larger population of subjects upon which to test for potential preventive activity.

Some new research findings have come from a recent placebo-controlled trial testing the exercise-induced immunological effects of *E. purpurea* aboveground fresh plant juice (Echinacin®) on 42 male athletes (Berg et al., 1998). The echinacea group had marked changes in concentration of the cytokines interleukin 6 (IL-6) and soluble interleukin 2 receptor (sIL-2R), proteins that stimulate various immune functions, in serum and urine and significantly increased serum. Exercise-induced cortisol usually lowers natural killer (NK) cell levels and inhibits macrophage activity, two variables of immune function. The echinacea group did not demonstrate a significant decrease in NK cells one hour after competition, suggesting that echinacea may counteract the immune suppressant effect of cortisol. However, another result of this study was that none of the echinacea group experienced URI, while 3 of 13 in the magnesium group and 4 of 13 in the placebo group developed URI. A total of six in both the magnesium and placebo groups reported symptoms of other infections, while none on echinacea did. The authors concluded that preventive treatment of athletes with the *E. purpurea* juice preparation counteracts the immunosuppressant effects of exhaustive exercise and reduces risk of URI in athletes.

There is evidence to suggest that echinacea is a reliable supportive therapy for people with recurring candidiasis, particularly when antifungal therapy is failing (Brown, 1996). The positive effect of *E. purpurea* leaf juice was demonstrated in a study of 203 women with recurrent vaginal yeast infections (Coeugniet and Kühnast, 1986). All the women were being treated with a topical econazole nitrate cream (a commonly prescribed antifungal/antiyeast medication). Women using the econazole nitrate alone experienced a 60.5% recurrence rate, while the women taking echinacea (oral Echinacin®) had a recurrence rate lowered to 16.7%.

In a study in the United States the pharmacological basis for the immunological activity of echinacea was investigated by researchers at the Department of Medicine, University of California at Irvine Medical Center at Orange (See et al., 1997). Extracts of both *E. purpurea* (plant part not noted) and *Panax ginseng* root were tested for their capacity to stimulate cellular immune function by peripheral blood mononuclear cells (PBMC) from normal individuals and patients with either chronic fatigue syndrome or acquired immunodeficiency syndrome. Results indicated that the extracts enhanced cellular immune function of PBMC from both normal individuals and patients with depressed cellular immunity.

Bauer and Wagner note that various preparations of echinacea enhance leukocyte activity, have antibacterial properties, inhibit the enzyme hyaluronidase (thus retarding breakdown of hyaluronic acid, a gelatinous component of intercellular spaces), provide an interferon-like effect on viruses, and have (relatively mild) anti-inflammatory properties (Bauer and Wagner, 1991). Another potential use of echinacea preparations is for the treatment of otitis media in small children, an application that is gaining a small number of adherents among some pediatricians and naturopathic physicians in the United States (Blumenthal, 1993).

The monograph on *E. pallida* root is an example of a case where specifications based on a proprietary extract of an herb were approved. This preparation consists of a tincture (1:5) with 50% (v/v) ethanol from native dry extract (50% ethanol, 7–11:1) corresponding to 900 mg of the herb, i.e., dried root. A placebo-controlled, double-blind trial conducted on 160 adults indicated that a daily dose of 900 mg of the extract of *E. pallida* root was effective in shortening the duration of URIs (sinusitis, cough, pharyngitis) in infected adults, whether of bacterial or viral origin (Dorn et al., 1997).

There has been some confusion regarding the contraindications and side effects listed in the monographs, most of which are for injectible preparations. The contraindications noted below for echinacea preparations in cases of HIV and AIDS, tuberculosis, leukosis, collagenosis, and multiple sclerosis have been misinterpreted to mean that echinacea use can exacerbate such conditions; however, there is no clinical evidence to support this concern. The reason for the Commission's caution was based on theoretical concerns and because such conditions are not amenable to self-medication. A cogent argument by an Australian phytotherapist suggests that there is no rational basis for this contraindication and in fact, current clinical practice, previous prolonged use by Eclectic physicians in the United States in the latter nineteenth and early twentieth centuries, and proper evaluation of modern scientific data support long-term use of echinacea preparations for autoimmune disorders (Bone, 1997–1998).

Regarding the issue of Commission E's contraindication of echinacea preparations for various types of autoimmune disorders, Professor Bauer, the world's leading researcher on echinacea, writes, "As far as I know, these contraindications have only been included because of theoretical considerations. There is a paper by Shohan (1985) in which the possible risks of immunostimulating agents in general are discussed. These recommendations for Echinacea are as far as I know not based on any reported adverse effect in such indications. There is a recent paper by Parnham (1996) which reports that long-term treatment, e.g., with the expressed juice of *E. purpurea*, is well-tolerated" (Bauer, 1999b).

It should also be noted that in Germany, physicians previously had access to injectable (parenteral) drug products made from either a monopreparation of E. *purpurea* herb juice or a fixed combination that contained E. *pallida*. Thus, the monographs for E. *purpurea* herb and E. *pallida* root both note adverse side effects associated with injectable forms of these echinacea products.

Despite safety concerns with injectable echinacea, there are few significant adverse events reported for echinacea products taken orally. One such event was a case of anaphylaxis reported with ingestion of an echinacea preparation made of E. *angustifolia* (whole plant) and E. *purpurea* root (Mullins, 1998). Animal toxicology studies indicate a high degree of safety for echinacea: in experiments using oral (greater than 15 g per kg) or intravenous (greater than 5 g per kg) administration, it was impossible to kill rats or mice (Hoheisel et al., 1997). Thus, an average lethal dose has not been determinable. Rats and mice given prolonged (4 weeks) doses of an E. *purpurea* preparation up to 8 g per kg did not exhibit adverse effects on numerous end points measured (blood lipids, liver enzymes, weight loss, etc.) (Mengs et al., 1991).

Based on the data presented above, there are sufficient pharmacological and clinical research studies to support the safety and probable efficacy of preparations made from both the aerial parts of E. *purpurea* and the roots of at least two and possibly three species of echinacea (E. *pallida* and E. *purpurea*, and possibly, E. *angustifolia*).

ECHINACEA ANGUSTIFOLIA HERB AND ROOT/ PALLIDA HERB

Latin Name:
Echinacea angustifolia/E. pallida

Pharmacopeial Name:
Echinaceae angustifoliae/pallidae herba; Echinaceae angustifoliae radix

Other Names:
Kansas snake root, narrow-leaved echinacea, narrow-leaved purple coneflower

Description
The fresh or dried roots, or the fresh or dried aboveground parts collected at the time of flowering, of *Echinacea angustifolia* D.C. [Fam. Asteraceae] and their preparations in effective dosage. The fresh or dried aboveground parts, collected at the time of flowering, of E. *pallida* (Nutt.) Nutt., and their preparations in effect dosage. On the market, preparations of E. *pallida* are to some extent incorrectly labeled as "*Echinacea angustifolia.*"

Chemistry and Pharmacology
Echinacea angustifolia herb contains caffeic acid derivatives such as cichoric acid, echinacoside, verbascoside, chlorogenic acid, and isochlorogenic acid; flavonoids of the quercetin and kaempferol type in free and glycoside forms, including rutoside, luteolin, kaempferol, quercetin, apigenin, and isorhamnetin; alkamides, mainly of the undeca-2,4-diene type with the isomeric mixture of dodeca-2E,4E,8Z,10E/Z-tetraenoic acid isobutylamides; polysaccharides; and < 0.1% essential oil (Bauer, 1998; Bauer and Liersch, 1993; Leung and Foster, 1996; Pietta et al.,

1998); trideca-1-en-3,5,7,9,11-pen-tayne and ponticaepoxide have been detected in the flowerbuds (Bauer and Liersch, 1993).

Echinacea angustifolia root contains caffeic acid derivatives, mainly echina-coside (0.3–1.7%) followed by chloro-genic acid, an isochlorogenic acid, and its characteristic constituent cynarin (1.5-O-Dicaffeoyl-quinic acid); polysac-charides, including inulin (5.9%) and fructans; glycoproteins comprised of approximately 3% protein of which the dominant sugars are arabinose (64–84%), galactose (1.9–5.3%) and glucosamines (6%); 0.01–0.15% alka-mides, mainly derived from undeca- and dodeca-noic acid, primarily the iso-meric dodeca-2E,4E,8Z,10E/Z-tetraenoic acid isobutylamides; and <0.1% essential oil (Bauer, 1998; Bauer, 1999a; Bauer and Liersch, 1993; Pietta et al., 1998).

Echinacea pallida herb contains caf-feic acid derivatives, including cichoric acid, caftaric acid, echinacoside, verbas-coside, chlorogenic acid, and isochloro-genic acid; flavonoids mainly rutoside; alkamides, mainly of the 2,4-diene type with the isomeric mixture of dodeca-2E,4E,8Z,10E/Z-tetraenoic acid isobutylamides; and <0.1% essential oil (Bauer, 1998; Bauer and Liersch, 1993; Leung and Foster, 1996; Pietta et al., 1998).

Animal experiment: In the carbon clearance test, alcoholic root extracts as well as extracts of the aboveground herb show a rate increase in elimination of carbon particles.

In vitro: Alcoholic root extracts show an increase in phagocytic elements of 23% when tested in granulocyte smears. Experiments reported in older publications cannot be definitely assigned to either of these species.

Uses

Preparations of E. angustifolia are used to support and promote the natural powers of resistance of the body, espe-cially in infectious conditions (influenza and colds, etc.) in the nose and throat, as an alterative in influenza, inflamma-tory and purulent wounds, abscesses, furuncles, indolent leg ulcers, herpes simplex, inflammation of connective tissue, wounds, headaches, metabolic disturbances, and as a diaphoretic and antiseptic. According to the Commis-sion E, when the monograph was pub-lished in August, 1992, efficacy for the uses listed above has not been docu-mented scientifically, although, as noted previously, recent investigations suggest possible beneficial activity of E. angusti-folia root preparations (Galea and Thacker, 1996), although published studies are not available. The Commis-sion E noted that since the activity of the various parts of the herbs for the conditions listed above has not been substantiated, their therapeutic use could not be recommended. Because of the risks, the use of parenteral (i.e., injectable) preparations is not justified. Parenteral preparations of echinacea species are no longer approved in Ger-many.

However, the World Health Organi-zation (WHO) conducted a more recent review of the literature, including new research conducted since the Commis-sion E monograph was published in 1992, and concluded that the following uses for E. angustifolia root (not aerial parts) are supported by clinical data: supportive therapy for colds and infec-tions of the respiratory and urinary tracts (WHO, 1999).

Contraindications

Internal use: Commission E cautioned that echinacea preparations are not to be used in systemic diseases such as tuberculosis, leukosis, collagenosis, multiple sclerosis, AIDS, HIV infection, and other autoimmune diseases. (As noted above, these cautions were made based on theoretical considerations and not on any reports of adverse findings.)

Side Effects

Parenteral use: Depending upon the dosage, chills, short-term fever reac-tions, and nausea and vomiting may occur. In rare cases immediate allergic reactions may occur. If there is a tendency for allergy, especially against Asteraceae, and during pregnancies, do not apply parenterally. (Parenteral use of echinacea preparations is no longer approved in Germany.)

Warning: The metabolic condition in diabetics can decline upon parenteral application.

Use During Pregnancy and Lactation

No restrictions known.

Interactions with Other Drugs

None known.

Dosage and Administration

Echinacea angustifolia root: Unless otherwise prescribed: 1 g cut root several times daily, for teas and other galenical preparations for internal use.
Decoction: Boil 1 g root in 150 ml water for 10 minutes, three times daily (Bradley, 1992).
Infusion: Steep 1 g root in 150 ml boiled water for at least 10 minutes, several times daily between meals (Bauer and Liersch, 1993; Wichtl and Bisset, 1994).
Fluidextract 1:1 (g/ml), 45% ethanol: 0.5–1.0 ml, three times daily (Bradley, 1992).
Tincture 1:5 (g/ml), 45% ethanol: 2–5 ml, three times daily (Bradley, 1992).

ECHINACEA PALLIDA ROOT

Latin Name:
Echinacea pallida

Pharmacopeial Name:
Echinaceae pallidae radix

Other Names:
pale-flowered echinacea, pale purple coneflower root

Description

Echinacea pallida root, consisting of fresh or dried root of *E. pallida* (Nutt.) Nutt. [Fam. Asteraceae] and its preparations in effective dosage.

Chemistry and Pharmacology

Echinacea pallida root contains caffeic acid derivatives, mainly echinacoside (0.7–1.0%), followed by isochlorogenic acid, 6-O-caffeoylechinacoside, and chlorogenic acid; 0.2–2.0% essential oil composed mainly of ketoalkynes and ketoalkenes (pentadeca-8Z-en-2-one, pentadeca-1,8Z-diene, and 1-pentadecene); polyacetylenes (trideca-1-en-3,5,7,9,11-pentayne and ponticaepoxide); polysaccharides; and glycoproteins (Bauer, 1999a; Bauer and

Liersch, 1993; ESCOP, 1999; Pietta et al., 1998).

The Commission E reported that in a carbon clearance test, alcohol root extracts showed an increase in the elimination of carbon particles by a factor of 2.2. In an *in vitro* test: Alcohol root extracts showed an increase in phagocytic elements by 23% when tested in granulocyte smears at a concentration of 10:4–10:2 mg/ml.

Uses

The Commission E approved the internal use of *E. pallida* root as supportive therapy for influenza-like infections. The German Standard License for infusion of *E. pallida* root recommends it to strengthen resistance to infectious conditions in the upper respiratory tract (Wichtl and Bisset, 1994).

The WHO approved *E. pallida* root as supportive therapy for colds and infections of the respiratory and urinary tracts (WHO, 1999).

Contraindications

Commission E cautioned that echinacea preparations are not to be used when progressive systemic diseases such as the following exist: tuberculosis, leukosis, collagenosis, multiple sclerosis, AIDS, HIV infection, and other autoimmune diseases. (As noted above, these cautions were made based on theoretical considerations and not on any reports of adverse findings.)

Side Effects

None known.

Use During Pregnancy and Lactation

No restrictions known.

Interactions with Other Drugs

None known.

Dosage and Administration

Unless otherwise prescribed: 900 mg of root per day in liquid forms for oral administration for a period of not longer than eight weeks.

Tincture 1:5 (g/ml) with 50% (v/v) ethanol prepared from native dry extract (50% ethanol, 7–11:1): 90 drops (Bauer and Liersch, 1993; ESCOP, 1999).

Decoction: Boil 1 g in 150 ml water for 10 minutes, three times daily (Newall et al., 1996).

ECHINACEA PURPUREA HERB

Latin Name:
Echinacea purpurea

Pharmacopeial Name:
Echinaceae purpureae herba

Other Names:
echinacea, coneflower, purple coneflower, purple echinacea

Description

Purple coneflower herb consists of fresh, aboveground parts, harvested at flowering time, of *Echinacea purpurea* (L.) Moench [Fam. Asteraceae], and its preparations in effective dosage.

Chemistry and Pharmacology

Echinacea purpurea herb contains caffeic acid derivatives, mainly cichoric acid (1.2–3.1% in the flowers), caftaric acid and chlorogenic acid; 0.001–0.03% alkamides, mainly isomeric dodeca-2E,4E,8Z,10E/Z-tetraenoic acid isobutylamides; water soluble polysaccharides, including PS I

(a 4-0-methylglucoronylarabinoxylan) and PS II (an acidic rhamnoarabinogalactan), fructans; 0.48% flavonoids of quercetin and kaempferol type (e.g., rutoside); 0.08–0.32% essential oil composed of borneol, bornyl acetate, pentadeca-8-en-2-one, palmitic acid, and others (Bauer, 1999a; Bauer and Liersch, 1993).

The Commission E reported that in human and animal experiments, *E. purpurea* preparations given internally or parenterally have shown immunostimulant effects. Among others, the number of white blood cells and spleen cells is increased, the capacity for phagocytosis by human granulocytes is activated, and the body temperature is elevated. Echinacea has been studied for nonspecific stimulation of the immune system, involving an overall increase in phagocytosis by macrophages and granulocytes.

Oral dosage is as effective as parenteral dosage, though slower acting. The combined action of multiple constituents is apparently responsible for the immunostimulatory activity of both alcoholic and aqueous extracts of echinacea. The immunostimulant activity of alcoholic echinacea extracts is largely due to the lipophilic amides (alkylamides), as well as the polar caffeic acid derivatives (e.g., cichoric acid), whereas the water soluble polysaccharides are implicated in the expressed juice or aqueous preparations of *E. purpurea*. Expressed juice of fresh flowering *E. purpurea* applied topically on local tissues inhibits hyaluronidase, thereby stimulating wound healing (Bauer and Wagner, 1990, 1991).

Uses

The Commission E approved the internal use of *E. purpurea* herb as supportive therapy for colds and chronic infections of the respiratory tract and lower urinary tract. The Commission E approved external use for poorly healing wounds and chronic ulcerations.

The WHO supports the findings of Commission E regarding internal and external uses of *E. purpurea* herb. WHO added "treatment of inflammatory skin conditions" to external use (WHO, 1999).

Contraindications

External: None known.
Internal: Progressive systemic diseases, such as tuberculosis, leukosis, collagenosis, and multiple sclerosis. (As noted above, these cautions were made based on theoretical considerations and not on any reports of adverse findings.)

No parenteral administration in case of tendencies to allergies, especially allergies to members of the Compositae (Asteraceae), as well as in pregnancy. (Parenteral use is no longer approved in Germany.)

Warning: The metabolic condition in diabetics can decline upon parenteral application.

Side Effects

Internal and external application: None known.
Parenteral application: Depending upon dosage, short-term fever reactions, and nausea and vomiting can occur. In individual cases, immediate allergic reactions are possible.

Use During Pregnancy and Lactation

No restrictions known.

Interactions with Other Drugs

None known.

Dosage and Administration

Unless otherwise prescribed: **Internal:** 6–9 ml expressed juice of fresh plant or equivalent preparations, per day. **External:** Semi-solid preparations containing at least 15% pressed juice. Preparations for internal and external use: Not longer than eight weeks.
Internal: Succus, in 25% solution (95% ethanol): 6–9 ml (Bauer and Liersch, 1993; Commission E; ESCOP, 1999).
Infusion: 1 g in 150 ml water.
Fluidextract 1:1 (g/ml): 1 ml.
Tincture 1:5 (g/ml): 5 ml.
External: Ointment: Semi-solid preparation containing at least 15% pressed juice in a base of petroleum jelly or anhydrous lanolin and vegetable oil applied locally.
Poultice: Semi-solid paste or plaster containing at least 15% pressed juice applied locally.
Parenteral: Depends on kind and seriousness of condition as well as the nature of the preparation. Parenteral application requires a gradation of dosage, especially for children; the manufacturer is required to show this information for the particular preparation. Preparations for parenteral use: Not longer than three weeks. (No longer approved in Germany.)

ECHINACEA PURPUREA ROOT

Latin Name:
Echinacea purpurea

Pharmacopeial Name:
Echinaceae purpureae radix

Other Names:
echinacea root, purple coneflower root

Description

Echinacea purpurea root, consisting of fresh or dried root of *Echinacea purpurea* (L.) Moench [Fam. Asteraceae] and its preparations.

Chemistry and Pharmacology

Echinacea purpurea root contains 0.6–2.1% caffeic acid derivatives, mainly cichoric acid and caftaric acid, plus caffeic acid and chlorogenic acid; 0.01–0.04% alkamides, mainly of the undeca-2,4-diene type with the isomeric mixture of dodeca-2E,4E,8Z,10E/Z-tetraenoic acid isobutylamides; polyacetylene derivatives; polysaccharides (fructosans, mainly of polymerization grade 4); glycoproteins comprised of approximately 3% protein, of which the dominant sugars are arabinose (64–84%), galactose (1.9–5.3%), and glucosamines (6%); up to 0.2% essential oil (e.g., caryophyllene, humulene, caryophyllene epoxide) (Bauer, 1998, 1999; Bauer and Liersch, 1993; ESCOP, 1999; Pietta et al., 1998).

According to the Commission E, alcoholic root extracts demonstrated a rate increase in the elimination of carbon particles in the carbon clearance test. *In vitro*, alcoholic extracts show an increase in phagocytic elements when tested in granulocyte smears. Acute toxicity of *E. purpurea* root extract was measured on NMRI-mice using oral application. The toxicity was greater than 3,000 mg/kg body weight. More information concerning the kind of extract is not given. Extrapolation to the herb (i.e., aboveground parts) or other preparations is not possible.

Uses

[The Component Characteristic monographs have a different format; the primary herb is listed with various potential combinations with other herbs and other natural products, reflecting some of the proprietary products sold in Germany at the time of the Commission E evaluation. Commission E did not approve the following uses as they were *not* supported by clinical studies.]

Combinations with up to 5 components:

a) Echinacea purpurea root, coneflower root, arbor vitae tips, indigo weed rhizome.
Nonspecific irrigation therapy, prophylaxis and therapy for infectious diseases, common infections (virus, influenza), leukopenia after radiation therapy or cytostatic therapy, support of anti-infectious chemotherapy.

b) Echinacea purpurea root, beta-sitosterol, alpha-tocopherol acetate.
Prostatic syndrome (hypertrophy, adenoma), disturbances of bladder functions and urination, chronic inflammation of bladder lining.

c) Echinacea purpurea root, witch hazel leaves, horse chestnut seeds, esculin.
Varicose symptoms, ulcus cruris, thrombophlebitis, varicose veins, edema, hemorrhoids, varicose stasis, paresthesia, dysmenorrhea.

d) Echinacea purpurea root, 1 homeopathic preparation.

Disturbances of hair growth, loss of hair, hair damage, for improved sheen and elasticity of the hair, seborrhea, brittleness of nails.

e) Echinacea purpurea root, onion, pumpkin seed, poplar buds, pareira root.

Prostatitis syndrome, irritated bladder condition in men and women, abacterial chronic and recurrent prostatitis, bacterial chronic and recurrent prostatitis—needed in combination with a targeted antibacterial therapy, vegetatively fixed prostatitis, catarrhal adnexitis, symptomatic therapy for radiation-damaged bladder, support of antibiotic therapy of acute bacterial prostatitis by removal of inflamed and vegetative components of this disease form, and by its additive antibacterial effect.

f) Echinacea purpurea root, onion, pumpkin seed, poplar buds, pareira root.

Functional, hormonal, radiogenic micturition disturbances, cystitis, infections of the bladder, prophylaxis and therapy of infections in the urinary system after urologic and gynecologic surgery.

Combinations with more than 5 components:

g) Echinacea purpurea root, peppermint leaves, turmeric root, buckthorn bark, milk thistle fruit, dandelion whole plant, tetterwort, madder root.

Diseases of the liver-gall system, recidivous prophylaxis for gallstones, cholecystitis, cholangiitis, gall spasms, postcystectomic syndrome, posthepatic syndrome, hypotonic-asthenic dyskinesia.

h) Echinacea purpurea root, fennel, caraway, coriander fruit, hawthorn leaves, hawthorn flowers, hawthorn herb, mistletoe, melissa, eleuthero ginseng root.

For stress symptoms, fatigue, unrest, tiredness, exhaustion, convalescence.

i) Echinacea purpurea root, hawthorn flowers, valerian root, lily-of-the-valley herb, arnica flowers, large-flowered cereus flowers, arborvitae tips.

For coronary circulation problems, inflammation of the peri- and endocardium, neurosis of the circulatory system.

According to the Commission E, since the effectiveness of the claimed applications was not documented at the time of publication of the monograph (August, 1992), therapeutic use could not be recommended. The Commission also stated that the application of parenteral (injectable) preparations was not justifiable because of various risks (see below). However, subsequent to the publication of the monograph on *E. purpurea* root by the Commission E, a double-blind, placebo-controlled trial examined the effectiveness of a hydroalcoholic extract made from the root of *E. purpurea* (1:5, 55% ethanol) in relieving the symptoms and duration of flu-like infections in 180 volunteers (Bräunig et al., 1992). Subjects were divided into three groups of 60 and administered the echinacea at 450 mg/dose, 900 mg/dose, or placebo. Those who received only 450 mg/dose showed improvement only comparable to the placebo. Those receiving 900 mg/dose showed a statistically significant improvement. An effect from the higher dose was seen after three to four days, but the full effect was not seen for 8 to 10 days. This trial is frequently referred to as plausible evidence of the efficacy of preparations of *E. purpurea* root preparations for the treatment of symptoms of URIs associated with colds and flu (Melchart et al., 1994; Barrett et al., 1999).

Contraindications

External: None known.

Internal: Commission E noted the following: progressive systemic diseases such as tuberculosis, leukosis, collagenosis, multiple sclerosis, AIDS, HIV infection, and other autoimmune diseases. (As noted above, these cautions were made based on theoretical considerations and not on any reports of adverse findings.)

In case of tendency for allergies, especially from Asteraceae, and during pregnancy, no parenteral application to be used.

Warning: The metabolic condition of diabetics can decline upon parenteral application. (Parenteral preparations are no longer approved in Germany.)

Side Effects

Parenteral use:
Depending upon dosage, chills, short-term fever reactions, and nausea and vomiting may occur. In single cases, immediate allergic reactions are possible. (These effects were noticed with injectable preparations only and do not apply to oral use.)

Use During Pregnancy and Lactation

No parenteral application during pregnancy.

Interactions with Other Drugs

None known.

Dosage and Administration

Unless otherwise prescribed: 0.9 g cut root several times daily, for teas and other galenical preparations for internal use.
Infusion: Steep 0.9 g root in 150 ml boiled water for 10 minutes, several times daily between meals.
Tincture 1:5 (g/ml), ethanol 55% V/V: 30–60 drops, three times daily (Bauer and Liersch, 1993; ESCOP, 1999).

References

Barrett, B., M. Vohmann, C. Calabrese. 1999. Echinacea for upper respiratory tract infection. *J Fam Pract* 48(8):628–635.

Bauer, R. 1999a. Chemistry, analysis and immunological investigations of *Echinacea* phytopharmaceuticals. In: Wagner, H. (ed.). *Immunomodulatory Agents from Plants*. Basel, Switzerland: Birkhäuser Verlag. 41–88.

———. 1999b. Personal communication to M. Blumenthal. Jan. 21; Feb. 4.

———. 1998. *Echinacea*: Biological Effects and Active Principles. In: Lawson, L. and R. Bauer (eds.). *Phytomedicines of Europe: Chemistry and Biological Activity*. Washington, D.C.: American Chemical Society. 140–157.

———. 1996. Echinacea-Drogen—Wirkungen und Wirksubstanzen [Echinacea drugs—effects and active ingredients (Review). *Z Arztl Fortbild (Jena)* 90(2):111–115.

Bauer, R. and R. Liersch. 1993. Echinacea. In: Hänsel, R., K. Keller, H. Rimpler, G. Schneider (eds.). *Hagers Handbuch der Pharmazeutischen Praxis*, 5th ed. Vol. 5. Drogen E–O. New York: Springer Verlag. 1–34.

Bauer, R. and H. Wagner. 1991. Echinacea species as potential immunostimulatory drugs. In: Wagner, H. and N.R. Farnsworth (eds.). 1991. *Economic and Medicinal Plants Research*, Vol. 5. New York: Academic Press. 253–321.

———. 1990. *Echinacea: Ein Handbuch für Ärzte, Apotheker, und andere Naturwissenschaftler*. Stuttgart: Wissenschaftliche Verlagsgesellschaft.

Berg, A. et al. 1998. Influence of Echinacin (EC31) treatment on the exercise-induced immune response in athletes. *J Clin Res* 1:367–380.

Blumenthal, M. 1993. Echinacea Highlighted as Cold and Flu Remedy. *HerbalGram* 29:8–9.

Bone, K. 1997–1998. Echinacea: When Should it be Used? *Eur J Herb Med* 3(3):13–17.

Bradley, P.R. (ed.). 1992. *British Herbal Compendium*, Vol. 1. Bournemouth: British Herbal Medicine Association.

Bräunig, B., M. Dorn, E. Knick. 1992. *Echinacea purpurea* radix for strengthening the immune response in flu-like infections. *Z Phytotherapie* 13:7–13.

Brinkeborn, R.M, D.V. Shah, S. Geissbuhler, F.H. Degenring. 1998. Echinaforce® in the treatment of acute colds. *Schweiz Zschr Ganzheits Med* 10:26–29.

Brown, D.J. 1996. *Herbal Prescriptions for Better Health*. Rocklin, CA: Prima Publishing. 63–68.

Coeugniet, E. and R. Kühnast. 1986. Recurrent candidiasis: Adjutant immunotherapy with different formulations of Echinacin®. *Therapiewoche* 36:3352–3358.

Dorn, M., E. Knick, G. Lewith. 1997. Placebo-controlled, double-blind study of Echinacea pallidae radix in upper respiratory tract infections. *Complement Ther Med* 5:40–42.

ESCOP. 1999. "Echinacea—Proposal for the Summary of Product Characteristics." *Monographs on the Medicinal Uses of Plant Drugs*. Exeter, U.K.: European Scientific Cooperative on Phytotherapy.

Galea, S. and K. Thacker. 1996. Double-blind prospective trial investigating the effectiveness of a commonly prescribed herbal remedy in altering the duration, severity and symptoms of the common cold. Unpublished.

Grimm, W. and H.H. Müller. 1999. A randomized controlled trial of the effect of fluid extract of *Echinacea purpurea* on the incidence and severity of colds and respiratory infections. *Am J Med* 106(2):138–143.

Hobbs, C. 1994. Echinacea: A literature review. *HerbalGram* 30:33–48.

Hoheisel, O., M. Sandberg, S. Bertram, M. Bulitta, M. Schäfer. 1997. Echinagard treatment shortens the course of the common cold: a double-blind, placebo-controlled clinical trial. *Eur J Clin Res* 9:261–269.

Leung, A.Y. and S. Foster. 1996. *Encyclopedia of Common Natural Ingredients Used in Food, Drugs, and Cosmetics*, 2nd ed. New York: John Wiley & Sons, Inc.

Melchart, D. and K. Linde. 1999. Clinical investigations of Echinacea phytopharmaceuticals. In: Wagner, H. (ed.). *Immunomodulatory Agents from Plants*. Basel: Birkhauser Verlag.

Melchart, D. et al. 1995. Results of five randomized studies on the immunomodulatory activity of preparations of *Echinacea*. *J Altern Complement Med* 1(2):145–160.

Melchart, D., K. Linde, F. Worku, R. Bauer, H. Wagner. 1994. Immunomodulation with *Echinacea*—A systematic review of controlled clinical trials. *Phytomed* 1:245–254.

Melchart, D., E. Walther, K. Linde, R. Brandmaier, C. Lersch. 1998. Echinacea root extracts for the prevention of upper respiratory tract infections: a double-blind, placebo-controlled randomized trial. *Arch Fam Med* 7(6):541–545.

Mengs, U., C.B. Clare, J.A. Poiley. 1991. Toxicity of *Echinacea purpurea*. *Arzneimforsch/Drug Res* 41(10): 1076–1081.

Mullins, R.J. 1998. Echinacea-associated anaphylaxis [letter]. *Med J Aust* 168(4):584.

Newall, C.A., L.A. Anderson, J.D. Phillipson. 1996. *Herbal Medicines: A Guide for Health-Care Professionals*. London: The Pharmaceutical Press.

Parnham, M.J. 1996. Benefit-risk assessment of the squeezed sap of the purple coneflower (*Echinacea purpurea*) for long-term oral immunostimulation. *Phytomed* 3(1):95–102.

Pietta, P., P. Mauri, R. Bauer. 1998. MEKC analysis of different *Echinacea* species. *Planta Med* 64:649–652.

Richman, A. and J.P. Witkowski. 1996. A Wonderful Year for Herbs. *Whole Foods* Oct:52–60.

———. 1997. Herbs…By the Numbers. *Whole Foods* Oct:20–28.

———. 1998. Herb Sales Still Strong. *Whole Foods* Oct:19–26.

Schilcher, H. 1997. Personal communication to M. Blumenthal, Dec. 30.

Schöneberger, D. 1992. The influence of immune-stimulating effects of pressed juice from *Echinacea purpurea* on the course and severity of colds. *Forum Immunol* 8:2–12.

See, D.M., N. Broumand, L. Sahl, J.G. Tilles. 1997. *In vitro* effects of echinacea and ginseng on natural killer and antibody-dependent cell cytotoxicity in healthy subjects and chronic fatigue syndrome or acquired immunodeficiency syndrome patients. *Immunopharmacology* 35(3):229–235.

Shohan, J. 1985. Specific safety problems of inappropriate immune responses to immunostimulating agents. *TIPS* 6:178–182.

Wagner, H. 1997. Herbal immunostimulants for the prophylaxis and therapy of colds and influenza. *Eur J Herbal Med* 3(1).

WHO. See World Health Organization.

Wichtl, M. and N.G. Bisset (eds.). 1994. *Herbal Drugs and Phytopharmaceuticals*. Stuttgart: Medpharm Scientific Publishers.

World Health Organization (WHO). 1999. "Herba Echinaceae Purpureae Radix Echinacea" and "Radix Echinaceae." *WHO Monographs on Selected Medicinal Plants*, Vol. 1. Geneva: World Health Organization. 136–144; 125–135.

Additional Resources

Bauer, R. 1997. Echinacea—Pharmazeutische Qualität und therapeutischer Wert. *Z Phytother* 18:207–214.

———. 1993. Neue Ergebnisse zur frage der wirksubstanzen von *Echinacea*-drogen. *Natur und G Med* 6:32–40.

Bauer, R. and H. Wagner. 1988. Echinacea—Der Sonnenhut—Stand der Forschung. *Z Phytother* 9(5):151–159.

Bauer, R., I.A. Khan, H. Wagner. 1988. TLC and HPLC analysis of *Echinacea pallida* and *E. angustifolia* roots. *Planta Med* 54:426–430.

Bauer, R., P. Remiger, H. Wagner. 1988. Echinacea-vergleichende DC- und HPLC-analyse der Herba-Drogen von *Echinacea purpurea*, Echinacea pallida und Echinacea angustifolia. *DAZ* 128:174–180.

Bauer, R., K. Jurcic, J. Puhlmann, H. Wagner. 1988. Immunologische in-vivo und in-vitro untersuchungen mit *Echinacea* extrakten [Immunologic *in vivo* and *in vitro* studies on *Echinacea* extracts]. *Arzneimforsch* 38(2):276–281.

Bauer, R. et al. 1987. Two acetylenic compounds from Echinacea pallida roots. *Phytochem* 26:1198–1200.

Bodinet, C., I. Willigmann, N. Beuscher. 1996. Host-resistance increasing activity of root extracts from *Echinacea* species. Poster: Schaper and Brümmer, D-38251 Salzgitter, F.R.G.

Bone, K. 1999. Echinacea: Fact and Mythology. *HerbalGram* 49 (in press).

Bradley, P.R. (ed.). 1992. *British Herbal Compendium*, Vol. 1. Bournemouth: British Herbal Medicine Association. 81–83.

Brinkeborn, R.M., D.V. Shah, F.H. Degenring. 1999. Echinaforce® and other *Echinacea* fresh plant preparations in the treatment of the common cold. A randomized, placebo-controlled, double-blind clinical trial. *Phytomedicine* 6(1):1–6.

Bruneton, J. 1995. *Pharmacognosy, Phytochemistry, Medicinal Plants*. Paris: Lavoisier Publishing.

Burger, R.A., A.R. Torres, R.P. Warren, V.D. Caldwell, B.G. Hughes. 1997. Echinacea-induced cytokine production by human macrophages. *Int J Immunopharmacol* 19(7):371–379.

Der Marderosian, A. (ed.). 1999. *The Review of Natural Products*. St. Louis: Facts and Comparisons.

Dorn, M., E. Knick, G. Lewith. 1997. Placebo-controlled, double-blind study of Echinaceae pallidae radix in upper respiratory tract infections. *Complement Ther Med* 3:40–42.

Dorn, M. 1989. Mitigation of flu-like effects by means of a plant immunostimulant. *Natur und Ganzheitsmedizin* 2:314–319.

Dorsch, W. 1996. Klinische anwendung von extrakten aus *Echinacea purpurea* oder Echinacea pallida. Kritische wertung kontrollierter klinischer
studien. *Z Arztl Fortbild (Jena)* 90(2):117, 122.

Gallo, M., W.A. Koren, G. Koren. 1998. The safety
of *Echinacea* use during pregnancy: a prospective controlled cohort study. Proceedings of the
11th International Conference of the Organization of Teratology: San Diego, June 19–21. *Teratology* 57:283.

Hänsel, R., K. Keller, H. Rimpler, G. Schneider
(eds.). 1992–1994. *Hagers Handbuch der Pharmazeutischen Praxis,* 5th ed. Vol. 4–6. Berlin-
Heidelberg: Springer Verlag.

List, P.H. and L. Hörhammer (eds.). 1973–1979.
Hagers Handbuch der Pharmazeutischen Praxis,
Vols. 1–7. New York: Springer Verlag.

McGuffin, M., C. Hobbs, R. Upton, A. Goldberg.
1997. American Herbal Product Association's
Botanical Safety Handbook. Boca Raton: CRC
Press.

Schulthess, B.H., E. Giger, T.W. Baumann. 1991.
Echinacea: anatomy, phytochemical pattern, and
germination of the achene. *Planta Med*
57(4):384–388.

Shalaby, A.S. et al. 1997. Response of *Echinacea* to
some agricultural practices. *J Herbs Spices Med
Plants* 4(4):59–67.

Skwarek, T., Z. Tynecka, K. Glowniak, E.
Lutostanksa. 1996. Echinacea L. Inducer of
interferons. *Herba Polonica* 42(2):110–117.

Snow, J.M. 1997. *Echinacea* (Moench) spp. Asteraceae. *Protocol J Botan Med* 2(2):18–24.

Wichtl, M. (ed.). 1997. *Teedrogen,* 4th ed.
Stuttgart: Wissenschaftliche Verlagsgesellschaft.

Wood, H.C. et al. *The Dispensatory of the United
States of America,* Centennial (22nd) ed.
Philadelphia: J.B. Lippincott Co. 1:402.

The echinacea angustifolio herb and root/pallida herb, echinacea pallida root, and echinacea purpurea root
monographs, published by the Commission E in 1992, were modified based on new scientific research.
They contain more extensive pharmacological and therapeutic information taken directly from the Commission E.

This material was adapted from *The Complete German Commission E Monographs—Therapeutic Guide to
Herbal Medicines.* M. Blumenthal, W.R. Busse, A. Goldberg, J. Gruenwald, T. Hall, C.W. Riggins, R.S. Ris-
ter (eds.) S. Klein and R.S. Rister (trans.). 1998. Austin: American Botanical Council; Boston: Integrative
Medicine Communications.

1) The Overview section is new information.
2) Description, Chemistry and Pharmacology, Uses, Contraindications, Side Effects, Interactions with
   Other Drugs, and Dosage sections have been drawn from the original work. Additional information has
   been added in some or all of these sections, as noted with references.
3) The dosage for equivalent preparations (tea infusion, fluidextract, and tincture) have been provided
   based on the following example:
   Unless otherwise prescribed: 2 g per day of [powdered, crushed, cut or whole] [plant part]
   Infusion: 2 g in 150 ml of water
   Fluidextract 1:1 (g/ml): 2 ml
   Tincture 1:5 (g/ml): 10 ml
4) The References and Additional Resources sections are new sections. Additional Resources are not cited
   in the monograph but are included for research purposes.

ELDER FLOWER

Latin Name:
Sambucus nigra

Pharmacopeial Name:
Sambuci flos

Other Names:
black elder flower, European elder flower

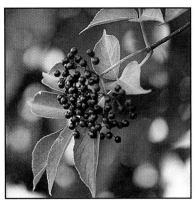
©1999 Steven Foster

Overview

Elder is a small tree native throughout Europe, western and central Asia, and North Africa, naturalized in the United States (Leung and Foster, 1996; Wichtl and Bisset, 1994). Elder is one of Germany's more important medicinal plant crops (Lange and Schippmann, 1997). The material of commerce, however, is mostly collected from the wild, mainly from the former U.S.S.R., former Yugoslavia, Bulgaria, Hungary, Romania, and the United Kingdom (BHP, 1996; Wichtl and Bisset, 1994). The Roman naturalist Pliny the Elder (ca. 23–79 b.c.) wrote of its uses, as did the Swiss alchemist and physician Paracelsus (1493–1541) (Grieve, 1979; Nadkarni, 1976). Its current therapeutic use as a diaphoretic in Germany and the United States stems from traditional Greek medicine. Its same indications for use in traditional Greek medicine have spread to India where it has been introduced into Ayurvedic medicine (Karnick, 1994; Nadkarni, 1976). It is used in Belgium and France as a diuretic (Bradley, 1992; Bruneton, 1995).

Well-designed human clinical studies have not been conducted on elder flower (Newall et al., 1996). The approved modern therapeutic applications for elder flower are supportable based on a combination of factors, including its long history of use in well established systems of traditional medicine, *in vitro* and *in vivo* studies in animals, and phytochemical investigations.

In Germany, elder flower is a standard medicinal tea used as a diaphoretic for feverish common colds. In both the United States and Germany it is also used as a component of compounds for cold and flu in dosage forms, including teas, alcoholic fluidextract or tincture, and native extract in solid dosage forms such as dragées (coated tablets) (Bradley, 1992; Leung and Foster, 1996; Wichtl and Bisset, 1994). In the United States and Canada it is often combined with yarrow flower and peppermint leaf in formulas intended to relieve fevers associated with colds.

Pharmacopeial grade dried elder flower must contain not less than 0.8% total flavonoids, calculated as isoquercitrin (DAB 1997; Ph.Eur.3, 1998). The *Pharmacopoeia of Switzerland* requires not less than 0.7% flavonoids (Ph.Helv.VII, 1987). The dried flower should also contain not less than 25% water-soluble extract (Bradley, 1992).

Description

Elder flower consists of the dried, sifted inflorescence of *Sambucus nigra* L. [Fam. Caprifoliaceae] as well as its preparations in effective dosage.

Chemistry and Pharmacology

Elder flower contains flavonoids (up to 3%) composed mainly of flavonol glycosides (astragalin, hyperoside, isoquercitrin, and rutin up to 1.9%) and free aglycones (quercetin and kaempferol); minerals (8–9%), mainly potassium; phenolic compounds (approx. 3% chlorogenic acid); triterpenes (approx. 1%) including α- and β-amyrin; triterpene acids (approximately 0.85% ursolic and oleanolic acids); sterols (approximately 0.11%); volatile oils (0.03–0.3%) composed of approx. 66% free fatty acids (linoleic, linolenic, and palmitic acids) and approx. 7% alkanes; mucilage; pectin; plastocynin (protein); sugar; tannins (Bradley, 1992; Leung and Foster, 1996; List and Hörhammer, 1973–1979; Newall et al., 1996; Wichtl and Bisset, 1994).

The Commission E reported diaphoretic and increased bronchial secretion activity.

The *British Herbal Compendium* reported diaphoretic and diuretic actions (Bradley, 1992). The mechanism of action is not fully understood. Its flavonoids and phenolic acids may contribute to the diaphoretic effect (Bradley, 1992). It has demonstrated anti-inflammatory, antiviral, and diuretic actions in *in vitro* studies. The flavonoids and triterpenes appear to be the main biologically active constituents (Newall et al., 1996).

Uses

The Commission E approved the internal use of elder flower for colds. The *British Herbal Compendium* lists its uses for common cold, feverish conditions, and as a diuretic (Bradley, 1992). The German Standard License for elder flower tea calls it a diaphoretic medicine for the treatment of feverish common colds or catarrhal complaints (Braun et al., 1997).

Contraindications

None known.

Side Effects

None known.

Use During Pregnancy and Lactation

No restrictions known.

Interactions with Other Drugs

None known.

Dosage and Administration

Internal: Unless otherwise prescribed: 10–15 g whole flower per day (3–5 g, three times daily).

Infusion: 3–4 g in 150 ml water, 1–2 cups sipped several times daily, as hot as may be taken safely.

Fluidextract 1:1 (g/ml): 1.5–3 ml (Erg.B.6).

Tincture 1:5 (g/ml): 2.5–7.5 ml (Erg.B.6).

Native soft extract 4.0–5.0:1 (w/w): 2–3.75 g (0.7–1.25 g three times daily).

References

Bradley, P.R. (ed.). 1992. *British Herbal Compendium*, Vol. 1. Bournemouth: British Herbal Medicine Association.

Braun, R. et al. 1997. *Standardzulassungen für Fertigarzneimittel—Text and Kommentar*. Stuttgart: Deutscher Apotheker Verlag.

British Herbal Pharmacopoeia (BHP). 1996. Exeter, U.K.: British Herbal Medicine Association.

Bruneton, J. 1995. *Pharmacognosy, Phytochemistry, Medicinal Plants*. Paris: Lavoisier Publishing.

Deutsches Arzneibuch (DAB 1997). 1997. Stuttgart: Deutscher Apotheker Verlag.

Ergänzungsbuch zum Deutschen Arzneibuch, 6th ed. (Erg.B.6). 1953. Stuttgart: Deutscher Apotheker Verlag.

Europäisches Arzneibuch, 3rd ed. 1st suppl. (Ph.Eur.3). 1998. Stuttgart: Deutscher Apotheker Verlag. 442–444.

Grieve, M. 1979. *A Modern Herbal*. New York: Dover Publications, Inc.

Lange D. and U. Schippmann. 1997. *Trade Survey of Medicinal Plants in Germany—A Contribution to International Plant Species Conservation*. Bonn: Bundesamt für Naturschutz. 32–33.

Leung, A.Y. and S. Foster. 1996. *Encyclopedia of Common Natural Ingredients Used in Food, Drugs, and Cosmetics*, 2nd ed. New York: John Wiley & Sons, Inc.

List, P.H. and L. Hörhammer (eds.). 1973–1979. *Hagers Handbuch der Pharmazeutischen Praxis*, Vols. 1–7. New York: Springer Verlag.

Nadkarni, K.M. 1976. *Indian Materia Medica*. Bombay: Popular Prakashan. 1097.

Newall, C.A., L.A. Anderson, J.D. Phillipson. 1996. *Herbal Medicines: A Guide for Health-Care Professionals*. London: The Pharmaceutical Press.

Pharmacopoeia Helvetica, 7th ed. Vol. 1–4. (Ph.Helv.VII). 1987. Bern: Office Central Fédéral des Imprimés et du Matériel.

Ph.Eur.3. See Europäisches Arzneibuch.

Wichtl, M. and N.G. Bisset (eds.). 1994. Herbal Drugs and Phytopharmaceuticals. Stuttgart: Medpharm Scientific Publishers.

Additional Resources

British Pharmaceutical Codex (BPC). 1949. London: The Pharmaceutical Press.

Davidek, J. 1961. Isolation of Chromatographically Pure Rutin from Flowers of Elder. Nature 189:487–488.

Deutscher Arzneimittel-Codex (DAC). 1986–1991. Stuttgart: Deutscher Apotheker Verlag.

Hajkova, I.I. and V. Brazdova. 1963. [The content of some principals in Sambucus nigra flowers and fruits in the course of vegetation] [In Czech]. Farm Obzor 32:343–347.

Hänsel, R. and M. Kussmaul. 1975. Zwei Triterpene aus den Holunderblüten [Two triterpenes from the flowers of the elder]. Arch Pharm (Weinheim) 308(10):790–792.

Karnick, C.R. 1994. Pharmacopoeial Standards of Herbal Plants, Vol. 2. Delhi: Sri Satguru Publications. 49.

Kolodynska, M. and W. Pasieczna. 1967. Oznaczanie rutyny i kwercetyny w wybranych preparatach galenowych z kwiatow bzu czarnego (Sambucus nigra) [The determination of rutin and quercetin in selected galenic preparations of Sambucus nigra flowers] [In Polish]. Ann Univ Mariae Curie Sklodowska [Med] 22:127–130.

Lamaison J.L., C. Petitjean-Freytet, A. Carnat. 1991. Presence de 3-glucoside et de 3-rutinoside d'isorhamnetine dans les fleurs de Sambucus nigra L. [Presence of isorhamnetin 3-glucoside and 3-rutinoside in Sambucus nigra L. flowers]. Ann Pharm Fr 49(5):258–262.

Liefertova, I., J. Kudrnacova, V. Brazdova. 1971. [Substances contained in flowers and fruit of Sambucus during the growth period] [In Russian]. Acta Fac Pharm Univ Comeniana 20:57–82.

Lukash, L.L. et al. 1997. Vliianie lektina sotsvetii Sambucus nigra na spontannyi i indutisrovannyi alkiliruiushchim agentom mutagenez v somaticheskikh kletkakh mlekopitaiushchikh [The effect of the lectin from Sambucus nigra inflorescences on spontaneous and alkylating agent-induced mutagenesis in mammalian somatic cells]. Tsitol Genet 31(5):52–60.

McGuffin, M., C. Hobbs, R. Upton, A. Goldberg. 1997. American Herbal Product Association's Botanical Safety Handbook. Boca Raton: CRC Press.

Pharmacopée Française Xe Édition (Ph.Fr.X.). 1983–1990. Moulins-les-Metz: Maisonneuve S.A.

Pietta, P., A. Bruno, P. Mauri, A. Rava. 1992. Separation of flavonol-2-O-glycosides from Calendula officinalis and Sambucus nigra by high-performance liquid and micellar electrokinetic capillary chromatography. J Chromatogr 593(1–2):165–170.

Radu, A., M. Tamas, A. Otlacan. 1976. [Comparative study of flavones in indigenous Elder flowers (Sambucus nigra L., S. ebulus L., S. racemosa L.)] [In Romanian]. Farmacia (Bucharest) 24:9–15.

Reynolds, J.E.F. (ed.). 1993. Martindale: The Extra Pharmacopoeia, 30th ed. London: The Pharmaceutical Press.

Richter, W. and G. Willuhn. 1977. Zur Kenntnis der Inhaltsstoffe von Sambucus nigra L.III. Bestimmung des Ursol- und Oleanolsäure-, des Amyrin- und Steringehaltes der Flores Sambuci DAB 7. Pharm Ztg 122:1567–1570.

Schmersahl, K.J. 1964. Über die Wirkstoffe der diaphoretischen Drogen des DAB 6. Naturwissenschaften 51:361.

Serkedjieva, J. et al. 1990. Antiviral activity of the infusion (SHS-174) from flowers of Sambucus nigra L., aerial parts of Hypericum perforatum L., and roots of Saponaria officinalis L. against influenza and herpes simplex viruses. Phytotherapy Res 4:97.

Steinegger, E. and R. Hänsel. 1988. Lehrbuch der Pharmakognosie und Phytopharmazie. Berlin-Heidelberg; New York: Springer Verlag.

Taylor, M. 1998. Elderflower. Canadian Journal of Herbalism 6–7.

Toulemonde, B. and H.M.J. Richard. 1983. Volatile constituents of dry elder (Sambucus nigra L.) flowers. J Agric Food Chem 31:365–370.

This material was adapted from The Complete German Commission E Monographs—Therapeutic Guide to Herbal Medicines. M. Blumenthal, W.R. Busse, A. Goldberg, J. Gruenwald, T. Hall, C.W. Riggins, R.S. Rister (eds.) S. Klein and R.S. Rister (trans.). 1998. Austin: American Botanical Council; Boston: Integrative Medicine Communications.

1) The Overview section is new information.

2) Description, Chemistry and Pharmacology, Uses, Contraindications, Side Effects, Interactions with Other Drugs, and Dosage sections have been drawn from the original work. Additional information has been added in some or all of these sections, as noted with references.

3) The dosage for equivalent preparations (tea infusion, fluidextract, and tincture) have been provided based on the following example:
   Unless otherwise prescribed: 2 g per day of [powdered, crushed, cut or whole] [plant part]
   Infusion: 2 g in 150 ml of water
   Fluidextract 1:1 (g/ml): 2 ml
   Tincture 1:5 (g/ml): 10 ml

4) The References and Additional Resources sections are new sections. Additional Resources are not cited in the monograph but are included for research purposes.

ELEUTHERO ROOT

Latin Name:
Eleutherococcus senticosus
(syn. *Acanthopanax senticosus*)

Pharmacopeial Name:
Eleutherococci radix

Other Names:
Siberian ginseng, Ussurian thorny
pepperbush, Taiga root

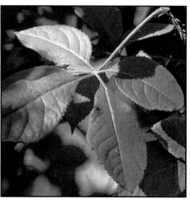

© 1999 Steven Foster

Overview

Eleuthero is sold in the United States as "Siberian Ginseng" (*E. senticosus* (Rupr. et Maxim.) Maxim., family Araliaceae). It is known in China as *ci wu jia*. The plant is a spiny-stemmed shrub found in northeast Asia and Japan, and is presently prescribed for medicinal use in France, Germany, Russia, and China. The part used consists of the dried roots and root bark. Eleuthero has been used in China as a folk remedy for bronchitis, heart ailments, and rheumatism, and as a tonic to restore vigor, improve general health, restore memory, promote healthy appetite, and increase stamina (Foster, 1996). The term "adaptogen" was coined by a Soviet researcher to describe eleuthero's ability to increase "non-specific" resistance in an organism and to help modulate stress and improve performance under stressful conditions. Much of the scientific literature published in China still employs the former Latin binomial *Acanthopanax senticosus*.

There is a relatively small number of controlled clinical trials performed with eleuthero. A single-blind, placebo-controlled, crossover trial lasting eight days investigated the effect of eleuthero extract (2 ml, twice daily) on working capacity and fatigue of six male athletes, ages 21–22. Oxygen uptake, heart rate, total work, and exhaustion time were measured. Significant results were observed in all parameters, particularly the 23.3% increase in total work noted in the eleuthero test group compared with 7.5% of the placebo group (Asano et al., 1986).

An eight-week double-blind, placebo-controlled study evaluated the efficacy of eleuthero extract (3.4 ml daily) on submaximal and maximal exercise performance of 20 highly trained distance runners. No significant difference was observed between test and control groups in heart rate, oxygen consumption, expired minute volume, respiratory exchange ratio, perceived exertion, and serum lactate levels (Dowling et al., 1996).

A randomized, placebo-controlled, double-blind, crossover study compared cognitive function measurements in 24 subjects who took eleuthero (625 mg twice daily), *Ginkgo biloba* (28.2 mg flavonolglycosides daily), or placebo. At the end of each three-month dose period, concentration, selective memory, cognitive function, and well-being were measured. Significant improvements in selective memory of the eleuthero group versus the placebo group (p<0.02) were demonstrated. For those taking ginkgo, results were significant only in those subjects over age 48 (p<0.05). No change in concentration was discovered in any group. Significant effects from eleuthero were also noted in feelings of well-being and levels of activity (Winther et al., 1997).

Several studies were conducted to evaluate the effects of eleuthero on eye conditions and color distinction. One study evaluated the pre- and post-operative effects of eleuthero extract (1.5 ml twice daily) on 282 male or female patients suffering from primary glaucoma (102 cases) and eye burns (58 cases). Beneficial effects were noted in both treatments. Eleuthero was also found beneficial in 122 cases of myopia treatment (Zaikova et al., 1968).

In 50 patients with normal trichromatic vision a single dose of eleuthero extract (2 ml) stimulated color distinction (red and green) within 30 to 60 minutes after ingestion. Maximum effect was reached in six to seven hours and persisted for a minimum of 29 hours (Sosnova, 1969).

Description

Eleuthero consists of the dried roots and rhizome of *Eleutherococus senticosus* Rupr. et Maxim. [syn. *A. senticosus* (Rupr. et Maxim. ex Maxim. Harms)] [Fam. Araliaceae] and their preparations in effective dosage. The root contains lignans and coumarin derivatives.

Chemistry and Pharmacology

Eleuthero contains phenolics, polysaccharides, and eleutherosides A-G, the total content ranging between 0.6–0.9% (Bradley, 1992). Eleutherosides B, B1, and E are representative of three classes of compounds collectively called eleutherosides. Other constituents include phenylpropanoids, lignans, coumarins, polysaccharides, and sugars (Bradley, 1992). A review of the chemistry of eleuthero with 29 chemical structures has been published (Tang and Eisenbrand, 1992).

The Commission E reported that in the immobilization test and the coldness test, the endurance of rodents was enhanced. In addition, the lymphocyte count in healthy volunteers, especially T-lymphocytes, increased following intake of fluidextracts.

Eleuthero has demonstrated adaptogenic and endurance-enhancing effects (Wagner et al., 1985; Leung and Foster, 1996), immunomodulatory effects (Bradley, 1992; Bohn et al., 1987), immunostimulatory effects (Fang et al., 1985), hypoglycemic activity (Hikino et al., 1986), platelet aggregation-inhibiting effects (Yun-Choi et al., 1987), and antiproliferative effects on leukemia cells *in vitro* (Bradley, 1992; Hacker and Medon, 1984). However, one *in vivo* experiment that evaluated the effect of eleuthero on stamina and longevity found no significant difference between mice given eleuthero and control mice (Lewis et al., 1983). In animal and *in vitro* studies, eleuthero has demonstrated effects of radiation protection (Yonezawa et al., 1989) and stress reduction (Takasugi et al., 1985).

Uses

Commission E approved eleuthero as a tonic in times of fatigue and debility, declining capacity for work or concentration, and during convalescence. Other uses for eleuthero are for chronic inflammatory conditions and traditionally for functional asthenia (Bruneton, 1995).

Contraindications

The Commission E notes a contraindication for hypertension. Eleuthero is generally considered by most herbalists in the United States to be milder in activity than the more stimulating root of Asian ginseng (*Panax ginseng*). There at least two studies in which it is recommended that eleuthero not be given to persons with a blood pressure in excess of 180/90 mm Hg (Farnsworth, 1985). Presumably, this information prompted the Commission to note this possible adverse effect in some people. However, the glycosides contained in eleuthero have been shown to lower blood pressure (McGuffin et al., 1997).

Side Effects

None known.

Use During Pregnancy and Lactation

No restrictions known.

Interactions with Other Drugs

None known.

Dosage and Administration

Unless otherwise prescribed: 2–3 g per day of powdered or cut root for teas for up to three months, as well as aqueous alcoholic extracts for internal use. A repeated course is feasible.
Infusion: 2–3 g in 150 ml of water.
Fluidextract 1:1 (g/ml): 2–3 ml.
Tincture 1:5 (g/ml): 10–15 ml.

References

Asano, K. et al. 1986. Effect of *Eleutherococcus senticosus* extract on human physical working capacity. *Planta Med* 3:175–177.

Bohn, B., C. Nebe, C. Birr. 1987. Flow-cytometric studies with *E. senticoccus* extract as an immunomodulatory agent. *Arzneimforsch* 37(10):1193–1196.

Bradley, P.R. (ed.). 1992. *British Herbal Compendium*, Vol. 1. Bournemouth: British Herbal Medicine Association.

Bruneton, J. 1995. *Pharmacognosy, Phytochemistry, Medicinal Plants*. Paris: Lavoisier Publishing.

Dowling, E.A., et al. 1996. Effect of *Eleutherococcus senticosus* on submaximal and maximal exercise performance. *Med Sci Sports Exerc* 28(4):482–499.

Fang, J. et al. 1985. Immunologically active polysaccharides of *E. senticosus*. *Phytochem* 24:2619–2622.

Farnsworth, N.R. 1985. *Siberian Ginseng (Eleutherococcus senticosus)*: Current Status as an Adaptogen. In Wagner, H., H. Hikino, N.R. Farnsworth (eds.). *Economic and Medicinal Plant Research*, Vol. I. London: Academic Press.

Foster, S. 1996. Siberian Ginseng—*Eleutherococcus senticosus*. Botanical Booklet Series, No. 302. Austin: American Botanical Council.

Hacker, B. and P. Medon. 1984. Cytotoxic effects of *E. senticosus* aqueous extract against L1210 leukemia cells. *J Pharm Sci* 73(2):270–272.

Hikino, H. et al. 1986. Isolation and hypoglycemic activity of Eleutherans A–G: glycans of *E. sentococcus* roots. *J Nat Prod* 49(2):293–297.

Leung, A.Y. and S. Foster. 1996. *Encyclopedia of Common Natural Ingredients Used in Food, Drugs, and Cosmetics*, 2nd ed. New York: John Wiley & Sons, Inc.

Lewis, W.H., V.E. Zenger, R.G. Lynch. 1983. No adaptogen response of mice to ginseng and *Eleutherococcus* infusions. *J Ethnopharmacol* 8(2):209–214.

McGuffin, M., C. Hobbs, R. Upton, A. Goldberg. 1997. American Herbal Product Association's *Botanical Safety Handbook*. Boca Raton: CRC Press.

Sosnova, T. 1969. [The effect of *E. spinosus* upon the color-distinction function of the optic analyzer in persons with normal trichromatic vision] [In Russian]. *Vestn Oftalmol* 82(5):59–61.

Takasugi, N. et al. 1985. Effect of *Eleutherococcus senticosus* and its components on rectal temperature, body and grip tones, motor coordination, and exploratory and spontaneous movements in acute stressed mice. *Shoyakugaku Zasshi* 39(3):232–237.

Tang, W. and G. Eisenbrand. 1992. *Chinese Drugs of Plant Origin: Chemistry, Pharmacology, and Use in Traditional and Modern Medicine*. New York: Springer Verlag.

Wagner, H., H. Hikino, N.R. Farnsworth. 1985. *Economic and Medicinal Plant Research*. London; Orlando, FL: Academic Press. 155–215.

Winther, K. et al. 1997. Russian root (Siberian ginseng) improves cognitive functions in middle aged people, whereas *Gingko biloba* seems effective only in the elderly. (XVI World Congress of Neurology, Buenos Aires) *J Neurologic Sciences* 150:S90.

This material was adapted from *The Complete German Commission E Monographs—Therapeutic Guide to Herbal Medicines*. M. Blumenthal, W.R. Busse, A. Goldberg, J. Gruenwald, T. Hall, C.W. Riggins, R.S. Rister (eds.) S. Klein and R.S. Rister (trans.). 1998. Austin: American Botanical Council; Boston: Integrative Medicine Communications.

1) The Overview section is new information.

2) Description, Chemistry and Pharmacology, Uses, Contraindications, Side Effects, Interactions with Other Drugs, and Dosage sections have been drawn from the original work. Additional information has been added in some or all of these sections, as noted with references.

3) The dosage for equivalent preparations (tea infusion, fluidextract, and tincture) have been provided based on the following example:
   Unless otherwise prescribed: 2 g per day of [powdered, crushed, cut or whole] [plant part]
   Infusion: 2 g in 150 ml of water
   Fluidextract 1:1 (g/ml): 2 ml
   Tincture 1:5 (g/ml): 10 ml

4) The References and Additional Resources sections are new sections. Additional Resources are not cited in the monograph but are included for research purposes.

Yonezawa, M. et al. 1989. Radiation protection by Shigoka extract on split dose irradiation in mice. *J Radiation Res* 30(3):247–254.

Yun-Choi, H., J. Kim, J. Lee. 1987. Potential inhibitors of platelet aggregation from plant sources, III. *J Nat Prod* 50(6):1059–1064.

Zaikova, M., A. Verba, M. Snegireva. 1968. [*Eleutherococcus* in ophthalmology] [In Russian]. *Vestn Oftalmol* 81(3):70–74.

Additional Resources

Kaloeva, Z.D. 1986. [Effect of the glycosides of *Eleutherococcus senticosus* on the hemodynamic indices of children with hypotensive states] [In Russian]. *Farmakol Toksikol* 49(5):73.

Medon, P.J., P. Ferguson, C. Watson. 1984. Effects of *Eleutherococcus senticosus* extracts on hexobarbital metabolism *in vivo* and *in vitro*. *J Ethnopharmacol* 10(2):235–241.

EPHEDRA

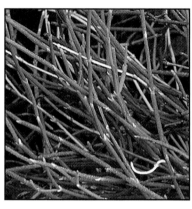

© 1999 Steven Foster

Latin Name:
Ephedra sinica

Pharmacopeial Name:
Ephedrae herba

Other Names:
Chinese ephedra, mahuang, cao mahuang

Overview

Ephedra is a dioecious, perennial, evergreen subshrub native to central Asia, widely distributed throughout China, Tibet, India, Pakistan, Japan, and Southern Siberia, also cultivated extensively (Bruneton, 1995; Budavari, 1996; Grieve, 1979; Leung and Foster, 1996).

In Oriental medicines, ephedra is the chief drug for treatment of asthma and bronchitis. It has been used for thousands of years in traditional Chinese medicine (TCM) as a primary component of multi-herb formulas prescribed to treat bronchial asthma, cold and flu, cough and wheezing, fever, chills, lack of perspiration, headache, and nasal congestion. It is listed in the oldest comprehensive materia medica, *Shen Nong Ben Cao Jing*, among the "middle class" herbs, used to induce perspiration and as an anti-allergy agent (Blumenthal and King, 1995; Bruneton, 1995; Der Marderosian, 1999; Huang, 1999; Leung and Foster, 1996; Weiss, 1988). Today, ephedra is official in the national pharmacopeias of China, Germany, and Japan. In India, ephedra herb is listed in the Ayurvedic pharmacopoeia. Only its isolated derivatives ephedrine and ephedrine hydrochloride are official in the *Indian Pharmacopoeia* (DAB 1998; IP, 1996; JP XII, 1993; Karnick, 1994; Tu, 1992). The Chinese pharmacopeia indicates its use for common cold with wind-cold syndrome (marked by chilliness and mild fever, headache, stuffy and runny nose, general aching, but no sweating), and for bronchial asthma (Tu, 1992). The Ayurvedic pharmacopeia lists ephedra for asthma, spasms, hayfever, and allergic symptoms (Karnick, 1994). In China, ephedra is a major component of a cold medication used to relieve headache, body ache, coughing, and to lower fever by increasing perspiration. The formula is an aqueous decoction containing ephedra herb, cinnamon twig, licorice root, and almond (Huang, 1999).

In Germany, ephedra is official in the *German Pharmacopoeia* and is an approved herb in the Commission E monographs. It is used as a primary component of licensed prepared respiratory medicines (BAnz, 1998; DAB 1998). In the United States, the herb ephedra is regulated as a dietary supplement under the Dietary Supplement Health and Education Act of 1994 (DSHEA) in aqueous infusion, alcoholic tincture, and dry extract in capsules or tablets. Ephedra is used in TCM herbal teas and prepared professional products prescribed to patients by licensed acupuncturists and naturopathic physicians. The alkaloids (and their salts) from ephedra—i.e., ephedrine and pseudoephedrine—are approved by the Food and Drug Administration (FDA) as over-the-counter (OTC) drug ingredients for common cold, flu, and allergies.

Modern human studies in China have investigated its clinical uses for treatment of bronchial asthma, chronic bronchitis, pneumonia of children, and whooping cough (Chang and But, 1986; Liu, 1989). Human studies in the West have focused on its pharmacokinetics (Gurley et al., 1998; Pickup et al., 1976), cardiovascular effects in healthy adults (White et al., 1997), and potential in weight loss (Nasser et al., 1999).

One clinical study reported that therapeutic effects were achieved in patients suffering from chronic asthmatic bronchitis who were treated with TCM formula "San Ao Decoction" [ephedra stem (*Ephedra sinica* Stapf.), bitter apricot seed (*Prunus armeniaca* L. var. ansu Maxim.), licorice root (*Glycyrrhiza uralensis* Fisch.), perilla fruit (*Perilla frutescens* (L.) Britt.), and ground dragon body (*Pheretima aspergillum* (Perier) or *Allolobophora caliginosa* (Savigny) *trapezoides* (Ant. Duges)] modified to suit individual manifestations (Chang and But, 1986). Another clinical study reported that satisfactory results were obtained in 288 cases of whooping cough in children, mostly between 3 and 5 years old, treated with the TCM formula "Ephedra-Prunus-Gypsum-Glycyrrhiza Decoction" [ephedra stem (*Ephedra sinica* Stapf.), bitter apricot seed (*Prunus armeniaca* L. var. ansu Maxim.), gypsum plaster stone (hydrated calcium sulfate), Chinese licorice root (*Glycyrrhiza uralensis* Fisch.), stemona root tuber (*Stemona sessilifolia* (Miq.) Miq., pepperweed seed (*Descurainia sophia* (L.) Webb ex Prantl.), Chinese date fruit (*Ziziphus jujuba* Mill.), and maltose (malt sugar)]. The authors reported it to be effective in catarrhal and spastic stages (Chang and But, 1986).

The approved modern therapeutic applications for ephedra are supportable based on its history of clinical use in well established systems of traditional and conventional medicines, extensive phytochemical investigations, pharmacological studies in animals, and human clinical studies.

Ephedra became controversial in the 1980–1990s due to its popularity as a major ingredient in herbal dietary supplements in the United States. Regulators and health officials were becoming increasingly concerned about its use for various purposes that were not approved for OTC drug use by the FDA, e.g., in products intended as diet aids for weight loss, for stimulation of the central nervous system, for enhancement of athletic performance, and briefly, as substitutes for illegal street drugs (Blumenthal and King, 1995; Blumenthal, 1996b). The FDA and state regulatory officials repeatedly voiced concerns about adverse reaction reports—in some cases, fatalities—that were claimed, but not always confirmed, to be associated with the ingestion of herbal supplement products containing ephedra, as well as products containing the ephedrine alkaloids (e.g., pure ephedrine). Consequently, federal and state regulatory agencies attempted to limit the uses of ephedra in supplements, the level of alkaloids per dose and per day, and, in some states, access to ephedrine-containing products (Anon., 1996; Blumenthal et al., 1995; Blumenthal 1996a, 1997a, 1997b, 1997c; Blumenthal and Dickinson, 1996).

Concerned about the potential risks associated with ephedra, herb industry groups established standards for ephedra products, including daily intake limits of 25 mg total alkaloids per dose and 100 mg total daily consumption. In 1994 the American Herbal Products Association issued a label warning statement for all ephedra products stating, "Seek advice from a healthcare practitioner prior to use if you are pregnant or nursing, or if you have high blood pressure, heart or thyroid disease, diabetes, difficulty in urination due to prostate enlargement, or if taking a MAO inhibitor or any other prescription drug. Reduce or discontinue use if nervousness, tremor, sleeplessness, loss of appetite, or nausea occur. Not intended for use by persons under 18 years of age. Keep out of the reach of children" (McGuffin, 1997). The industry warning and dose limits have been adopted by several states and have become the standard for labeling for ephedra products.

In June 1997 the FDA issued proposed regulations on ephedra-containing dietary supplements that would limit the level of total ephedra alkaloids in herbal preparations to no more than 8 mg per dose, with no more than 24 mg total ingestion per day. The proposed rule would ban the combination with other stimulants like caffeine or caffeine-containing herbs (e.g., cola (*Cola nitida*), guarana (*Paullinia cupana*), maté (*Ilex paraguariensis*), and others) in ephedra-containing herbal products; would prohibit the sale of ephedra products for use in weight loss or for athletic performance; would restrict use of ephedra herbal products to no more than seven days duration; and would require strict warnings on all ephedra product labels. The proposal would ban so-called "street drug knockoffs" containing ephedra or ephedrine alkaloids (FDA, 1997; Blumenthal, 1997c).

In August 1999 the U.S. General Accounting Office (GAO), the government agency that monitors accountability of all federal agencies, issued a 68-page report, *Dietary Supplements: Uncertainties in Analyses Underlying FDA's Proposed Rule on Ephedrine Alkaloids* (GAO, 1999). The report reveals deficiencies in the FDA's proposed rules on ephedra. GAO acknowledged that the FDA was justified in its concern about the safety of ephedra herbal products, based on the adverse event reports (AERs) it had received. However, GAO questioned the reliability of many of these AERs and also criticized the apparent lack of science employed in formulating the proposed dosage limits of alkaloids. The GAO also commented on the FDA's failure to comply with standard methods for cost-benefit analysis, including the failure to address whether there was any need for an FDA regulation in light of state requirements, and the failure to establish a benefit to the proposed actions.

Recent research suggests that ephedra as a single herb can be used safely in persons with normal blood pressure levels. A small clinical study of 12 healthy men and women between the ages of 23 and 40 employed four capsules twice daily, each containing 375 mg of powdered ephedra herb (Solaray brand, Ogden, Utah) (White et al., 1997). After blood pressure baselines were recorded, during the treatment phase four capsules were taken with breakfast and again nine hours later, with dinner. No additional herbal ingredients were present in the capsules, nor did they contain added ephedra extracts. Alkaloid levels of the capsules were measured by high-performance liquid chromatography (HPLC); the average level for each four-capsule dose was 19.4 mg ephedrine, 4.9 mg pseudoephedrine, and 1.2 mg methylephedrine. (By comparison, an over-the-counter cold capsule or tablet contains 25 mg ephedrine in the hydrochloride or sulfate forms.) Blood pressure was monitored every 15 minutes during the treatment phase. None of the 12 subjects experienced adverse effects during the study. Six experienced statistically significant increases in mean 12-hour heart rate after taking the herb, three had minor increases, and three showed no change. During the first three hours of treatment, four had significant increases in systolic pressure and two had significant decreases in diastolic pressure. The authors did not consider these effects clinically significant. They concluded that "pharmacodynamic aspects of ingestion of ma-huang in a normotensive, young population were fairly benign." They cautioned about the use of ephedra with other stimulants or in high doses. The weakness of this trial is the obvious small sample and lack of data on how the weight of each subject may have affected the results (Leigh, 1998).

The primary use for ephedra in dietary supplements—other than for athletic performance—is for weight loss and thermogenesis (burning of fatty tissue). Much of the industry-generated promotion for this purpose is based on research on a formula containing the alkaloid ephedrine, combined with caffeine and aspirin (Astrup et al., 1997; Astrup et al., 1992; Daley et al., 1993; Pardoe et al., 1993; Toubro et al., 1993). However, one unpublished study conducted at the Obesity Research Center, St. Luke's-Roosevelt Hospital Center, and Columbia University in New York tested a combination of ephedra herb with guarana, a natural source of caffeine (Nasser et al., 1999). The herbal combination (Metabolife 356®) was used in a double-blind, placebo-controlled eight-week trial on healthy subjects ages 25 to 55 years. The total daily intake of ephedrine alkaloids was 72 mg; caffeine, 240 mg (equivalent to 2 to 3 average cups of coffee). Of the 48 subjects completing the study (67 had initially been randomized), 24 taking the herbal product had greater weight reduction (−8.7±7.5 lbs.) versus the placebo group (1.8±5.4 lbs.), lower percentage of body fat, and lower serum triglyceride levels. The authors concluded that the herbal formula promotes weight loss but may also produce undesirable side effects in some subjects (dry mouth, heart palpitations, changes in blood pressure, and insomnia). The researchers suggest further study to determine long-term safety of the product.

Chinese pharmacopeial grade ephedra must be composed of the dried herbaceous stem collected in autumn, containing not less than 0.8% total alkaloids, calculated as ephedrine. Botanical identity must be confirmed by thin-layer chromatography (TLC) as well as by macroscopic and microscopic examinations (Tu, 1992). The *Japanese Pharmacopoeia* requires a minimum of only 0.6% total alkaloids but has additional purity requirements, including not more than 5% woody stems and the absence of stems of *Equisetaceae or Gramineae* plants (JP XII, 1993). The *German Pharmacopoeia* requires not less than 1% total alkaloids as well as identity, purity, and quality requirements comparable to those of the Chinese and Japanese monographs (DAB, 1997; DAB, 1998).

Description

Ephedra consists of the dried, young branchlets, harvested in the fall, of *Ephedra sinica* Stapf, *E. shennungiana* Tang [Fam. Ephedraceae], or other equivalent *Ephedra* species, and their equivalent preparations in effective dosage. The herb contains alkaloids; main alkaloids are ephedrine and pseudoephedrine. Ed. Note: The species listed by the Commission E are quite rare in U.S. commerce. Many species of ephedra are used in commerce, including *E. equisetina* Bge (Leung, 1999).

Chemistry and Pharmacology

Ephedra herb contains alkaloids (approx. 1.3%) mostly composed of l-ephedrine (50–90%), d-pseudoephedrine, l-norephedrine, d-norpseudoephedrine, l-N-methylephedrine and d-N-methylpseudoephedrine; flavonoid glycosides; glycans (ephedrans); citric, malic, and oxalic acids; proanthocyanidins (condensed tannins); and tannins and volatile oils (l-α-te-rpineol, limonene, and linalool) (Bruneton, 1995; Budavari, 1996; Leung and Foster, 1996).

The Commission E reported antitussive actions in animal experiments. Ephedrine acts by indirectly stimulating the sympathomimetic and central nervous systems. Bacteriostatic activity is also reported.

A diaphoretic action in humans has been reported for the aqueous decoction and volatile oil forms, and antiallergic effects *in vitro* have been demonstrated for the decoction and alcoholic extract forms of ephedra herb (Leung and Foster, 1996).

The pure alkaloid ephedrine acts as an indirect sympathomimetic. It is structurally similar to adrenaline. It stimulates cardiac automaticity with a positive inotropic action. It accelerates and increases the intensity of respiration and functions as a bronchodilator (Bruneton, 1995; Robbers and Tyler, 1999). *The Merck Index* lists the therapeutic category of l-ephedrine as bronchodilator and d-pseudoephedrine as decongestant (Budavari, 1996).

Uses

The Commission E approved the internal use of ephedra herb for diseases of the respiratory tract with mild bronchospasms in adults and children over the age of 6.

The World Health Organization has found the following uses of ephedra preparations to be supported by clinical data: treatment of nasal congestion due to hay fever, allergic rhinitis, acute coryza (rhinitis), common cold, sinusitis, and as a bronchodilator in treatment of bronchial asthma (WHO, 1999).

In Oriental medicine, ephedra herb, known as *mahuang*, is the primary drug used in treatment of asthma and bronchitis (Bruneton, 1995). *Mahuang* has been used for more than two thousand years to treat bronchial asthma, cold and flu, fever, chills, lack of perspiration, headache, nasal congestion, aching joints and bones, and cough and wheezing (Leung and Foster, 1996; Morton, 1977).

Contraindications
Anxiety and restlessness, high blood pressure, glaucoma, impaired circulation of the cerebrum, adenoma of prostate with residual urine accumulation, pheochromocytoma, thyrotoxicosis.

Side Effects
Insomnia, motor restlessness, irritability, headaches, nausea, vomiting, disturbances of urination, tachycardia. In higher dosage: Drastic increase in blood pressure, cardiac arrhythmia, development of dependency.

Use During Pregnancy and Lactation
Not recommended (McGuffin et al., 1997).

Interactions with Other Drugs
In combination with:
Cardiac glycosides or halothane: Disturbance of heart rhythm.
Guanethidine: Enhancement of the sympathomimetic effect.
MAO-inhibitors: Greatly raising the sympathomimetic action of ephedrine.
Secale alkaloid derivatives or oxytocin: Development of hypertension.

Dosage and Administration
Unless otherwise prescribed:
Adults: 1.2–2.3 g of cut herb containing approximately 1.3% (13 mg/g) total alkaloids.
Children: 0.04 g (40 mg) of cut herb per kg of body weight (Single dose for a 30 kg child, 1.2 g of cut herb).
Single dosage:
Adults: Herb preparations corresponding to 15–30 mg total alkaloid (=1.2–2.3 g of cut herb), calculated as ephedrine.
Children: Herb preparations corresponding to 0.5 mg total alkaloid (=0.04 g of cut herb) per kg of body weight.
Infusion or decoction: 1.2–2.3 g in 150 ml water.
Fluidextract 1:1 (g/ml): 1.2–2.3 ml.
Tincture 1:5 (g/ml): 5.75–11.5 ml.
Native extract 3.5–4.5:1 (w/w): 0.25–0.65 g.
Maximum daily dosage:
Adults: Herb preparations corresponding to 300 mg total alkaloid (=23 g of cut herb), calculated as ephedrine.
Children: 2 mg total alkaloid (=0.15 g of cut herb) per kg of body weight.
Duration of administration:
Commission E recommended that ephedra preparations should only be used short-term because of tachyphylaxis and danger of addiction.
Note: When the monograph was published in January, 1991, the Commission E stated that ephedrine-containing preparations are listed as addictive by the International Olympic Committee and the German Sports Association. However, a more recent analysis of the available U.S. health and safety data compiled by Edgar H. Adams, M.S., Sc.D., former Director of the Division of Epidemiology and Statistical Analysis at the U.S. National Institute on Drug Abuse, indicates that there is no evidence of significant abuse of, or addiction to, ephedra, despite decades of widespread use, establishing that any potential for addiction is low and does not rise to the level of regulatory concern to the extent that it warrants scheduling (as is done with addictive narcotic drugs) (Adams, 1999).

References
Adams, E.H. 1999. Statement to U.S. FDA. FDA Docket No. 98N-0148, cmt. 28, tab A. Feb 10.
Astrup, A., S. Toubro, S. Cannon, P. Hein, J. Madsen. 1997. Thermogenic synergism between ephedrine and caffeine in healthy volunteers: A double-blind, placebo-controlled study. *Metabolism* 40(3):323–329.

Astrup, A., L. Breum, S. Toubro, P. Hein, F. Quaade. 1992. The effect and safety of an ephedrine/caffeine compound compared to ephedrine, caffeine, and placebo in obese subjects on an energy restricted diet. A double blind trial. *Intl J Obesity Relat Metab Disord* 16(4):269–277.

Anon. 1996. Nebraska Law Criminalizes Ma Huang. *HerbalGram* 38:30.

BAnz. See *Bundesanzeiger*.

Blumenthal, M. 1996a. FDA Holds Expert Advisory Committee Hearing on Ma Huang. *HerbalGram* 36:21–23, 73.

———. 1996b. The Agony of the Ecstasy: Herbal High Products Get Media Attention. *HerbalGram* 37: 20–24, 32, 49.

———. 1997a. Ma Huang Update: Ohio Amends Ephedrine Ban: Herb Products Allowed with Limited Alkaloid Levels. *HerbalGram* 39:25.

———. 1997b. Texas Pulls Back Proposed Regulations Banning Ephedra. *HerbalGram* 39:25.

———. 1997c. FDA Proposes Warnings and Dose Limits on Ephedra: Government Proposal Comes Three Years After Industry Warning. *HerbalGram* 40:26–27.

Blumenthal, M. and A. Dickinson. 1996. FDA Hearing Portends Uncertain Future for Ma Huang: Members of FDA Panel Divided on Fate of Controversial Herb. *HerbalGram* 38:28–31.

Blumenthal, M. and P. King. 1995. Ma Huang: Ancient Herb, Modern Medicine, Regulatory Dilemma. A Review of the Botany, Chemistry, Medicinal Uses, Safety Concerns, and Legal Status of Ephedra and its Alkaloids. *HerbalGram* 34:22–26, 43, 56–57.

Blumenthal, M., G. Webb, P. King. 1995. Ma Huang Update: Industry Group Submits Ma Huang Safety Data to Texas Department of Health. *HerbalGram* 35:21–22.

Bruneton, J. 1995. *Pharmacognosy, Phytochemistry, Medicinal Plants*. Paris: Lavoisier Publishing.

Budavari, S. (ed.). 1996. *The Merck Index: An Encyclopedia of Chemicals, Drugs, and Biologicals*, 12th ed. Whitehouse Station, N.J.: Merck & Co, Inc.

Bundesanzeiger (BAnz). 1998. Monographien der Kommission E (Zulassungs- und Aufbereitungskommission am BGA für den humanmed. Bereich, phytotherapeutische Therapierichtung und Stoffgruppe). Köln: Bundesgesundheitsamt (BGA).

Chang, H.M. and P.P.H. But (eds.). 1986. *Pharmacology and Applications of Chinese Materia Medica*, Vol. 2. Philadelphia: World Scientific. 1119–1124.

Daley, P.A. et al. 1993. Ephedrine, caffeine and aspirin: safety and efficacy for the treatment of human obesity. *Intl J Obesity* 17(suppl):S73–78.

Der Marderosian, A. (ed.). 1999. *The Review of Natural Products*. St. Louis: Facts and Comparisons.

Deutsches Arzneibuch (DAB 1997). 1997. Stuttgart: Deutscher Apotheker Verlag.

Deutsches Arzneibuch (DAB 1998). 1998. Stuttgart: Deutscher Apotheker Verlag.

Food and Drug Administration (FDA). 1997. Dietary Supplements Containing Ephedrine Alkaloids: Proposed Rule. *Federal Register* Vol. 62, No. 107, Jun 4:30678–30717.

General Accounting Office (GAO). 1999. Dietary Supplements: Uncertainties in Analyses Underlying FDA's Proposed Rule on Ephedrine Alkaloids. Washington, DC: United States General Accounting Office; July.

Grieve, M. 1979. *A Modern Herbal*. New York: Dover Publications, Inc.

Gurley, B.J., S.F. Gardner, L.M. White, P.L. Wang. 1998. Ephedrine pharmacokinetics after the ingestion of nutritional supplements containing *Ephedra sinica* (Ma Huang). *Ther Drug Monit* 20(4):439–445.

Huang, K.C. 1999. *The Pharmacology of Chinese Herbs*, 2nd ed. Boca Raton: CRC Press. 292–295.

Indian Pharmacopoeia, Vol. 1. (IP 1996). 1996. Delhi: Government of India Ministry of Health and Family Welfare—Controller of Publications. 282–285.

Japanese Pharmacopoeia, 12th ed. (JP XII). 1993. Tokyo: Government of Japan Ministry of Health and Welfare—Yakuji Nippo, Ltd. 107–108.

Karnick, C.R. 1994. *Pharmacopoeial Standards of Herbal Plants*. Delhi: Sri Satguru Publications. 121–122.

Leigh, E. 1998. Cardiovascular effects of Ephedra in normal volunteers. *HerbalGram* 43:22.

Leung, A. 1999. Personal communication. July 7th.

Leung, A.Y. and S. Foster. 1996. *Encyclopedia of Common Natural Ingredients Used in Food, Drugs, and Cosmetics*, 2nd ed. New York: John Wiley & Sons, Inc.

Liu, X.X. 1989. [Pharmacologic action and clinical use of herbal Ephedrae] [In Chinese]. *Chung Hsi I Chieh Ho Tsa Chih* 9(4):255–256.

McGuffin, M., C. Hobbs, R. Upton, A. Goldberg. 1997. American Herbal Product Association's *Botanical Safety Handbook*. Boca Raton: CRC Press.

Morton, J.F. *Major Medicinal Plants: Botany, Culture and Uses*. Springfield, IL: Charles C. Thomas.

Nasser, J.A. et al. 1999. Efficacy trial for weight loss of an herbal supplement of Ma Huang and guarana. *FASEB J* 13(5).

Pardoe, A.U., D.K.J. Gorecki, D. Jones. 1993. Ephedrine alkaloid patterns in herbal products based on Ma Huang (*Ephedra sinica*). *Intl J Obesity* 17(suppl):S82.

Pickup, M.E., C.S. May, R.S. Senadagrie, J.W. Patterson. 1976. The pharmacokinetics of ephedrine after oral dosage in asthmatics receiving acute and chronic treatment. *Br J Clin Pharmacol* 3(1):123–134.

Robbers, J.E. and V.E. Tyler. 1999. *Tyler's Herbs of Choice: The Therapeutic Use of Phytomedicinals*. New York: Haworth Herbal Press. 112–116.

Toubro, S., A.V. Astrup, L. Breum, F. Quaade. 1993. Safety and efficacy of long-term treatment with ephedrine, caffeine, and an ephedrine/caffeine mixture. *Intl J Obesity Relat Metab Disord* 17 (suppl. 1):S69–S72.

Tu, G. (ed.). 1992. *Pharmacopoeia of the People's Republic of China* (English Edition 1992). Beijing: Guangdong Science and Technology Press. 99–100.

Weiss, R.F. 1988. *Herbal Medicine*. Beaconsfield, England: Beaconsfield Publishers.

White, L.M. et al. 1997. Pharmacokinetics and cardiovascular effects of ma-huang (Ephedra sinica) in normotensive adults. *J Clin Pharmacol* 37:116–122.

World Health Organization (WHO). 1999. Herba Ephedrae. *WHO Monographs on Selected Medicinal Plants*, Vol. 1. Geneva: World Health Organization. 145–153.

Additional Resources

Bensky, D. and A. Gamble. 1986 and 1993. *Chinese Herbal Medicine*. Seattle: Eastland Press, Inc.

Chen, K.H. and C.F. Schmidt. 1925. Chinese Materia Medica: Ma Huang. *China Med J* 39:982–989.

Chinese Pharmacopoeia (CHP). 1990. Beijing: Chinese Ministry of Health—People's Health Publications.

Cui, J.F., T.H. Zhou, J.S. Zhang, Z.C. Lou. 1991. Analysis of alkaloids in Chinese Ephedra species by gas chromatographic methods. *Phytochemical Analysis* 2:116–119.

Cui, J.F., C.Q. Niu, J.S. Zhang. 1991. [Determination of six *Ephedra* alkaloids in Chinese Ephedra (Ma Huang) by gas chromatography] [In Chinese]. *Yao Hsueh Hsueh Pao* 26(11):852–857.

Hsu, H. 1986. *Oriental Materia Medica, A Concise Guide*. Long Beach: Oriental Healing Arts.

Kimura, et al. 1973. [Determination of crude drugs in the Japanese pharmacopoeia. III. Determination of Ephedra alkaloids] [In Japanese]. *Yakugaku Zasshi* 93(3):364–368.

Konno, C., T. Mizuno, H. Hikino.1985. Isolation and hypoglycemic activity of ephedrans A, B, C, D, and E, glycans of Ephedra distachya herbs. *Planta Med* (2):162–163.

Ling, M., S. J. Piddlesden, B.P. Morgan. 1995. A component of the medicinal herb ephedra blocks activation in the classical and alternative pathways of complement. *Clin Exp Immunol* 102(3):582–588.

Liu, Y.M. et al. 1993. A comparative study on commercial samples of Ephedrae Herba. *Planta Med* 59:376–378.

Liu, X.X. 1989. [Pharmacologic action and clinical use of herbal Ephedrae] [In Chinese]. *Chung Hsi I Chieh Ho Tsa Chih* 9(4):255–256.

McCaleb, R.S. 1995. Perspective on Ephedra, Ephedrine, and Caffeine Products. *HerbalGram* 35:27.

Ming, O. (ed.). 1989. *Chinese-English Manual of Common-Used in Traditional Chinese Medicine*. Hong Kong: Joint Publishing (H.K.) Co., Ltd. 492–493.

Nadkarni, K.M. 1976. *Indian Materia Medica*. Bombay: Popular Prakashan. 486–503.

Oujiangcha Commune Health Center. 1960. *Jiangxi Zhongyiyao (Jiangxi Journal of Traditional Chinese Medicine)*. Yiyang, Hunan: Research Group of Oujiangcha Commune Health Center. (10):25.

Pharmacopée Française Xe Édition (Ph.Fr.X.). 1983–1990. Moulins-les-Metz: Maisonneuve S.A.

Portz, B.S., K.C. Faul, J.C. Pensoneau, J.A. Hurlbut. Revised Method for HPLC/UV Determination and SPE Cleanup of Ephedra Alkaloids in Dietary Products and Herbal Preparations. U.S. F.D.A. Laboratory Information Bulletin (LIB) No. 4053. 1–18.

Tang, W. and G. Eisenbrand. 1992. *Chinese Drugs of Plant Origin: Chemistry, Pharmacology, and Use in Traditional and Modern Medicine*. New York: Springer Verlag.

Yen, K.Y. 1992. *The Illustrated Chinese Materia Medica—Crude and Prepared*. Taipei: SMC Publishing, Inc. 190.

Yeung, H. 1985. *Handbook of Chinese Herbs and Formulas*, Vol. 1. Los Angeles: Institute of Chinese Medicine.

This material was adapted from *The Complete German Commission E Monographs—Therapeutic Guide to Herbal Medicines*. M. Blumenthal, W.R. Busse, A. Goldberg, J. Gruenwald, T. Hall, C.W. Riggins, R.S. Rister (eds.) S. Klein and R.S. Rister (trans.). 1998. Austin: American Botanical Council; Boston: Integrative Medicine Communications.

1) The Overview section is new information.

2) Description, Chemistry and Pharmacology, Uses, Contraindications, Side Effects, Interactions with Other Drugs, and Dosage sections have been drawn from the original work. Additional information has been added in some or all of these sections, as noted with references.

3) The dosage for equivalent preparations (tea infusion, fluidextract, and tincture) have been provided based on the following example:

Unless otherwise prescribed: 2 g per day of [powdered, crushed, cut or whole] [plant part]
Infusion: 2 g in 150 ml of water
Fluidextract 1:1 (g/ml): 2 ml
Tincture 1:5 (g/ml): 10 ml

4) The References and Additional Resources sections are new sections. Additional Resources are not cited in the monograph but are included for research purposes.

Zhang, J.S., S.H. Li, Z.C. Lou. 1989. [Morphological and histological studies of Chinese Ephedra *mahuang*. I. Seven species produced in north China] [In Chinese]. *Yao Hsueh Hsueh Pao* 24(12):937–948.

Zhou, J.H. and J.M. Wang (eds.). 1986. *Pharmacology of Chinese Materia Medica*. Shanghai: Shanghai Scientific and Technical Publications.

EUCALYPTUS:

EUCALYPTUS LEAF
(page 119)

EUCALYPTUS OIL
(page 120)

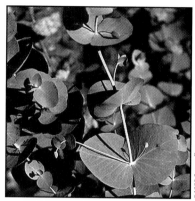

©1999 Steven Foster

Overview

Eucalyptus is a tall evergreen tree native to Australia and Tasmania, successfully introduced worldwide, now extensively cultivated in Mediterranean and subtropic regions, including Australia, China, India, Portugal, Spain, Egypt, Algeria, the southern United States, and South America (Bruneton, 1995; Budavari, 1996; Grieve, 1979; Leung and Foster, 1996; Nadkarni, 1976). The material of commerce comes mainly from Australia, Morocco, Spain, and the former U.S.S.R. (BHP, 1996; Wichtl and Bisset, 1994). It is known as *Malee* in Australia and is used in traditional Australian Aboriginal medicines (Bown, 1995; Budavari, 1996). The genus name *Eucalyptus* comes from Greek *eucalyptos*, meaning "well-covered," and refers to its flowers that, in bud, are covered with a cup-like membrane (Grieve, 1979). Though native to Australia, its therapeutic uses have been introduced and integrated into traditional medicine systems, including Chinese, Indian Ayurvedic, and Greco-European.

Its volatile oil is obtained by steam distillation and rectification from the fresh leaves or the fresh terminal branches (IP, 1996; Ph.Eur.3, 1998). The major oil producing countries include Australia, Brazil, Portugal, and Spain (Leung and Foster, 1996). Commercial production of eucalyptus oil first began in 1860 in Victoria, Australia (Bown, 1995). Oil production is of economic importance in New South Wales and Victoria, where about 25 different species of Eucalyptus are used (Grieve, 1979). Eucalyptus oil is official in the *Indian Pharmacopoeia* as a counter-irritant and mild expectorant (IP, 1996), and official in the Chinese pharmacopeia as a skin irritant used in nerval pain (Tu, 1992). The present *Ayurvedic Pharmacopoeia* indicates its topical application for headache due to colds (Karnick, 1994).

One study reported the successful treatment of chronic suppurative otitis with a compound alcoholic tincture that contained eucalyptus leaf. Its efficacy was attributed to the antibacterial and anti-inflammatory actions of the combined herbs (Newall et al., 1996; Shaparenko et al., 1979). Other studies have investigated use of the volatile oil for catarrh as an inhalant, and topically as a rubefacient (Newall et al., 1996).

In Germany, eucalyptus leaf is licensed as a standard medicinal tea, used for bronchitis and inflammation of the throat. It is sometimes also used as a component of herbal cough mixtures (Leung and Foster, 1996; Wichtl and Bisset, 1994). In the United States, it is used mainly as a component of decongestant compounds, available in galenical dosage forms including aqueous infusion, alcoholic fluidextract or tincture, inhalants, essential oil, and native extract in solid dosage forms. In both the United States and Germany, eucalyptus oil is used extensively as an expectorant component of cough and cold compounds in various oral dosage forms, including lozenges and syrups, and as an inhalant in vapor baths. It is also used externally for percutaneous absorption in dosage forms, including the essential oil, liniment, and ointment (Duke, 1997; Leung and Foster, 1996; Lust, 1974; Wichtl and Bisset, 1994).

The modern therapeutic applications for eucalyptus leaf and oil are supportable based on its history of use in well established systems of traditional medicine, phytochemical investigations, and *in vitro* and *in vivo* studies in animals.

Pharmacopeial grade dried eucalyptus leaf must contain at least 2.0% (v/m) volatile oil, composed mainly of 1,8-cineole (Bruneton, 1995; DAB, 1997; Ph.Fr.X, 1983–1990; Wichtl and Bisset, 1994). Pharmacopeial grade eucalyptus oil must contain at least 70.0% w/w of 1,8-cineole (eucalyptol) and it must be freely soluble in 5 parts by volume ethanol 70% v/v (Bruneton, 1995; DAB, 1997; Karnick, 1994; Ph.Eur.3, 1998; Ph.Fr.X, 1983–1990; Tu, 1992; Wichtl and Bisset, 1994). [Note: The *Indian Pharmacopoeia* requires not less than 60% w/w of cineole (IP, 1996).]

EUCALYPTUS LEAF

Latin Name:
Eucalyptus globulus

Pharmacopeial Name:
Eucalypti folium

Other Names:
Australian fever tree leaf, blue gum tree leaf, fever tree leaf, malee, Tasmanian blue gum leaf

Description
Eucalyptus leaf consists of the dried, mature leaves from older trees of *Eucalyptus globulus* Labillardiere [Fam. Myrtaceae] and other preparations in effective dosage. The leaves contain essential oil, which consists mainly of 1,8-cineol and tannins.

Chemistry and Pharmacology
Eucalyptus leaf contains tannins (up to 11%) and associated phenolic acids (caffeic, ferulic, gallic, gentisic, and protocatechuic acids); flavonoids (eucalyptrin, hyperin, hyperoside, quercetin, quercitrin, and rutin); volatile oils (1.0–3.5%), of which 54–95% is 1,8-cineole (=eucalyptol); triterpenes (2–4%) which are ursolic acid derivatives; monoterpenes (α- and β-pinene, D-limonene, and P-cymene); sesquiterpenes; aldehydes (myrtenal); and ketones (carvone) (Bruneton, J., 1995; Budavari, 1996; Leung and Foster, 1996; List and Hörhammer, 1973–1979; Newall et al., 1996; Wichtl and Bisset, 1994).

The Commission E reported secretomotory, expectorant, and weakly antispasmodic activity.

The *British Herbal Pharmacopoeia* reported antiseptic action (BHP, 1996). Antiseptic, febrifuge, and expectorant actions have been reported from traditional medicine usage (Leung and Foster, 1996). A compound herbal tincture containing eucalyptus has been used successfully to treat chronic suppurative otitis, apparently due to the antibacterial and anti-inflammatory actions of the herbs in the formula (Shaparenko et al., 1979).

Uses

The Commission E approved the internal use of eucalyptus leaf for catarrhs of the respiratory tract.

In France, eucalyptus leaf preparations are traditionally used to treat acute benign bronchial disease (oral route and local use), and applied locally, to relieve nasal congestion due to the common cold (Bruneton, 1995). The German Standard License for tea infusion of eucalyptus leaf recommends its use for catarrhal conditions of the upper respiratory tract and bronchitis (Braun et al., 1997). Eucalyptus leaf tea is used to treat bronchitis and inflammation of the throat (Wichtl and Bisset, 1994). *The Merck Index* reports it as an aid for flavor (Budavari, 1996).

Contraindications

Inflammation of the gastrointestinal tract and the bile ducts; serious liver diseases. Eucalyptus preparations should not be applied to the face, especially the nose, of babies and very young children.

Side Effects

In rare cases, after taking eucalyptus preparations nausea, vomiting, and diarrhea may occur.

Use During Pregnancy and Lactation

No restrictions known.

Interactions with Other Drugs

None known.

Note: Eucalyptus oil induces the enzyme system of the liver involved in the detoxification process. Therefore, the effects of other drugs can be weakened and/or shortened.

Dosage and Administration

Internal: Unless otherwise prescribed: 4–6 g per day of chopped leaf for infusions and other galenical preparations.
Infusion: 2–3 g in 150 ml water, twice daily.
Fluidextract 1:1 (g/ml): 2–3 ml, twice daily.
Tincture 1:5 (g/ml): 10–15 ml, twice daily.
Tincture: Daily dosage 3–9 g (Erg.B.6).
Native extract 4.5–5.5:1 (w/w): 0.36–0.67 g, twice daily.
External: Unless otherwise prescribed: 4–6 g per day of chopped leaf for infusions and other galenical preparations.
Inhalant: Deeply inhale the steam vapor of hot aqueous infusion.

EUCALYPTUS OIL

Latin Name:
Eucalyptus

Pharmacopeial Name:
Eucalypti aetheroleum

Other Names:
n/a

Description

Eucalyptus oil is the volatile oil from cineol-rich species of *Eucalyptus*, such as *Eucalyptus globulus* Labillardiere, *E. fructicetorum* F. Von Mueller (syn. *E. polybractea* R.T. Baker), and *E. smithii* R.T. Baker [Fam. Myrtaceae] and their preparations in effective dosage. The oil is obtained by steam distillation, followed by rectification of the fresh leaves and branch tops, and contains at least 70% (w/w) 1,8-cineol.

Chemistry and Pharmacology

Eucalyptus oil contains 70–85% 1,8-cineole (=eucalyptol); plus triterpenes (ursolic acid derivatives); monoterpenes (α- and β-pinene, D-limonene, p-cymene); sesquiterpenes (aromadendrene, alloaromadendrene, globulol); aldehydes (myrtenal); and ketones (carvone) (Bruneton, 1995; Budavari, 1996; Leung and Foster, 1996; List and Hörhammer, 1973–1979; Newall et al., 1996; Wichtl and Bisset, 1994).

The Commission E reported secretomotory, expectorant, mildly antispasmodic, and mild local hyperemic activity.

Eucalyptus oil, at a daily dosage of 0.05–0.2 ml, has demonstrated expectorant and mucolytic actions, as well as stimulation of the bronchial epithelium (Bruneton, 1995). Antiseptic, expectorant (secretolytic and secretomotor), deodorant, and cooling actions have been reported (Wichtl and Bisset, 1994). Both eucalyptus oil and eucalyptol have demonstrated strong antibacterial action against several strains of *Streptococcus*, as well as expectorant activity (Leung and Foster, 1996). Oral ingestion of eucalyptus oil can be toxic unless diluted appropriately (Leung and Foster, 1996; Newall et al., 1996; Reynolds, 1989).

Uses

The Commission E approved the internal use of eucalyptus oil for catarrhs of the respiratory tract and its external use for rheumatic complaints.

Eucalyptus oil is used in inhalants and also in products intended for percutaneous (through the skin) absorption (Wichtl and Bisset, 1994). Eucalyptus oil is ingested orally to treat catarrh, used as an inhalant, and applied topically as a rubefacient (Newall et al., 1996; Reynolds, 1989).

Contraindications

Internal: Inflammatory diseases of the gastrointestinal tract and bile ducts, severe liver diseases.
External: Eucalyptus preparations should not be applied to the face, especially the nose, of infants and young children.

Side Effects

In rare cases, nausea, vomiting and diarrhea may occur after ingestion of eucalyptus preparations.

Use During Pregnancy and Lactation

No restrictions known.

Interactions with Other Drugs

The Commission E notes that eucalyptus oil induces the enzyme system of the liver involved in the detoxification process. Therefore, the effects of other drugs can be weakened and/or shortened.

Dosage and Administration

Internal: Unless otherwise prescribed: 0.3–0.6 g per day essential oil or other equivalent galenical preparations.
External: Essential oil: Several drops rubbed into the skin. (This may be diluted at 30 ml essential oil to 500 ml of a suitable carrier such as vegetable oil.)
Ointment: Semi-solid preparation containing 5–20% essential oil (in a base of paraffin, petroleum jelly, or vegetable oil) for local application.
Tincture: Aqueous-alcoholic preparation containing 5–10% essential oil for local application.
Inhalant: Add a few drops of essential oil to hot water or to a vaporizer; deeply inhale the steam vapor.

References

Bown, D. 1995. *Encyclopedia of Herbs and Their Uses*. New York: DK Publishing, Inc. 280.

Braun, R. et al. 1997. *Standardzulassungen für Fertigarzneimittel—Text and Kommentar.* Stuttgart: Deutscher Apotheker Verlag.

British Herbal Pharmacopoeia (BHP). 1996. Exeter, U.K.: British Herbal Medicine Association. 77-78.

Bruneton, J. 1995. *Pharmacognosy, Phytochemistry, Medicinal Plants.* Paris: Lavoisier Publishing.

Budavari, S. (ed.). 1996. *The Merck Index: An Encyclopedia of Chemicals, Drugs, and Biologicals,* 12th ed. Whitehouse Station, N.J.: Merck & Co, Inc.

Deutsches Arzneibuch (DAB 1997). 1997. Stuttgart: Deutscher Apotheker Verlag.

Duke, J.A. 1997. *The Green Pharmacy.* Emmaus, PA: Rodale Press. 94.

Europäisches Arzneibuch, 3rd ed. 1st suppl. (Ph.Eur.3). 1998. Stuttgart: Deutscher Apotheker Verlag. 400–401.

Grieve, M. 1979. *A Modern Herbal.* New York: Dover Publications, Inc.

Indian Pharmacopoeia, Vol. 1. (IP 1996). 1996. Delhi: Government of India Ministry of Health and Family Welfare—Controller of Publications. 310.

Karnick, C.R. 1994. *Pharmacopoeial Standards of Herbal Plants.* Delhi: Sri Satguru Publications. 51.

Leung, A.Y. and S. Foster. 1996. *Encyclopedia of Common Natural Ingredients Used in Food, Drugs, and Cosmetics,* 2nd ed. New York: John Wiley & Sons, Inc.

List, P.H. and L. Hörhammer (eds.). 1973–1979. *Hagers Handbuch der Pharmazeutischen Praxis,* Vols. 1–7. New York: Springer Verlag.

Lust, J.B. 1974. *The Herb Book.* New York: Bantam Books. 184–185.

Nadkarni, K.M. 1976. *Indian Materia Medica.* Bombay: Popular Prakashan. 512-516.

Newall, C.A., L.A. Anderson, J.D. Phillipson. 1996. *Herbal Medicines: A Guide for Health-Care Professionals.* London: The Pharmaceutical Press.

Ph.Eur.3. See *Europäisches Arzneibuch.*

Pharmacopée Française Xe Édition (Ph.Fr.X.). 1983–1990. Moulins-les-Metz: Maisonneuve S.A.

Reynolds, J.E.F. (ed.). 1989. *Martindale: The Extra Pharmacopoeia,* 29th ed. London: The Pharmaceutical Press.

Shaparenko, B.A., A.B. Slivko, O.V. Bazarova, E.N. Vishnevetskaia, G.T. Selezneva. 1979. [Use of medicinal plants for the treatment of chronic suppurative otitis] [In Russian]. *Zh Ushn Nos Gorl Bolezn* (3):48–51.

Tu, G. (ed.). 1992. *Pharmacopoeia of the People's Republic of China* (English Edition 1992). Beijing: Guangdong Science and Technology Press. 129.

Wichtl, M. and N.G. Bisset (eds.). 1994. *Herbal Drugs and Phytopharmaceuticals.* Stuttgart: Medpharm Scientific Publishers.

Additional Resources

Belzner, S. 1997. Eukalyptusol-Kompresse bei Harnverhalten. [Eucalyptus oil dressings in urinary retention] [In German]. *Pflege Aktuell* 51(6):386-387.

Brieskorn, C.H. and W. Schlicht. 1976. Quantitative bestimmung von cineol in eucalyptusol als cineol-eisenrhodanid-komplex [Quantitative determination of cineol in eucalyptus oil as cineol-iron-thiocyanate-complex]. *Pharm Acta Helv* 51(5):133–137.

British Pharmaceutical Codex (BPC). 1973. London: The Pharmaceutical Press.

Burrow, A, R. Eccles, A.S. Jones. 1983. The effects of camphor, eucalyptus and menthol vapour on nasal resistance to airflow and nasal sensation. *Acta Otolaryngol* (Stockh) 96(1–2):157–161.

Cai, Z, X. Li, X. Xu. 1990. [Determination of eucalyptole in eucalyptus oil by gas chromatography.] *Chung Kuo Chung Yao Tsa Chih* 15(5):298–299, 319.

Council of Europe. 1981. *Flavouring Substances and Natural Sources of Flavourings,* red ed. Strasbourg: Maisonneuve.

De Smet, P.A. et al. (eds.). 1992. *Adverse Effects of Herbal Drugs,* Vol. 1. New York: Springer Verlag.

Duke, J.A. 1992. *Handbook of Phytochemical Constituents of GRAS Herbs and Other Economic Plants.* Boca Raton: CRC Press. 249.

This material was adapted from *The Complete German Commission E Monographs—Therapeutic Guide to Herbal Medicines.* M. Blumenthal, W.R. Busse, A. Goldberg, J. Gruenwald, T. Hall, C.W. Riggins, R.S. Rister (eds.) S. Klein and R.S. Rister (trans.). 1998. Austin: American Botanical Council; Boston: Integrative Medicine Communications.

1) The Overview section is new information.

2) Description, Chemistry and Pharmacology, Uses, Contraindications, Side Effects, Interactions with Other Drugs, and Dosage sections have been drawn from the original work. Additional information has been added in some or all of these sections, as noted with references.

3) The dosage for equivalent preparations (tea infusion, fluidextract, and tincture) have been provided based on the following example:

Unless otherwise prescribed: 2 g per day of [powdered, crushed, cut or whole] [plant part]

Infusion: 2 g in 150 ml of water

Fluidextract 1:1 (g/ml): 2 ml

Tincture 1:5 (g/ml): 10 ml

4) The References and Additional Resources sections are new sections. Additional Resources are not cited in the monograph but are included for research purposes.

Food Chemicals Codex, 3rd ed. (FCC III). 1981. Washington, D.C.: National Academy of Sciences.

Formacék, V. and K.H. Kubeczka. 1982. *Essential oils analysis by capillary chromatography and carbon-13 NMR spectroscopy*. New York: John Wiley & Sons, Inc.

Gobel, H., G. Schmidt, D. Soyka. 1994. Effect of peppermint and eucalyptus oil preparations on neurophysiological and experimental algesimetric headache parameters. *Cephalalgia* 14(3):182; 228–234.

Hänsel, R., K. Keller, H. Rimpler, G. Schneider (eds.). 1992–1994. *Hagers Handbuch der Pharmazeutischen Praxis*, 5th ed. Vol. 4–6. Berlin-Heidelberg: Springer Verlag.

Ioffe, T.P. 1960. [The treatment of hypertension with infusion of eucalyptus in polyclinical conditions.] *Sovet Med* 24:106–107.

Iwu, M.M. 1990. *Handbook of African Medicinal Plants*. Boca Raton: CRC Press. 180–181.

Jori, A., E. Di Salle, R. Pescador. 1972. On the inducing activity of eucalyptol. *J Pharm Pharmacol* 24(6):646–649.

Kumar, A. et al. 1988. Antibacterial properties of some *Eucalyptus* oils. *Fitoterapia* 59:141–144.

McGuffin, M., C. Hobbs, R. Upton, A. Goldberg. 1997. American Herbal Product Association's *Botanical Safety Handbook*. Boca Raton: CRC Press.

National Formulary (NF), 16th ed. 1985. Washington, D.C.: American Pharmaceutical Association.

Osawa, K. et al. 1996. Macrocarpals H, I, and J from the Leaves of *Eucalyptus globulus*. *J Nat Prod* 59(9):823–827.

Whitman, B.W. and H. Ghazizadeh. 1994. Eucalyptus oil: therapeutic and toxic aspects of pharmacology in humans and animals [letter; comment]. *J Paediatr Child Health* 30(2):190–191.

Wichtl, M. (ed.). 1997. *Teedrogen*, 4th ed. Stuttgart: Wissenschaftliche Verlagsgesellschaft.

Zaianchkovskii, I.F. 1966. Primenenie nastoiki evkalipta v akushersko-ginekologicheskoi praktike [The use of eucalyptus tincture in obstetric-gynecologic practice]. *Veterinariia* 43(7):82–83.

FENNEL:

FENNEL OIL
(page 125)

FENNEL SEED
(page 126)

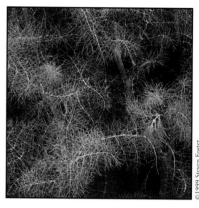

© 1999 Steven Foster

Overview

Fennel is a tall perennial herb native to the Mediterranean region, now widely cultivated as an annual or perennial in Bulgaria, Romania, Hungary, Greece, Turkey, Italy, France, Germany, Egypt, India, and China (Bruneton, 1995; Grieve, 1979; Leung and Foster, 1996; Wichtl and Bisset, 1994). Fennel is one of Germany's more important medicinal plant crops (Lange and Schippmann, 1997). The material of commerce comes mainly from Bulgaria, Hungary, Romania, Egypt, and China (BHP, 1996; Wichtl and Bisset, 1994).

Its modern therapeutic uses in Germany and the United States stem from traditional Greek medicine as practiced by Hippocrates and later by Dioscorides. It is still widely used in traditional Arabian medicine as a diuretic, appetizer, and digestive (Tanira et al., 1996). Its original Greek genus name was *Marathron*, from *maraino*, meaning to grow thin. Its current genus name, *Foeniculum*, was assigned by the Romans, derived from the Latin word *foenum*, meaning hay (Grieve, 1979). Fennel's therapeutic uses have been introduced and integrated into many other systems of traditional medicine, including Ayurvedic, Chinese, and Japanese Kampo. For example, the present *Ayurvedic Pharmacopoeia* recommends it in dried fruit or fluidextract form, for flatulent dyspepsia, anorexia, and flatulent colic in children (Karnick, 1994). Its indications for use in the present Chinese pharmacopoeia include for distending pain in the epigastrium with anorexia, dysmenorrhea with lower abdominal pain and cold sensation, vomiting, and diarrhea (Tu, 1992).

The modern therapeutic applications for fennel seed and oil are supportable based on their history of use in well established systems of traditional medicine, phytochemical investigations, and *in vitro* and *in vivo* studies in animals.

In Germany, fennel seed is licensed as a standard medicinal tea for dyspepsia. It is also used in cough syrups and honeys (antitussives and expectorants), and stomach and bowel remedies, especially in pediatrics, as aqueous infusion, water (Aqua Foeniculi), *dragée* (lozenge), juice, and syrup. It is often used in combination with aniseed (Leung and Foster, 1996; Wichtl and Bisset, 1994). In the United States, it is also used as a component of galactagogue preparations. Indications for use of fennel oil are similar to those for fennel seed. In Germany and the United States, fennel oil is used as an expectorant component of cough remedies, and also as a carminative component of stomach and bowel remedies in dosage forms including honey and syrup. Traditionally, it is combined with laxative or purgative herbs to counteract or modify their harsh griping effects in the bowels (ESCOP, 1997; Leung and Foster, 1996; Nadkarni, 1976; Wichtl and Bisset, 1994). The Commission E limits the use of fennel seed and fennel oil for up to two weeks and then recommends consulting a physician.

Pharmacopeial grade bitter fennel seed must contain not less than 4% (v/m) total volatile oils, calculated with reference to the anhydrous drug, as determined by the

European Pharmacopoeia (Ph.Eur.3) method 2.8.12. Its volatile oil must be composed of not less than 60% anethole, not less than 15% fenchone, and maximum 5% estragole, as determined by Ph.Eur.3 GC method 2.2.28 (DAB 10, 1991; ESCOP, 1997; Ph.Eur.3, 1997). The *Austrian Pharmacopoeia* requires not less than 3.5% volatile oil (ÖAB, 1981–1983).

The official fennel oil of the *European Pharmacopoeia* is derived from bitter fennel (var. *vulgare*) as opposed to sweet fennel (var. *dulce*). Pharmacopeial grade fennel oil must be composed of not less than 60% anethole, not less than 15% fenchone, and no more than 5% estragole, as determined by Ph.Eur.3 GC method 2.2.28 (Ph.Eur.3, 1997). The relative proportions of its main constituents determine its overall bitterness or sweetness. Fenchone has a disagreeable bitter taste; anethole is sweet (Bown, 1995; Grieve, 1979). The relative ratios of these components and their yields vary somewhat by strain and region. Historically, the strains yielding oils most suitable for pharmaceutical use have been Russian, Saxon, Galician, and Romanian (Bown, 1995; Grieve, 1979; Nadkarni, 1976). As the ratio of its main components determine the pharmaceutical quality of the oil, long-term studies investigated the production—the biological and structural regularities of essential oil accumulation in developing fruits of bitter fennel. In a study of 13 different plant populations, representing three different chemovarieties (e.g., cv. "Soroksári"), the presence and ratio of anethole, methyl-chavicol, and fenchone were analyzed and found to be stable throughout nine stages of flowering and fruiting (Bernáth et al., 1998).

FENNEL OIL

Latin Name:
Foeniculum vulgare

Pharmacopeial Name:
Foeniculi aetheroleum

Other Names: bitter fennel oil

Description
Fennel oil is the essential oil obtained from the dried, ripe fruits of *Foeniculum vulgare* Miller var. *vulgare* (Miller) Thellung [Fam. Apiaceae] by steam distillation and its preparations in effective dosage. Fennel oil contains anethole, fenchone, and not more than 5% estragole.

Chemistry and Pharmacology
Fennel essential oil contains trans-anethole (50–70%), (+)-fenchone (9–22%), and estragole [methyl chavicol] (2–5%). Other compounds in the oil include anisaldehyde, camphene, fenchyl alcohol, limonene, p-anisic acid, 3-carene, p-cymene, α-fenchene, β-myrcene, α-pinene, β-pinene, α-phellandrene, sabinene, α- and β-terpinene, γ-terpinene, terpinolene, α-thujene, cis- and trans-ocimenes, trans-1,8-terpin (Bruneton, 1995; ESCOP, 1997; Leung and Foster, 1996; Wichtl and Bissett, 1994).

The Commission E reported stimulation of gastrointestinal motility activity that, in higher concentrations, was antispasmodic. Experimentally, anethole and fenchone have shown a secretolytic action on the respiratory tract. *In vitro*, fennel oil has demonstrated antimicrobial activity.

Volatile oil of fennel seed has demonstrated carminative and stimulant activities as well as spasmolytic actions on the smooth muscles of experimental animals (Leung and Foster, 1996). Fennel syrup and fennel honey reduced spasms induced by acetylcholine and barium chloride *in vitro* in isolated guinea pig ileum though weaker than the effects of an aqueous infusion of bitter fennel seed (ESCOP, 1997).

Uses

The Commission E approved the internal use of fennel oil preparations for peptic discomforts, such as mild, spastic disorders of the gastrointestinal tract, feeling of fullness, and flatulence; and also for catarrhs of the upper respiratory tract. Fennel honey was recommended for catarrhs of the upper respiratory tract in children.

ESCOP approves the use of fennel syrup or fennel honey for catarrh of the upper respiratory tract in children (ESCOP, 1997).

Contraindications

Fennel honey: None known.
Other preparations: Pregnancy. Not to be used for infants and toddlers.

Side Effects

In rare cases, allergic reactions affecting skin and respiratory system.

Use During Pregnancy and Lactation

No restrictions known for fennel honey. Other fennel oil preparations not recommended during pregnancy. No restrictions known during lactation.

Interactions with Other Drugs

None known.

Dosage and Administration

Unless otherwise prescribed: 0.1–0.6 ml essential oil or equivalent galenical preparations for internal use.
Essential oil: 0.1–0.6 ml.
Fennel honey or fennel syrup with 0.5 g fennel oil/kg [=0.5:1000 (w/w)]:
Adult: 10–20 g.
Children 4–10 years: 6–10 g.
Children 1–4 years: 3–6 g.
Duration of administration: Unless otherwise advised by a physician or pharmacist, one should not consume fennel oil for an extended period (several weeks).
Note: Fennel syrup, fennel honey: Diabetics must consider sugar content of bread exchange units according to manufacturer's information.

FENNEL SEED

Latin Name:
Foeniculum vulgare

Pharmacopeial Name:
Foeniculi fructus

Other Names:
bitter fennel, common fennel

Description

Fennel seed consists of the dried, ripe fruits of *Foeniculum vulgare* Miller var. *vulgare* (Miller) Thellung [Fam. Apiaceae] and their preparations in effective dosage. The seeds contain at least 4% essential oil with not more than 5% estragole.

Chemistry and Pharmacology

Fennel seed contains essential oils (4–6%), of which 50–70% is *trans*-anethole, 9–22% (+)-fenchone, 2–5% estragole (methyl chavicol), plus α- and β-pinene, α-phellandrene, limonene, camphene, and others; fixed oil (17–20%), of which 60–75% is petroselinic acid; the flavonoids kaempferol, quercetin, isoquercitrin, and rutin; protein (16–20%); minerals (relatively high in calcium and potassium); sugars; and vitamins (Bruneton, 1995; ESCOP, 1997; Leung and Foster, 1996; Wichtl and Bissett, 1994).

The Commission E reported that fennel seed promotes gastrointestinal motility and in higher concentrations acts as an antispasmodic. In experiments, anethole and fenchone have been shown to have a secretolytic action in the respiratory tract. In the frog, aqueous fennel extracts raise the mucociliary activity of the ciliary epithelium.

The *British Herbal Pharmacopoeia* reported its action as carminative (BHP, 1996). Aqueous infusion of bitter fennel seed increased the transport velocity of the isolated ciliated epithelium of a frog esophagus by 12% (ESCOP, 1997; Leung and Foster, 1996; Müller-Limmroth and Fröhlich, 1980). Fennel administered orally increased the spontaneous movement of the unanesthetized rabbit stomach and taken intravenously reduced the inhibition of stomach movement by sodium pentobarbitone (Niiho et al., 1977). A bitter fennel infusion reduced spasms induced by acetylcholine and barium chloride *in vitro* in isolated guinea pig ileum and inhibited *in situ* ileum spasms *in vivo* in cats (ESCOP, 1997).

Uses

The Commission E approved the internal use of fennel seed preparations for dyspepsias such as mild, spastic gastrointestinal afflictions, fullness, and flatulence. It is also approved for catarrh of the upper respiratory tract. Fennel syrup and fennel honey are used for catarrh of the upper respiratory tract in children.

In France, fennel seed is allowed the same indications for use as the star anise seed or aniseed (Bruneton, 1995). The German Standard License for infusion of fennel seed reports its use against flatulence and cramp-like pains in the gastrointestinal tract, especially in infants and small children, and to dissolve mucus in the respiratory tract (Braun et al., 1997). ESCOP lists fennel seed for dyspeptic complaints such as mild, spasmodic gastrointestinal complaints, bloating, and flatulence, for catarrh of the upper respiratory tract, and fennel syrup or fennel honey for catarrh of the upper respiratory tract in children (ESCOP, 1997).

Contraindications

Herb for infusions and preparations containing an equivalent amount of the essential oil:
None known.
Other preparations:
Pregnancy.

Side Effects

In individual cases allergic reactions of skin and respiratory tract.

Use During Pregnancy and Lactation

No restrictions known for the seed used in infusions and preparations containing an equivalent amount of the essential oil. Other fennel seed preparations not recommended during pregnancy. No restrictions known during lactation.

Interactions with Other Drugs

None known.

Dosage and Administration

Unless otherwise prescribed: 5–7 g per day crushed or ground seeds for teas, tea-like products, and other galenical preparations for internal use.
Fennel syrup or honey: 10–20 g (Erg.B.6).
Compound fennel tincture: 5–7.5 g (=5–7.5 ml).
Equivalent preparations:
Infusion: 1–3 g in 150 ml water, two to three times daily between meals.
Fluidextract 1:1 (g/ml): 1–3 ml, two to three times daily between meals.
Tincture 1:5 (g/ml): 5–15 ml, two to three times daily between meals.

Native dry extract 3.9–4.9:1 (w/w): 0.2–0.7 g, two to three times daily between meals.
Duration of administration: Fennel preparations should not be used on a prolonged basis (several weeks) without consulting a physician or pharmacist.
Note: Fennel syrup, fennel honey: Diabetics must consider sugar content of bread exchange units according to manufacturer's information.

References

Bernáth, J. et al. 1998. Production-biological and structural regularities of essential oil accumulation in developing fruits of fennel (*Foeniculum vulgare* Mill.). Budapest: UHFI Department of Medicinal Plant Production.

Bown, D. 1995. *Encyclopedia of Herbs and Their Uses.* New York: DK Publishing, Inc. 283–284.

Braun, R. et al. 1997. *Standardzulassungen für Fertigarzneimittel—Text und Kommentar.* Stuttgart: Deutscher Apotheker Verlag.

British Herbal Pharmacopoeia (BHP). 1996. Exeter, U.K.: British Herbal Medicine Association.

Bruneton, J. 1995. *Pharmacognosy, Phytochemistry, Medicinal Plants.* Paris: Lavoisier Publishing.

Deutsches Arzneibuch, 10th ed. (DAB 10). 1991. (With subsequent supplements through 1996.) Stuttgart: Deutscher Apotheker Verlag.

ESCOP. 1997. "Foeniculi aetheroleum" and "Foeniculi fructus." *Monographs on the Medicinal Uses of Plant Drugs.* Exeter, U.K.: European Scientific Cooperative on Phytotherapy.

Europäisches Arzneibuch, 3rd ed. (Ph.Eur.3). 1997. Stuttgart: Deutscher Apotheker Verlag. 939-941.

Grieve, M. 1979. *A Modern Herbal.* New York: Dover Publications, Inc.

Karnick, C.R. 1994. *Pharmacopoeial Standards of Herbal Plants,* Vols. 1–2. Delhi: Sri Satguru Publications. Vol. 1:139–141; Vol. 2:71.

Lange, D. and U. Schippmann. 1997. *Trade Survey of Medicinal Plants in Germany—A Contribution to International Plant Species Conservation.* Bonn: Bundesamt für Naturschutz. 32–33.

Leung, A.Y. and S. Foster. 1996. *Encyclopedia of Common Natural Ingredients Used in Food, Drugs, and Cosmetics,* 2nd ed. New York: John Wiley & Sons, Inc.

Müller-Limmroth, W. and H.H. Fröhlich. 1980. Wirkungsnachweis einiger phytotherapeutischer Expektorantien auf den mukoziliaren Transport [Proof of efficacy of some phytotherapeutic expectorants on mucociliary transport]. *Fortschr Med* 98:95–101.

Nadkarni, K.M. 1976. *Indian Materia Medica.* Bombay: Popular Prakashan. 557–559.

Niiho, Y., I. Takayanagi, K. Takagi. 1977. Effects of a combined stomachic and its ingredients on rabbit stomach motility *in situ. Jpn J Pharmacol* 27:177–179.

Ph.Eur.3. See *Europäisches Arzneibuch.*

Österreichisches Arzneibuch, Vols. 1–2, 1st suppl. (ÖAB). 1981–1983. Wien: Verlag der Österreichischen Staatsdruckerei.

Tanira, M.O.M. et al. 1996. Pharmacological and toxicological investigations on *Foeniculum vulgare* dried fruit extract in experimental animals. *Phytother Res* 10:33–36.

Tu, G. (ed.). 1992. *Pharmacopoeia of the People's Republic of China* (English Edition 1992). Beijing: Guangdong Science and Technology Press. 70.

Wichtl, M. and N.G. Bisset (eds.). 1994. *Herbal Drugs and Phytopharmaceuticals.* Stuttgart: Medpharm Scientific Publishers.

Additional Resources

Betts, T.J. 1968. Anethole and fenchone in the developing fruits of *Foeniculum vulgare* Mill. *J Pharm Pharmacol* 20(6):469–472.

Boyd, E.M. and E.P. Sheppard. 1968. The effect of steam inhalation of volatile oils on the output and composition of respiratory tract fluid. *J Pharmacol Exp Ther* 163(1):250–256.

———. 1971. An autumn-enhanced mucotropic action of inhaled terpenes and related volatile agents. *Pharmacology* 6(2):65–80.

Deutsches Arzneibuch, 10th ed. Vol. 1–6. (DAB 10). 1991. Kommentar. Stuttgart: Wissenschaftliche Verlagsgesellschaft mbH.

Food Chemicals Codex, 2nd ed. (FCC II). 1972. Washington, D.C.: National Academy of Sciences.

Hänsel, R., K. Keller, H. Rimpler, G. Schneider (eds.). 1993. *Hagers Handbuch der Pharmazeutischen Praxis*, 5th ed. Vol. 5. Berlin-Heidelberg: Springer Verlag. 156-181.

Kapoor, L.D., A. Singh, S.L. Kapoor, S.N. Srivastava. 1969. Survey of Indian plants for saponins, alkaloids and flavonoids. *Lloydia* 32(3):297–304.

Kapoor, L.D. 1990. *Handbook of Ayurvedic Medicinal Plants.* Boca Raton: CRC Press. 189.

List, P.H. and L. Hörhammer (eds.). 1973–1979. *Hagers Handbuch der Pharmazeutischen Praxis*, Vols. 1–7. New York: Springer Verlag.

Madaus, G. 1976. *Lehrbuch der Biologischen Heilmittel.* Vol. 2. Hildesheim; New York: Georg Olms. 1354–1361.

Marsh, A.C. et al. 1977. *Composition of Foods, Spices, and Herbs: Raw, Processed, Prepared.* Agriculture Handbook No. 8–2. Washington, D.C.: Agricultural Research Service, U.S. Department of Agriculture.

Maruzzella, J.C. and M. Freundlich. 1959. Antimicrobial substances from seeds. *J Am Pharm Assoc* 48:356–358.

Maruzzella J.C. and N.A. Sicurella. 1960. Antibacterial activity of essential oil vapors. *J Am Pharm Assoc* 49:692–694.

McGuffin, M., C. Hobbs, R. Upton, A. Goldberg. 1997. American Herbal Product Association's *Botanical Safety Handbook.* Boca Raton: CRC Press.

Pharmacopée Française Xe Édition (Ph.Fr.X.). 1983–1990. Moulins-les-Metz: Maisonneuve S.A.

Ramadan, F.M., R.T. El-Zanfaly, F.A. El-Wakeil, M. Alian. 1972. On the antibacterial effects of some essential oils. I. Use of agar diffusion method. *Chem Mikrobiol Technol Lebensm* 2:51–55.

Reynolds, J.E.F. (ed.). 1993. *Martindale: The Extra Pharmacopoeia*, 30th ed. London: The Pharmaceutical Press. 1369–1370.

Steinegger, E. and R. Hänsel. 1992. *Pharmakognosie*, 5th ed. Berlin-Heidelberg: Springer Verlag.

Weiss, R.F. 1991. *Lehrbuch der Phytotherapie*, 7th ed. Stuttgart: Hippokrates. 107–108.

Yen, K.Y. 1992. *The Illustrated Chinese Materia Medica—Crude and Prepared*. Taipei: SMC Publishing, Inc. 133.

This material was adapted from *The Complete German Commission E Monographs—Therapeutic Guide to Herbal Medicines*. M. Blumenthal, W.R. Busse, A. Goldberg, J. Gruenwald, T. Hall, C.W. Riggins, R.S. Rister (eds.) S. Klein and R.S. Rister (trans.). 1998. Austin: American Botanical Council; Boston: Integrative Medicine Communications.

1) The Overview section is new information.

2) Description, Chemistry and Pharmacology, Uses, Contraindications, Side Effects, Interactions with Other Drugs, and Dosage sections have been drawn from the original work. Additional information has been added in some or all of these sections, as noted with references.

3) The dosage for equivalent preparations (tea infusion, fluidextract, and tincture) have been provided based on the following example:

Unless otherwise prescribed: 2 g per day of [powdered, crushed, cut or whole] [plant part]

Infusion: 2 g in 150 ml of water

Fluidextract 1:1 (g/ml): 2 ml

Tincture 1:5 (g/ml): 10 ml

4) The References and Additional Resources sections are new sections. Additional Resources are not cited in the monograph but are included for research purposes.

FENUGREEK SEED

Latin Name:
Trigonella foenum-graecum

Pharmacopeial Name:
Foenugraeci semen

Other Names:
Greek hay, trigonella

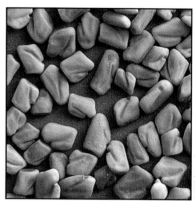

©1999 Steven Foster

Overview

Fenugreek is an annual herb native to the Mediterranean region, the Ukraine, India, and China, now widely cultivated in these areas. The material of commerce comes exclusively from cultivated plants mainly from Morocco, Turkey, India, and China (BHP, 1996; Bruneton, 1995; Budavari, 1996; Leung and Foster, 1996; Wichtl and Bisset, 1994). It was brought under cultivation in ancient Assyria during the seventh century B.C.E. (Bown, 1995). Its present genus name, *Trigonella*, comes from Greek, meaning "three-angled," from the form of its corolla. Its species name *foenum-graecum* means "Greek hay." Fenugreek was once used to scent inferior hay (Grieve, 1979).

Its recorded use dates back to ancient Egyptian medicine, first mentioned in the Ebers papyri (ca. 1500 B.C.E.) as an herb to induce childbirth. It has been used therapeutically for millennia in traditional Arabian, Greek, and Indian (Ayurvedic, Siddha, and Unani) medicines. Its use eventually spread eastward to China, where it was introduced into Chinese medicine during the Sung Dynasty in the eleventh century (Bown, 1995; Grieve, 1979; Leung and Foster, 1996; Nadkarni, 1976). It is official in the present-day Chinese pharmacopeia for pain and "coldness" in the lower abdomen, hernia, and weakness and edema of the legs caused by "cold-damp" (Tu, 1992). In the United States, it was a key ingredient in Lydia Pinkham's famous "Vegetable Compound," a popular nineteenth century patent medicine for menstrual pain and postmenopausal vaginal dryness (Duke, 1997).

Modern clinical studies have investigated its hypocholesterolemic and hypo-glycemic actions in normal and diabetic humans (Bruneton, 1995; Newall et al., 1996). One study reported hypoglycemic activity in healthy individuals who ingested whole seed extracts. Improved plasma glucose and insulin responses and reduced 24-hour urinary glucose concentrations were reported after chronic ingestion for 21 days. In two diabetic insulin-dependent subjects, daily administration of 25 g fenugreek seed powder reduced fasting plasma-glucose profile, glycosuria, and daily insulin requirements (56 to 20 units) after eight weeks. Significant reductions in serum-cholesterol concentrations were also reported (Sharma, 1986). A subsequent study investigated the lipid-lowering activity of fenugreek seeds in 60 non-insulin dependent diabetic subjects. Isocaloric diets without and with fenugreek were given for seven days and 24 weeks, respectively. Ingestion of an experimental diet containing 25 g fenugreek seed powder daily resulted in a significant reduction of total cholesterol, low density and very low density lipoprotein cholesterol, and triglyceride levels. The effect on lipid levels was sustained and lasting. Because it also affects glucose and insulin levels, the authors concluded that it should be considered a useful dietary supplement for prevention of hyperlipidemia and athero-sclerosis in diabetic subjects (Sharma et al., 1996).

In Germany, fenugreek seed is usually used externally, prepared as an aqueous paste for poultices to reduce inflammation. Occasionally it is used internally as a component of cholagogue and gastrointestinal remedy compounds (Leung and Foster, 1996; Wichtl and Bisset, 1994). In the United States, it is used similarly and also in traditional galactagogue preparations (Duke, 1997).

The approved modern therapeutic applications for fenugreek seed are supportable based on its long history of use in well established systems of traditional medicine, phytochemical investigations, *in vitro* and *in vivo* studies in animals, and some clinical studies.

Pharmacopeial grade fenugreek seed is not presently defined on the basis of a specific chemical composition quantitatively, but rather on a number of tests, including positive identification by thin-layer chromatography (TLC), organoleptic evaluations, macroscopical and microscopical authentication, and certain quantitative standards. For example, it should contain not less than 30% water-soluble extractive (BHP, 1996; DAB 10, 1994; Tu, 1992).

Description

Fenugreek consists of the ripe, dried seed of *Trigonella foenum-graecum* L. [Fam. Fabaceae], as well as its preparations in effective dosage. The preparation contains mucilage and bitter principles.

Chemistry and Pharmacology

Fenugreek seed contains 45–60% carbohydrates, mainly mucilaginous fiber (galactomannans); 20–30% proteins high in lysine and tryptophan; 5–10% fixed oils (lipids); pyridine-type alkaloids, mainly trigonelline (0.2–0.36%), choline (0.5%), gentianine, and carpaine; the flavonoids apigenin, luteolin, orientin, quercetin, vitexin, and isovitexin; free amino acids, such as 4-hydroxyisoleucine (0.09%), arginine, histidine, and lysine; calcium and iron; saponins (0.6–1.7%); glycosides yielding steroidal sapogenins on hydrolysis (diosgenin, yamogenin, tigogenin, neotigogenin); cholesterol and sitosterol; vitamins A, B_1, C, and nicotinic acid; and 0.015% volatile oils (n-alkanes and sesquiterpenes) (Bruneton, 1995; Budavari, 1996; Leung and Foster, 1996; Newall et al., 1996; Wichtl and Bisset, 1994).

The Commission E reported secretolytic, hyperemic, and mild antiseptic activity.

The *British Herbal Pharmacopoeia* reported its actions as demulcent and hypoglycemic (BHP, 1996). Fenugreek seeds are reported to have antidiabetic, blood cholesterol-lowering, and blood lipid-lowering actions as demonstrated experimentally by decreased post-prandial glycemia in the diabetic rat and dog (Bruneton, 1995). Hypoglycemic activity in healthy individuals has been reported for whole seed extracts. A significant reduction in serum-cholesterol concentrations in diabetic patients was also reported (Sharma, 1986). Fenugreek infusion has hypoglycemic effects in animals (Leung and Foster, 1996). *The Merck Index* reported its veterinary medicine therapeutic category as emollient (Budavari, 1996).

Uses

The Commission E approved internal use of fenugreek seed for loss of appetite and external use as a poultice for local inflammation. Traditionally, fenugreek is used internally to treat anorexia, dyspepsia, gastritis, and convalescence, and topically for furunculosis, myalgia, lymphadenitis, gout, wounds, and leg ulcers. It is indicated for use externally as an emollient for treating furuncles, boils, inflamed indurations, and eczema, applied as a poultice (Duke, 1997; Newall et al., 1996; Wichtl and Bisset, 1994).

Contraindications

None known.

Side Effects

Repeated external applications can result in undesirable skin reactions.

Use During Pregnancy and Lactation

Not recommended during pregnancy (McGuffin et al., 1997).

Interactions with Other Drugs

None known.

Dosage and Administration

Internal: Cut or crushed seed: 6 g per day; equivalent preparations.
Infusion: Macerate 0.5 g cut seed in 150 ml cold water for 3 hours, strain, and add honey if desired. Drink several cups daily.
Fluidextract 1:1 (g/ml): 6 ml.
Tincture 1:5 (g/ml): 30 ml.
Native extract 3–4:1 (w/w): 1.5–2 g.
External: Bath additive: Mix 50 g powdered seed with 1/4 liter water. Add to hot bath.
Inhalant: Inhale deeply the steam vapor of the hot aqueous infusion.
Liniment: Liquid preparation containing infusion or tincture in vegetable oil emulsion or alcohol, applied locally by rubbing.
Ointment: Semi-solid preparation containing infusion or tincture in a base of petroleum jelly or anhydrous lanolin and vegetable oil, applied locally.
Oil infusion: Maceration of powdered seed in vegetable oil, grain alcohol, and ammonia water, applied locally.
Poultice: Semi-solid paste prepared from 50 g powdered seed per 1 liter hot water, applied locally.

References

Bown, D. 1995. *Encyclopedia of Herbs and Their Uses.* New York: DK Publishing, Inc. 364.
British Herbal Pharmacopoeia (BHP). 1996. Exeter, U.K.: British Herbal Medicine Association.
Bruneton, J. 1995. *Pharmacognosy, Phytochemistry, Medicinal Plants.* Paris: Lavoisier Publishing.
Budavari, S. (ed.). 1996. *The Merck Index: An Encyclopedia of Chemicals, Drugs, and Biologicals,* 12th ed. Whitehouse Station, N.J.: Merck & Co, Inc.
Deutsches Arzneibuch, 10th ed. (DAB 10). 1991. (With subsequent supplements through 1996.) Stuttgart: Deutscher Apotheker Verlag.
Duke, J.A. 1997. *The Green Pharmacy.* Emmaus, PA: Rodale Press. 88–89
Grieve, M. 1979. *A Modern Herbal.* New York: Dover Publications, Inc.
Leung, A.Y. and S. Foster. 1996. *Encyclopedia of Common Natural Ingredients Used in Food, Drugs, and Cosmetics,* 2nd ed. New York: John Wiley & Sons, Inc.
McGuffin, M., C. Hobbs, R. Upton, A. Goldberg. 1997. American Herbal Product Association's *Botanical Safety Handbook.* Boca Raton: CRC Press.
Nadkarni, K.M. 1976. *Indian Materia Medica.* Bombay: Popular Prakashan. 1240–1243.
Newall, C.A., L.A. Anderson, J.D. Phillipson. 1996. *Herbal Medicines: A Guide for Health-Care Professionals.* London: The Pharmaceutical Press.
Sharma, R.D. 1986. Effect of fenugreek seeds and leaves on blood glucose and serum insulin responses in human subjects. *Nutr Res* 6:1353–1364.
Sharma, R.D. et al. 1996. Hypolipidaemic effect of fenugreek seeds: a chronic study in non-insulin dependent diabetic patients. *Phytotherapy Res* 10:332–334.
Tu, G. (ed.). 1992. *Pharmacopoeia of the People's Republic of China* (English Edition 1992). Beijing: Guangdong Science and Technology Press. 236.
Wichtl, M. and N.G. Bisset (eds.). 1994. *Herbal Drugs and Phytopharmaceuticals.* Stuttgart: Medpharm Scientific Publishers.

Additional Resources

Ali, L. et al. 1995. Characterization of the hypoglycemic effect of *Trigonella foenum graecum* seed [letter]. *Planta Med* 61(4):358–360.
British Herbal Pharmacopoeia (BHP). 1983. Keighley, U.K.: British Herbal Medicine Association.
British Pharmaceutical Codex (BPC). 1949. London: The Pharmaceutical Press.
Der Marderosian, A. (ed.). 1999. *The Review of Natural Products.* St. Louis: Facts and Comparisons.
Duke, J.A. 1985. *Handbook of Medicinal Herbs.* Boca Raton: CRC Press.
Gupta, R.K. et al. 1986. Minor steroidal sapogenins from fenugreek seeds, *Trigonella foenum-graecum. J Nat Prod* 49:1153.
Gupta, R.K., D.C. Thain, R.S. Thakur. 1986. Two furostanol saponins from *Trigonella foenum-graecum. Phytochem* 25:2205–2207.

Hänsel, R., K. Keller, H. Rimpler, G. Schneider (eds.). 1992–1994. *Hagers Handbuch der Pharmazeutischen Praxis,* 5th ed. Vol. 4–6. Berlin-Heidelberg: Springer Verlag.

Hardman, R. and F.R. Fazli. 1972. Labelled steroidal sapogenins and hydrocarbons from *Trigonella foenumgraecum* by acetate, mevalonate and cholesterol feeds to seeds. *Planta Med* 21(2):188–195.

———. 1972. Methods of screening the genus *Trigonella* for steroidal sapogenins in genus *Trigonella. Planta Med* 21(2):131–138.

———. 1972. Studies in the steroidal sapogenin yield from *Trigonella foenumgraecum* seed. *Planta Med* 21(3):322–328

Hardman, R. and K.R. Brain. 1972. Variations in the yield of total and individual 25 - and 25 - sapogenins on storage of whole seed of *Trigonella foenumgraecum* L. *Planta Med* 21(4):426–430.

Hoffmann, D.L. Health World Online—Herbal Materia Medica. Available at www.healthy.net/hwlibrarybooks/hoffman/materiamedica/fenugreek.htm

Iwu, M.M. 1990. *Handbook of African Medicinal Plants.* Boca Raton: CRC Press. 253–254.

Kapoor, L.D. 1990. *Handbook of Ayurvedic Medicinal Plants.* Boca Raton: CRC Press. 327.

List, P.H. and L. Hörhammer (eds.). 1973–1979. *Hagers Handbuch der Pharmazeutischen Praxis,* Vols. 1–7. New York: Springer Verlag.

Madaus, G. 1979. *Lehrbuch der Biologischen Heilmittel.* Bde 1–3, Nachdruck. Hildesheim: Georg Olms.

Marsh, A.C. et al. 1977. *Composition of Foods, Spices, and Herbs: Raw, Processed, Prepared.* Agriculture Handbook No. 8–2. Washington, D.C.: Agricultural Research Service, U.S. Department of Agriculture.

Opdyke, D.L.J. 1978. Fenugreek absolute. *Food Cosmet Toxicol* 16(suppl.1):755–756.

Reynolds, J.E.F. (ed.). 1989. *Martindale: The Extra Pharmacopoeia,* 29th ed. London: The Pharmaceutical Press.

Rosengarten, F., Jr. 1969. *The Book of Spices.* Wynnewood, PA: Livingston.

Sharma, R.D. 1986. An evaluation of hypocholesterolemic factor of fenugreek seeds (*T. foenum graecum*) in rats. *Nutr Rep Int* 33:669–677.

Sharma, R.D., T.C. Raghuram, N.S. Rao. 1990. Effect of fenugreek seeds on blood glucose and serum lipids in type I diabetes. *Eur J Clin Nutr* 44(4):301–306.

Stark, A. and Z. Madar. 1993. The effect of an ethanol extract derived from fenugreek (*Trigonella foenum-graecum*) on bile acid absorption and cholesterol levels in rats. *Br J Nutr* 69(1):277–287.

Steinegger, E. and R. Hänsel. 1992. *Pharmakognosie,* 5th ed. Berlin-Heidelberg: Springer Verlag.

Yeung, H. 1985. *Handbook of Chinese Herbs and Formulas,* Vol. 1. Los Angeles: Institute of Chinese Medicine.

This material was adapted from *The Complete German Commission E Monographs—Therapeutic Guide to Herbal Medicines.* M. Blumenthal, W.R. Busse, A. Goldberg, J. Gruenwald, T. Hall, C.W. Riggins, R.S. Rister (eds.) S. Klein and R.S. Rister (trans.). 1998. Austin: American Botanical Council; Boston: Integrative Medicine Communications.

1) The Overview section is new information.

2) Description, Chemistry and Pharmacology, Uses, Contraindications, Side Effects, Interactions with Other Drugs, and Dosage sections have been drawn from the original work. Additional information has been added in some or all of these sections, as noted with references.

3) The dosage for equivalent preparations (tea infusion, fluidextract, and tincture) have been provided based on the following example:

Unless otherwise prescribed: 2 g per day of [powdered, crushed, cut or whole] [plant part]
Infusion: 2 g in 150 ml of water
Fluidextract 1:1 (g/ml): 2 ml
Tincture 1:5 (g/ml): 10 ml

4) The References and Additional Resources sections are new sections. Additional Resources are not cited in the monograph but are included for research purposes.

FLAXSEED

Latin Name:
Linum usitatissimum

Pharmacopeial Name:
Lini semen

Other Names:
flax, linseed

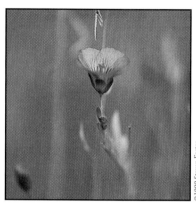

©1999 Steven Foster

Overview

Flax is an annual herb believed to be a native of Egypt. It has been cultivated worldwide for so many centuries that its geographical origin is uncertain. The material of commerce in Europe comes from Argentina, Morocco, Turkey, India, and other countries (BHP, 1996; Grieve, 1979; Nadkarni, 1976; Wichtl and Bisset, 1994). Flaxseed used in Chinese medicine is produced mainly in Inner Mongolia, Heilongjiang, Liaoning, and Jilin provinces (Yen, 1992) and that used in Indian medicine is extensively cultivated throughout India, mostly in Bengal, Bihar, and the United provinces (Kapoor, 1990; Karnick, 1994; Nadkarni, 1976). Flaxseed is one of the oldest cultivated plants worldwide (Wichtl and Bisset, 1994). Flaxseed, and cloth woven from flax, has been found in Egyptian tombs. The Bible mentions in Exodus 28 that the Jewish high priests wore garments made from flax (Grieve, 1979).

Its present-day therapeutic uses in Asia, Europe, and North America can be traced to ancient Roman medicine and probably back even further to ancient Greek and Egyptian medicines. Pliny the Elder (ca. 23–79 C.E.) cited 30 remedies using flaxseed, including oral ingestion as a mild laxative and topical application as a poultice for local inflammation (Carlson, 1998). It is still official in the Chinese pharmacopeia for constipation and dry itching skin (Tu, 1992). The *Ayurvedic Pharmacopoeia* specifically approves its external use as a poultice for boils and carbuncles and its internal use as a demulcent or laxative (Karnick, 1994). Flaxseed poultices are used for inflammations, abscesses, and relief of pain in American conventional medicine (Taber, 1962) and as an emollient in modern veterinary medicine (Budavari, 1996).

In Germany, flaxseed is usually taken as a laxative, whole or freshly crushed with water. It is also prepared as a mucilage or gruel for demulcent action. Externally it is applied as a hot moist cataplasm, compress, or poultice to reduce inflammation (ESCOP, 1997; Wichtl and Bisset, 1994). In the United States, it is used in the same way, though American consumers are more likely to take flaxseed as a component of a health food or nutraceutical product (e.g., baked goods, breads, bars, breakfast cereals, granolas).

The approved modern therapeutic applications for flaxseed are supportable based on its multi-thousand year history of clinical use in well established systems of traditional medicine, *in vitro* and *in vivo* studies in animals, nutrient composition and dietary value studies, and numerous human studies.

Recent clinical studies suggest significant potential beyond the current, well-documented uses of flaxseed. Flaxseed preparations have had experimental success as anticarcinogens (Serraino and Thompson, 1991,1992a, 1992b) and in treating lupus nephritis (Clark et al., 1995); reducing atherogenic risk in hyperlipemic patients (Bierenbaum et al., 1993) and improving arterial function in obese subjects

(Nestel et al., 1997); and positively affecting platelet composition and function (Allman et al., 1995) and nutritional health in humans (Cunnane et al., 1993).

Three animal studies showed the dietary addition of flaxseed to reduce cancer incidence in rats. In the first, test animals were given 5 or 10% flax flour supplementation to high-fat diets and researchers found mammary tissue reductions in epithelial cells (39–55%) and nuclear aberrations (59–66%) (Serraino and Thompson, 1991). In the second, test animals were injected with a carcinogen (7,12-dimethylbenz(a) anthracene) before being fed a high-fat diet mixed with 5% flax flour. Tumor size was reduced by 67% (Serraino and Thompson, 1992a). The third study used a single injection of the carcinogen azoxymethane and 5 and 10% flax flour diets and saw a 50% reduction in colon cancer. Preventative effects are apparently due to flaxseed's high levels of lignans. Other studies examined effects of pure lignans (secoisolariciresinol diglucoside) on tumor growth (Serraino and Thompson, 1992b).

One small, preliminary study reported that flaxseed supplementation may slow the progression of kidney disease associated with lupus. Nine lupus nephritis patients were enrolled, eight of whom completed the study. After the baseline studies, patients were given 15, 30, and 45 g of flaxseed/day sequentially at four-week intervals, followed by a five-week washout period. Compliance, disease activity, blood pressure, plasma lipids, rheology, PAF-induced platelet aggregation, renal function, and serum immunology were assessed. The 30 g dose performed the best. It significantly reduced total and LDL cholesterol, and blood viscosity. The 30 g/day dose was well tolerated and determined to be beneficial in terms of renal function as well as inflammatory and atherogenic mechanisms important in the pathogenesis of lupus nephritis (Clark et al., 1995).

One three-month feeding trial investigated reducing atherogenic risk with flaxseed supplementation. The researchers reported the effects on serum lipids of a flaxseed supplement consisting of three slices of flaxseed-containing bread and 15 g of ground flaxseed in 15 hyperlipemic subjects on long-term intake of vitamin E (800 IU/day). Serum total and LDL cholesterol levels were reduced significantly; HDL cholesterol did not change during flaxseed consumption. Thrombin-stimulated platelet aggregation decreased with the supplement. Serum lipid oxidation products decreased significantly during the washout period (Bierenbaum et al., 1993).

Another study investigated nutritional properties in humans ingesting high-alpha-linolenic acid flaxseed. Healthy female volunteers consumed test meals containing 50 g ground, raw flaxseed/day for four weeks, which provided 12–13% of energy intake (24–25 g/100 g total fat). The study concluded that up to 50 g high-alpha-linolenic acid flaxseed/day is palatable, safe, and may be nutritionally beneficial in humans by raising long chain n-3 fatty acids in plasma and erythrocytes and by decreasing postprandial glucose responses. The flaxseed supplementation also lowered serum total cholesterol by 9% and LDL cholesterol by 18% (Cunnane et al., 1993).

Pharmacopeial grade flaxseed is not presently defined on the basis of a specific chemical composition, but rather on a number of identity and quality tests, including organoleptic evaluation, macroscopic and microscopic authentication, and certain quantitative standards. For example, its swelling index should be not less than 4 for the whole seed and 4.5 for the powdered seed (Bruneton, 1995; Ph.Eur.3, 1997; Ph.Fr.X, 1990; Tu, 1992; Wichtl and Bisset, 1994).

Description

Flaxseed consists of the dried, ripe seed of the collective variations of *Linum usitatissimum* L. [Fam. Linaceae], as well as its preparations in effective dosage. The cultivars of *L. usitatissimum* (L.) Vav. et Ell. are equally acceptable for the indications listed in this monograph. The seeds contain: fiber (hemicellulose, cellulose, and lignin), fatty oil with 52–76% linolenic acid esters, albumin, linustatin, and linamarin.

Chemistry and Pharmacology

Flaxseed contains fixed oil (30–45%); triglycerides of linolenic, linoleic, oleic, stearic, palmitic, and myristic acids; proteins (20–25%); mucilage (3–10%), composed of neutral and acidic polysaccharides which after hydrolysis yield galactose (8–10%), arabinose (9–12%), rhamnose (13–29%), xylose (25–27%), and galacturonic and mannuronic acids (approx. 30%); sterols and triterpenes (cholesterol, campesterol, stigmasterol, and sitosterol); cyanogenic glycosides (0.1–1.5%), mostly linustatin and neolinustatin and the monoglycosides linamarin and lotaustralin; and secoisolariciresinol glycoside (a precursor of lignans in mammals) (Bruneton, 1995; Budavari, 1996; ESCOP, 1997; Wichtl and Bissett, 1994).

The Commission E reported laxative effects due to increase in volume and consequent initiation of intestinal peristalsis due to stretching reflexes. A protective effect on the mucosa has been observed because of flaxseed's coating action.

The *British Herbal Pharmacopoeia* reported its actions as bulk-forming laxative and demulcent (BHP, 1996). A decrease in transit time and increase of stool weight in patients suffering from constipation was demonstrated in two multicentric studies (ESCOP, 1997). Linseed binds with water and swells to form a demulcent gel in the intestine, thus softening the feces and increasing the volume of the bowel content (ESCOP, 1997).

In a recent overview of clinical trials, flaxseed's high levels of α-linolenic acid, an essential fatty acid, and the lignan secoisolariciresinol diglucoside (SDG) are suggested as anti-carcinogenic and as beneficial in treating systemic lupus erythematosus (SLE), hyperlipidemia, and perhaps malaria and rheumatoid arthritis. Flaxseed contains more (between 75 and 800 times) of the beneficial phytochemical SDG when compared to other food sources (Haggerty, 1999).

Uses

The Commission E approved the internal use of flaxseed for chronic constipation, for colons damaged by abuse of laxatives, irritable colon, diverticulitis, and as mucilage for gastritis and enteritis. External use is approved as a cataplasm for local inflammation.

ESCOP reports its internal use for constipation, irritable bowel syndrome, diverticular disease and for symptomatic short-term treatment of gastritis and enteritis, and external use for painful skin inflammations (ESCOP, 1997). The German Standard License for whole or freshly crushed linseed lists it as a bulk laxative for the treatment of constipation and functional bowel complaints (irritable colon) and as a demulcent preparation for the supportive treatment of inflammatory gastrointestinal complaints (Wichtl and Bisset, 1994). *The Merck Index* indicates its use externally as an emollient (Budavari, 1996). Its mucilage content justifies its use like psyllium seed, as an adjunctive therapy for pains related to spasmodic colitis (Bruneton, 1995).

Popular herbal use of flaxseed includes coughs, sore throats, hardening of the arteries, and rheumatoid arthritis. External indications include abscesses, ulcers, and, when mixed with white mustard seeds, a poultice for chest complaints (Bown, 1995).

Contraindications

Ileus of any origin.

Side Effects

If directions are observed, i.e., especially if the concomitant administration of sufficient amounts of liquid (1:10) is observed, there are no known side effects.

Use During Pregnancy and Lactation

No restrictions known.

Interactions with Other Drugs

As with any other mucilage, the absorption of other drugs may be negatively affected.

Dosage and Administration

Internal: Unless otherwise prescribed: As seed, as cracked or coarsely ground seed, in which only the cuticle and mucilage epidermis are damaged; as flaxseed mucilage (gruel) and other galenical preparations.

Bruised or whole seed: Take 1 tablespoon whole or "bruised" seed (not ground) with 150 ml of liquid two to three times daily. [Note: 1 tablespoon = 10 g seed].

Mucilage (gruel): Soak 2–3 tablespoons of milled flaxseed in 200–300 ml water, strain after 30 minutes.

External: Unless otherwise prescribed: As flaxseed flour or flaxseed expellent.

Cataplasm: Semi-solid paste containing 30–50 g flaxseed flour for a moist-heat direct application to the skin used like a poultice as a counterirritant drawing blood to the surface to remove deep-seated inflammation.

Note: Flaxseed meal is traditionally mixed with mustard seed powder in this application.

Compress or fomentation: Saturate a stupe with hot semi-solid preparation containing 30–50 g flaxseed flour; fold and apply firmly for a moist-heat direct application to the skin to relieve pain or inflammation.

References

Allman, M.A., M.M. Pena, D. Pang. 1995. Supplementation with flaxseed oil versus sunflowerseed oil in healthy young men consuming a low fat diet: effects on platelet composition and function. *Eur J Clin Nutr* 49(3):169–178.

Bierenbaum, M.L., R. Reichstein, T.R. Watkins. 1993. Reducing atherogenic risk in hyperlipemic humans with flax seed supplementation: a preliminary report. *J Am Coll Nutr* 12(5):501–504.

Bown, D. 1995. *Encyclopedia of Herbs and Their Uses.* New York: DK Publishing, Inc. 304.

British Herbal Pharmacopoeia (BHP). 1996. Exeter, U.K.: British Herbal Medicine Association.

Bruneton, J. 1995. *Pharmacognosy, Phytochemistry, Medicinal Plants.* Paris: Lavoisier Publishing.

Budavari, S. (ed.). 1996. *The Merck Index: An Encyclopedia of Chemicals, Drugs, and Biologicals,* 12th ed. Whitehouse Station, N.J.: Merck & Co, Inc.

Carlson, C. 1998. The Benefits of Flax. *Herbs for Health* Sept/Oct:63–65.

Clark, W.F. et al. 1995. Flaxseed: A potential treatment of lupus nephritis. *Kidney Int* 48(2):475–480.

Cunnane, S.C. et al. 1993. High alpha-linolenic acid flaxseed (*Linum usitatissimum*): some nutritional properties in humans. *Br J Nutr* 69(2):443–453.

ESCOP. 1997. "Lini semen." *Monographs on the Medicinal Uses of Plant Drugs.* Exeter, U.K.: European Scientific Cooperative on Phytotherapy.

Europäisches Arzneibuch, 3rd ed. (Ph.Eur.3). 1997. Stuttgart: Deutscher Apotheker Verlag.

Grieve, M. 1979. *A Modern Herbal.* New York: Dover Publications, Inc.

Haggerty, W. 1999. *Flax: Ancient Herb and Modern Medicine. HerbalGram* 45:51–56.

Kapoor, L.D. 1990. *Handbook of Ayurvedic Medicinal Plants.* Boca Raton: CRC Press. 217.

Karnick, C.R. 1994. *Pharmacopoeial Standards of Herbal Plants,* Vols. 1–2. Delhi: Sri Satguru Publications. Vol. 1:228–229; Vol. 2:55

Nadkarni, K.M. 1976. *Indian Materia Medica.* Bombay: Popular Prakashan. 743–746.

Nestel, P.J. et al. 1997. Arterial compliance in obese subjects is improved with dietary plant n-3 fatty acid from flaxseed oil despite increased LDL oxidizability. *Arterioscler Thromb Vasc Biol* 17(6):1163–1170.

Ph.Eur.3. See *Europäisches Arzneibuch.*

Pharmacopée Française Xe Édition (Ph.Fr.X.). 1983–1990. Moulins-les-Metz: Maisonneuve S.A.

Serraino, M. and L.U. Thompson. 1991. The effect of flaxseed supplementation on early risk markers for mammary carcinogenesis. *Cancer Lett* 60(2):135–142.

———. 1992a. The effect of flaxseed supplementation on the initiation and promotional stages of mammary tumorigenesis. *Nutr Cancer* 17(2):153–159.

————. 1992b. Flaxseed supplementation and early markers of colon carcinogenesis. *Cancer Lett* 63(2):159–165.

Taber, C.W. 1962. *Taber's Cyclopedic Medical Dictionary*, 9th ed. Philadelphia: F.A. Davis Company. F-21.

Tu, G. (ed.). 1992. *Pharmacopoeia of the People's Republic of China* (English Edition 1992). Beijing: Guangdong Science and Technology Press.

Wichtl, M. and N.G. Bisset (eds.). 1994. *Herbal Drugs and Phytopharmaceuticals*. Stuttgart: Medpharm Scientific Publishers.

Yen, K.Y. 1992. *The Illustrated Chinese Materia Medica—Crude and Prepared*. Taipei: SMC Publishing, Inc. 174.

Additional Resources

Cunnane, S.C. et al. 1995. Nutritional attributes of traditional flaxseed in healthy young adults. *Am J Clin Nutr* 61(1):62–68.

Gilman, A.G., T.W. Rall, A.S. Nies, P. Taylor (eds.). 1990. *The Pharmacological Basis of Therapeutics*. New York: Pergamon Press. 915–918.

Jenab, M. and L.U. Thompson. 1996. The influence of flaxseed and lignans on colon carcinogenesis and beta-glucuronidase activity. *Carcinogenesis* 17(6):1343–1348.

Jens, R., R. Nitsch-Fitz, H. Wutzl, H. Maruna. 1981. Ergebnisse einer Praxisstudie mit einer Leinsamen-Kombination zur Behebung der chronischen Obstipation bei 114 Patienten aus dem Raum Wien. *Der Praktische Arzt* 35:80.

Kurth, W. 1976. Therapeutische Wirksamkeit, Verträglichkeit und Akzeptabilität von Linusit in der Praxis. *Der Kassenarzt* 16:3546.

McGuffin, M., C. Hobbs, R. Upton, A. Goldberg. 1997. American Herbal Product Association's *Botanical Safety Handbook*. Boca Raton: CRC Press.

Obermeyer, W.R., C. Warner, R.E. Casey, S.M. Musser. 1993. Flaxseed lignans. Isolation, metabolism and biological effects (Abstract 4985). *Experimental Biol* 93

Obermeyer, W.R. et al. 1995. Chemical studies of phytoestrogens and related compounds in dietary supplements: flax and chaparral (43824). *Proc Soc Exp Biol Med* 208(1):6–12.

Schilcher, H. 1979. Zyanidvergiftung durch Leinsamen? *Dtsch Ärzteblatt* 76:955–956.

Schilcher, H. and A. Nissler. 1980. Pflanzliche Öle—ihre Analytik und diätetische Verwendung. *Phys Med u Reh* 21:141–156.

Schilcher, H, V. Schulz, A. Nissler. 1986. Zur Wirksamkeit und Toxikologie von Semen Lini. *Z Phytotherapie* 7:113–117.

Schilcher, H. and M. Wilkens-Sauter. 1986. Quantitative Bestimmung cyanogener Glykoside in *Linum usitatissimum* mit Hilfe der HPLC. *Fette Seifen Anstrichmittel* 88:287–290.

Steinegger, E. and R. Hänsel. 1988. *Lehrbuch der Pharmakognosie und Phytopharmazie*, 4th ed. Berlin-Heidelberg: Springer Verlag.128–129.

Thompson, L.U., P. Robb, M. Serraino, F. Cheung. 1991. Mammalian lignan production from various foods. *Nutr Cancer* 16(1):43–52.

Thompson, L.U. et al. 1996. Flaxseed and its lignan and oil components reduce mammary tumor growth at a late stage of carcinogenesis. *Carcinogenesis* 17(6):1373–1376.

Wagner, H., W. Budweg, M.A. Iyengar, O. Volk, M. Sinn. 1972. Linosid A und B, zwei neue flavon-C-glykoside aus Linum maritimum [Linoside A and B, two new flavone-C-glycosides from *Linum maritimum* L]. *Z Naturforsch B* 27(7):809–812.

Wagner, H. 1980. *Pharmazeutische Biologie*, Vol. 2. Drogen und ihre Inhaltsstoffe. Stuttgart-New York: Gustav Fischer. 261–262.

Weiss, R.F. 1991. *Lehrbuch der Phytotherapie*, 7th ed. Stuttgart: Hippokrates.131–133.

Weiss, S.G., M. Tin-Wa, R.E. Perdue, N.R. Farnsworth. 1975. Potential anticancer agents II: antitumor and cytotoxic lignans from *Linum album* (Linaceae). *J Pharm Sci* 64(1):95–98.

Willuhn, G. 1989. *Teedrogen*, 2nd ed. Stuttgart: Wissenschaftliche Verlagsgesellschaft. 306–308.

Yan, L., J.A. Yee, D. Li, M.H. McGuire, L.U. Thompson. 1998. Dietary flaxseed supplementation and experimental metastasis of melanoma cells in mice. *Cancer Lett* 124(2):181–186.

This material was adapted from *The Complete German Commission E Monographs—Therapeutic Guide to Herbal Medicines*. M. Blumenthal, W.R. Busse, A. Goldberg, J. Gruenwald, T. Hall, C.W. Riggins, R.S. Rister (eds.) S. Klein and R.S. Rister (trans.). 1998. Austin: American Botanical Council; Boston: Integrative Medicine Communications.

1) The Overview section is new information.

2) Description, Chemistry and Pharmacology, Uses, Contraindications, Side Effects, Interactions with Other Drugs, and Dosage sections have been drawn from the original work. Additional information has been added in all or some of these sections, as noted with references.

3) The dosage for equivalent preparations (tea infusion, fluidextract, and tincture) have been provided based on the following example:

Unless otherwise prescribed: 2 g per day of [powdered, crushed, cut or whole] [plant part]
Infusion: 2 g in 150 ml of water
Fluidextract 1:1 (g/ml): 2 ml
Tincture 1:5 (g/ml): 10 ml

4) The References and Additional Resources sections are new sections. Additional Resources are not cited in the monograph but are included for research purposes.

GARLIC

Latin Name:
Allium sativum

Pharmacopeial Name:
Allii sativi bulbus

Other Names:
garlic clove

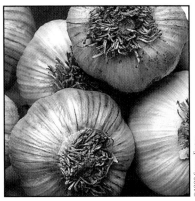

© 1999 Steven Foster

Overview

In the United States and Western Europe, garlic is one of the most popular substances used to reduce various risks associated with cardiovascular disease. Most of its popularity is based on the herb's strong folkloric familiarity and awareness that scientist research suggests cardiovascular benefits associated with ingestion of the herb as a conventional food and as a dietary supplement.

Uses for garlic and its preparations cover cardiovascular effects (lipid, blood pressure and blood sugar lowering, and fibrinolytic activity); chemoprevention; antimicrobial, antifungal, antiprotozoal, and antioxidant activities; and immunologic activity, among others. By 1996 there were at least 1,808 scientific studies (chemical, pharmacological, clinical, and epidemiological) investigating the activities of garlic. Pharmacological and clinical studies have been published in the following areas: antimicrobial effects (252 pharmacological/35 clinical), anticancer effects (221/2, plus 10 epidemiological studies), effect on blood sugar levels (28/3), immune stimulation (15/3), anti-inflammatory (11/1), and antioxidant (60/4), as well as additional studies researching other areas (Lawson, 1998a). In the areas of cardiovascular effects, the studies break down as follows: blood lipids (179/62, plus 2 epidemiological studies), blood pressure (78/18), blood fibrinolysis, coagulation, and flow (51/18), platelet aggregation (76/6), and atherosclerosis (23/2) (Lawson, 1998a). A comprehensive and detailed review of the therapeutic aspects of garlic and its preparations is provided in a recent book dealing with the history, chemistry, and medical aspects of the herb (Koch and Lawson, 1996). Numerous studies are outlined—all conducted on garlic as a food or in dietary supplement or pharmaceutical preparations. Also cited are 9 epidemiological studies correlating cancer prevention and garlic consumption as food.

Clinical studies conducted on garlic to measure cardiovascular effects have been performed with both healthy persons and patients with hyperlipidemia and hypercholesterolemia. In recognition of the clinical trials suggesting the low-density lipoprotein (LDL) cholesterol-lowering ability of garlic preparations, garlic received a positive evaluation by the Commission E. Garlic is the subject of a monograph by the European Scientific Cooperative on Phytotherapy (ESCOP), a western European group of scientists developing harmonized drug monographs on phytomedicines for the European Union (ESCOP, 1997). Additionally, the World Health Organization (WHO) has prepared a monograph on standards and therapeutic uses of garlic (WHO, 1999). (See Uses section, below.)

Meta-analyses of clinical trials have documented its use for lowering cholesterol in hyperlipidemia (Silagy and Neil, 1994a; Warshafsky et al., 1993) and in treating hypertension (Silagy and Neil, 1994b). Another study has investigated garlic's effectiveness in treating peripheral arterial occlusive disease, as measured by pain-free walking distance (Kiesewetter et al., 1993b). Research on garlic treatment for hyperlipidemic pediatric patients, however, has yielded insignificant results (McCrindle et al., 1998). Garlic has also been shown to be effective in respiratory infections and catarrhal conditions (Bradley, 1992; ESCOP, 1997).

The primary objective of a significant number (104) of clinical trials conducted on garlic has been to evaluate its ability to regulate serum lipid levels, i.e., total cholesterol (TC), and in particular, LDL cholesterol. There is much evidence to support such an application. The influence of garlic on atherogenic LDL has been investigated in at least 9 clinical studies, with 7 reporting a significant decrease (mean decrease of 16%) (Koch and Lawson, 1996).

In 40 studies that investigated the effect of various garlic preparations on the TC levels of 43 groups of patients and volunteers, the mean decrease in serum choles-terol levels was 10.6%, with the treatment lasting from three weeks to several months. The 13 placebo-controlled studies with alliin/allicin-standardized garlic powder tablets on 427 treatment patients showed an average decrease of 10.3%. Serum triglyceride levels were also measured in 32 of the 40 studies, with an aver-age decrease of 13.4%—the 12 placebo-controlled studies with garlic powder tablets resulted in an 8.5% decrease in the 406 treatment patients. Most European clinical trials measuring cardiovascular activity of garlic used garlic powder tablets (the German brand Kwai®, Lichtwer Pharma, Berlin), which has long been stan-dardized on 1.3/0.6% of the alliin/allicin-yield (Brown, 1996; Koch and Lawson, 1996).

Two meta-analyses have analyzed the results of clinical studies on the effect of garlic on serum TC (Warshafsky et al., 1993; Silagy and Neil, 1994a). They indi-cated that over a one- to three-month period, the administration of garlic powder in a dietary supplement form (tablets: usually 100 mg each; dosage: 600–900 mg daily) resulted in an average reduction in serum TC of 9 to 12% (range, 6 to 21%); triglyceride levels fell from 8 to 27%, mean 13% (Silagy and Neil, 1994a).

The goal of the Warshafsky study was to assess the range and consistency of gar-lic's effect on serum TC in persons with cholesterol levels greater than 5.17 mmol/l (200 mg/dl). Five of 28 clinical trials were selected for review; all were randomized and placebo-controlled, with at least 75% of the patients having cholesterol levels greater than 200 mg/dl. Patients treated with garlic consistently showed a greater decrease in TC levels than those receiving placebo. Meta-analysis of homogeneous trials estimated a net cholesterol decrease attributable to garlic of 0.59 mmol/l. The study concluded that the best available evidence suggests that garlic, in an amount approximating one-half to one clove per day, decreased serum TC levels by about 9% in the groups of patients studied (Warshafsky et al., 1993).

To determine the effect of garlic on serum lipids and lipoproteins relative to placebo or to other lipid-lowering agents, the Silagy and Neil meta-analysis reviewed randomized, controlled trials of garlic preparations of at least 4 weeks duration. Sixteen trials with data from 952 subjects were included. The mean dif-ference in reduction of TC between garlic-treated subjects and those receiving placebo (or avoiding garlic in their diet) was –0.77 mmol/l. These changes repre-sent a 12% reduction with garlic therapy beyond the final levels achieved with placebo alone. In the commercial preparations made from dried garlic powders, in which the allicin yield is purportedly standardized, there was no significant differ-ence in the size of the reduction across the dose range of 600–900 mg daily. Dried garlic powder preparations also significantly lowered serum triglyceride by 0.31 mmol/l compared to placebo (Silagy and Neil, 1994a).

A 12-week study compared the effect of standardized garlic powder tablets (Kwai®) with that of bezafibrate, the most commonly prescribed blood lipid-lower-ing drug in Germany (Holzgartner et al., 1992). This multicenter, double-blind study involved 98 patients with primary hyperlipoproteinemia, and cholesterol and/or triglyceride values exceeding 250 mg/dl. The daily doses of the active sub-stances were 900 mg of garlic powder (standardized to 1.3% alliin) and 600 mg of bezafibrate, respectively. In the course of the treatment, decreases in TC, LDL choles-terol, and triglyceride levels were statistically significant, with no differences between the effects of garlic and bezafibrate. High-density lipoprotein (HDL) cholesterol val-ues also increased significantly, with no differences between the two regimens.

However, a dissenting 12-week randomized, double-blind, placebo-controlled, parallel treatment study could not confirm previous reports that standardized garlic powder tablets (Kwai®) were effective in lowering cholesterol levels in patients with hypercholesterolemia. Twenty-eight patients received 300 mg of Kwai® three times daily for 12 weeks. There were no significant lipid or lipoprotein changes in either the placebo- or garlic-treated groups and no significant difference between changes in the placebo-treated group compared with changes in the garlic-treated patients (Isaacsohn et al., 1998).

An eight-week randomized, double-blind, placebo-controlled clinical trial again disputed garlic as therapy for hypercholesterolemia by concluding that Kwai® had no significant effect on cardiovascular risk factors in pediatric patients with familial hyperlipidemia. The 30 hypercholesterolemic children were given 300 mg of Kwai® three times daily for eight weeks and tested for absolute and relative changes in fasting lipid parameters. Researchers found no significant reduction attributable to garlic extract therapy in cardiovascular risk factors, with the excep-tion of a small increase in apolipoprotein A-I levels. Authors note that adult studies have yielded positive results. It is management of hyperlipidemia in children that remains controversial (McCrindle et al., 1998).

A likely reason for the failure of these two trials (Isaacsohn et al., 1998 and McCrindle et al., 1998) to show an effect on serum cholesterol while many prior studies with the same brand (Kwai®) gave positive effects is that the Kwai® tablets used in these negative studies appear to have released only one-third as much allicin as the Kwai® tablets used in older trials under simulated gastrointestinal con-ditions, as has been shown with Kwai® tablets made at the same time as the trials were conducted (Lawson, 1998c).

In a study that received significant media attention, 25 patients with moderate hypercholesterolemia were studied in a randomized, double-blind, placebo-con-trolled trial (Berthold et al., 1998). Five mg of steam-distilled garlic oil preparation (Tegra®, Hermes, Munich, Germany) was given to patients twice daily for 12 weeks. The product studied did not influence serum lipoproteins, cholesterol absorption, or cholesterol synthesis and the authors concluded that garlic cannot be recommended for hypercholesterolemia. This study was criticized for using garlic oil bound to β-cyclodextrin to form a solid slow-release tablet, which was found to greatly reduce the total absorption of the garlic oil compared to liquid oil. Thus, the results of this trial are not applicable to other forms of garlic (Lawson, 1998b).

A six-week randomized, placebo-controlled, double-blind study investigated the efficacy of a standardized garlic powder preparation (brands Kwai® and Sapec®, 900 mg daily) on alimentary hypertriglyceridemia after intake of a standardized fatty test meal containing 100 g of butter (Rotzsch et al., 1992). (Sapec® is also made by Lichtwer. It is the same material as Kwai®, but in a larger tablet, 300 mg compared to 100 mg for Kwai®.) The 24 volunteers had low plasma HDL2-choles-terol concentrations of less than 10 mg/dl (men) and 15 mg/dl (women). Control measurements were made on the 1st, 22nd, and 43rd day of treatment, at 0, 3, and 15 hours after the meal. The increase in plasma triglycerides was reduced by up to 35% after garlic consumption in comparison with the placebo group. The regular intake of the garlic preparation over the six weeks also showed a significant lower-ing of the fasting values of triglycerides in comparison to placebo.

In another study using brands Kwai® and Sapec®, the effect of standardized gar-lic powder tablets in the treatment of hyperlipidemia was investigated (Mader, 1990). This multicenter, placebo-controlled, randomized study had 261 patients with TC and/or triglyceride values more than 200 mg/dl. Patients were given a daily dose of 800 mg (standardized to 1.3% of alliin content) for 16 weeks. There was a 12% decrease in mean serum cholesterol levels, and a 17% decrease in mean triglyceride values.

In one of only two trials on garlic conducted in the United States, researchers assessed the effects of standardized garlic powder tablets (Kwai®) on serum lipids and lipoproteins, glucose, and blood pressure (Jain et al., 1993). Forty-two healthy adult patients, with a serum TC level of 220 mg/dl or greater, received a daily dose of 900 mg or placebo. After 12 weeks of treatment, the baseline serum TC level of 262 mg/dl was reduced to 247 mg/dl. The placebo group went from 276 to 274 mg/dl. LDL cholesterol was reduced 11% by garlic treatment and 3% by placebo. The study concluded that treatment with standardized garlic (900 mg/day) produced a significantly greater reduction in serum TC and LDL cholesterol than placebo.

In addition to the cholesterol-lowering action documented above, other clinical studies conducted on garlic preparations have examined their effects on plaque-reduction and blood pressure lowering actions (Auer et al., 1990), as well as on garlic's reputed antibiotic, anticancer, antioxidant, and immunomodulatory effects (Brown, 1996; Koch and Lawson, 1996). Other clinical studies have concluded that garlic is helpful in lessening pain in patients with intermittent claudication (Kiesewetter et al., 1993b).

In the longest clinical trial on garlic to date, garlic's ability to prevent and possibly reverse atherosclerosis was tested in a randomized, double-blind, placebo-controlled, four-year study in which 152 men and women were given 900 mg garlic powder as tablets (Kwai®) per day (Koscielny et al., 1999). The subjects were chosen because they possessed significant plaque buildup and at least one additional cardiovascular risk factor (e.g., high LDL cholesterol levels, hypertension, diabetes, and/or history of smoking). Increased plaque volume is correlated with increased risk of heart attack or stroke. The amount of plaque in both carotid and femoral arteries was determined by ultrasound and was shown to be reduced over the four year period, as measured at 16, 36, and 48 months. After the four years, those in the garlic group had an average 2.6% reduction in plaque volume while the plaque in the placebo group increased 15.6%. Researchers concluded: "These results substantiated that not only a preventive but possibly also a curative role in arteriosclerosis therapy (plaque regression) may be ascribed to garlic remedies."

In a Danish multicenter study on Kwai® garlic tablets the effects of the tablets on blood lipids and blood pressure were measured. A total of 48 patients (with TC levels over 6.5 mmol/l) were treated with a daily dose of 600 mg (standardized on 1.3% alliin, equal to 0.6% allicin) for a period of 18 weeks. Mean serum cholesterol levels dropped 8%. LDL cholesterol dropped 5% while HDL cholesterol rose 5%. These changes improved the HDL-LDL cholesterol ratio 12%, from 6.6 to 5.9. Also, triglyceride levels were reduced by 11%. Of the patients, 23 with mild hypertension (diastolic blood pressure greater than 95 mmHg) showed reductions in both systolic and diastolic blood pressure. Systolic blood pressure dropped 7%, from 158 to 147 mmHg, while diastolic blood pressure dropped 4%, from 96 to 92 mmHg (Grünwald et al., 1992).

One hypertension study found that when 47 non-hospitalized patients with mild hypertension were administered either 600 mg of a garlic powder preparation or placebo for 12 weeks, after 8 weeks blood pressure was significantly reduced from 171/102 mmHg to 155/91 mmHg (Auer et al., 1990). A double-blind, placebo-controlled study of 60 patients with constantly elevated spontaneous platelet aggregation who were given 800 mg of a standardized garlic powder preparation for four weeks, resulted in the reduction of the spontaneous platelet aggregation by 56.3% with no significant change in the placebo group (Kiesewetter et al., 1992 in Koch and Lawson , 1996).

A double-blind crossover study comparing the effect of an odorless, aged garlic extract (AGE, Wakunaga, Japan) to a placebo on blood lipids was performed on a group of 41 moderately hypercholesteremic men (220–290 mg/dl). After a four-week baseline period in which the subjects were told to maintain a National Cholesterol Education Program Step I diet, the verum group was given 7.2 g of AGE (capsules: 800 mg each; dosage: 9 capsules daily) for six months. The garlic and placebo group then crossed over for four months without a washout period. TC levels were lowered 6.1 or 7.0% compared to placebo period or baseline, respectively. LDL cholesterol was decreased by 4.0% compared to average baseline values and 4.6% compared to placebo period levels. There was also a 5.5% decrease in systolic blood pressure and "modest" reduction of diastolic pressure in the AGE group (Steiner et al., 1996).

Regarding anticancer effects, epidemiological evidence suggests the possibility that garlic and other members of the genus *Allium* can reduce incidence of risk of certain types of cancer. In their comprehensive book on garlic, Koch and Lawson (1996) cite at least 15 statistical studies and review articles that correlate garlic consumption to low cancer rates in Europe, Egypt, India, China, and other Third World countries "where the favorable effects of garlic for cancer are well known" (Koch and Lawson, 1996). They also include data from 10 epidemiological studies on cancer and consumption of raw or cooked garlic cloves. Two comparison studies in China concluded that dietary garlic inhibited formation of carcinogenic nitroso compounds (Mei et al., 1982). Another study involving 564 patients with stomach cancer and 1,131 controls in an area of China with a high incidence of gastric cancer revealed a significant reduction in stomach cancer risk with increased consumption of *Allium* vegetables (garlic, onions, leeks, shallots, and chives) (You et al., 1989).

By the end of 1996, of the 221 anticancer studies conducted on garlic, 72 had been conducted on fresh whole garlic (including the 10 epidemiological studies), 82 had been conducted with the allyl sulfides (garlic oil components), and 19 had been conducted on AGE. This garlic preparation is processed in a proprietary manner to produce a chemically distinct product that does not contain these intermediate sulfur-based compounds (e.g., allicin), which tend to further decompose into other sulfur compounds. AGE is the material formerly used for research by the National Cancer Institute for its Designer Foods Program. By 1996 there were at least 90 research papers and meeting abstracts published on various aspects of AGE (Koch and Lawson, 1996).

U.S. pharmacopeial grade garlic consists of the fresh or dried compound bulbs of *Allium sativum* L. It must contain not less than 0.5% alliin, as determined by liquid chromatography, calculated on a dry weight basis. Botanical identity must be confirmed by a thin-layer chromatography (TLC) test as well as macroscopic and microscopic examinations. USP powdered garlic consists of garlic that has been cut, freeze-dried or dried at a temperature not greater than 65° C, then powdered. It must contain not less than 0.3% alliin, calculated on the dried basis (USP 24–NF 19, 1999). The difference in values reflects a potential loss of 40% of the alliin due to the powdering process. European pharmacopeial grade garlic powder has identity and purity test requirements closely comparable to the USP monograph, though it must *yield* (does not *contain*) not less than 0.45% allicin calculated with reference to the dried drug (Ph.Eur., 1999). The ESCOP garlic powder monograph requires that the material comply with the quality requirements of the *European Pharmacopoeia* (ESCOP, 1997). The *British Herbal Pharmacopoeia* contains separate quantitative standards for powdered garlic from Egypt and from China. Powdered garlic from Egypt is typically produced from the entire bulbs (cloves, skins, and roots). It may contain not more than 12% total ash and must contain not less than 70% water-soluble extractive, calculated with reference to the oven-dried material. Powdered garlic from China, however, is typically produced from the cloves only (skins peeled). It may contain not more than 5% total ash and must contain not less than 80% water-soluble extractive (BHP, 1996). The *Ghana Herbal Pharmacopoeia* includes a monograph for the fresh, whole, intact garlic bulb for manufacture of an alcoholic tincture preparation (GHP, 1992).

Description

Garlic, fresh or carefully dried, consists of the main bulb with several secondary bulbs (cloves) of *A. sativum* L. [Fam. Alliaceae] and its preparations in effective dosage. Garlic contains alliin and its transformation products and sulfur-containing essential oil.

Chemistry and Pharmacology

Garlic contains a large number of compounds, but only the thiosulfinates (allicin) have been found to have significant activity at levels representing normal garlic consumption (3–5 g/day). Allicin has been shown to be essential to most of the antimicrobial and hypocholesterolemic effects of garlic and probably to most of the antithrombotic and antioxidant effects. The anticancer effects appear to be shared about equally between allicin and other unidentified compounds (Lawson, 1998a).

Garlic contains about 1% alliin, which converts to allicin in the presence of the enzyme alliinase (ESCOP, 1997). Pharmacological research on garlic has shown for the thiosulfinates free radical scavenging, inhibition of lipid peroxidation (Harris et al., 1995; Phelps and Harris, 1993), inhibition of platelet aggregation (Barrie et al., 1987; Kiesewetter et al., 1993a), stimulation of fibrinolysis (Kiesewetter et al., 1990), and reduction of serum cholesterol and lipid levels Brosche et al., 1990; Bordia, 1981; Jain et al,., Mader, 1990; Rotzsch et al., 1992).

Garlic bulbs contain about 65% water, 28% carbohydrates (mainly fructans), 2.3% organosulfur compounds, 2% protein (mainly alliinase), 1.2% free amino acids (mainly arginine), 1.5% fiber, 0.15% lipids, and small amounts of phytic acid (0.08%), saponins (0.07%), and β-sitosterol (0.0015%). No vitamin or mineral are sufficiently abundant to meet 2% of the U.S. RDA for a 3–5 g clove. The main organosulphur compounds in whole garlic are the S-(+)-alkyl-L-cysteine sulfoxides [alliin (1%), methiin (0.12%), isoalliin (0.06%), and cycloalliin (0.1%)] and the γ-L-glutamyl-S-alkyl-L-cysteines [γ-glutamyl-S-trans-1-propenylcysteine (0.6%) and γ-glutamyl-S-allylcysteine (0.4%)]. Upon disrupting the cells by bruising, crushing, chewing, or mincing the bulb, the enzyme alliinase comes into contact with the amino acid alliin, causing its rapid transformation into allylsulphenic acid, and subsequent conversion to allicin. One mg of alliin produces 0.458 mg of allicin. Allicin potentially becomes the main precursor of various other transformation compounds found in commercially produced garlic oils, such as allyl sulfides, ajoenes, and vinyldithiins, depending on the method of processing (Lawson 1998a, Block, 1985; Bradley, 1992; Budavari, 1996; ESCOP, 1997).

According to some chemical reviews, aging garlic to produce the odorless aged garlic extract (AGE) reduces the content of all sulfur compounds. Thus, AGE contains 3% of the alliin and 6% of the γ-glutamylcysteines found in fresh garlic. Its most abundant sulfur compound is S-allylcysteine, representing about 21% of the γ-glutamyl-S-allyl-cysteine from which it is derived (Lawson, 1998a).

The Commission E reported antibacterial, antimycotic, lipid-lowering, inhibiting of platelet aggregation, prolonging of bleeding and clotting time, and enhancing of fibrinolytic activity. *In vitro* and *in vivo* animal studies have also demonstrated garlic's ability to inhibit tumor formation (Belman, 1983; Weisberger and Pensky, 1958) and reduce blood pressure (Elbl, 1991; Koch, 1992). Garlic powder, fresh garlic, aged garlic, and garlic oil have been found to exhibit anti-aggregative, antibacterial, antimycotic, antiviral, and antihepatotoxic action *in vitro* and *in vivo*. Other *in vitro* studies have concluded that garlic possesses direct anti-atherosclerosis effects and inhibition of cholesterol biosynthesis by allicin and ajoene. *In vivo* studies in animals have concluded that garlic powder, fresh garlic, and garlic oil reduced experimentally induced hyperlipidemia and atherosclerosis (ESCOP, 1997). Gamma-glutamylpeptides, scordinins, steroids, triterpenoids, flavonoids, and fructans also possess pharmacological activity and are believed to contribute to these hypotensive and anticancer effects (Koch and Lawson, 1996). (Despite extensive and persistent popular beliefs in Transylvania and Wallachia (Romania), both the Commission E and the editors of this volume were unable to document scientific data to confirm the anti-vampiral activity of garlic.)

Uses

Commission E approved the use of garlic as a support to dietary measures at elevated levels of lipids in the blood and as a preventive measure for age-dependent vascular changes.

Based on clinical studies, ESCOP recognizes the following indications for garlic: "Prophylaxis of atherosclerosis. Treatment of elevated blood lipid levels insufficiently influenced by diet. Improvement of blood flow in arterial vascular disease" (ESCOP, 1997). ESCOP also noted that garlic has been used traditionally for relief of cough, colds, catarrh, and rhinitis, although clinical trials are not as abundant to support such uses.

WHO notes in the "Uses supported by clinical data" section of its garlic monograph: "As an adjuvant to dietetic management in the treatment of hyperlipidaemia, and in the prevention of atherosclerotic (age-dependent) vascular changes. The drug may be useful in the treatment of mild hypertension" (WHO, 1999).

Contraindications

The Commission E reported that none were known. Some sources suggest that substantial amounts of garlic should not be consumed prior to surgery, since it can prolong bleeding time (Burnham, 1995). WHO notes that garlic is contraindicated in those individuals who have a known allergy to garlic (WHO, 1999).

Side Effects

In rare instances there may be gastrointestinal symptoms, changes to the flora of the intestine, or allergic reactions. Note: The odor of garlic may pervade the breath and skin.

Use During Pregnancy and Lactation

Not recommended during lactation (Chadha, 1988; McGuffin et al., 1997).

Interactions with Other Drugs

In 1988, Commission E reported that none were known. ESCOP notes that "none [are] reported" (ESCOP, 1997). Garlic consumption substantially increases the anticoagulant effects of warfarin (Sunter, 1991). WHO notes that, "Patients with on warfarin therapy should be warned that garlic supplements may increase bleeding times. Blood clotting times have been reported to double in patients taking warfarin and garlic supplements" (WHO, 1999).

Dosage and Administration

Internal:
Unless otherwise prescribed: 4 g per day of fresh, minced garlic bulb.
Infusion: 4 g in 150 ml of water.
Fluidextract 1:1 (g/ml): 4 ml.
Tincture 1:5 (g/ml): 20 ml.

References

Auer, W. et al. 1990. Hypertension and hyperlipi-daemia: garlic helps in mild cases. *Br J Clin Pract Suppl* 44(suppl.69):3–6.

Barrie, S.A., J.V. Wright, J.E. Pizzorono. 1987. Effects of garlic oil on platelet aggregation, serum lipids and blood pressure in humans. *J Orthomolec Med* 2:15–21.

Belman, S. 1983. Onion and garlic oils inhibit tumor promotion. *Carcinogenesis* 4(8):1063–1065.

Berthold, H.K., T. Sudhop, K. von Bergmann. 1998. Effect of a garlic oil preparation on serum lipoproteins and cholesterol metabolism: a ran-domized controlled trial. *JAMA* 279(23):1900–1902.

BHP. See *British Herbal Pharmacopoeia.*

Block, E. 1985. The chemistry of garlic and onions. *Sci Am* 252(3):114–119.

Bordia, A. 1981. Effect of garlic on blood lipids in patients with coronary heart disease. *Am J Clin Nutr* 34(10):2100–2103.

Bradley, P.R. (ed.). 1992. *British Herbal Com-pendium,* Vol. 1. Bournemouth: British Herbal Medicine Association. 105–108.

British Herbal Pharmacopoeia (BHP). 1996. Exeter, U.K.: British Herbal Medicine Association. 85–86.

Brosche, T., D. Platt, H. Dorner. 1990. The effect of a garlic preparation on the composition of plasma lipoproteins and erythrocyte membranes in geriatric subjects. *Br J Clin Pract Suppl* 44(suppl.69):12–19.

Brown, D.J. 1996. *Herbal Prescriptions for Better Health.* Rocklin, CA: Prima Publishing. 97–109.

Budavari, S. (ed.). 1996. *The Merck Index: An Encyclopedia of Chemicals, Drugs, and Biologi-cals,* 12th ed. Whitehouse Station, N.J.: Merck & Co, Inc. 741.

Burnham, B.E. 1995. Garlic as a possible risk for postoperative bleeding. *Plast Recontr Surgery* 95(1):213.

Chadha, Y.R. et al. (eds.). 1952–1988. *The Wealth of India (Raw Materials),* Vols. 1–11. New Delhi: Publications and Information Directorate, CSIR.

Elbl, G. 1991. Chemisch-biologische Untersuchun-gen pflanzlicher Inhibitoren des Angiotensin I-converting Enzyms (ACE), insbesondere die der Arzneipflanzen Lespedeza capitata (Michx.) und *Allium ursinum* (L.). Dissertation, University of Munich (Abstract).

Europäisches Arzneibuch (Ph.Eur.). 1999. Stuttgart: Deutscher Apotheker Verlag. 754–755.

ESCOP. 1997. "Allii sativi bulbus." *Monographs on the Medicinal Uses of Plant Drugs.* Exeter, U.K.: European Scientific Cooperative on Phytother-apy.

Ghana Herbal Pharmacopoeia (GHP). 1992. Accra, Ghana: Policy Research and Strategic Planning Institute (PORSPI). 59–61.

Grünwald, J. et al. 1992. Effects of garlic powder tablets on blood lipids and blood pressure. The Danish Multicenter Kwai® Study. *Eur J Clin Res* 3:179–186.

Harris, W.S., S.L. Windsor, J. Lickteig. 1995. Garlic and lipoprotein resistance to oxidation. *Z Phy-tother Abstr* 16:15.

Holzgartner H., U. Schmidt, U. Kuhn. 1992. Com-parison of the efficacy and tolerance of a garlic preparation vs. bezafibrate. *Arzneimforsch* 42(12):1473–1477.

Isaacsohn, J.L. et al. 1998. Garlic powder and plasma lipids and lipoproteins: a multicenter, randomized, placebo-controlled trial. *Arch Intern Med* 158(11):1189–1194.

Jain, A.K., R. Vargas, S. Gotzkowsky, F.G. McMahon. 1993. Can garlic reduce levels of serum lipids? A controlled clinical study. *Am J Med* 94(6):632–635.

Kiesewetter, H. et al. 1993a. Effect of garlic on platelet aggregation in patients with increased risk of juvenile ischaemic attack. *Eur J Clin Phar-macol* 45(4):333–336.

Kiesewetter, H. et al. 1993b. Effects of garlic coated tablets in peripheral arterial occlusive dis-ease. *Clin Investig* 71(5):383–386.

Kiesewetter, H. et al. 1990. Effects of garlic on blood fluidity and fibrinolytic activity: a ran-domised, placebo-controlled, double-blind study. *Br J Clin Pract Suppl* 44(suppl.69):24–29.

Koch, H.P. 1992. "Hormonwirkungen" bei Allium-arten: historische berichte und moderne wis-senschaftliche erkenntnisse. *Z Phytother* 13:177–188.

Koch, H.P. and L.D. Lawson (eds.). 1996. *Garlic: The Science and Therapeutic Application of* Allium sativum *L. and Related Species,* 2nd ed. Baltimore: Williams & Wilkins Publishing Co.

Koscielny, J. et al. 1999. The antiatherosclerotic effect of *Allium sativum.* Atherosclerosis 144(1):237–249.

Lawson, L.D. 1998a. Garlic: A Review of its Medi-cinal Effects and Indicated Active Compounds. In: Lawson, L.D. and R. Bauer (eds.). *Phytomed-icines of Europe: Chemistry and Biological Activ-ity.* Washington, DC: American Chemical Society. 176–209.

———. 1998b. Effect of garlic on serum lipids (let-ter). *JAMA* 280(18):1568.

———. 1998c. Garlic powder for hyperlipi-demia—analysis of recent negative results. *Quart Rev Nat Med* 187–189.

Mader, F.H. 1990. Treatment of hyperlipidemia with garlic-powder tablets. Evidence from the German Association of General Practitioners' multicentric placebo-controlled double-blind study. *Arzneimforsch* 40(10):1111–1116.

McCrindle, B.W., E. Helden, W.T. Conner. 1998. Garlic extract therapy in children with hyper-cholesterlemia. *Arch Pediatr Adolesc Med* 152(11):1089–1094.

McGuffin, M., C. Hobbs, R. Upton, A. Goldberg. 1997. American Herbal Product Association's *Botanical Safety Handbook.* Boca Raton: CRC Press.

Mei, X. et al. 1982. Garlic and gastric cancer: the influence of garlic on the level of nitrate and nitrite in gastric juice. *Acta Nutr Sin* 4:53–56.

Phelps, S. and W.S. Harris. 1993. Garlic supplementation and lipoprotein oxidation susceptibility. *Lipids* 28(5):475–477.

Ph.Eur. See *Europäisches Arzneibuch.*

Rotzsch W., V. Richter, F. Rassoul, A. Walper. 1992. [Postprandial lipemia under treatment with *Allium sativum.* Controlled double-blind study of subjects with reduced HDL2-cholesterol] [In German]. *Arzneimforsch* 42(10):1223–1227.

Silagy, C.A. and H.A. Neil. 1994a. Garlic as a lipid lowering agent—a meta-analysis. *J R Coll Physicians Lond* 28(1):39–45.

———. 1994b. A meta-analysis of the effect of garlic on blood pressure. *J Hypertens* 12(4):463–468.

Steiner, M., A.H. Khan, D. Holbert, R.I. Lin. 1996. A double-blind crossover study in moderately hypercholesterolemic men that compared the effect of aged garlic extract and placebo administration on blood lipids. *Am J Clin Nutr* 64(6):866–870.

Sunter, W.H. 1991. Warfarin and garlic. *Pharmaceut J* 246:722.

United States Pharmacopeia, 24th rev. and *National Formulary,* 19th ed. (USP 24–NF19). 1999. Rockville, MD: United States Pharmacopeial Convention, Inc. 2455–2456.

Warshafsky S., R.S. Kamer, S.L. Sivak. 1993. Effect of garlic on total serum cholesterol. *Ann Intern Med* 119(7 pt 1):599–605.

Weisberger, A.S. and J. Pensky. 1958. Tumor inhibition by a sulfhydryl-blocking agent related to an active principle of garlic. *Cancer Res* 18:1301–1308.

World Health Organization (WHO). 1999. "Allii Sativi Bulbus." *WHO Monographs on Selected Medicinal Plants,* Vol. 1. Geneva: World Health Organization. 5–15.

You, W.C. et al. 1989. *Allium* vegetables and reduced risk of stomach cancer. *J Natl Cancer Inst* 81(2):162–164.

Additional Resources

Anon. 1997. *Aged Garlic Extract™. 1997's Research Excerpts from Peer Reviewed Scientific Journals & Scientific Meetings.* Mission Viejo, CA: Wakunaga of America Co., Ltd.

Anon. 1998. *Nutritional and Health Benefits of Garlic as a Supplement.* Presented at the Recent Advances on the Benefits Accompanying the Use of Garlic as a Supplement Conference. University Park, PA: Pennsylvania State University; Nov. 14–17.

Abdullah, T.H., O. Kandil, A. Elkadi, J. Carter. 1988. Garlic revisited: therapeutic for the major diseases of our times? *J Nat Med Assoc* 80(4):439–445.

Almeida Santos, O. and J. Grünwald. 1993. Effect of garlic powder tablets on blood lipids and blood pressure. A six month placebo-controlled double blind study. *Br J Clin Res* 4:37–44.

Blumenthal, M. 1997. Herbal Monographs Initiated by Numerous Groups: WHO, USP, ESCOP, ABC, and AHP all working toward similar goals. *HerbalGram* 40:30–38.

Bordia, A. et al. 1977. Effect of essential oil of onion and garlic on experimental atherosclerosis in rabbits. *Atherosclerosis* 26(3):379–386.

Brewitt, B. and B. Lehmann. 1991. Lipidregulierung durch standardisierte Naturarzneimittel. Multizentrische Langzeitstudie an 1209 Patienten. *Der Kassenarzt* 5:47–55.

Brosche, T. and D. Platt. 1990. Knoblauch als pflanzlicher Lipidsenker. Neuere untersuchungen mit einem standardisierten knoblauchtrockenpulver-präparat [Garlic as phytogenic antilipemic agent. Recent studies with a standardized dry garlic powder substance]. *Fortschr Med* 108(36):703–706.

Ernst, E., T. Weihmayr, A. Matrai. 1985. Garlic and blood lipids. *Br Med J (Clin Res Ed)* 291(6488):139.

Fulder, S. 1989. Garlic and the prevention of cardiovascular disease. *Cardiology in Practice* 7:30–35.

Gebhardt, R. 1991. Inhibition of cholesterol biosynthesis by a water-soluble garlic extract in primary cultures of rat hepatocytes. *Arzneimforsch* 41(8):800–804.

———. 1993. Multiple inhibitory effects of garlic extracts on cholesterol biosynthesis in hepatocytes. *Lipids* 28(7):613–619.

Harenberg J., C. Giese, R. Zimmermann. 1988. Effect of dried garlic on blood coagulation, fibrinolysis, platelet aggregation and serum cholesterol levels in patients with hyperlipoproteinemia. *Artherosclerosis* 74(3):247–249.

Heinle, H. and E. Betz. 1994. Effects of dietary garlic supplementation in a rat model of atherosclerosis. *Arzneimforsch* 44(5):614–617.

Jain, R.C. and D.B. Konar. 1978. Effect of garlic oil in experimental cholesterol atherosclerosis. *Atherosclerosis* 29(2):125–129.

Jung, F. and H. Kiesewetter. 1991. Einfluss einer fettbelastung auf plasmalipide und kapilläre hautdurchblutung unter knoblauch. *Med Welt* 42:14–17.

Kiesewetter, H. et al. 1991. Effect of garlic on thrombocyte aggregation, micro-circulation and other risk factors. *Int J Clin Pharmacol Ther Toxicol* 29(4):151–155.

Kleijnen, J., P. Knipschild, G. ter Riet. 1989. Garlic, onions and cardiovascular risk factors. A review of the evidence from human experiments with emphasis on commercially available preparations. *Br J Clin Pharmacol* 28(5):535–544.

Koch, H.P. and G. Hahn. 1988. *Knoblauch: Grundlagen der therapeutischen Anwendung von* Allium sativum L. *[Garlic-Fundamentals of the Therapeutic Application of* Allium sativum L.*]* Munich: Urban and Schwarzenberg.

Kümmel, B. 1991. Lipidsenkender Effekt von Knoblauch-Ölmazerat-Kapseln. *Med Welt* 42:20.

Leung, A.Y. and S. Foster. 1996. *Encyclopedia of Common Natural Ingredients Used in Food, Drugs, and Cosmetics,* 2nd ed. New York: John Wiley & Sons, Inc. 260–264.

Mand, J.K., P.P. Gupta, G.L. Soni, R. Singh. 1985. Effect of garlic on experimental atherosclerosis in rabbits. *Indian Heart J* 37(3):183–188.

McMahon, F.G. et al. 1992. Clinical effects of a garlic powder preparation on various cardiovascular risk factors. *Eur J Clin Res* 3a:8–9.

Orekhov, A.N., V.V. Tertov, I.A. Sobenin, E.M. Pivovarova. 1995. Direct anti-atherosclerosis-related effects of garlic. *Ann Med* 27(1):63–65.

Reuter, H.D. 1991. *Spektrum* Allium sativum *L.* Zug: Aesopus Verlag.

Schulz, V., R. Hänsel, V.E. Tyler. 1998. *Rational Phytotherapy: A Physicians' Guide to Herbal Medicine.* New York: Springer.

Steinmetz, K.A., L.H. Kushi, R.M. Bostick, A.R. Folsom, J.D. Potter. 1994. Vegetables, fruit, and colon cancer in the Iowa Women's Health Study. *Am J Epidemiol* 139(1):1–15.

Tang W. and G. Eisenbrand. 1992. *Chinese Drugs of Plant Origin: Chemistry, Pharmacology, and Use in Traditional Modern Medicine.* New York: Springer Verlag. 79–86.

Tsai, Y. et al. 1985. Antiviral properties of garlic: in vitro effects on influenza B, herpes simplex and coxsackie viruses. *Planta Med* 51:460–461.

Vorberg, G. and B. Schneider. 1990. Therapy with garlic: results of a placebo-controlled, double-blind study. *Br J Clin Pract Suppl* 44(69):7–11.

Yeh, Y.Y. and S.M. Yeh. 1994. Garlic reduces plasma lipids by inhibiting hepatic cholesterol and triacylglycerol synthesis. *Lipids* 29(3):189–193.

This material was adapted from *The Complete German Commission E Monographs—Therapeutic Guide to Herbal Medicines.* M. Blumenthal, W.R. Busse, A. Goldberg, J. Gruenwald, T. Hall, C.W. Riggins, R.S. Rister (eds.) S. Klein and R.S. Rister (trans.). 1998. Austin: American Botanical Council; Boston: Integrative Medicine Communications.

1) The Overview section is new information.

2) Description, Chemistry and Pharmacology, Uses, Contraindications, Side Effects, Interactions with Other Drugs, and Dosage sections have been drawn from the original work. Additional information has been added in some or all of these sections, as noted with references.

3) The dosage for equivalent preparations (tea infusion, fluidextract, and tincture) have been provided based on the following example:
   Unless otherwise prescribed: 2 g per day of [powdered, crushed, cut or whole] [plant part]
   Infusion: 2 g in 150 ml of water
   Fluidextract 1:1 (g/ml): 2 ml
   Tincture 1:5 (g/ml): 10 ml

4) The References and Additional Resources sections are new sections. Additional Resources are not cited in the monograph but are included for research purposes.

GENTIAN ROOT

Latin Name:
Gentiana lutea

Pharmacopeial Name:
Gentianae radix

Other Names:
gentiana, wild gentian,
yellow gentian

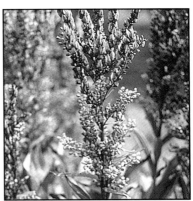

Overview

Gentian is a perennial herb native to the high pastures of central and southern
Europe and western Asia, most often at elevations between 1,000–2,500 meters.
The roots become mature and ready for harvesting after 7 to 10 years in the
ground (Bruneton, 1995; Budavari, 1996; Grieve, 1979; Leung and Foster, 1996).
The material of commerce is obtained from wild plants in the mountains of France,
Spain, and the Balkans (BHP, 1996; Bruneton, 1995; Wichtl and Bisset, 1994).
Wild gentian is almost depleted from many locations and is now under protected
status in Germany, Yugoslavia, and many other countries. In Germany, gentian is
listed in Annex 1 of the German Federal Ordinance on the Conservation of Species
(BArtSchV) and a permit is necessary for both import and export of any wild col-
lected material. There is a small amount under cultivation in France and Germany,
though Germany imports most of its requirements from Yugoslavia, France, and
Romania (Bruneton, 1995; Lange and Schippmann, 1997; Menkovic et al., 1998;
Wichtl and Bisset, 1994).

The genus name *Gentiana* is derived from Gentius, king of ancient Illyria
(180–167 B.C.E.), who discovered its therapeutic values according to Pliny the
Elder (ca. 23–79 C.E.) and Dioscorides, author of *De Materia Medica* in the first
century C.E. (Grieve, 1979). Its present-day therapeutic uses date at least back to
ancient Roman and Greek medicines. Though native to Europe, this species and
related Indian species *G. chirata* and *G. chirayita* are included in the *Ayurvedic
Pharmacopoeia*, which indicates their use for anorexia, atonic dyspepsia, and gastrointestinal atony. It classifies gentian's actions as bitter, gastric stimulant, siala-
gogue, and cholagogue (Karnick, 1994).

In Germany, gentian is licensed as a standard medicinal tea. Gentian infusions
and other equivalent preparations, including percolate, tincture, strong bitter
(Amarum purum), and dry extracts in solid dosage forms, are used in gastrointestinal and cholagogue formulas for appetite loss, flatulence, and insufficient production of gastric juices (Bradley, 1992; Leung and Foster, 1996; Wichtl and Bisset,
1994). In the United States, it is less common because its wild populations in
Europe are protected and little is cultivated. Its use in the United States is comparable to Germany as a bitter tonic and more often as a component in digestive preparations. Gentian was official in the *United States Pharmacopoeia* from 1820 to
1950 (Boyle, 1991; Budavari, 1996; Leung and Foster, 1996; Taber, 1962).

Few modern human studies have been done. One pharmacological study
involved radiological examinations of the effects of bitters on digestive organs in
humans. Secretion of gastric juice in 10 healthy individuals was stimulated after
one oral dose of an alcoholic gentian root fluidextract. Using X-ray contrast,
increased and prolonged emptying of the gall bladder was also observed, which

was interpreted as a cholagogic effect. No adverse effects to the treatment were reported (ESCOP, 1997; Glatzel and Hackenberg, 1967).

Therapeutic applications for gentian root are supportable based on its history of use in well established systems of traditional medicine, *in vitro* studies, *in vivo* studies in animals, the known properties of its bitter principles, and some pharmacological and clinical human studies.

Pharmacopoeial grade gentian root must have a bitterness value of not less than 10,000 and must also contain not less than 33% water soluble extractive (Bruneton, 1995; DAB 10, 1994; Ph.Eur.3, 1997; Ph.Fr.X, 1990; Wichtl and Bisset, 1994).

Description

Gentian root consists of the dried, unfermented roots and rhizome of *Gentiana lutea* L. [Gentianaceae], and its preparations in effective dosage. The preparation contains bitter principles (amarogentin, gentiopicroside) and the bitter-tasting gentiobiose.

Chemistry and Pharmacology

Gentian root contains secoiridoid bitter principles gentiopicroside (2–4%) and amarogentin (0.025–0.084%) [bitterness value=58,000,000]; oligosaccharides gentianose and gentiobiose (2.5–8.0%); (gentisic, caffeic, and protocatechuic) phenolic acids; phytosterols; polysaccharides inulin and pectin; tannin; lupeol and β-amyrin triterpenes; xanthones (approximately 0.1%), mainly gentisin, isogentisin, gentisein, and gentioside; and traces of volatile oil. (Bradley, 1992; Bruneton, 1995; ESCOP, 1997; Leung and Foster, 1996; Newall et al., 1996; Wichtl and Bisset, 1994).

The Commission E reported that the essential active principles are the bitter substances contained in the herb. These bring about a reflex excitation of the taste receptors, leading to increased secretion of saliva and the digestive juices. Therefore, gentian root is considered to be not only a pure bitter, but also a roborant and tonic. In animal experimentation there are indications that bronchial secretion is increased.

The *British Herbal Compendium* reported its actions as bitter and as a digestive stimulant (Bradley, 1992). Its secoiridoid bitter principles, particularly amarogentin, stimulate gustatory receptors in the taste buds, causing a reflex promotion of saliva, gastric juice and bile secretion, thereby stimulating appetite (Hartke and Mutschler, 1987; Schmid, 1966). One oral dose of gentian root fluidextract stimulated gastric juice secretion and increased and prolonged emptying of the gall bladder in healthy individuals (Glatzel and Hackenberg, 1967).

Uses

The Commission E approved the internal use of gentian root for digestive disorders, such as loss of appetite, fullness, and flatulence.

The *British Herbal Compendium* approves gentian for lack of appetite, anorexia, atonic dyspepsia, gastrointestinal atony, and as a tonic and antiemetic (Bradley, 1992). The German Standard License for gentian root tea indicates its use for digestive problems, such as insufficient production of gastric juice (Braun et al., 1997). ESCOP indicates its use for anorexia following illness and dyspepsia (ESCOP, 1997).

Contraindications

Gastric and duodenal peptic ulcers.

Side Effects

Especially sensitive persons may occasionally experience headaches.

Use During Pregnancy and Lactation

No restrictions known.

Interactions with Other Drugs

None known.

Dosage and Administration

Unless otherwise prescribed: 2–4 g per day cut root or dried extract.
Fluidextract: 2–4 g (Erg.B.6).
Tincture: 1–3 g (Erg.B.6).
Root: 2–4 g.
Equivalent preparations:
Infusion or decoction: 1–2 g in 150 ml boiled water, two to three times daily, one hour before meals.
Cold maceration: 1–2 g in 150 ml cold water for at least 8 to 10 hours, then boil.
Fluidextract 1:1 (g/ml): 1–2 ml, two to three times daily, one hour before meals.
Native dry extract 3.5–4.5:1 (w/w): 0.2–0.4 g, two to three times daily, one hour before meals.

References

Boyle, W. 1991. *Official Herbs: Botanical Substances in the United States Pharmacopoeias 1820–1990*. East Palestine, OH: Buckeye Naturopathic Press.

Bradley, P.R. (ed.). 1992. *British Herbal Compendium*, Vol. 1. Bournemouth: British Herbal Medicine Association.

Braun, R. et al. 1997. *Standardzulassungen für Fertigarzneimittel—Text and Kommentar*. Stuttgart: Deutscher Apotheker Verlag.

British Herbal Pharmacopoeia (BHP). 1996. Exeter, U.K.: British Herbal Medicine Association.

Bruneton, J. 1995. *Pharmacognosy, Phytochemistry, Medicinal Plants*. Paris: Lavoisier Publishing.

Budavari, S. (ed.). 1996. *The Merck Index: An Encyclopedia of Chemicals, Drugs, and Biologicals*, 12th ed. Whitehouse Station, N.J.: Merck & Co, Inc.

Deutsches Arzneibuch, 10th ed. (DAB 10). 1991. (With subsequent supplements through 1996.) Stuttgart: Deutscher Apotheker Verlag.

ESCOP. 1997. "Gentianae radix." *Monographs on the Medicinal Uses of Plant Drugs*. Exeter, U.K.: European Scientific Cooperative on Phytotherapy.

Europäisches Arzneibuch, 3rd ed. (Ph.Eur.3). 1997. Stuttgart: Deutscher Apotheker Verlag.

Glatzel, H. and K. Hackenberg. 1967. Röntgenologische Untersuchungen der Wirkungen von Bittermitteln auf die Verdauungsorgane [Roentgenological studies of the effect of bitters on digestive organs]. *Planta Med* 15(3):223–232.

Grieve, M. 1979. *A Modern Herbal*. New York: Dover Publications, Inc.

Hartke, K. and E. Mutschler (eds.). 1987. *DAB 9—Kommentar: Deutsches Arzneibuch*, 9. Band 2.: Monographien A-L. Stuttgart: Wissenschaft Verlagsges 1546–1550.

Karnick, C.R. 1994. *Pharmacopoeial Standards of Herbal Plants*, Vols. 1–2. Delhi: Sri Satguru Publications. Vol. 1:228–229; Vol. 2:154–155.

Lange, D. and U. Schippmann. 1997. *Trade Survey of Medicinal Plants in Germany—A Contribution to International Plant Species Conservation*. Bonn: Bundesamt für Naturschutz. 32–33, 93, 115–121.

Leung, A.Y. and S. Foster. 1996. *Encyclopedia of Common Natural Ingredients Used in Food, Drugs, and Cosmetics*, 2nd ed. New York: John Wiley & Sons, Inc.

Menkovic, N.R., K.P. Savikin-Fodulovic, D.V. Grubisic, I. Momcilovic. 1998. Secondary Products in *Gentiana lutea in vitro* Culture. Belgrade, Yugoslavia: Institute for Medicinal Plant Research.

Newall, C.A., L.A. Anderson, J.D. Phillipson. 1996. *Herbal Medicines: A Guide for Health-Care Professionals*. London: The Pharmaceutical Press.

Ph.Eur.3. See *Europäisches Arzneibuch*.

Pharmacopée Française Xe Édition (Ph.Fr.X.). 1983–1990. Moulins-les-Metz: Maisonneuve S.A.

Schmid, W. 1966. Zur Pharmakologie der Bittermittel [On the Pharmacology of Gentian]. *Planta Med* 14(Suppl):34–41.

Taber, C.W. 1962. *Taber's Cyclopedic Medical Dictionary*, 9th ed. Philadelphia: F.A. Davis Company. G-16.

Wichtl, M. and N.G. Bisset (eds.). 1994. *Herbal Drugs and Phytopharmaceuticals*. Stuttgart: Medpharm Scientific Publishers.

Additional Resources

Atkinson, J.E., P. Gupta, J.R. Lewis. 1969. Some phenolic constituents of *Gentiana lutea*. *Tetrahedron* 25(7):1507–1511.

British Pharmacopoeia (BP). 1988. (With subsequent Addenda up to 1992.) London: Her Majesty's Stationery Office.

British Herbal Pharmacopoeia (BHP). 1983. Keighley, U.K.: British Herbal Medicine Association.

Bricout, J. 1974. Identification et dosage des constituants amers des racines de *Gentiana lutea* L. *Phytochem* 13:2819–2823.

Burret, F., A.J. Chulia, A.M. Debelmas. 1979. Contribution a l'étude du genre *Gentiana*. 2'-O-glucosides d'ísoorientine et d'ísovitexine chez *Gentiana lutea* L. [Contribution to the study of the genus gentian: 2'-O-glucosides of isoorientine and isovitexine in *Gentiana lutea* L.]. *Planta Med* 36(2):178–179.

Council of Europe. 1981. *Flavouring Substances and Natural Sources of Flavourings*, 3rd ed. Strasbourg: Maisonneuve.

Der Marderosian, A. (ed.). 1999. *The Review of Natural Products*. St. Louis: Facts and Comparisons.

Duke, J.A. 1985. *Handbook of Medicinal Herbs.* Boca Raton: CRC Press. 207–208.

Hänsel, R., K. Keller, H. Rimpler, G. Schneider (eds.). 1993. *Hagers Handbuch der Pharmazeutischen Praxis,* 5th ed. Vol. 5. Berlin-Heidelberg: Springer Verlag. 227–247.

Inouye, H., T. Yoshida, Y. Nakamura, S. Tobita. 1968. Die Stereochemie einiger Secoiridoidglucoside und die Revision der Strukter des Gentiopicrosids. *Tetrahedron Lett* 4429–4432.

Karrer, W. 1958. *Konstitution und Vorkommen der Organischen Pflanzenstoffe (exclusive Alkaloide).* Basel: Birkhäuser Verlag.

List, P.H. and L. Hörhammer (eds.). 1973–1979. *Hagers Handbuch der Pharmazeutischen Praxis,* Vols. 1–7. New York: Springer Verlag.

Luckner, M., O. Bessler, P. Schroder. 1965. Vorschlage für den Drogenteil des DAB 7. 5. Radix *Gentianae* [Suggestions for the drug section of the *DAB 7. 5.* Radix Gentianae]. *Pharmazie* 20(1):16–19.

Madaus, G. 1979. *Lehrbuch der biologischen Arzneimittel,* Vols. 1–3, reprinting. Hildesheim: Georg Olms Verlag.

Matzkies, F. and B. Webs. 1983.Wirkung eines pflanzlichen Kombinationspraparats auf die gastrointestinale Transitzeit und die Gallensauren-Ausscheidung [Effect of a plant extract combination preparation on gastrointestinal transit time and bile acid excretion]. *Fortschr Med* 101(27–28):1304–1306.

McGuffin, M., C. Hobbs, R. Upton, A. Goldberg. 1997. American Herbal Product Association's *Botanical Safety Handbook.* Boca Raton: CRC Press.

Reynolds, J.E.F. (ed.). 1993. *Martindale: The Extra Pharmacopoeia,* 30th ed. London: The Pharmaceutical Press.

Steinegger, E. and R. Hänsel. 1988. *Lehrbuch der Pharmakognosie und Phytopharmazie,* 4th ed. Berlin-Heidelberg: Springer Verlag.

Sticher, O. and B. Meier. 1978. Identifizierung der bitterstoffe von radix *Gentianae* mit hochleistungs-flussigkeitschromatographie (HPLC) [Identification of bitter substances in radix gentianae with high pressure liquid chromatography]. *Pharm Acta Helv* 53(2):40–45.

———. 1980. Quantitative determination of the bitter principles in the roots of *Gentiana lutea* and *Gentiana purpurea* with HPLC. *Planta Med* 40:55–67.

Takino, Y. et al. 1980. Quantitative determination of bitter components in Gentianaceous plants. Studies on the evaluation of crude drugs VIII. *Planta Med* 38:344–350.

Verotta, L. 1985. Isolation and HPLC determination of the active principles of *Rosmarinus officinalis* and *Gentiana lutea. Fitoterapia* 56:25–29.

Wagner, H. et al. 1983. *Plant Drug Analysis.* Berlin-Heidelberg: Springer Verlag.

Wagner, H. and M. Wiesenauer. 1995. *Phytotherapie. Phytopharmaka und Pflanzliche Homöopathika.* Stuttgart: Fischer Verlag.

Weiss, R.F. 1991. *Lehrbuch der Phytotherapie,* 7th ed. Stuttgart: Hippokrates Verlag. 74–79.

Wichtl, M. (ed.). 1997. *Teedrogen,* 4th ed. Stuttgart: Wissenschaftliche Verlagsgesellschaft.

Wichtl, M. and M. Schäfer-Korting. 1994. *DAB 10—Kommentar.* Stuttgart: Wissenschaftliche Verlagsgesellschaft. II/2:Monograph E8.

This material was adapted from *The Complete German Commission E Monographs—Therapeutic Guide to Herbal Medicines.* M. Blumenthal, W.R. Busse, A. Goldberg, J. Gruenwald, T. Hall, C.W. Riggins, R.S. Rister (eds.) S. Klein and R.S. Rister (trans.). 1998. Austin: American Botanical Council; Boston: Integrative Medicine Communications.

1) The Overview section is new information.

2) Description, Chemistry and Pharmacology, Uses, Contraindications, Side Effects, Interactions with Other Drugs, and Dosage sections have been drawn from the original work. Additional information has been added in some or all of these sections, as noted with references.

3) The dosage for equivalent preparations (tea infusion, fluidextract, and tincture) have been provided based on the following example:

Unless otherwise prescribed: 2 g per day of [powdered, crushed, cut or whole] [plant part]
Infusion: 2 g in 150 ml of water
Fluidextract 1:1 (g/ml): 2 ml
Tincture 1:5 (g/ml): 10 ml

4) The References and Additional Resources sections are new sections. Additional Resources are not cited in the monograph but are included for research purposes.

GINGER ROOT

Latin Name:
Zingiber officinale

Pharmacopeial Name:
Zingiberis rhizoma

Other Names:
ginger rhizome

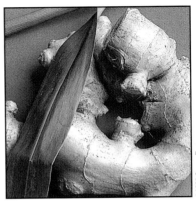

© 1999 Steven Foster

Overview

Ginger is a large tuberous perennial plant native to southern Asia, now cultivated extensively in almost all tropical and subtropical countries, especially China, India, Nigeria, Australia, Jamaica, and Haiti (Bruneton, 1995; Budavari, 1996; Grieve, 1979; Leung and Foster, 1996; Reineccius, 1994). China and India are the world's leading producers of ginger. The material of commerce is supplied in "completely scraped" (peeled), "partially scraped," or "unpeeled" rhizomes. Peeled rhizomes ("white" ginger) are produced in Jamaica, while unpeeled rhizomes ("black" ginger) are mainly from China and Sierra Leone. Partially scraped rhizomes come from India, Bengal, Nigeria, Australia, and Japan (BHP, 1996; Felter and Lloyd, 1983; Reineccius, 1994; Wichtl and Bisset, 1994). Ginger became naturalized in the Caribbean and Central America early in the sixteenth century when Spaniards brought it from the East Indies and began to cultivate it on a large scale for export to Europe (Grieve, 1979).

Ginger has been used as a medicine since ancient times, recorded in early Sanskrit and Chinese texts and ancient Greek, Roman, and Arabic medical literature (Bone, 1997). In Asian medical practices, dried ginger has been used as a drug to treat stomachache, diarrhea, and nausea for thousands of years. It is traditionally prepared in aqueous decoctions and infusions (Bruneton, 1995; But et al., 1997; Kapoor, 1990; Leung and Foster, 1996). In Africa, dried ginger is used much as it is in Asia (GHP, 1992; Iwu, 1990). Today, ginger is official in the national pharmacopeias of Austria, China, Egypt, Germany, Great Britain, Japan, and Switzerland (BP, 1988; Bradley, 1992; DAB, 1997; JP XII, 1993; Newall et al., 1996; ÖAB, 1981; Ph.Helv.VII, 1987; Tu, 1992). The Chinese pharmacopeia lists ginger for epigastric pain with cold feeling, vomiting and diarrhea accompanied by cold extremities and faint pulse, dyspnea, and cough with copious frothy expectoration (Tu, 1992). The *Ayurvedic Pharmacopoeia* specifically recommends ginger for flatulent intestinal colic (Karnick, 1994).

In Germany, ginger is an economically important herb, imported on a large scale (Lange and Schippmann, 1997). It is official in the *German Pharmacopoeia*, approved in the Commission E monographs, and used as a component of antiemetic stomach medicines (BAnz, 1998; DAB, 1997; Meyer-Buchtela, 1999; Wichtl and Bisset, 1994). In the United States, it is used singly and as a main component of digestive, antinausea, and cold and flu dietary supplements. It is also used extensively in Ayurvedic and traditional Chinese medicine herbal teas and by licensed acupuncturists and naturopathic physicians. Crude ginger, ginger fluidextract, and ginger oleoresin were formerly official in the *United States Pharmacopeia* (USP) and *National Formulary* as a carminative, aromatic, and stimulant. *King's American Dispensatory* indicated it for loss of appetite, flatulence, borborygmus (rumbling or gurgling sound of gas in the intestines), spasmodic gastric and intestinal contractions, and cool extremities (Felter and Lloyd, 1983; Leung and Foster, 1996; Taber, 1962).

The approved modern therapeutic applications for ginger are supportable based on its history of use in well established systems of traditional and conventional medicine, extensive phytochemical investigations, pharmacological studies in animals, and human clinical studies. In 1998, the USP issued a drug information monograph stating that despite its safety, the USP Advisory Panel did not recommend or support the use of ginger for prevention of motion sickness due to what it deemed a lack of sufficient quality studies (*USP Consumer Information*, 1998). Nonetheless, the data appear adequate to establish reasonable expectation of effectiveness, as documented in the following studies.

Modern human studies have investigated ginger as an anti-emetic (Bone et al., 1990; Phillips et al., 1993), anti-nausea treatment (Arfeen et al., 1995; Meyer et al., 1995; Pace, 1987), a prophylactic against motion sickness (Holtmann et al., 1989; Mowrey and Clayson, 1982; Riebenfeld and Borzone, 1986; Stewart et al., 1991; Stott et al., 1985; Wood et al., 1988) and/or seasickness (Grøntved et al., 1988; Schmid et al., 1994), a treatment for hyperemesis gravidarum (Fischer-Rasmussen et al., 1990), a treatment for vertigo (Grøntved and Hentzer, 1986), and for its effect on human platelet function (Lumb, 1994; Verma et al., 1993; Srivastava, 1989).

In a prospective, randomized, double-blind trial the incidence of postoperative nausea and vomiting was measured in 120 women presenting for elective laparoscopic gynecological surgery on a day-stay basis. Ginger (1 g oral) significantly (p=0.006) reduced postoperative nausea compared to placebo. Groups (n=40) were given either ginger (1 g), metoclopramide (10 mg), or placebo (1 g) postoperatively. The incidence of nausea and vomiting was similar in patients given metoclopramide and ginger (27% and 21%, respectively) and less than in those who received placebo (41%). The dosage requirement for postoperative anti-emetics was lower in those patients receiving ginger (15%) compared to the metoclopramide (32%) and placebo (38%) groups. The authors concluded that ginger is an effective and promising prophylactic anti-emetic that may be especially useful for day-case surgery (Phillips et al., 1993).

A double-blind randomized study tested the effectiveness of ginger (administered orally) as an anti-emetic agent, compared with placebo and metoclopramide (10 mg Maxolon® intravenously) in 60 women who had undergone major gynecological surgery. Patients were given 1 g of powdered ginger at the time of premedication before surgery. There were statistically significantly fewer incidents of nausea in the group that received ginger compared with placebo (p<0.05). The number of incidents of nausea in the groups (n=20) who received ginger or metoclopramide was comparable. Administration of post-operative anti-emetic was significantly less in the ginger and metoclopramide groups than in the placebo group (p<0.05) (Bone et al., 1990).

In one open study the use of ginger to prevent 8-MOP associated nausea was investigated. Eleven patients undergoing photophoresis therapy who regularly experienced nausea after ingestion of psoralen (8-MOP) were included in the study and acted as their own control. Patients undergoing photophoresis therapy are required to ingest psoralen before each treatment. This drug causes nausea. The authors reported that nausea was significantly reduced by ingesting three 530 mg capsules of ginger before taking psoralen (Meyer et al., 1995).

A double-blind, randomized, placebo-controlled trial tested the effect of powdered ginger rhizome on seasickness. Eighty naval cadets, unaccustomed to sailing in heavy seas, reported whether there were symptoms of seasickness every hour for four consecutive hours after ingestion of 1 g of the drug or placebo. The authors concluded that ginger reduced the tendency to vomiting and cold sweating significantly better than placebo (p<0.05) (Grøntved et al., 1988). In another double-blind, crossover, placebo trial, the effect of powdered ginger rhizome upon vertigo and nystagmus following caloric stimulation of the vestibular system (irrigation of the left ear with water at 44°C) was studied in eight healthy volunteers. In 3 out of 24 tests, nausea was present after placebo, but it did not occur after ingestion of ginger. The authors concluded that ginger reduced the induced vertigo significantly better than placebo (Grøntved and Hentzer, 1986).

Using the fact that ginger is approved by the Commission E as a nonprescription remedy for motion sickness in Germany, in 1995 the European-American Phytomedicine Coalition (EAPC) filed a citizens petition with the FDA for ginger to be reviewed as an OTC drug for anti-nausea and motion sickness in the United States (Pinco and Israelsen, 1995). The petition included clinical studies on ginger in experimental conditions as well as in situ (e.g., with first-time sailors at sea). It also contained extensive market data in Europe and other countries where ginger is employed as a medicine. The totality of the materials support the safety and efficacy of ginger as a medicine. By the summer of 1999 the FDA had not yet responded directly to this petition.

A standardized extract of ginger (Zintona®, Dalidar Pharma, Israel) has been approved as a nonprescription medicine for prevention of motion sickness in Germany, Switzerland, Austria, and Finland (Tenne, 1999).

Regarding quality control parameters, Chinese pharmacopeial grade ginger must be composed of the dried rhizome, removed from fibrous root, collected in winter, containing not less than 0.8% (ml/g) volatile oil. Botanical identity must be confirmed by macroscopic and microscopic examinations and organoleptic evaluation (Tu, 1992). Both the *Austrian Pharmacopoeia* and the *German Pharmacopoeia* require not less than 1.5% (m/v) volatile oil, botanical identity confirmation by thin-layer chromatography (TLC) and macroscopic and microscopic examinations, purity test for absence of bleaching agents (calcium carbonate), a test for absence of starch paste when boiled in water, and not less than 4% acetone-soluble extractive (DAB, 1997; ÖAB, 1981; Wichtl and Bisset, 1994). The *British Pharmacopoeia* requires not less than 10% water-soluble extractive and not less than 4.5% ethanol-soluble extractive (BP, 1980, 1988; Wichtl and Bisset, 1994). The ESCOP ginger monograph requires the material to comply with the *British Pharmacopoeia* (ESCOP, 1997). The *Ghana Herbal Pharmacopoeia* requires not less than 1% volatile oil, botanical identity confirmation by examination of characteristic macroscopic and microscopic features, purity tests for absence of sclerenchymatous cells, trichomes and crystals of calcium oxalate, and not less than 4% ethanol-soluble extractive (GHP, 1992).

Description

Ginger root consists of the peeled, finger-long, fresh or dried rhizome of *Zingiber officinale* Roscoe [Fam. Zingiberaceae] and its preparations in effective dosage. The rhizome contains essential oil and pungent principles.

Chemistry and Pharmacology

Ginger rhizome contains oleoresin (4.0–7.5%) composed of non-volatile pungent principles (phenols such as gingerols and their related dehydration products shogaols), non-pungent substances (fats and waxes), and volatile oils; volatile oil (1.0–3.3%), of which 30–70% are sesquiterpenes, mainly β-bisabolene, (–)-zingiberene, β-sesquiphellandrene, and (+)-ar-curcumene, and monoterpenes, mainly geranial and neral; carbohydrates, mainly starch (40–60%); proteins (9–10%); lipids (6–10%) composed of triglycerides, phosphatidic acid, lecithins, and free fatty acids; vitamins niacin and A; minerals; and amino acids (Bradley, 1992; Bruneton, 1995; Budavari, 1996; ESCOP, 1997; Leung and Foster, 1996; Newall et al., 1996; Wichtl and Bisset, 1994).

The Commission E reported antiemetic, positively inotropic, promoting secretion of saliva and gastric juices, and cholagogue activity. In animals: antispasmodic. In humans: increase in tonus and peristalsis in intestines.

The *British Herbal Compendium* reported its actions as carminative, anti-emetic, spasmolytic, peripheral circulatory stimulant, and anti-inflammatory (Bradley, 1992). Powdered ginger root taken by naval cadets as a prophylactic against seasickness significantly reduced the tendency to vomit and cold sweating compared to placebo (Grøntved et al., 1988).

Uses

The Commission E approved the internal use of ginger for dyspepsia and prevention of motion sickness.

The *British Herbal Compendium* indicates ginger for atonic dyspepsia, colic, prophylaxis of travel sickness, and vomiting of pregnancy. Other uses include for anorexia, bronchitis, and rheumatic complaints (Bradley, 1992). ESCOP indicates its use for prophylaxis of the nausea and vomiting of motion sickness and as a postoperative anti-emetic for minor day-case surgical procedures (ESCOP, 1997).

Contraindications

With gallstones, first consult a physician.

Side Effects

None known.

Use During Pregnancy and Lactation

Not recommended (McGuffin et al., 1997).
Note: The Commission E contraindicates ginger as a remedy for morning sickness during pregnancy. However, there is no evidence that the therapeutic dosage for antinauseant activity cited by Commission E (1 gram of dried root) produces any harm to either the fetus or the mother. The Commission E presumably based its caution on two studies published in the 1980s in Japan on

6-gingerol, one of the compounds isolated from ginger rhizome. *In vitro* tests indicated that the gingerol had mutagenic activity *in vitro* at high doses (Namakura and Yamamoto, 1982; Nagabhushan et al., 1987). However, other compounds in ginger have been found to exhibit anti-mutagenic activity (Kada et al., 1978). Ginger is also widely used in traditional Chinese medicine (traditional Chinese medicine), but without contraindications in pregnancy. "On the contrary, ginger has been traditionally used for nausea and vomiting in pregnancy, though as in typical traditional Chinese medicine usage, rarely by itself. There is no lack of remedies for these conditions using ginger. Also, there is no contraindication of ginger in any of the recent issues of the *Pharmacopoeia of the People's Republic of China* (newest edition, 1995); the dosage is 3–9 grams for both fresh and dried ginger" (Leung, 1998). A literature review of all available clinical studies on ginger could find no scientific or medical evidence for Commission E's contraindication during pregnancy (Fulder and Tenne, 1996). Professor Schilcher, vice president of Commission E, agrees with this assessment of ginger's presumed safety during pregnancy (Schilcher, 1998).

Interactions with Other Drugs

None known.

Dosage and Administration

Unless otherwise prescribed: 2–4 g per day cut rhizome or dried extract.
Powdered rhizome: 0.25–1.0 g, three times daily.
Infusion or decoction: 0.25–1.0 g in 150 ml boiled water, three times daily.
Fluidextract 1:1 (g/ml): 0.25–1.0 ml, three times daily.
Tincture 1:5 (g/ml): 1.25–5.0 ml, three times daily.
[Note: A standardized ginger extract (Zintona®) is dosed in 250 mg capsules, recommended at two capsules 30 minutes before expected onset of symptoms, then two capsules every four

hours "to ease discomfort of digestive upset (or motion sickness)" (Tenne, 1999).]

References

Arfeen, Z. et al. 1995. A double-blind randomized controlled trial of ginger for the prevention of postoperative nausea and vomiting. *Anaesth Intensive Care* 23(4):449–452.

BAnz. See *Bundesanzeiger.*

Bone, K. 1997. Ginger. *Brit J Phytother* 4(3):110–120.

Bone, M.E., D.J. Wilkinson, J.R. Young, J. McNeil, S. Charlton. 1990. Ginger root—a new antiemetic. The effect of ginger root on postoperative nausea and vomiting after major gynaecological surgery. *Anaesthesia* 45:669–671.

Bradley, P.R. (ed.). 1992. *British Herbal Compendium*, Vol. 1. Bournemouth: British Herbal Medicine Association.

British Herbal Pharmacopoeia (BHP). 1996. Exeter, U.K.: British Herbal Medicine Association.

British Pharmacopoeia (BP). 1980. London: Her Majesty's Stationery Office. 209–210.

———. 1988. (With subsequent Addenda up to 1992.) London: Her Majesty's Stationery Office.

Bruneton, J. 1995. *Pharmacognosy, Phytochemistry, Medicinal Plants*. Paris: Lavoisier Publishing.

Budavari, S. (ed.). 1996. *The Merck Index: An Encyclopedia of Chemicals, Drugs, and Biologicals,* 12th ed. Whitehouse Station, N.J.: Merck & Co, Inc.

Bundesanzeiger (BAnz). 1998. Monographien der Kommission E (Zulassungs- und Aufberitungskommission am BGA für den humanmed. Bereich, phytotherapeutische Therapierichtung und Stoffgruppe). Köln: Bundesgesundheitsamt (BGA).

But, P.P.H. et al. (eds.). 1997. *International Collation of Traditional and Folk Medicine.* Singapore: World Scientific. 210–211.

Deutsches Arzneibuch (DAB 1997). 1997. Stuttgart: Deutscher Apotheker Verlag.

ESCOP. 1997. "Zingiberis rhizoma." *Monographs on the Medicinal Uses of Plant Drugs.* Exeter, U.K.: European Scientific Cooperative on Phytotherapy.

Felter, H.W. and J.U. Lloyd. 1983. *King's American Dispensatory*, 18th ed., 3rd rev. Portland, OR: Eclectic Medical Publications [reprint of 1898 original]. 2109–2112.

Fischer-Rasmussen, W., S.K. Kjaer, C. Dahl, U. Asping. 1990. Ginger treatment of hyperemesis gravidarum. *Eur J Obstet Gynecol Reprod Biol* 38(1):19–24.

Fulder, S. and M. Tenne. 1996. Ginger as an Antinausea Remedy in Pregnancy: The Issue of Safety. *HerbalGram* 38:47–50.

Ghana Herbal Pharmacopoeia (GHP). 1992. Accra, Ghana: Policy Research and Strategic Planning Institute (PORSPI).

Grieve, M. 1979. *A Modern Herbal.* New York: Dover Publications, Inc.

Grøntved, A. and E. Hentzer. 1986. Vertigo-reducing effect of ginger root. A controlled clinical study. *ORL J Otorhinolaryngol Relat Spec* 48(5):282–286.

Grøntved, A., T. Brask, J. Kambskard, E. Hentzer. 1988. Ginger root against seasickness. A controlled trial on the open sea. *Acta Otolaryngol (Stockh)* 105(1–2):45–49.

Holtmann, S., A.H. Clarke, H. Scherer, M. Hohn. 1989. The anti-motion sickness mechanism of ginger. A comparative study with placebo and dimenhydrinate. *Acta Otolaryngol (Stockh)* 108(3–4):168–174.

Iwu, M.M. 1990. *Handbook of African Medicinal Plants.* Boca Raton: CRC Press. 263–265.

Japanese Pharmacopoeia, 12th ed. (JP XII). 1993. Tokyo: Government of Japan Ministry of Health and Welfare—Yakuji Nippo, Ltd. 125–126.

Kada, T., K. Morita, T. Inoue. 1978. Anti-mutagenic action of vegetable factors on the mutagenic principle of tryptophan pyrolysate. *Mutat Res* 53(3):351–353.

Kapoor, L.D. 1990. *Handbook of Ayurvedic Medicinal Plants.* Boca Raton: CRC Press. 341–342.

Karnick, C.R. 1994. *Pharmacopoeial Standards of Herbal Plants*, Vol. 1. Delhi: Sri Satguru Publications. 347–348.

Lange, D. and U. Schippmann. 1997. *Trade Survey of Medicinal Plants in Germany—A Contribution to International Plant Species Conservation.* Bonn: Bundesamt für Naturschutz. 83–84.

Leung, A.Y. 1998. Personal communication to Mark Blumenthal. Mar. 2.

Leung, A.Y. and S. Foster. 1996. *Encyclopedia of Common Natural Ingredients Used in Food, Drugs, and Cosmetics*, 2nd ed. New York: John Wiley & Sons, Inc.

Lumb, A.B. 1994. Effect of dried ginger on human platelet function. *Thromb Haemost* 71(1):110–111.

McGuffin, M., C. Hobbs, R. Upton, A. Goldberg. 1997. American Herbal Product Association's *Botanical Safety Handbook.* Boca Raton: CRC Press.

Meyer, K., J. Schwartz, D. Crater, B. Keyes. 1995. *Zingiber officinale* (ginger) used to prevent 8-MOP associated nausea. *Dermatol Nurs* 7(4):242–244.

Meyer-Buchtela, E. 1999. *Tee-Rezepturen—Ein Handbuch für Apotheker und Ärzte.* Stuttgart: Deutscher Apotheker Verlag.

Mowrey, D.B. and D.E. Clayson. 1982. Motion sickness, ginger, and psychophysics. *Lancet* 1(8273):655–657.

Nagabhushan, M., A.J. Amonkar, S.V. Bhide. 1987. Mutagenicity of gingerol and shogaol and antimutagenicity of zingerone in Salmonella/microsome assay. *Cancer Lett* 36(2):221–223.

Namakura, H. and T. Yamamoto. 1982. Mutagen and anti-mutagen in ginger, *Zingiber officinale. Mutat Res* 103(2):119–126.

Newall, C.A., L.A. Anderson, J.D. Phillipson. 1996. *Herbal Medicines: A Guide for Health-Care Professionals.* London: The Pharmaceutical Press.

Österreichisches Arzneibuch, Vols. 1–2, 1st suppl. (ÖAB). 1981–1983. Wien: Verlag der Österreichischen Staatsdruckerei.

Pace, J.C. 1987. Oral ingestion of encapsulated ginger and reported self-care actions for the relief of chemotherapy-associated nausea and vomiting. *Diss Abstr Int (Sci)* 47(8):3297.

Pharmacopoeia Helvetica, 7th ed. Vol. 1–4. (Ph.Helv.VII). 1987. Bern: Office Central Fédéral des Imprimés et du Matériel.

Phillips, S., R. Ruggier, S.E. Hutchinson. 1993. *Zingiber officinale* (ginger)—an anti-emetic for day case surgery. *Anaesthesia* 48(8):715–717.

Pinco, R.G. and L.D. Israelsen. 1995. European-American Phytomedicines Coalition Citizen Petition to Amend FDA's OTC Drug Review Policy Regarding Foreign Ingredients. Jul. 24.

Reineccius, G. (ed.). 1994. *Source Book of Flavors*, 2nd ed. New York; London: Chapman & Hall. 295–299.

Riebenfeld, D. and L. Borzone. 1986. Randomised double-blind study to compare the activities and tolerability of Zintona® and dimenhydrinate in 60 subjects with motion sickness. (Unpublished report, *Pharmaton*, Lugano, Switz.)

Schilcher, H. 1998. The Present State of Phytotherapy in Germany. *Deutsche Apotheker Zeitung* 138 Jahrgang, No. 3, Jan. 15:144–149.

Schmid, R., T. Schick, R. Steffen, A. Tschopp, T. Wilk. 1994. Comparison of Seven Commonly Used Agents for Prophylaxis of Seasickness. *J Travel Med* 1(4):203–206.

Srivastava, K.C. 1989. Effect of onion and ginger consumption on platelet thromboxane production in humans. *Prostaglandins Leukot Essent Fatty Acids* 35(3):183–185.

Stewart, J.J., M.J. Wood, C.D. Wood, M.E. Mims. 1991. Effects of ginger on motion sickness susceptibility and gastric function. *Pharmacology* 41(2):111–120.

Stott, J.R.R., M.P. Hubble, M.B. Spencer. 1985. A double-blind comparative trial of powdered ginger root, Hyosine (sic) Hydrobromide and Cinnarizinein the prophylaxis of motion sickness induced by cross coupled stimulation. Advisory Group for Aerospace Research and Development, Conference Proceedings. 372, 39:1–6.

Taber, C.W. 1962. *Taber's Cyclopedic Medical Dictionary*, 9th ed. Philadelphia, PA: F.A. Davis Company. G–18.

Tenne, M. 1999. Personal communication to Alicia Goldberg, May 25.

Tu, G. (ed.). 1992. *Pharmacopoeia of the People's Republic of China* (English Edition 1992). Beijing: Guangdong Science and Technology Press. 215–216.

United States Pharmacopeia (USP) *Consumer Information*. 1998. U.S. Rockville, MD: U.S. Pharmacopoeial Convention. Available at: www.usp.org

Verma, S.K., J. Singh, R. Khamesra, A. Bordia. 1993. Effect of ginger on platelet aggregation in man. *Indian J Med Res* 98:240–242.

Wichtl, M. and N.G. Bisset (eds.). 1994. *Herbal Drugs and Phytopharmaceuticals*. Stuttgart: Medpharm Scientific Publishers.

Wood, C.D., J.E. Manno, M.J. Wood, B.R. Manno, M.E. Mims. 1988. Comparison of efficacy of ginger with various antimotion sickness drugs. *Clin Res Pract Drug Reg Aff* 6:129–136.

Additional Resources

British Pharmaceutical Codex (BPC). 1973. London: The Pharmaceutical Press.

Connel, D.W. and M.D. Sutherland. 1969. A re-examination of gingerol, shogaol and zingerone, the pungent principles of ginger (*Zingiber officinale* Roscoe). *Austr J Chem* 22:1033–1043.

Connel, D.W. 1969. The extraction of ginger. *Food Technol Austr* 21:570.

———. 1970. The chemistry of the essential oil and oleoresin of ginger (*Zingiber officinale* Roscoe). *Flavour Industry* 1:677–693.

Council of Europe. 1981. *Flavouring Substances and Natural Sources of Flavourings*, 3rd ed. Strasbourg: Maisonneuve.

List, P.H. and L. Hörhammer (eds.). 1973–1979. *Hagers Handbuch der Pharmazeutischen Praxis*, Vols. 1–7. New York: Springer Verlag.

Marsh, A.C. et al. 1977. *Composition of Foods, Spices, and Herbs: Raw, Processed, Prepared*. Agriculture Handbook No. 8–2. Washington, D.C.: Agricultural Research Service, U.S. Department of Agriculture.

This material was adapted from *The Complete German Commission E Monographs—Therapeutic Guide to Herbal Medicines*. M. Blumenthal, W.R. Busse, A. Goldberg, J. Gruenwald, T. Hall, C.W. Riggins, R.S. Rister (eds.) S. Klein and R.S. Rister (trans.). 1998. Austin: American Botanical Council; Boston: Integrative Medicine Communications.

1) The Overview section is new information.

2) Description, Chemistry and Pharmacology, Uses, Contraindications, Side Effects, Interactions with Other Drugs, and Dosage sections have been drawn from the original work. Additional information has been added in some or all of these sections, as noted with references.

3) The dosage for equivalent preparations (tea infusion, fluidextract, and tincture) have been provided based on the following example:
   Unless otherwise prescribed: 2 g per day of [powdered, crushed, cut or whole] [plant part]
   Infusion: 2 g in 150 ml of water
   Fluidextract 1:1 (g/ml): 2 ml
   Tincture 1:5 (g/ml): 10 ml

4) The References and Additional Resources sections are new sections. Additional Resources are not cited in the monograph but are included for research purposes.

Ming, O. (ed.). 1989. *Chinese-English Manual of Common-Used in Traditional Chinese Medicine.* Hong Kong: Joint Publishing (H.K.) Co., Ltd. 162–163, 341, 498–499.

Nadkarni, K.M. 1976. *Indian Materia Medica.* Bombay: Popular Prakashan. 1308–1315.

Reynolds, J.E.F. (ed.). 1989. *Martindale: The Extra Pharmacopoeia,* 29th ed. London: The Pharmaceutical Press.

———. 1993. *Martindale: The Extra Pharmacopoeia,* 30th ed. London: The Pharmaceutical Press.

Rosengarten, F., Jr. 1969. *The Book of Spices.* Wynnewood, PA: Livingston.

Shoji, N., A. Iwasa, T. Takemoto, Y. Ishida, Y. Ohizumi. 1982. Cardiotonic principles of ginger (*Zingiber officinale* Roscoe). *J Pharm Sci* 71(10):1174–1175.

Srivastava, K.C. and T. Mustafa. 1989. Ginger (*Zingiber officinale*) and rheumatic disorders. *Med Hypotheses* 29(1):25–28.

Suekawa, M. et al. 1984. Pharmacological studies on ginger. I. Pharmacological actions of pungent constituents, [6]-gingerol and [6]-shogaol. *J Pharmacobiodyn* 7(11):836–848.

Suekawa, M. et al. 1986. [Pharmacological studies on ginger. V. Pharmacological comparison between [6]-shogaol and capsaicin] [In Japanese]. *Nippon Yakurigaku Zasshi* 88(5):339–347.

Trease, G.E. and W.C. Evans. 1989. *Trease and Evans' Pharmacognosy,* 13th ed. London; Philadelphia: Baillière Tindall. 466.

Witchl, M. 1989. Ingwer. In: Wichtl, M. (ed.). *Teedrogen,* 2nd ed. Stuttgart: Wissenschaftliche Verlagsgesellschaft. 249–251.

Wood, A.B. 1987. Determination of the pungent principles of chilies and ginger by reversed-phase high-performance liquid chromatography with use of a single standard substance. *Flavour Fragrance J* 2:1–12.

GINKGO BILOBA
LEAF EXTRACT

Latin Name:
Ginkgo biloba L.

Pharmacopeial Name:
Ginkgo folium

Other Names:
duck foot tree, maidenhair tree,
silver apricot

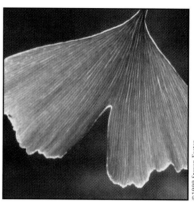

©1999 Steven Foster

Overview

There have been over four hundred scientific studies conducted on proprietary
standardized extracts of the leaf of ginkgo in the past 30 years. Ginkgo is the
world's most ancient extant tree, originating two hundred million years ago. Primary research was conducted by the W. Schwabe Co. of Karlsruhe, Germany, producer of the proprietary extract EGb 761. Ginkgo extract is a good example of a
phytomedicine that must be standardized in order to deliver the intended benefits;
the scientific literature does not support the clinical benefits of other dosage forms
of crude ginkgo leaf or low-concentration extracts made from the leaf. The dry
extract is pharmaceutically prepared to a 35–67:1 ratio of dried leaves to final
extract; standardization is carried out to 24% ginkgo flavonol glycosides (based on
flavones like quercetin, kaempferol, and isorhamnetin) and 6% terpene lactones
(ginkgolides and bilobalide). A comprehensive, almost exhaustive, 401 page book
reviewing the chemistry, pharmacology, toxicology, and all clinical studies conducted on EGb761 in various areas of clinical application has been published
(DeFeudis, 1998).

Ginkgo biloba extract (GBE) has been popular in Europe and now is popular in
the United States and other parts of the world for its neuroprotective properties
and ability to aid circulatory problems in the elderly, especially cerebral insufficiency and the consequent cognitive effects, peripheral circulatory impairment,
particularly intermittent claudication (poor circulation to the lower legs), and vertigo and tinnitus. New uses for protection against altitude sickness and to mediate
erectile dysfunction in males have also been investigated.

Clinical studies demonstrate that daily doses of 120 to 240 mg of GBE can lead
to an improvement in the symptoms associated with cerebral insufficiency, such as
memory loss, depression, and tinnitus, within 8 to 12 weeks (Vorberg, 1985; Rai et
al., 1991). An early review of 20 clinical studies concluded that many categories of
elderly patients could benefit from GBE (Warburton, 1988). All of these trials used
EGb 761.

In a later critical review of 40 ginkgo trials, the authors looked for evidence of
the efficacy of GBE in cerebral insufficiency (Kleijnen and Knipschild, 1992a,
1992b). Four gingko preparations were used in the trials: Tebonin®, Tanakan®,
rökan®, and Kaveri®. The first three are different names for EGb 761, the
Schwabe product. Kaveri® (LI 1370; Lichtwer Pharma, Germany) is standardized
in comparable percentages (25 and 6%). In accordance with German regulatory
requirements, both products are purified to contain less than 5 parts per million
ginkgolic acids. The standard dose was 120 mg/day for at least four to six weeks.
Of the 40 trials, eight were deemed well performed. Shortcomings in the other tri-

als included small patient numbers, inadequate description of randomization proce-dures, patient characteristics, effect measurement, and data presentation. In no trial was double-blindness checked. Virtually all trials reported positive results, and no serious side effects were reported in any trial. In a comparison of ginkgo with co-dergocrine, registered for the same indication, no marked differences were found in the quality of the evidence of the efficacy of ginkgo in cerebral insufficiency compared with co-dergocrine. The authors concluded that positive results have been reported for ginkgo in the treatment of cerebral insufficiency, but further studies should be conducted for a more detailed assessment of its efficacy.

In a meta-analysis of 11 placebo-controlled, randomized, double-blind trials in aged patients with cerebral insufficiency (Hopfenmüller, 1994), eight comparable trials were examined, most using a daily dose of 150 mg. Seven of the studies con-firmed the effectiveness of ginkgo compared to placebo in cerebral insufficiency, while one study was inconclusive. Another double-blind trial tested the efficacy of LI 1370 on 90 patients with cerebral insufficiency caused by old age (Vesper and Hänsgen, 1994). A daily dose of 150 mg was administered for 12 weeks, with the ginkgo group showing significant improvement compared to placebo.

A recent meta-analysis (Oken et al., 1998) systematically reviewed over 50 clini-cal studies on GBE for treatment of dementia and cognitive functions associated with Alzheimer's disease (AD). Only four studies met the inclusion criteria for the evaluation, because in many of the trials patients did not have a clear diagnosis of dementia and AD. There were 212 patients each in the ginkgo and placebo groups of the four studies. Based on a quantitative analysis of these trials, the researchers concluded that administration of 120 mg to 240 mg GBE (EGb 761, Tanakan®; Ipsen, France) for three to six months had a small but significant effect on objective measures of cognitive function in AD, without significant adverse effects in formal clinical trials.

Until recently, market claims for the application of ginkgo for Alzheimer's dis-ease were viewed as exaggerated and unfounded. However, three studies have sug-gested potential benefits in this area. Ginkgo has shown therapeutic potential in slowing some of the symptoms associated with early stages of Alzheimer's disease. In a randomized, double-blind, placebo-controlled study of 40 patients with senile dementia of the Alzheimer type, a daily dose of 240 mg of EGb 761 was given to the treatment group (Hofferberth, 1994). Battery tests were administered at base-line, one, two, and three months, with a significant improvement in memory and attention in the ginkgo group after only one month. No side effects were reported, and improvement continued over the three-month study.

Another study also suggests ginkgo's benefits for early stages of Alzheimer's (Kanowski et al., 1996, 1997). A randomized, double-blind, placebo-controlled study of 156 patients with presenile or senile primary degenerative dementia of the Alzheimer's type or multi-infarct dementia was conducted for 24 weeks using EGb 761. Seventy-nine subjects received 240 mg ginkgo extract per day; 77 received placebo. The ginkgo group was observed to have responded at a rate of 28% to three primary variables compared to only 10% for the placebo group. The authors concluded that GBE is "of clinical efficacy in the treatment of outpatients with dementia" of the two types noted.

Of considerable interest was the recent study published in *JAMA* on ginkgo's effects in preventing symptoms associated with Alzheimer's (Le Bars et al., 1997). This involved a placebo-controlled, double-blind, randomized, multicenter trial with 202 men and women 45 years of age or older, diagnosed with mild to moder-ately severe dementia. The trial lasted 52 weeks, with 97 subjects given 120 mg per day of EGb 761, and 105 given placebo. Using standardized assessment scales, patients were evaluated at baseline and at three-month intervals for cognitive func-tion, daily living skills, social behavior, and overall impairment. Compared to placebo, the ginkgo group showed either improvement or a delay in progression of the disease with every assessment tool except that used for evaluation of overall impairment. The researchers concluded that EGb 761 was safe and appeared capable of stabilizing and, in a substantial number of cases, improving the cognitive performance and the social functioning of demented patients for six months to one year.

In an editor's note published with the Le Bars study, *JAMA* senior editor Margaret Winker, M.D., acknowledged that "Few treatments for Alzheimer's disease (AD) have been found to be both effective and acceptable to patients and their caregivers" (Winker, 1997). She noted the increase in popularity of natural substances for various conditions and lamented the lack of controlled clinical trials (presumably focusing on American medical journals) to test these products and the fact that, as natural products, their chemistry of "active ingredients" is variable. Dr. Winker stated that this trial used EGb 761, the chemically defined, standardized extract for treatment of dementia. She pointed out, "While the effect size was modest, EGb 761 reduced patients' cognitive decline and manifestations of dementia rated by the caregiver as compared with placebo, particularly for patients with a diagnosis of AD. The mechanism of action is unclear but it is postulated to be related to the agent's antioxidant properties. Only a single dose was studied, dropout rates were high, and longer-term follow-up will be important; but this agent is an intriguing addition to the drugs thought to be helpful for patients with AD."

A recent review compared ginkgo with two conventional nootropic (cognitive-activating) medications (Letzel et al., 1996). Forty-four randomized, double-blind, placebo-controlled clinical trials were reviewed in which ginkgo extract, nimodipine, and tacrine were tested. Statistically significant results were obtained at three levels of efficacy (psychopathological, psychometric, and behavioral) for all three substances. The authors compared 25 studies on ginkgo, 9 on nimodipine, and 10 on tacrine. They noted that frequency of adverse events was lowest with ginkgo, confirming the previously established relative safety of ginkgo extract. They also compared study design to new standards set in Germany and the European Community, reporting that progress in the methodology of the studies has improved in the last decade and that "the efficacy of *Ginkgo biloba* special extract and tacrine has already been demonstrated according to the strictest criteria."

Another recent review investigated the use of ginkgo for dementia (Alzheimer type, multi-infarct dementia, or mixed types) (Ernst and Pittler, 1999). Eighteen double-blind, randomized, placebo-controlled trials were identified by the authors after extensive search on major databases. Nine were excluded, eight because patients were assessed with "cerebral insufficiency" and one due to assessment of cerebro-organic syndome. The authors concluded that the majority of randomized controlled trials support the idea that GBE is "efficacious in delaying the clinical deterioration of patients with dementia or in bringing about symptomatic improvement." The authors noted that none of the current studies were "flawless and ultimately convincing" but that the safety and tolerability profile of ginkgo is "reassuring." They called for more research to answer many questions that remain about ginkgo's efficacy.

A review of controlled studies on GBE in the treatment of intermittent claudication reported on 10 trials, finding most of poor methodological quality. All studies implied gingko was an effective therapy for intermittent claudication. The author recommended further trials with meticulous methodology, including studies on whether ginkgo can be usefully combined with walking exercise (Ernst, 1996). The Commission E reviewed some of these studies and concluded that there was sufficient evidence for approval for this indication. A recent trial on 111 patients with angiographically proven peripheral arterial disease and intermittent claudication was published on EGb 761 (Peters et al., 1998). A significant increase in pain-free walking distance was observed in the group taking 120 mg ginkgo extract over a 24-week study conducted in five centers. However, because Doppler index values did not change to indicate an increase in total circulation to the legs, the authors of this study speculated that the improvement in walking distance may be due to improved nutrition to tissues and microcirculation, rather than changes in macro-circulatory parameters.

The use of GBE (EGb 761) was examined for the treatment of peripheral arterial occlusive disease in a randomized, placebo-controlled, double-blind study. Forty patients suffering from Fontaine stage IIb were given two 80 mg tablets per day and the difference in pain-free walking distance was measured after eight, sixteen, and twenty-four weeks of treatment. By twenty-four weeks, the changes in the mean pain-free walking distance were +47.7% and +14.3% (p=0.021). The study concluded that the tolerability of GBE was good and that it had demonstrated clinical efficacy for peripheral arterial occlusive disease (Blume et al., 1998).

An analysis of twelve placebo-controlled, randomized, double-blind studies (five on GBE, seven on pentoxifylline) found a relative increase in pain-free walking distance of 45% for GBE (EGb 761) and 57% for pentoxifylline, the most-frequently prescribed synthetic treatment for peripheral occlusive arterial disease (Letzel and Schoop, 1992).

A meta-analysis of EGb 761 in the treatment of peripheral arterial disease examined five placebo-controlled trials with similar design and inclusion criteria (Schneider, 1992). In all studies, treatment effect was quantified by the increase of walking distance measured in a standard treadmill exercise. The analysis revealed a highly significant therapeutic effect of EGb 761 for the treatment of peripheral arterial disease, based on a mean increase in walking distance of 0.75 times (of the standard deviation) higher than that achieved by placebo. A daily dose of 120 mg for six months was successful in the treatment of intermittent claudication in 79 patients (Bauer, 1984). The randomized, placebo-controlled, double-blind study found significant improvement in the ginkgo group compared to placebo after 24 weeks.

The results of studies on ginkgo's effectiveness in tinnitus (ringing of the ears) have been mixed. A recent study failed to substantiate ginkgo's efficacy in treating this condition. Eighty patients were given ginkgo in this open trial, with 21 patients reporting improvements. Twenty of the 21 patients reporting improvements were then included in a double-blind, placebo-controlled, crossover study, with discouraging results. Seven patients believed ginkgo effective, seven preferred placebo, and the other six found no difference between placebo and ginkgo. The authors concluded that while statistical group analysis in this study did not support the use of ginkgo for tinnitus, it is possible that GBE has an effect on some patients (Holgers et al, 1994). However, this study was not performed using the GBE EGb 761, and the dose was 29.2 mg of extract per day instead of the usual dose of 120–240 mg per day. The Commission E approved GBE for tinnitus of "vascular and involutive origin."

In a randomized, double-blind, placebo-controlled study on tinnitus, 99 patients were given a 40 mg tablet of GBE (EGb 761), 3 times daily for 12 weeks. Improvement in the sound volume (5 to 10 dB) of the ear with the worst tinnitus was shown after 8 and 12 weeks in the GBE group, while the placebo group remained unchanged. Statistically significant differences were not observed in the other measured parameters: the contralateral ear, click-evoked otoacoustic emissions, subjective assessment of intensity, or hearing loss (Morgenstern and Biermann, 1997).

An interesting study of mountain climbers was conducted in the Himalayas using EGb 761 (Tanakan®) (Roncin et al., 1996). This randomized, controlled study was based on 44 healthy men who had experienced symptoms of altitude sickness on previous climbs. Over a period of eight days, they ascended to a base camp at about 14,700 feet elevation, with periodic ascents to higher points. The daily dose for the ginkgo group was two tablets twice per day (160 mg total). According to the assessment of cerebral symptoms, none of the climbers in the ginkgo group experienced acute mountain sickness (headache, dizziness, shortness of breath, nausea, vomiting), compared to 41% of the placebo group. In the assessment by respiratory parameters, 14% of the ginkgo climbers experienced altitude sickness, compared to 82% in the placebo group. Ginkgo was also rated significantly more effective in preventing cold-related circulatory problems (numbness, tingling, aching, and swelling of extremities), based on evaluations of the functional disabilities and results obtained by plethysmography (measurement extremity circulation). Also, 18% of the ginkgo climbers reported moderate or severe impairment of diuresis, compared to 77% on placebo.

In a somewhat novel application of ginkgo, researchers have studied its benefits in assisting patients suffering from anti-depression-induced sexual dysfunction, caused predominantly by selective serotonin reuptake inhibitors (SSRIs) (Cohen and Bartlik, 1998). The study was conducted in response to a case of a geriatric patient using *Ginkgo biloba* for memory enhancement who reported improved erections. The open study on 63 subjects found that women (33) were more responsive to the sexually enhancing effects than men (30), with relative success rates of 91% compared to 76% for the men. The ginkgo (product brand not noted) was given at a dosage range of 60 to 120 mg twice daily, within the normal range for the usual applications of ginkgo. The ginkgo reportedly had a positive effect on all four phases of the sexual response cycle: desire, excitement (erection and lubrication), orgasm, and resolution (afterglow). The authors note that the mechanism of action for this application is not yet clear. Postulated mechanisms include enhanced circulation to genitals by inhibition of PAF, direct effect on prostaglandins, known to enhance erectile function, and yet-to-be described norepinephrine receptor-induced effects on the brain.

In sum, there is a considerable degree of evidence from clinical trials to support the present use of GBE for a range of cognitive and peripheral vascular conditions. This conclusion was reinforced by the recent publication of a monograph on ginkgo by the World Health Organization (see Uses, below) (WHO, 1999).

Although most commercial ginkgo products sold as dietary supplements in the United States appear to be standardized to similar parameters (i.e., concentrated 50–1, standardized to 65 terpenes and 24% flavonol glycosides), it is possible that there may be differences in the biological activity of various brands. One study compared three commercial products in humans by measuring dynamic mapping of brain wave activity by computer-aided EEG (Itil and Mortorano, 1995). All three products increased alpha activity and decreased delta, theta, and beta waves. The study demonstrated that one product (Ginkgold®, Nature's Way, Utah; equivalent to EGb 761) was observed in all areas of the brain, while the effects of the others were limited to specific areas: one brand was limited to the temporal area and the other was limited primarily to the frontal area and slightly in the left posterior temporal area. The authors concluded that Ginkgold® produced the most homogeneous central nervous system effects in healthy subjects, with 9 out of 12 showing central nervous system effects correlated with cognitive activating drugs, e.g., tacrine.

In 1994, the Commission E published a negative (unapproved) monograph for various types of ginkgo preparations that did not conform to the parameters for the approved dried standardized preparation (made with acetone and water). These unapproved preparations include crude ginkgo leaf and related preparations, plus non-standardized extracts and fluidextracts from ginkgo leaf made with water and ethanol or methanol. The approved monograph clearly focuses on a specific type of preparation; the two commercial extracts of this type being the preparations on which almost all the scientific and clinical studies on the effectiveness of GBE have been carried out (as noted above). Thus, only the specified acetone-water extract of ginkgo was approved.

In May 1997, the German Federal Institute for Drugs and Medical Devices (BfArM) sent a letter to manufacturers of ginkgo extracts and other preparations regarding the levels of ginkgolic acids in these products. The letter stated that, based on the present level of knowledge, the BfArM considered it necessary to reduce the content of ginkgolic acids in finished ginkgo preparations to a maximum level of five parts per million. If proof of this level cannot be documented, "the registration for these pharmaceuticals will be cancelled since in this case, there is the well-founded suspicion that the pharmaceuticals—when used in accordance with the instructions [in the monographs]—produce damaging effects which exceed a justifiable degree according to the knowledge of medical science" (Thiele, 1997).

Pharmacopeial grade ginkgo leaf, for use in manufacturing the standardized extracts described in this monograph, consists of the dried leaf of *Ginkgo biloba* L. The raw material may contain no more than 3.0% stems and not more than 2.0% other foreign organic matter. It must contain not less than 0.8% flavonol glycosides as determined by liquid chromatography. Botanical identity must be confirmed by a thin-layer chromatography (TLC) test, as well as macroscopic and microscopic examinations (USP 24–NF19, 1999). Additionally, the *British Herbal Pharmacopoeia* requires that the dried leaf contain not less than 18% water-soluble extractive (BHP, 1996).

Description

A dry extract from the dried leaf of *Ginkgo biloba* L. manufactured using acetone-water and subsequent purification steps without addition of concentrates or isolated ingredients. The preparation/extract ratio is 35–67:1, on average 50:1. The extract is characterized by: 22–27% flavonone glycosides, determined as quercetin and kaempferol, including isorhamnetin (via HPLC) and calculated as flavones with a molar mass of $MM_r = 756.7$ (quercetin glycosides) and $M_r = 740.7$ (kaempferol glycosides); 5–7% terpene lactones, of which approximately 2.8–3.4% consists of ginkgolides A, B, and C, as well as approximately 2.6–3.2% bilobalide; below 5 ppm ginkgolic acids. The given ranges include manufacturing and analytical variances.

Chemistry and Pharmacology

Ginkgo leaf contains diterpenes including ginkgolide A, ginkgolide B, ginkgolide C (Budavari, 1996), plus ginkgolide J, and the sesquiterpene bilobalide; flavonols, including kaempferol, quercetin, and isorhamnetin; flavones, including luteolin and tricetin; biflavones, mainly bilobetin, ginkgetin, isoginkgetin (Huang, 1999; Leung and Foster, 1996), and sciadopitysin (Gobbato et al., 1996); catechins; proanthocyanidins; sterols (Leung and Foster, 1996); and 6-hydroxykynurenic acid (6-HKA) (Gräsel and Reuter, 1998).

According to the Commission E, the following pharmacological effects have been established experimentally:

Improvement of hypoxic tolerance, particularly in the cerebral tissue.

Inhibition of the development of traumatically or toxically induced cerebral edema, and acceleration of its regression.

Reduction of retinal edema and of cellular lesions in the retina.

Inhibition in age-related reduction of muscarinergic cholinoceptors and alpha-adrenoceptors as well as stimulation of choline uptake in the hippocampus.

Increased memory performance and learning capacity.

Improvement in the compensation of disturbed equilibrium.

Improvement of blood flow, particularly in the region of microcirculation.

Improvement of the rheological properties of the blood.

Inactivation of toxic oxygen radicals (flavonoids).

Antagonism of the platelet-activating factor (PAF) (ginkgolides).

Neuroprotective effect (ginkgolides A and B, bilobalide).

The pharmacokinetics have been investigated both in animal experiments and in trials involving humans. An absorption rate of 60% was found in rats for a radioactively labeled extract (as specified under the Description section, above). In humans, after application of an extract specified as above, absolute bioavailability was 98–100% for ginkgolide A, 79–93% for ginkgolide B, and at least 70% for bilobalide.

Both the acute and the chronic toxicity of an extract as specified under Description is very low; accordingly, the LD50 in the mouse was 7725 mg/kg body weight after oral application and 1100 mg/kg body weight after intravenous application.

Investigations with this extract as specified above showed no effects which were either mutagenic, carcinogenic, or toxic to reproduction (DeFeudis, 1998).

No evaluation was performed on the transferability of the experimental results to extracts other than those investigated.
[Ed. note: This statement refers to the fact that only a few proprietary ginkgo extracts were used in the studies upon which this monograph is based. Whether these results can be extrapolated to other ginkgo extracts is uncertain.]

The vaso- and tissue-protective actions of ginkgo extract include the properties of relaxing blood vessels in spastic conditions, increasing tone of abnormally relaxed vessels, protecting against capillary permeability, inhibiting platelet aggregation and antithrombotic activity, and anti-ischemic and anti-edematous properties. The flavonoids present in GBE may be responsible for the cognitive-enhancing action of ginkgo extract. These flavonoids may enhance the release of catecholamines and other neurotransmitters, inhibit biogenic amine uptake, protect catechol-O-methyltransferase and monoamine oxidase, and protect endothelial-derived relaxing factor mechanisms in the brain (Van Beek et al., 1998).

Uses

The Commission E approved the internal use of ginkgo for the following conditions:

(a) For symptomatic treatment of disturbed performance in organic brain syndrome within the regimen of a therapeutic concept in cases of dementia syndromes with the following principal symptoms: memory deficits, disturbances in concentration, depressive emotional condition, dizziness, tinnitus, and headache. The primary target groups are dementia syndromes, including primary degenerative dementia, vascular dementia, and mixed forms of both.

Note: Before starting treatment with ginkgo extract, clarification should be obtained as to whether the pathological symptoms encountered are not based on an underlying disease requiring a specific treatment.

(b) Improvement of pain-free walking distance in peripheral arterial occlusive disease in Stage II according to Fontaine (intermittent claudication) in a regimen of physical therapeutic measures, in particular walking exercise.

(c) Vertigo and tinnitus (ringing in the ear) of vascular and involutional origin.

The World Health Organization reiterated the Commission E approved uses noted above, adding the following specific conditions to peripheral arterial occlusive disease: Raynaud's disease (intermittent blue coloring of extremities due to restricted blood flow with no known direct cause, i.e., idiopathic, other than possible cold or emotion), acrocyanosis (i.e., Crocq's disease: persistently poor circulation to hands and sometimes the feet, resulting in cold, blue, sweaty condition), and post phlebitis syndrome (painful swelling of veins) (WHO, 1999).

Contraindications

The Commission E noted hypersensitivity to ginkgo preparations.

The product data sheet of the leading ginkgo preparation (EGb 761) notes that the 120 mg dosage (Tebonin® intens 120 mg) should not be used in children under 12. "Since Ginkgo extracts have not yet been sufficiently investigated in case of depressive mood and headache not occurring in relation with demential syndromes, [this product] may only be applied in these symptoms when taking into consideration all necessary precautionary measures" (Schwabe, 1999).

Side Effects

Very seldom cases of stomach or intestinal upsets, headaches, or allergic skin reaction.

Use During Pregnancy and Lactation

No restrictions known.

Interactions with Other Drugs

Commission E reported that none were known (based on data available before publication of the monograph in July, 1994).

The Tebonin® product data sheet notes, "The effect of platelet-aggregation inhibitors may be enhanced. The case of a spontaneous hyphema after combined intake of a Ginkgo-biloba-containing pharmaceutical and aspirin has been documented" (Schwabe, 1999).

Dosage and Administration

Unless otherwise prescribed: 120–240 mg standardized dry extract in liquid or solid pharmaceutical form for oral intake, given in two or three daily doses to treat indication (a) listed above in the Use section. Indications (b) and (c) require 120–160 mg native dry extract, given in two or three daily doses.

References

Bauer, U. 1984. Six-month double-blind randomized clinical trial of Ginkgo biloba extract versus placebo in two parallel groups of patients suffering from peripheral arterial insufficiency. Arzneimforsch 34(6):716–720.

Blume, J., M. Kieser, U. Hölscher. 1998. [Efficacy of Ginkgo biloba special extract EGb 761 in peripheral arterial occlusive disease] [In German]. Fortschr Med 116:137-143.

British Herbal Pharmacopoeia (BHP). 1996. Exeter, U.K.: British Herbal Medicine Association. 87–88.

Budavari, S. (ed.). 1996. The Merck Index: An Encyclopedia of Chemicals, Drugs, and Biologicals, 12th ed. Whitehouse Station, N.J.: Merck & Co, Inc. 751.

Cohen, A.J. and B. Bartlik. 1998. Ginkgo Biloba for antidepressant-induced sexual dysfunction. J Sex Marital Ther 24(2):139–143.

DeFeudis, F.V. 1998. Ginkgo biloba extract (EGb 761): From Chemistry to the Clinic. Weisbaden, Germany: Ullstein Medical Verlagsgesellschaft.

Ernst, E. 1996. [Ginkgo biloba in treatment of intermittent claudication. A systematic research based on controlled studies in the literature] [In German]. Fortschr Med 114(8):85–87.

Ernst, E. and M.H. Pittler. 1999. Ginkgo biloba Dementia: A systematic review of double-blind, placebo-controlled trials. Clin Drug Invest 17(4):301–308.

Gobbato, S., A. Griffini, E. Lolla, F. Peterlongo. 1996. HPLC quantitative analysis of biflavones in Ginkgo biloba leaf extracts and their identification by thermospray liquid chromatography-mass spectrometry. Fitoterapia 67(2):152–158.

Gräsel, I. and G. Reuter. 1998. Analysis of 6-hydroxykynurenic acid in Ginkgo biloba and Ginkgo preparations. Planta Med 64:566–570.

Hofferberth, B. 1994. The efficacy of EGb 761 in patients with senile dementia of the Alzheimer type: A double-blind, placebo-controlled study on different levels of investigation. Hum Psychopharmacol 9:215–222.

Holgers K., A. Axelsson, I. Pringle. 1994. Ginkgo biloba extract for the treatment of tinnitus. Audiology 33(2):85–92.

Hopfenmüller, W. 1994. [Proof of the therapeutic effectiveness of a Ginkgo biloba special extract. Meta-analysis of 11 clinical trials in aged patients with cerebral insufficiency] [In German]. Arzneimforsch 44(9):1005–1013.

Huang, K.C. 1999. The Pharmacology of Chinese Herbs. Boca Raton: CRC Press. 97–99.

Itil, T. and D. Martorano. 1995. Natural substances in psychiatry (Ginkgo biloba in dementia). Psychopharm Bull 31(1):147–158.

Kanowski, S., W.M. Hermann, K. Stephan, W. Wierich, R. Horr. 1997. Proof of the efficacy of the Ginkgo biloba special extract EGb 761 in outpatients suffering from mild to moderate dementia of the Alzheimer's type or multi-infarct dementia. Phytomedicine 4(1):3–13.

Kanowski, S., W.M. Hermann, K. Stephan, W. Wierich, R. Horr. 1996. Proof of efficacy of the Ginkgo biloba special extract EGb 761 in outpatients suffering from mild to moderate primary degenerative dementia of the Alzheimer type or multi-infarct dementia. Pharmacopsychiatry 29:47–56.

Kleijnen, J. and P. Knipschild. 1992a. Ginkgo biloba for cerebral insufficiency. Br J Clin Pharmacol 34(4):352–358.

———. 1992b. Ginkgo biloba. Lancet 340(8828):1136–1139.

Le Bars, P.L. et al. 1997. A placebo-controlled, double-blind, randomized trial of an extract of *Ginkgo biloba* for dementia. *JAMA* 278(16):1327–1332.

Letzel, H., J. Haan, W.B. Feil. 1996. Nootropics: Efficacy and tolerability of products from three active substance classes. *J Drug Dev Clin Pract* 8:77–94.

Letzel, H. and W. Schoop. 1992. *Ginkgo biloba* extract EGb 761 and pentoxifylline in intermittent claudicaton: Secondary analysis of clinical efficacy studies. *Vasa* 21(4):403–410.

Leung, A.Y. and S. Foster. 1996. *Encyclopedia of Common Natural Ingredients Used in Food, Drugs, and Cosmetics*, 2nd ed. New York: John Wiley & Sons, Inc.

Morgenstern, C. and E. Biermann. 1997. *Ginkgo biloba* special extract EGb 761 in the treatment of tinnitus aurium: Results of a randomized, double-blind, placebo-controlled study. *Fortschr Med* 115(4):7–11.

Oken, B.S., D.M. Storzbach, J.A. Kaye. 1998. The efficacy of *Ginkgo biloba* on cognitive function in Alzheimer disease. *Arch Neurol* 55(11):1409–1415.

Peters, H., M. Kieser, U. Holscher. 1998. Demonstration of the efficacy of *Ginkgo biloba* special extract EGb 761 on intermittent claudication—a placebo-controlled, double-blind multicenter trial. *Vasa* 27(2):105–110.

Rai, G.S., C. Shovlin, K.A. Wesnes. 1991. A double-blind, placebo controlled study of *Ginkgo biloba* extract (Tanakan) in elderly out-patients with mild to moderate memory impairment. *Curr Med Res Opin* 12(6):350–355.

Roncin, J.P., F. Schwartz, P. D'Arbigny. 1996. EGb 761 in control of acute mountain sickness and vascular reactivity to cold exposure. *Aviat Space Environ Med* 67(5):445–52.

Schneider, B. 1992. *Ginkgo biloba* extract in peripheral arterial diseases. Meta-analysis of controlled clinical studies. *Arzneimforsch* 42(4):428–436.

Thiele, A. 1997. Averting of drug-induced risks, grade II: pharmaceuticals containing *Ginkgo biloba* leaves. Communication to Dr. Willmar Schwabe GmbH & Co., May 27.

United States Pharmacopeia, 24th rev. and *National Formulary*, 19th ed. (USP 24–NF19). 1999. Rockville, MD: United States Pharmacopeial Convention, Inc. 2458–2459.

Van Beek, T.A., E. Bombardelli, P. Morazzoni, F. Peterlongo. 1998. *Ginkgo biloba* L. *Fitoterapia* 49(3):195–244.

Schwabe. 1999. Tebonin® intens 120 mg Data Sheet. Karlsruhe, Germany: Willmar Schwabe Arzneimittel GmbH & Co.

Vesper, J. and K.D. Hänsgen. 1994. Efficacy of *Ginkgo biloba* in 90 outpatients with cerebral insufficiency caused by old age. *Phytomedicine* 1:9–16.

Vorberg, G. 1985. *Ginkgo biloba* extract (GBE): A long-term study of chronic cerebral insufficiency in geriatric patients. *Clin Trials J* 22:149–157.

Warburton, D.M. 1988. Clinical psychopharmacology of *Ginkgo biloba* extract. In: Funfgeld, E.W. (ed.). *Rokan (Ginkgo biloba): Recent Results in Pharmacology and Clinic*. Berlin: Springer Verlag. 327–345.

Winker, M.A. 1997. Aging: A global issue [Editor's Note]. *JAMA* 278(16):1378b.

World Health Organization (WHO). 1999. Ginkgo folium. *WHO Monographs on Selected Medicinal Plants*, Vol. 1. Geneva: World Health Organization.

Additional Resources

Ahlemeyer, B. and J. Kriglstein. 1998. Neuroprotective Effects of *Ginkgo biloba* Extract. In: L.D. Lawson and R. Bauer (eds.). *Phytomedicines of Europe: Chemistry and Biological Activity*. Washington, DC: American Chemical Society. 210–220.

Auguer, M. et al. 1994. *Advances in Ginkgo biloba Extract Research*, Vol. 3. Elsevier: Paris. 31–37.

Blume J., M. Kieser, U. Hölscher. 1996. [Placebo-controlled double-blind study on the efficacy of *Ginkgo biloba* special extract EGb 761 in maximum-level-trained patients with intermittent claudication] [In German]. *Vasa* 25(3):265–274.

Bone, K. 1996. Ginkgo—Recent Research. *Can J Herbalism* Spring:29–41.

Braquet, P. 1987. The ginkgolides: potent platelet-activating factor antagonists isolated from *Ginkgo biloba* L.: Chemistry, pharmacology and clinical applications. *Drugs of the Future* (12):643–699.

Brown, D. 1997. Ginkgo Biloba Extract for Age-Related Cognitive Decline and Early-stage Dementia—A Clinical Overview. *Quarterly Rev Nat Med* Summer:91–96.

Bruneton, J. 1995. *Pharmacognosy, Phytochemistry, Medicinal Plants*. Paris: Lavoisier Publishing.

Chatterjee, S.S. et al. 1985. *Effects of Ginkgo Biloba Extract on Organic Cerebral Impairment*. London: John Libbey Eurotext, Ltd.

Chung, K.F. et al. 1987. Effect of a ginkgo-like mixture (BN 52063) in antagonizing skin and platelet responses to platelet activating factor in man. *Lancet* (1):218–219.

DeFeudis, F.V. 1991. *Ginkgo biloba extract (EGb 761): Pharmacological Activities and Clinical Applications*. Elsevier Editions Scientifiques: Paris. 50–51.

Della Loggia, R. et al. 1996. Anti-inflammatory activity of some *Ginkgo biloba* constituents and their phospholipid-complexes. *Fitoterapia* 67(3):257–264.

Foster, S. 1991. *Ginkgo biloba. Botanical Booklet Series*, No. 304. Austin, TX: American Botanical Council.

Guinot, P., E. Caffrey, R. Lambe, A. Darragh. 1989. Tanakan inhibits platelet-activating-factor-induced platelet aggregation in healthy male volunteers. *Haemostasis* 19(4):219–223.

Haguenauer, J.P., F. Cantenot, H. Koskas, H. Pierart. 1988. Treatment of disturbed equilibrium with Ginkgo Biloba extract: Multicenter double-blind study versus placebo. In: Füngfeld, E.W. (ed.). *Rökan (Ginkgo Biloba). Recent Results in Pharmacology and Clinic.* New York: Springer Verlag.

Itil, T.M., E. Erlap, E. Tsambis, K.Z. Itil, U. Stein. 1996. Central nervous system effect of Ginkgo Biloba, a plant extract. *Am J Therapeutics* 3(63):63–73.

Itil, T.M., S.H. Kornhauser, I. Ahmed. 1996. Early diagnosis and treatment of memory disturbances. *Am J Electromed* Jun:81–85.

Janssens, D. et al. 1995. Protection of hypoxia-induced ATP decrease in endothelial cells by *Ginkgo biloba* extract and bilobalide. *Biochem Pharmacol* 50(7):991–999.

Jung, F., C. Mrowietz, H. Kiesewetter, E. Wenzel. 1990. Effect of Gingko Biloba on fluidity of blood and peripheral microcirculation in volunteers. *Arzneimforsch* 40(5):589–593.

Maurer, K., R. Ihl, T. Dierks, L. Frolich. 1997. Clinical efficacy of Gingko biloba special extract EGb 761 in dementia of the Alzheimer type. *J Psychiatr Res* 31(6):645–655.

Meyer, B. 1988. A multicenter randomized double-blind study of *Ginkgo biloba* extract versus placebo in the treatment of tinnitus. In: Fünfgeld, E.W. (ed.). *Rökan (Ginkgo Biloba). Recent Results in Pharmacology and Clinic.* New York: Springer Verlag.

Pietri, S., J.R. Seguin, P. d'Arbigny, K. Drieu, M. Culcasi. 1997. Gingko biloba extract (EGb 761) pretreatment limits free radical-induced oxidative stress in patients undergoing coronary bypass surgery. *Cardiovasc Drugs Ther* 11(2):121–131.

Pincemail, J. and C. Deby. 1986. Propietes anti-radiclaites de l'extraite de *Ginkgo biloba* [Antiradical properties of *Ginkgo biloba* extract]. *Presse Med* 15(31):1475–1479.

Pincemail, J. et al. 1989. Superoxide anion scavenging effect and superoxide dismutase activity of *Ginkgo biloba* extract. *Experientia* 45:708–712.

Robben Batre, P. et al. 1996. Phase II study with 5-FU plus Gingko biloba extract (GBE 761 ONC) in 5-FU pretreated patients with advanced colorectal cancer. (Annual Congress of the German and the Austrian Society of Hematology) *Ann Hematol* 73(2):A73.

Schulz, V., R. Hänsel, V.E. Tyler. 1998. *Rational Phytotherapy: A Physicians' Guide to Herbal Medicine.* New York: Springer. 38-50.

Scorolli, L. et al. 1997. Evolution of color vision in early diabetic retinopathy treated by *Ginkgo biloba* extract. *Ann Ottalmol Clin Ocul* 123(6–8):245–251.

Smith, P.F., K. Maclennan, C.L. Darlington. The neuroprotective properties of *Ginkgo biloba* leaf: a review of the possible relationship to platelet-activating factor. 1996. *J Ethnopharmacol* 50(3):131–139.

Soholm, B.1998. Clinical improvement of memory and other cognitive functions by Gingko biloba: Review of relevant literature. *Adv Ther* 15(1):54–65.

Tang, W. and G. Eisenbrand. 1992. *Chinese Drugs of Plant Origin: Chemistry, Pharmacology, and Use in Traditional and Modern Medicine.* New York: Springer Verlag.

Wesnes, K.A. et al. 1997. The cognitive, subjective, and physical effects of a *Ginkgo biloba/Panax ginseng* combination in healthy volunteers with neurasthenic complaints. *Psychopharmacol Bull* 33(4):677–683.

This monograph, published by the Commission E in 1994, was modified based on new scientific research. It contains more extensive pharmacological and therapeutic information taken directly from the Commission E.

This material was adapted from *The Complete German Commission E Monographs—Therapeutic Guide to Herbal Medicines.* M. Blumenthal, W.R. Busse, A. Goldberg, J. Gruenwald, T. Hall, C.W. Riggins, R.S. Rister (eds.) S. Klein and R.S. Rister (trans.). 1998. Austin: American Botanical Council; Boston: Integrative Medicine Communications.

1) The Overview section is new information.

2) Description, Chemistry and Pharmacology, Uses, Contraindications, Side Effects, Interactions with Other Drugs, and Dosage sections have been drawn from the original work. Additional information has been added in some or all of these sections, as noted with references.

3) The dosage for equivalent preparations (tea infusion, fluidextract, and tincture) have been provided based on the following example:
Unless otherwise prescribed: 2 g per day of [powdered, crushed, cut or whole] [plant part]
Infusion: 2 g in 150 ml of water
Fluidextract 1:1 (g/ml): 2 ml
Tincture 1:5 (g/ml): 10 ml

4) The References and Additional Resources sections are new sections. Additional Resources are not cited in the monograph but are included for research purposes.

GINSENG ROOT

Latin Name:
Panax ginseng

Pharmacopeial Name:
Ginseng radix

Other Names:
Asian Ginseng, Chinese ginseng, Korean ginseng, true ginseng

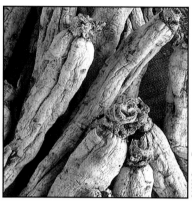

© 1999 Steven Foster

Overview

Ginseng is a slow-growing perennial herb native to the mountain forests of north-eastern China, Korea, and the far eastern regions of the Russian Federation. In China, the natural range for ginseng extends from Hebei Province to the three northeastern provinces of Liaoning, Jilin, and Heilongjiang. It is cultivated exten-sively in China, Japan, Korea, and Russia. The Changbai mountain range is report-edly the only area in China where wild ginseng still occurs naturally (Bone, 1998; Foster and Chongxi, 1992; Leung and Foster, 1996; Melisch et al., 1997; Wichtl and Bisset, 1994). It usually starts flowering at its fourth year and the roots take four to six years to reach maturity. "White" ginseng root (unprocessed) is some-times bleached and then dried and "red" ginseng is prepared from white ginseng by various processing methods, such as steaming the fresh root before drying. There are many types and grades of ginseng, depending on the origin, root maturity, parts of the root used, and methods of raw material preparation or processing (Bradley, 1992; Foster and Chongxi, 1992; Leung and Foster, 1996). In Russia, *Panax gin-seng* comes mostly from cultivation and partly from permitted or illegal harvest in the wild. Wild ginseng is listed under protected status in the *Russian Red Data Book* and, therefore, its harvest and trade is prohibited under Russian law. Under China's nationally protected species schedule, ginseng is subject to the Protection Category 1, comparable to its status in the Russian Federation (Melisch et al., 1997). In China, North and South Korea, and Japan, *P. ginseng* comes from culti-vated sources (Yen, 1992).

Ginseng's genus name *Panax* is derived from the Greek *pan* (all) *akos* (cure), meaning cure-all. The transliteration of the word gin (man) seng (essence) is derived from the Chinese ideogram for "crystallization of the essence of the earth in the form of a man" (Foster, 1991; Hu, 1976). Ginseng's therapeutic uses were recorded in the oldest comprehensive materia medica, *Shen Nong Ben Cao Jing*, written around two thousand years ago. In Asian medicine, dried ginseng is used as a tonic to revitalize and replenish vital energy (*qi*). The usual effect of replenishing *qi* is not to give an energy boost like that of caffeine or amphetamine (Dhar-mananda, 1999). It is traditionally used as an aid during convalescence and as a prophylactic to build resistance, reduce susceptibility to illness, and promote health and longevity. Its activity appears to be based on whole body effects, rather than particular organs or systems, which lends support to the traditional view that gin-seng is a tonic that can revitalize the functioning of the organism as a whole. There is no equivalent concept or treatment in Western conventional medicine. However, multivitamins are used in a similar manner. In traditional Chinese medicine it is usually prescribed in combination with other herbs and taken in an aqueous decoc-tion dosage form (Bone, 1998; Foster and Chongxi, 1992; Leung and Foster, 1996; Wichtl and Bisset, 1994). Today, ginseng is official in the national pharmacopeias of Austria, China, France, Germany, Japan, Switzerland, and Russia (Bradley, 1992; DAB 10, 1994; JP XII, 1993; ÖAB, 1981; Ph.Fr.X, 1990; Ph.Helv.VII, 1987; Tu, 1992; USSR X, 1973; Wichtl and Bisset, 1994). The *Pharmacopoeia of the People's Republic of China* indicates its use for prostration with impending collapse marked by cold limbs and faint pulse; diminished function of the spleen with loss of appetite; diabetes caused by "internal heat"; general weakness with irritability and insomnia in chronic diseases; impotence or frigidity; and heart failure and cardiogenic shock (Tu, 1992). [It should be noted that in traditional Chinese medicine, the term "spleen" does not correlate to the western anatomical definition of spleen but rather to the entire digestive system, with regard to its functions of digestion, transport and distribution of nutrients, blood flow, and reinforcement of vital energy (*qi*). "Diabetes caused by internal heat" is a specific condition with symptoms including excessive thirst and urination, and sometimes accompanied by excessive eating (Tu, 1992; Yen, 1992).]

In Germany, ginseng is one of a few economically important herbal drugs listed separately in the Foreign Trade Statistics. In 1992, Germany imported 174.6 tons, mainly from China and Hong Kong. A considerable amount of the roots are value-added in Germany and then exported mostly to France, Italy, and Argentina (Lange and Schippmann, 1997). Ginseng is official in the *German Pharmacopoeia*, approved in the Commission E monographs, and used in geriatric remedies, roborants (invigorating and strengthening medicines), and tonic preparations. The Commission E specifies powdered root or tea infusions (BAnz, 1998; Bradley, 1992; DAB 10, 1994; Meyer-Buchtela, 1999; Wichtl and Bisset, 1994). In the United States, it is used by itself and as a main ingredient in a wide range of tonic, energy, and immunostimulant dietary supplements. It is also used extensively in traditional Chinese medicine herbal teas and other fluid or solid forms prescribed to patients by licensed acupuncturists and naturopathic physicians.

During the past fifty years, numerous scientific studies of varying quality have been published on ginseng (Foster and Chongxi, 1992). Modern human studies have investigated its preventive effect on several kinds of cancer (Yun et al., 1993; Yun and Choi, 1995, 1998), its effect on newly diagnosed non-insulin-dependent diabetes mellitus patients (Sotaniemi et al., 1995), its long-term immunological effect on HIV patients (Cho et al., 1994; Cho et al., 1997; Sankary, 1989), its ability to treat "qi-deficiency" and blood-stasis syndrome of coronary heart disease and angina pectoris (Jiang et al., 1992), its ability to treat hepatotoxin-induced liver disease in the elderly (Zuin et al., 1987), its effect on cell-mediated immune functions in healthy volunteers (Scaglione et al., 1990), its ability to induce a higher immune response in vaccination against influenza (Scaglione et al., 1996), its effect on blood pressure in patients with hypertension (Han et al., 1998), its effect on alveolar macrophages from patients suffering with chronic bronchitis (Scaglione et al., 1994), its ability to treat severe chronic respiratory diseases (Gross et al., 1995), its use in the treatment of functional fatigue (Le Gal et al., 1996), its ability to improve quality-of-life in persons subjected to high stress (Caso Marasco et al., 1996), its effect on psychomotor performance in healthy volunteers (D'Angelo et al., 1986), its effect on physical performance during exercise (Pieralisi et al., 1991), its ability to treat erectile dysfunction (Choi et al., 1995), and its ability to treat male infertility (Salvati et al., 1996).

Some clinical trials have suggested the use of ginseng for fatigue and the improvement of physical and mental performance (Dorling and Kirchdorfer, 1980; Forgo et al., 1981). Ginseng has been studied for treatment of cerebrovascular insufficiency (Quiroga and Imbriano, 1979; Quiroga, 1982), psychophysical asthenia and depressive symptoms (Rosenfield, 1989), immunomodulation (Scaglione et al., 1990; Scaglione et al., 1996). Trials have also reported favorable results in treating post-menopausal symptoms (Reinold, 1990) and improving athletic performance (Forgo and Kirchdorfer, 1981, 1982). A review in a popular newsletter has raised questions regarding the design and results of some of these studies (Schardt, 1999). Several recent trials have reported negative results for improvement of performance during aerobic exercise (Allen et al., 1998; Morris et al., 1996; Engels and Wirth, 1997; Cherdrungsi et al., 1995) and in the secondary treatment of geriatric patients (Thommessen and Laake, 1996).

Many of the clinical studies published in the scientific literature have been conducted on a proprietary extract of *P. ginseng* standardized to 4% total ginsenosides (G115®, Ginsana®, Pharmaton, Lugano, Switzerland). There have been four studies conducted on G115 to measure the effect of ginseng on endurance and vitality (Dorling and Kirchdorfer, 1980; Forgo et al., 1981; Gross et al., 1995; Sandberg, 1980). Three studies have been conducted on psychoasthenia (Mulz et al., 1990; Rosenfeld, 1989; Gianoli and Riebenfeld, 1984). Ten clinical trials have attempted to determine if ginseng affects physical stress and psychomotor functions (Forgo and Kirchdorfer, 1981; Forgo and Kirchdorfer, 1982; Forgo, 1983; Forgo and Schimert, 1985; Van Schepdael, 1993; Pujol et al., 1996; Engels and Wirth, 1997; Engels et al., 1996; Collomp et al., 1996; D'Angelo et al., 1986). Two clinical trials have investigated cerebral blood flow deficits (Quiroga and Imbriano, 1979; Quiroga, 1982). Two studies on pharmacodynamics measured the immunomodulatory effects (Scaglione et al., 1990; Scaglione et al., 1994), oxygen uptake (von Ardenne and Klemm, 1987), doping substances in urine (Mulz and Degenring, 1989; Forgo, 1980), and serum glucose, serum cholesterol, and serum triglyceride levels (Cheah, 1994).

One double-blind placebo-controlled study investigated the effect of ginseng on newly diagnosed non-insulin-dependent diabetes mellitus (NIDDM) patients (Sotaniemi et al., 1995). Thirty-six NIDDM patients (20 women and 16 men) were recruited in five health centers and were treated for eight weeks. Patients were randomized to ingest one tablet daily containing 0 (placebo), 100, or 200 mg ginseng, presumably an extract, but the authors did not state the type of preparation used in the study (manufactured by Dansk Droge, Copenhagen). Effects on psychophysical tests, measurements of glucose balance, serum lipids, aminoterminalpropeptide (PIINP) concentration, and body weight were tested. Ginseng therapy elevated mood, improved psychophysical performance, and reduced fasting blood glucose (FBG) and body weight. The 200 mg dose of ginseng improved glycated hemoglobin, serum PIINP, and physical activity. The authors concluded that ginseng may be a useful therapeutic adjunct in the management of NIDDM, but because the active material was not adequately identified, it is difficult to draw meaningful conclusions from this study.

To test for possible anticancer effects, one case-controlled study, conducted at the Laboratory of Experimental Pathology at the Korea Cancer Center Hospital with 1,987 pairs of subjects, investigated the preventive effect of ginseng intake against various human cancers (Yun and Choi, 1995). In this study, those participants ingesting ginseng had a decreased risk for cancer compared with non-users. A decrease in risk with increased frequency and duration of ginseng ingestion was reported, showing a dose-response relationship. The preventive effect was reported with the ingestion of fresh undried root extract, white dried root extract, powdered white dried root, and red steamed root. Other ginseng dosage forms tested in this study did not show a decrease in cancer risk including fresh sliced root, fresh root juice, and white root tea. The authors concluded that their findings support the view that patients who take ginseng have a decreased risk for most cancers compared with those who do not.

In a subsequent prospective study the non-organ specific cancer preventive effects of ginseng were investigated in 4,634 people over 40 years old, residing in ginseng production areas, from August, 1987 to December, 1992 (Yun and Choi, 1998). Among ginseng preparations, fresh ginseng extract consumers were associated with a significantly decreased risk of gastric cancer. The authors concluded that their results strongly suggest that ginseng has a non-organ specific preventive effect against cancer, providing support for the previous case-control studies.

The approved modern therapeutic applications for ginseng appear to be generally supportable based on its history of use in well established systems of traditional medicine, extensive phytochemical investigations, pharmacological studies in animals, and human clinical studies. However, recent studies do not support results from earlier research. The World Health Organization (WHO) has issued a monograph reviewing standards and therapeutics of Asian ginseng, concluding that some general uses are warranted by clinical data (see Uses below) (WHO, 1999).

Chinese and Japanese pharmacopeial grade ginseng must be composed of the dried mature root, collected in autumn, from which the rootlets have been removed. Botanical identity must be confirmed by thin-layer chromatography (TLC) as well as by macroscopic and microscopic examinations and organoleptic evaluation. It must contain not less than 14% dilute ethanol-soluble extractive, among other quantitative purity standards (JP XII, 1993; Tu, 1992). The *British Herbal Pharmacopoeia* requirements are comparable to the Asian monographs with some exceptions, including not less than 20% ethanol-soluble extractive (70%), calculated with reference to the oven-dried material (BHP, 1996). The *German Pharmacopoeia* requires not less than 1.5% total ginsenosides calculated as ginsenoside Rg_1, botanical identification by TLC, macroscopic and microscopic examination, organoleptic evaluation, and some quantitative purity standards (DAB 10, 1994). The Swiss Pharmacopoeia requires not less than 2% total ginsenosides calculated as ginsenoside Rg_1 (Ph.Helv.VII, 1987).

Description

Ginseng root consists of the dried main and lateral root and root hairs of *P. ginseng* C.A. Meyer [Fam. Araliaceae] and their preparations in effective dosage. The root contains at least 1.5% ginsenosides, calculated as ginsenoside Rg_1.

Chemistry and Pharmacology

The biologically active constituents in *P. ginseng* are a complex mixture of triterpene saponins known as ginsenosides (Lewis, 1986; Ng and Yeung, 1986; Liu and Xiao, 1992). The root contains 2–3% ginsenosides of which Rg_1, Rc, Rd, Rb_1, Rb_2, and Rb_0 are quantitatively the most important.

At least 30 ginsenosides have been isolated and characterized (Ng and Yeung, 1986). The pharmacological actions of individual ginsenosides may work in opposition. For example, the two main ginsenosides, Rb_1 and Rg_1, respectively suppress and stimulate the central nervous system (Chong and Oberholzer, 1988). These opposing actions may contribute to the "adapto-

genic" description of ginseng and its purported ability to balance bodily functions. Ginseng's pharmacological activities may be multiple and complex, due not only to ginsenosides but to a variety of compounds such as panacene (a peptidoglycan), which has exhibited hypoglycemic activity (Konno et al., 1984), a peptide with insulinomimetic properties (Ando et al., 1980), and salicylate and vanillic acid, which showed antioxidant and antifatigue effects in animals (Han et al., 1983).

The Commission E reported that in various stress models such as immobilization test and coldness test, the resistance of rodents was enhanced. Ginseng is reported to possess hormone-like and cholesterol-lowering effects, promote vasodilatation, and act as an anxiolytic and antidepressant (Choi et al., 1995; Chong and Oberholzer, 1988). Many studies on animals have found ginseng extracts and ginsenosides to be effective in stimulating learning, memory, and physical capabilities (Petkov and Mosharrof, 1987), supporting radioprotection (Takeda et al., 1981; Takeda et al., 1982), providing resistance to infection (Singh et al, 1984), demonstrating antioxidant and antifatigue effects (Han et al., 1983; Saito et al., 1974), enhancing energy metabolism (Avakian et al., 1984), and reducing plasma total cholesterol and triglycerides while elevating HDL levels (Yamamoto et al., 1983). A recent study at Yale University has suggested that ginseng's vasodilatory action may be due to nitric oxide synthesis (Gillis, 1997).

Uses

The Commission E approved ginseng as a tonic for invigoration and fortification in times of fatigue and debility or declining capacity for work and concentration. Ginseng was also approved for use during convalescence.

The World Health Organization (WHO) monograph section on "uses supported by clinical data" re-affirms the Commission E approved uses: "… used as a prophylactic and restorative agent for enhancement of mental and physical capacities, in cases of weakness, exhaustion, tiredness, and loss of concentration, and during convalescence" (WHO, 1999).

Contraindications

Hypertension (Bradley, 1992).

Side Effects

None known.

Use During Pregnancy and Lactation

The Commission E reports no known restrictions on the use of ginseng during pregnancy and lactation. Although the *British Herbal Compendium* contraindicates ginseng during pregnancy, this is not substantiated by use in Asia or by the Commission E (McGuffin et al., 1997). However, controlled, long-term safety studies have not been conducted. WHO has also reiterated that the safety of ginseng use during pregnancy has not been established, although it noted that ginseng is not teratogenic (WHO, 1999).

Interactions with Other Drugs

The *British Herbal Compendium* contraindicates the use of ginseng with stimulants, including excessive use of caffeine (Bradley, 1992). The WHO monograph cites two cases of ginseng interaction with phenelzine, a monoamine oxidase inhibitor, although the clinical significance of this interaction was yet to be determined (WHO, 1999).

Dosage and Administration

Unless otherwise prescribed: 1–2 g of root per day for up to three months; a repeated course is feasible.
Decoction: 1–2 g in 150 ml of water.
Fluidextract 1:1 (g/ml): 1–2 ml.
Tincture 1:5 (g/ml): 5–10 ml.
Standardized extract (4% total ginsenosides): 100 mg twice daily.

References

Allen, J.D. J. McLung, A.G. Nelson, M. Welsch. 1998. Ginseng supplementation does not enhance healthy young adults' peak aerobic exercise performance. *J Am Coll Nutr* 17(5):462–466.

Ando, T., T. Muraoka, N. Yamasaki, H. Okuda. 1980. Preparation of anti-lipolytic substance from *Panax ginseng*. *Planta Med* 38(1):18–23.

Avakian, E.V., R.B. Sugimoto, S. Taguchi, S.M. Horvath. 1984. Effect of *Panax ginseng* extract on energy metabolism during exercise in rats. *Planta Med* 50(2):151–154.

BAnz. See *Bundesanzeiger*.

Bradley, P.R. (ed.). 1992. *British Herbal Compendium*, Vol. 1. Bournemouth: British Herbal Medicine Association.

British Herbal Pharmacopoeia (BHP). 1996. Exeter, U.K.: British Herbal Medicine Association.

Bone, K. 1998. Ginseng—The Regal Herb. *MediHerb Professional Review* (1):62:1–4; (2):63:1–4; (3):64:1–4.

Bundesanzeiger (BAnz). 1998. Monographien der Kommission E (Zulassungs- und Aufbereitungskommission am BGA für den humanmed. Bereich, phytotherapeutische Therapierichtung und Stoffgruppe). Köln: Bundesgesundheitsamt (BGA).

Caso Marasco, A., R. Vargas Ruiz, A. Salas Villagomez, C. Begoña Infante. 1996. Double-blind study of a multivitamin complex supplemented with ginseng extract. *Drugs Exp Clin Res* 22(6):323–329.

Cheah, J.S. 1994. Ginsana G115® versus placebo in patients with non-insulin dependent diabetes. Pharmaton in-house file.

Cherdrungsi, P. et al. 1995. Effects of a standardized ginseng extract and exercise training on aerobic and anaerobic exercise capacities in humans. *Korean J Ginseng Sci* 19:93–100.

Cho, Y.K. et al. 1994. The effect of red ginseng and Zidovudine on HIV patients. *Int Conf AIDS* 10(1):215. (Abstract No. PB0289).

Cho, Y.K., H.J. Lee, W.I. Oh, Y.K. Kim. 1997. Long term immunological effect of ginseng on HIV-infected patients. *Abstr Gen Meet Am Soc Microbiol* 97:247. (Abstract No. E44).

Choi, H.K., D.H. Seong, K.H. Rha. 1995. Clinical efficacy of Korean red ginseng for erectile dysfunction. *Int J Impot Res* 7(3):181–186.

Chong, S.K. and V.G. Oberholzer. 1988. Ginseng—is there a use in clinical medicine? *Postgrad Med J* 64(757):841–846.

Collomp, K. et al. 1996. Ginseng et exercice supramaximal. *Science et sports* 11:250–251.

D'Angelo, L. et al. 1986. A double-blind, placebo-controlled clinical study on the effect of a standardized Ginseng extract on psychomotor performance in healthy volunteers. *J Ethnopharmacol* 16(1):15–22.

Deutsches Arzneibuch, 10th ed. (DAB 10). 1991. (With subsequent supplements through 1996.) Stuttgart: Deutscher Apotheker Verlag.

Dharmananda, S. 1999. Personal communication to A. Goldberg, Jun 6.

Dorling, E. and A.M. Kirchdorfer. 1980. Do ginsenosides influence the performance? Results of a double-blind study. *Notabene Medici* 10(5):241–246.

Engels, H.J. and J.C. Wirth. 1997. No ergogenic effects of ginseng (*Panax ginseng* C.A. Meyer) during graded maximal aerobic exercise. *J Am Diet Assoc* 97(10):1110–1115.

Engels, H.J., J.M. Said, J.C.Wirth. 1996. Failure of chronic ginseng administration to affect work performance and energy metabolism in healthy adult females. *Nutr Res* 16:1295–1305.

Forgo, I. 1980. Doping control of top-ranking athletes after a 14-day treatment with Ginsana®. Report of the doping Commission of the International Amateur Boxing Association, Basle, Switzerland.

———. 1983. Effect of drugs on physical performance and hormone system of sportsmen. *Münchener Medizinische Wochenzeitschrift* 125(38):822–824.

Forgo, L., L. Kayasseh, J.J. Staub. 1981. Einfluss eines standardisierten Ginseng extraktes auf das allgemeinbefinden, die reaktionsfahigkeit, lungenfunktion und die gonadalen hormone [Effect of a standardized ginseng extract on general well-being, reaction time, pulmonary function and gonadal hormones.] *Med Welt* 32(19):751–756.

Forgo, I. and A.M. Kirchdorfer. 1981. On the question of influencing the performance of top sportsmen by means of biologically active substances. *Arztliche Praxis* 33(44):1784–1786.

———. 1982. The effect of different ginsenoside concentrations on physical work capacity. *Notabene Medici* 12(9):721–727.

Forgo, I. and G. Schimert. 1985. The duration of effect of the standardised ginseng extract G115® in healthy competitive athletes. *Notabene Medici* 15(9):636–640.

Foster, S. 1991. Asian Ginseng, *Panax ginseng*. *Botanical Booklet Series*, No. 303. Austin: American Botanical Council.

Foster, S. and Y. Chongxi. 1992. *Herbal Emissaries: Bringing Chinese Herbs to the West*. Rochester, VT: Healing Arts Press. 102–112.

Gianoli, A.C. and D. Riebenfeld. 1984. Doppelblind-Studie zur Beurteilung der Verträglichkeit und Wirkung des standardisierten Ginseng-Extraktes G115®. *Cytobiologische Revue* 8(3):177–186.

Gillis, C.N. 1997. *Panax ginseng* pharmacology: a nitrous oxide link? *Biochem Pharmacol* 54:1–8.

Gross, D., D. Krieger, R. Efrat, M. Dayan. 1995. Ginseng extract G115 for the treatment of chronic respiratory diseases. *Schweiz Zschr Ganzheits Medizin* 1:29–33.

Han, B.H. et al. 1983. Studies on the antioxidant components of Korean ginseng. III. Identification of phenolic acids. *Arch Pharmacol Res* 4:54–58.

Han, B.H. et al. 1998. Effect of red ginseng on blood pressure in patients with essential hypertension and white coat hypertension. *Am J Chin Med* 26(2):199–209.

Hu, S.Y. 1976. The genus *Panax* (ginseng) in Chinese medicine. *Econ Bot* 30(1):11–28.

Japanese Pharmacopoeia, 12th ed. (JP XII). 1993. Tokyo: Government of Japan Ministry of Health and Welfare—Yakuji Nippo, Ltd. 127–128.

Jiang, H.W., Z.H. Qian, W.L. Weng. 1992. [Clinical study in treating qi-deficiency and blood-stasis syndrome of angina pectoris with qi xue granule] [In Chinese]. *Chung Kuo Chung Hsi I Chieh Ho Tsa Chih* 12(11):663–665, 644.

Konno, C., K. Sugiyama, M. Kano, M. Takahashi, H. Hikino. 1984. Isolation and hypoglycaemic activity of panaxans A, B, C, D and E, glycans of *Panax ginseng* roots. *Planta Med* 50(5):434–436.

Lange, D. and U. Schippmann. 1997. *Trade Survey of Medicinal Plants in Germany—A Contribution to International Plant Species Conservation*. Bonn: Bundesamt für Naturschutz. 69–72.

Le Gal, M., P. Cathebras, K. Strüby. 1996. Pharmaton capsules in the treatment of functional fatigue: A double-blind study versus placebo evaluated by a new methodology. *Phytother Res* 10:49–53.

Leung, A.Y. and S. Foster. 1996. *Encyclopedia of Common Natural Ingredients Used in Food, Drugs, and Cosmetics*, 2nd ed. New York: John Wiley & Sons, Inc.

Lewis, W.H. 1986. Ginseng: A Medical Enigma. In: Etkin, N.L. (ed). *Plants in Indigenous Medicine and Diet: Biobehavioral Approaches*. Bedford Hills, N.Y.: Redgrave Publ. Co. 290–305.

Liu, C. and P.G. Xiao. 1992. Recent advances on ginseng research in China. *J Ethnopharmacol* 36(1):27–38.

McGuffin, M., C. Hobbs, R. Upton, A. Goldberg. 1997. American Herbal Product Association's *Botanical Safety Handbook*. Boca Raton: CRC Press.

Melisch, R., P. Fomenko, B. Hejda. 1997. The Status of *Panax ginseng* in the Russian Far East and Adjacent Areas: A Matter for Conservation Action. *Medicinal Plant Conservation* 4:11–13.

Meyer-Buchtela, E. 1999. *Tee-Rezepturen—Ein Handbuch für Apotheker und Ärzte*. Stuttgart: Deutscher Apotheker Verlag.

Morris, A.C. et al. 1996. No ergogenic effect of ginseng ingestion. *Int J Sport Nutr* 6(3):263–271.

Mulz, D. and F. Degenring. 1989. Doping control after a 14-day treatment. *Pharmazeutische Rundschau* 11:22.

Mulz, D., G. Scardigli, G. Jans, F.H. Degenring. 1990. Long term treatment of psycho-asthenia in the second half of life. *Pharmakologische Rundschau* 12:86.

Ng, T.B. and H.W. Yeung. 1986. Scientific basis of the therapeutic effects of ginseng. *Folk Med* 139–151.

Österreichisches Arzneibuch, Vols. 1–2. (ÖAB). 1981. Wien: Verlag der Österreichischen Staatsdruckerei.

Petkov, V.D. and A.H. Mosharrof. 1987. Effects of standarized ginseng extract on learning, memory, and physical capabilities. *Am J Chin Med* 15(1–2):19–29.

Pharmacopée Française Xe Édition (Ph.Fr.X). 1983–1990. Moulins-les-Metz: Maisonneuve S.A.

Pharmacopoeia Helvetica, 7th ed. Vol. 1–4. (Ph.Helv.VII). 1987. Bern: Office Central Fédéral des Imprimés et du Matériel.

Pieralisi, G., P. Ripari, L. Vecchiet. 1991. Effects of a standardized ginseng extract combined with dimethylaminoethanol bitartrate, vitamins, minerals, and trace elements on physical performance during exercise. *Clin Ther* 13(3):373–382.

Pujol P. et al. 1996. Effects of ginseng extract (G115®) alone and combined with other elements on free radical production and haemoglobin reoxygenation following a maximal stress test. Int Pre-Olympic Sci Cong: Dallas; July 10–14.

Quiroga, H.A. 1982. Comparative double-blind study of the effect of Ginsana G115 and Hydergin on cerebrovascular deficits. *Orientacion Medica* 1281:201–202.

Quiroga, H.A. and A.E. Imbriano. 1979. The effect of *Panax ginseng* extract on cerebrovascular deficits. *Orientacion Medica* 1208:86–87.

Reinold, E. 1990. The use of ginseng in gynecology. *Natur Ganzheits Med* 4:131–134.

Rosenfeld, M.S. 1989. Evaluation of the efficacy of a standardized ginseng extract in patients with psychophysical asthenia and neurological disorders. *Semana Med* 173(9):148–154.

Saito, H., Y. Yoshida, K. Takagi. 1974. Effect of *Panax ginseng* root on exhaustive exercise in mice. *Jpn J Pharmacol* 24(1):119–127.

Salvati, G. et al. 1996. Effects of *Panax ginseng* C.A. Meyer saponins on male fertility. *Panminerva Med* 38(4):249–254.

Sandberg, F. 1980. Vitality and senility—the effects of the ginsenosides on performance. *Svensk Farmaceutisk Tidskrift* 84(13):499–502.

Sankary, T. 1989. Controlled clinical trials of Anginlyc, Chinese herbal immune enhancer, in HIV seropositives. *Int Conf AIDS* 5:496. (Abstract No. B.596).

Scaglione, F., G. Cattaneo, M. Alessandria, R. Cogo. 1996. Efficacy and safety of the standardized ginseng extract G115 for potentiating vaccination against the influenza syndrome and protection against the common cold. *Drugs Exp Clin Res* 22(2):65–72. [Corrected; published erratum appears in 22(6):338.]

Scaglione, F. et al. 1990. Immunomodulatory effects of two extracts of *Panax ginseng* C.A. Meyer. *Drugs Exp Clin Res* 16(10):537–542.

Scaglione, F., R. Cogo, C. Cocuzza, M. Arcidiacono, A. Beretta. 1994. Immunomodulatory effects of *Panax ginseng* C.A. Meyer (G115) on alveolar macrophages from patients suffering with chronic bronchitis. *Int J Immunother* 10(1):21–24.

Schardt, D. 1999. Ginseng. *Nutrition Action Healthletter* May:10–11.

Singh, V.K., S.S. Agarwal, B.M. Gupta. 1984. Immunomodulatory activity of *Panax ginseng* extract. *Planta Med* 50(6):462–465.

Sotaniemi, E.A., E. Haapakoski, A. Rautio. 1995. Ginseng therapy in non-insulin-dependent diabetic patients. *Diabetes Care* 18(10):1373–1375.

State Pharmacopoeia of the Union of Soviet Socialist Republics, 10th ed. (USSR X). 1973. Moscow: Ministry of Health of the U.S.S.R.

Takeda, A., M. Yonezawa, N. Katoh. 1981. Restoration of radiation injury by ginseng. I. Responses of X-irradiated mice to ginseng extract. *J Radiat Res* (Tokyo). 22(3):323–335.

Takeda, A., N. Katoh, M. Yonezawa. 1982. Restoration of radiation injury by ginseng. III. Radioprotective effect of thermostable fraction of ginseng extract on mice, rats and guinea pigs. *J Radiat Res (Tokyo)*. 23(2):150–167.

Thommessen, B and K. Laake. 1996. No identifiable effect of ginseng (Gericomplex) as an adjuvant in the treatment of geriatric patients. *Aging (Milano)* 8(6):417–420.

Tu, G. (ed.). 1992. *Pharmacopoeia of the People's Republic of China* (English Edition 1992). Beijing: Guangdong Science and Technology Press. 163–164.

USSR X. See *State Pharmacopoeia of the Union of Soviet Socialist Republics*.

Van Schepdael, P. 1993. Les effets du ginseng G115® sur la capacité physique de sportifs d'endurance. *Acta Therapeutica* 19:337–347.

von Ardenne, M. and W. Klemm W. 1987. Measurements of the increase in the difference between the arterial and venous Hb-O2 saturation obtained with daily administration of 200 mg standardised ginseng extract G115® for four weeks. *Panminerva Med* 29(2):143–150.

Wichtl, M. and N.G. Bisset (eds.). 1994. *Herbal Drugs and Phytopharmaceuticals*. Stuttgart: Medpharm Scientific Publishers.

World Health Organization (WHO). 1999. "Ginseng radix." *WHO Monographs on Selected Medicinal Plants*, Vol. 1. Geneva: World Health Organization. 168–182.

Yamamoto, M., T. Uemura, S. Nakama, M. Uemiya, A. Kumagai. 1983. Serum HDL-cholesterol-increasing and fatty liver-improving actions of *Panax ginseng* in high cholesterol diet-fed rats with clinical affect on hyperlipidemia in man. *Am J Chin Med* 11(1–4):96–101.

Yen, K.Y. 1992. *The Illustrated Chinese Materia Medica—Crude and Prepared*. Taipei: SMC Publishing, Inc. 40.

Yun, T.K. and S.Y. Choi. 1998. Non-organ specific cancer prevention of ginseng: a prospective study in Korea. Int J Epidemiol 27(3):359–364.

———. 1995. Preventive effect of ginseng intake against various human cancers: a case-control study on 1,987 pairs. *Cancer Epidemiol Biomarkers Prev* 4(4):401–408.

Yun, T.K., S.Y. Choi, Y.S. Lee. 1993. Cohort study on ginseng intake and cancer for population over 40-year-old in ginseng production areas (a preliminary report). (Meeting Abstract (201993):132.) Second International Cancer Chemo Prevention Conference: Berlin.

Zuin, M., P.M. Battezzati, M. Camisasca, D. Riebenfeld, M. Podda. 1987. Effects of a preparation containing a standardized ginseng extract combined with trace elements and multivitamins against hepatotoxin-induced chronic liver disease in the elderly. *J Int Med Res* 15(5):276–281.

Additional Resources

Sorenson, H. and J.A. Sonne. 1996. Double-masked study of the effects of ginseng on cognitive functions. *Curr Ther Res* 57:959–968.

Sticher, O. 1998. Biochemical, Pharmaceutical, and Medical Perspectives of Ginseng. In: Lawson, L.D. and R. Bauer (eds.). 1998. *Phytomedicines of Europe: Chemistry and Biological Activity*. Washington, D.C.: American Chemical Society. 221–240.

Tang W. and G. Eisenbrand. *Panax ginseng* C.A. Mey. 1992. *Chinese Drugs of Plant Origin: Chemistry, Pharmacology, and Use in Traditional Modern Medicine*. New York: Springer Verlag. 711–737.

This material was adapted from *The Complete German Commission E Monographs—Therapeutic Guide to Herbal Medicines*. M. Blumenthal, W.R. Busse, A. Goldberg, J. Gruenwald, T. Hall, C.W. Riggins, R.S. Rister (eds.) S. Klein and R.S. Rister (trans.). 1998. Austin: American Botanical Council; Boston: Integrative Medicine Communications.

1) The Overview section is new information.

2) Description, Chemistry and Pharmacology, Uses, Contraindications, Side Effects, Interactions with Other Drugs, and Dosage sections have been drawn from the original work. Additional information has been added in some or all of these sections, as noted with references.

3) The dosage for equivalent preparations (tea infusion, fluidextract, and tincture) have been provided based on the following example:
Unless otherwise prescribed: 2 g per day of [powdered, crushed, cut or whole] [plant part]
Infusion: 2 g in 150 ml of water
Fluidextract 1:1 (g/ml): 2 ml
Tincture 1:5 (g/ml): 10 ml

4) The References and Additional Resources sections are new sections. Additional Resources are not cited in the monograph but are included for research purposes.

GOLDENROD

Latin Name:
Solidago virgaurea

Pharmacopeial Name:
Solidago, Virgaureae herba

Other Names:
European goldenrod

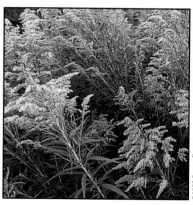

©1999 Steven Foster

Overview

European goldenrod (*Solidago virgaurea* L.) is a perennial plant native to Europe
that has spread throughout Europe, northern Africa, North America and parts of
Asia. Early goldenrod (*S. gigantea* Aiton) and Canadian goldenrod (*S. canadensis* L.)
are native in North America. Early goldenrod is now naturalized in Europe, where
it was introduced as an ornamental plant that later escaped cultivation (Wichtl,
1996; Wichtl and Bisset, 1994). The material of commerce is collected mainly from
the wild in southeast and eastern European countries, including Bulgaria, Hungary,
Poland, and the former Yugoslavia (BHP, 1996; Wichtl, 1996; Wichtl and Bisset,
1994). In commerce, early goldenrod is often substituted for European goldenrod
though they can be differentiated anatomically, chemically, and morphologically
(Wichtl, 1996). The genus name *Solidago* is derived from *soldare*, meaning "to
make whole," because it was used as a vulnerary drug (Grieve, 1979).

Goldenrod is classed as an aquaretic, increasing renal blood flow and increasing
the glomerular filtration rate without stimulating the loss of sodium and chloride.
Aquaretics are considered safer than many synthetic diuretics that promote the loss
of electrolytes (Tyler, 1994). Animal studies have investigated its effect on diuresis
and levels of electrolytes (Chodera et al., 1991), its anti-inflammatory, spasmolytic,
and diuretic effects (Leuschner, 1995), its effect on the metabolism of rabbit brain
slices (Dittmann, 1973), and its influence on respiration and glycolysis in brain
tumor sections (Ludt and Dittmann, 1972). Several *in vitro* and *in vivo* studies have
also investigated a combination aqueous/alcoholic extract composed of European
goldenrod herb, European ash (*Fraxinus excelsior* L.), and quaking aspen (*Populus
tremuloides* Michx.) for its effects on various myeloperoxidase systems (von Kruedener et al., 1996), its anti-inflammatory activity (el-Ghazaly et al., 1992; von
Kruedener et al., 1995), its antioxidative properties (Meyer et al., 1995) and its
effects on the inhibition of dihydrofolate reductase activity (Strehl et al., 1995).

The approved modern therapeutic applications for goldenrod herb are based on
its long history of use in well established systems of traditional medicine, numerous
in vitro and *in vivo* pharmacological studies, and on its well documented chemical
composition.

In Germany, goldenrod herb is official in the *German Pharmacopoeia*, listed in
the *German Drug Codex*, approved in the German Commission E monographs and
the tea form is official in the German Standard License monographs (BAnz, 1998;
Braun et al., 1997; DAB, 1997; DAC, 1986; Wichtl and Bisset, 1994). It is used as
an agent to increase the quantity of urine as a treatment for kidney and bladder
inflammation (Wichtl and Bisset, 1994). Goldenrod herb is commonly found as a
component in *Tee bei Blasen- und Nierenerkrankungen* (teas for bladder and kidney
disorders), typically in combination with java tea leaf (*Orthosiphon stamineus*),
birch leaf (*Betula alba*) and/or uva ursi leaf (*Arctostaphylos uva-ursi*) (Meyer-

Buchtela, 1999). In the United States, goldenrod is little used with the exception of its limited use by medical herbalists, naturopathic physicians, and aboriginal healers. For example, the Iroquois people prepare an infusion of Canadian goldenrod flowers as a gastrointestinal and liver aid (Moerman, 1998).

Pharmacopeial grade European goldenrod herb consists of the dried flowering tops of *S. virgaurea* L., collected during the flowering period, in whole or cut dried forms. It may contain no more than 5% brownish discolored fragments and maximum 2% other foreign matter. Botanical identity must be confirmed by thin-layer chromatography (TLC), macroscopic and microscopic examinations, and organoleptic evaluations (DAB, 1997). The German Standard License monograph requires not less than 1.5% flavonoids, calculated as rutoside with reference to the dried drug (Braun et al., 1997). The *British Herbal Pharmacopoeia* requires that it contain not less than 11% water-soluble extractive (BHP, 1996).

Pharmacopeial grade early goldenrod herb and/or Canadian goldenrod herb consists of the dried flowering tops of *S. gigantea* Ait. (early), *S. canadensis* L. (Canadian), and its hybrids or mixtures of these species, collected during the flowering period, in whole or cut dried forms. It must contain not less than 2.5% flavonoids calculated as hyperoside, with reference to the dried drug. It may contain no more than 5% discolored fragments and maximum 2% other foreign matter. Botanical identity must be confirmed by thin-layer chromatography (TLC), macroscopic and microscopic examinations, and organoleptic evaluations (DAB, 1997). For early goldenrod herb, the German Standard License monograph requires not less than 6.0% flavonoids calculated as rutin with reference to the dried drug (Braun et al., 1997; Wichtl and Bisset, 1994).

Description

European goldenrod herb consists of the aboveground parts of *S. virgaurea* L. [Fam. Asteraceae], gathered during the flowering season and dried carefully, as well as their preparations in effective dosage. Goldenrod herb consists of the aboveground parts of *S. serotina* Aiton (synonym *S. gigantea* Willdenow), *S. canadensis* L., and its hybrids, gathered during the flowering season and carefully dried, as well as their preparations in effective dosage. The herb contains flavonoids, saponins, and phenol glycosides.

Chemistry and Pharmacology

European goldenrod herb contains approximately 1.5% flavonoids, mainly rutin, plus quercitrin, isoquercitrin, astragalin, hyperoside, and nicotiflorin; approximately 10% catechin tannins; 2–6% triterpene saponins, of which more than 30% are bisdesmosidic polygala acid derivatives; 0.2–1.0% phenol glycosides, including leiocarposide and virgaureoside A; phenolic acids, including caffeic and chlorogenic acids; 0.4–0.5% essential oil; diterpenoid lactones of *cis*-clerodane type; and polysaccharides (ESCOP, 1997; Hänsel et al., 1992-1994; Meyer-Buchtela, 1999; Wichtl, 1996).

Early goldenrod herb contains minimum 2.4% flavonoids, including quercitrin and rutin; 9–12% triterpene saponins, mainly bayogenin glycosides; phenolic acids, including chlorogenic, hydroxycinnamic, and caffeic acids and their glucose esters; tannins; polysaccharides; diterpenes; and a small amount of essential oil (Wichtl, 1996; Wichtl and Bisset, 1994).

The Commission E reported diuretic, mildly antispasmodic, and antiphlogistic activity.

The *British Herbal Pharmacopoeia* reported diuretic, anticatarrhal, and diaphoretic actions (BHP, 1996). *In vitro* studies have shown a spermicidal effect on human sperm, possibly a result of the saponins of the β-amyrin type having a particular sequence of sugars at the 28-carboxyl function (Wichtl and Bisset, 1994). Fungicidic activity on *Candida albicans* has been shown using the triterpenoid glycosides (Bader et al., 1990).

Uses

The Commission E approved goldenrod herb as irrigation therapy for inflammatory diseases of the lower urinary tract, urinary calculi and kidney gravel, and as prophylaxis for urinary calculi and kidney gravel.

The German Standard License for goldenrod herb tea indicates its use to increase the amount of urine in inflammation of the kidneys and bladder (Braun et al., 1997; Wichtl and Bisset, 1994). ESCOP indicates its use for irrigation of the urinary tract, especially in cases of inflammation and renal gravel, and as an adjuvant in the treatment of bacterial infections of the urinary tract (ESCOP, 1997).

Contraindications

No irrigation therapy in case of edema due to impaired heart and kidney function.

Side Effects

None known.

Use During Pregnancy and Lactation

No restrictions known.

Interactions with Other Drugs

None known.

Dosage and Administration

Unless otherwise prescribed: 6–12 g of cut herb for teas and other galenical preparations for internal use.
Note: Observe copious intake of fluids.
Infusion: Steep 3 g in 150 ml boiled water for 10 to 15 minutes, two to four times daily between meals (Braun et al., 1997; ESCOP, 1997; Meyer-Buchtela, 1999; Weiss, 1991; Wichtl and Bisset, 1994) [Note: 21% of the potentially available O-glycoside bound flavonoids

are yielded into the tea infusion after 5 minutes of steeping and 28% are released after a 10 minute steep. 22% of the potentially available tannins are yielded after 5 minutes of steeping and 28% after a 10 minute steep (Meyer-Buchtela, 1999).
Cold macerate: Soak 1.2–2.4 g in 150 ml cold water for 10 to15 minutes then bring to a boil briefly before drinking, three to five times daily between meals (Wichtl and Bisset, 1994).
Fluidextract 1:1 (g/ml): 3 ml, two to four times daily between meals.

References

BAnz. See *Bundesanzeiger*.

Bader, G. et al. 1990. The antifungal action of polygalacic acid glycosides. *Pharmazie* 45(8):618–620.

Braun, R. et al. 1997. *Standardzulassungen für Fertigarzneimittel—Text and Kommentar*. Stuttgart: Deutscher Apotheker Verlag.

British Herbal Pharmacopoeia (BHP). 1996. Exeter, U.K.: British Herbal Medicine Association. 90–91.

Bundesanzeiger (BAnz). 1998. Monographien der Kommission E (Zulassungs- und Aufbereitungskommission am BGA für den humanmed. Bereich, phytotherapeutische Therapierichtung und Stoffgruppe). Köln: Bundesgesundheitsamt (BGA).

Chodera, A., K. Dabrowska, A. Sloderbach, L. Skrzypczak, J. Budzianowski. 1991. Wplyw frakcji flawonoidowych gatunkow rodzaju Solidago L. na diureze i ste~zenie elektrolitow [Effect of flavonoid fractions of *Solidago virgaurea* L on diuresis and levels of electrolytes] *Acta Pol Pharm* 48(5–6):35–37.

Deutsches Arzneibuch (DAB 1997). 1997. Stuttgart: Deutscher Apotheker Verlag.

Deutscher Arzneimittel-Codex (DAC). 1986. Stuttgart: Deutscher Apotheker Verlag.

Dittmann, J. 1973. Wirkungen von Extrakten aus *Solidago virgaurea* auf den Stoffwechsel von Kaninchen-Hirnschnitten [Effect of extracts from *Solidago virgaurea* on the metabolism of rabbit brain slices] (author's transl.). *Planta Med* 24(4):329–336.

ESCOP. 1997. "Virgaureae herba." *Monographs on the Medicinal Uses of Plant Drugs*. Exeter, U.K.: European Scientific Cooperative on Phytotherapy.

el-Ghazaly, M., M.T. Khayyal, S.N. Okpanyi, M. Arens-Corell. 1992. Study of the anti-inflammatory activity of *Populus tremula*, *Solidago virgaurea* and *Fraxinus excelsior*. *Arzneimforsch* 42(3):333–336.

Grieve, M. 1979. *A Modern Herbal*. New York: Dover Publications, Inc.

Hänsel, R., K. Keller, H. Rimpler, G. Schneider (eds.). 1992–1994. *Hagers Handbuch der Pharmazeutischen Praxis,* 5th ed. Vol. 4–6. Berlin-Heidelberg: Springer Verlag.

Leuschner, J. 1995. Anti-inflammatory, spasmolytic and diuretic effects of a commercially available *Solidago gigantea* Herb. extract. *Arzneimforsch* 45(2):165–168.

Ludt, H. and J. Dittmann. 1972. Rechnerische und graphische Auswertung von manometrischen Stoffwechselmessungen mit einer elektronischen Rechenanlage. Beispiel: Atmung und Glykolyse von Hirntumor-Schnitten unter dem Einfluss von *Solidago*-Extrakt [Mathematical and graphical evaluation of manometric measurements on metabolism using an electronic computer. Example: respiration and glycolysis in brain tumor sections, as influenced by *Solidago* extract]. *Z Med Labortech* 13(1):79–84.

Meyer-Buchtela, E. 1999. *Tee-Rezepturen—Ein Handbuch für Apotheker und Ärzte.* Stuttgart: Deutscher Apotheker Verlag.

Meyer, B., W. Schneider, E.F. Elstner. 1995. Antioxidative properties of alcoholic extracts from *Fraxinus excelsior, Populus tremula* and *Solidago virgaurea. Arzneimforsch* 45(2):174–176.

Moerman, D.E. 1998. *Native American Ethnobotany.* Portland, OR: Timber Press. 536–538.

Strehl, E., W. Schneider, E.F. Elstner. 1995. Inhibition of dihydrofolate reductase activity by alcoholic extracts from *Fraxinus excelsior, Populus tremula* and *Solidago virgaurea. Arzneimforsch* 45(2):172–173.

Tyler, V.E. 1994. *Herbs of Choice: The Therapeutic Use of Phytomedicinals.* New York: Pharmaceutical Products Press.

von Kruedener, S., W. Schneider, E.F. Elstner. 1995. A combination of *Populus tremula, Solidago virgaurea* and *Fraxinus excelsior* as an anti-inflammatory and antirheumatic drug. A short review. *Arzneimforsch* 45(2):169–171.

———. 1996. Effects of extracts from *Populus tremula* L., *Solidago virgaurea* L. and *Fraxinus excelsior* L. on various myeloperoxidase systems. *Arzneimforsch* 46(8):809–814.

Weiss, R.F. 1991. *Lehrbuch der Phytotherapie,* 7th ed. Stuttgart: Hippokrates. 304–306.

Wichtl, M. 1996. Monographien—Kommentar. In: Braun, R. et al. 1997. *Standardzulassungen für Fertigarzneimittel—Text and Kommentar.* Stuttgart: Deutscher Apotheker Verlag.

Wichtl, M. and N.G. Bisset (eds.). 1994. *Herbal Drugs and Phytopharmaceuticals.* Stuttgart: Medpharm Scientific Publishers.

Additional Resources

Boyle, W. 1995. Overview: History of Naturopathic Botanical Medicine. *Protocol J Botanical Med* 1(2):11–16.

Bruneton, J. 1995. *Pharmacognosy, Phytochemistry, Medicinal Plants.* Paris: Lavoisier Publishing.

Okpanyi, S.N., R. Schirpke-von Paczensky, D. Dickson. 1989. [Anti-inflammatory, analgesic and antipyretic effect of various plant extracts and their combinations in an animal model] [In German]. *Arzneimforsch* 39(6):698–703.

Priest, A.W. and L.R. Priest. 1982. *Herbal Medication, A Clinical and Dispensatory Handbook.* Essex, U.K.: L.N. Fowler & Co., Ltd.

Schatzle, M., M. Agathos, R. Breit. 1998. Allergic contact dermatitis from goldenrod (*Herba solidaginis*) after systemic administration. *Contact Dermatitis* 39(5):271–272.

This material was adapted from *The Complete German Commission E Monographs—Therapeutic Guide to Herbal Medicines.* M. Blumenthal, W.R. Busse, A. Goldberg, J. Gruenwald, T. Hall, C.W. Riggins, R.S. Rister (eds.) S. Klein and R.S. Rister (trans.). 1998. Austin: American Botanical Council; Boston: Integrative Medicine Communications.

1) The Overview section is new information.

2) Description, Chemistry and Pharmacology, Uses, Contraindications, Side Effects, Interactions with Other Drugs, and Dosage sections have been drawn from the original work. Additional information has been added in some or all of these sections, as noted with references.

3) The dosage for equivalent preparations (tea infusion, fluidextract, and tincture) have been provided based on the following example:
Unless otherwise prescribed: 2 g per day of [powdered, crushed, cut or whole] [plant part]
Infusion: 2 g in 150 ml of water
Fluidextract 1:1 (g/ml): 2 ml
Tincture 1:5 (g/ml): 10 ml

4) The References and Additional Resources sections are new sections. Additional Resources are not cited in the monograph but are included for research purposes.

HAWTHORN:

HAWTHORN BERRY
(page 185)

HAWTHORN FLOWER
(page 186)

HAWTHORN LEAF
(page 187)

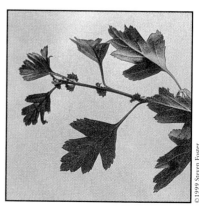

©1999 Steven Foster

HAWTHORN LEAF WITH FLOWER
(page 188)

Overview

There are approximately 280 known species of hawthorns in the genus *Crataegus*. The species referred to in this monograph is a spiny shrub native to the northern wooded temperate zones of Europe, from England to Latvia and from the Pyrenees Mountains (southern France) to northern Italy (Leung and Foster, 1996). It has become naturalized in parts of North America as a garden escape (Budavari, 1996; Leung and Foster, 1996). The material of commerce for the phytomedicine industry is obtained from the United Kingdom and other European countries (BHP, 1996), including Albania, Bulgaria, Romania, the former Yugoslavia, and Poland (Wichtl and Bisset, 1994).

Hawthorn has a long history of use, confirmed safety, and clinical evidence to support its cardiovascular benefits, especially cardiotonic activity. There is significant evidence to support its use in clinical cardiology and by the general public. The fruits (berries) of various species, long used in traditional European herbal medicine, are edible (Hedrick, 1972). Hawthorn is one of the oldest known medicinal plants used in European medicine; its cordial actions on the heart were first reported by first century Greek herbalist Dioscorides and later by Swiss physician Paracelsus (1493–1541) (Weihmayr and Ernst, 1996). Other sources state that its clinical use for heart disease and cardiovascular disorders did not begin in Europe until the nineteenth century (Anschutz, 1900; Hobbs and Foster, 1990).

In phytomedicine, hawthorn refers to the fruit, leaf, and/or flower of the genus *Crataegus* (usually *C. laevigata*, syn. *C. oxyacantha*) and *C. monogyna*. Commission E in 1984 published one monograph on hawthorn (often commonly referred to as crataegus, based on the Latin name of the genus) that included all of its aerial parts and was based on historical experience, many pharmacological studies on various preparations on the three different plant parts, about 20 open clinical studies, and many patient case reports (Schilcher, 1997). The original indications were for functional Stages I to II of the New York Heart Association (NYHA) assessment of the four stages of heart disease. Other indications included sensation of pressure in the chest, cardiac degeneration not yet requiring digitalis, and slight forms of bradycardic arrhythmias (Steinhoff, 1997).

In 1994, however, the original monograph was replaced by four: an approved monograph for hawthorn leaf with flower and three unapproved monographs for hawthorn fruit (berry), leaf, and flower, respectively. There was good reason for this change. When the first monograph had been produced, none of the scientific data on hawthorn included studies carried out according to good clinical practices (GCP). Both experimental and clinical studies that have been conducted since around 1991 have confirmed activity of hawthorn leaf with flower preparations. A subsequent review of clinical literature revealed the availability of pharmacodynamics (the effects of a substance on the physiological processes) of a 45% ethanol extract, or 70% methanol extract of flowering leaf tops with defined content of flavonoids and proanthocyanidins. The other three hawthorn components were re-evaluated and "the flowers, leaves, and fruits as single compounds received a negative assessment because there no longer seemed to be sufficient scientific evidence to justify their inclusion" (Steinhoff, 1993–1994). This also brought the monographs in line with the tenth edition of the French pharmacopeia, which specifies "dried flowering tops" of C. monogyna. The approval of the one hawthorn preparation based on the extract of leaf with flower is an example of the trend later adopted by the Commission to rely on new scientific data for evaluations and to re-assess and approve specific, well-defined extract preparations that are often proprietary commercial products. A recent monograph on hawthorn berry (fruit) acknowledges the lack of research on the cardioactivity of the berry (Upton, 1999a).

The literature review also resulted in a more precise indication for the approved monograph: "decreasing cardiac output according to functional Stage II of the NYHA." According to NYHA, Stage II is defined as "Patients with cardiac disease but without resulting limitations of physical activity. They are comfortable at rest. Ordinary physical activity results in fatigue, palpitation, dyspnea, or anginal pain" (NYHA, 1994). The use of hawthorn appears to be extremely safe; Commission E noted no contraindications or adverse side effects, nor have more recent reviews (e.g., Upton, 1999a, 1999b).

Hawthorn has been extensively studied in Germany. A review on hawthorn preparations used in cardiology found that hawthorn can be employed for indications for which digitalis is not yet indicated (Blesken, 1992). In a later review of its therapeutic effectiveness, the authors found that recent research supported its usefulness in congestive heart failure (CHF) (Weihmayr and Ernst, 1996). Rigorous clinical trials showed benefit concerning objective signs and subjective symptoms of Stage II NYHA congestive heart failure. No adverse drug reactions had been reported. The authors concluded that hawthorn is an effective and safe therapeutic alternative for CHF.

One placebo-controlled, randomized, double-blind study on 30 patients for eight weeks was performed with hawthorn leaf with flower extract WS 1442 (Crataegutt® forte; W. Schwabe, Germany) at a dose of 160 mg per day (Leuchtgens, 1993). The hawthorn group showed a statistically significant advantage over placebo in all parameters: Alteration in the pressure-x-rate product under standardized stationary bicycle endurance test, a score of subjective improvement of complaints elicited by a questionnaire, exercise tolerance, and changes in heart and arterial blood pressure (systolic and diastolic blood pressure was mildly reduced in both groups). No adverse reactions occurred.

Studies with early-stage CHF patients, using daily doses of leaf with flower extract ranging from 160 to 900 mg, showed improved heart function and exercise tolerance, and a lessening in shortness of breath and postexercise fatigue (Reuter, 1994; Zapfe et al., 1993). Schulz and co-authors cite 14 clinical studies published from 1981 to 1994 on the therapeutic efficacy of hawthorn preparations on a total of 808 patients (Schulz et al., 1998). A recent monograph on hawthorn leaf with flower extract cites 10 clinical studies on standardized preparations (3 open studies, 7 controlled) (Upton, 1997b). Reuter discussed 15 clinical trials on 872 patients given single preparations of Crataegus extracts (160–900 mg) standardized to 5% oligomeric proanthocyanidins (OPC), 19% OPC, and 2.2% flavonoids. Tolerability was generally very good, with higher dosages resulting in occasional mild side effects. Significant improvements in stress tolerance and anaerobic threshold occurred with daily doses of 300–900 mg over a four-week period, and to a greater extent after eight weeks. Subjective complaints, however, improved with much lower doses of 160–180 mg (Reuter, 1994).

An eight-week multicenter, placebo-controlled, double-blind trial using WS 1442 in 136 patients with Stage II NYHA cardiac insufficiency focused on changes in the blood pressure and heart rate output measured at the beginning and end of treatment (Weikl et al., 1996). A clear improvement in the performance of the heart in the treatment group was seen, while the placebo group progressively worsened. The therapeutic difference between the groups was statistically significant. Patient assessment of improvement in the main symptoms (reduced performance, shortness of breath, ankle edema, etc.) confirmed the superiority of hawthorn, with better quality of life and mental well-being reported. Tolerability was very good, with overall results confirming the extract to be an effective and low-risk phytotherapeutic form of treatment for patients with Stage II NYHA cardiac insufficiency.

Another study provided evidence that hawthorn extract can improve heart function in patients with chronic heart disease (Schmidt et al., 1994). This eight-week, multicenter, double-blind, placebo-controlled study tested the effects of 600 mg/day of Faros® 300, (LI 132, an extract manufactured by Lichtwer Pharma, Berlin). Seventy-eight patients with Stage II heart disease taking hawthorn had significant gains in their stamina and endurance (as measured by a stationary bicycle), had lower blood pressure and lower heart rates while exercising, and pumped more blood at lower pressure. Also, patients taking hawthorn had fewer overall symptoms, felt less fatigue, and experienced less shortness of breath.

Hawthorn extract (LI 132) at a dose of 900 mg daily was shown to compare favorably with the cardiac drug Captopril (37.5 mg daily) in the treatment of 132 Stage II cardiac insufficiency patients (Tauchert et al., 1994). Captopril is used to reduce resistance to blood flow in peripheral arteries. Hawthorn performed equally well, with the added benefit of working on the heart. Exercise tolerance significantly increased in both test groups, and the incidence and severity of symptoms decreased by 50%. There was no placebo control.

Another report evaluated the efficacy of high doses of hawthorn leaf with flower extract (900 mg daily of Faros® 300) in 1,476 patients with Stage I and Stage II cardiac insufficiency, with therapy lasting four and eight weeks (Loew et al., 1996). Treatment-related changes were evaluated for the typical symptoms of heart failure. The symptom score decreased by a mean of 66% at the conclusion of therapy, with the Stage I NYHA patients largely symptom-free. A subgroup of patients with symptoms including borderline hypertension showed decreases in systolic and diastolic pressure. This group also showed a drop in heart rate from 89 to 79 beats per minute, and arrhythmias were significantly reduced independently of heart failure.

Although the Commission E no longer recognizes this use, hawthorn berry preparations have been shown to combat angina, a condition resulting from insufficient blood flow to the heart muscle. In one study demonstrating the usefulness of a combined extract of hawthorn berry, leaf, and flower in the treatment of patients with stable angina pectoris (Hanack and Brückel, 1983), 60 angina patients were given either 180 mg of hawthorn berry-leaf-flower extract (Crataegutt® novo, W. Schwabe, Germany) or placebo for three weeks. The ECG measures improved in the hawthorn patients, and blood flow and oxygen delivery to the heart muscle rose. Hawthorn patients also exercised for longer periods of time without an angina attack.

A double-blind crossover study tested the effects of Crataegutt® novo hawthorn berry-leaf-flower extract in 36 patients, averaging 74 years in age, with Stage I or Stage II cardiac insufficiency (O'Connolly et al., 1986; O'Connolly et al., 1987). The study found that patients treated with this preparation had a decreased heart rate and improved cardiac output under resting and exercise conditions, which was ment in psychological assessment ratings and sleep behavior.

In Germany, hawthorn leaf with flower is official in the *German Pharmacopeia* (DAB, 1997), approved in the Commission E monographs, and the tea infusion dosage form is official in the German Standard License monographs (Braun et al., 1997). The alcoholic fluidextract dosage form is official in the *German Pharmacopeia*, tenth edition, third supplement (DAB 10, 1993). Hawthorn is used as a component in over 100 drug preparations, especially cardiotonics, coronary remedies, and antihypertensives, in various dosage forms, including the hydro-alcoholic native dry extract in *dragées* (coated tablets), fluidextract (drops) (Wichtl and Bisset, 1994), and aqueous infusion (Braun et al., 1997; Meyer-Buchtela, 1999).

German pharmacopeial grade hawthorn leaf with flower consists of the whole or cut, dried flower-bearing tips, up to about 7 cm long, of *C. monogyna* Jaquin emend. Lindman or *C. laevigata* (Poiret) de Candolle (syn: *C. oxyacantha* L.p.p. et auct.), and rarely some other European species such as *C. pentagyna* Waldstein et Kitaibel ex Willdenow, *C. nigra* Waldstein et Kitaibel, and/or *C. azarolus* L. It must contain not less than 0.7% flavonoids calculated as hyperoside. Botanical identity must be confirmed by a thin-layer chromatography (TLC) test, macroscopic and microscopic examinations, and organoleptic evaluations (DAB, 1997). Under proper storage conditions, the raw material shelf life is three years (Braun et al., 1997). It is interesting to note that the only form of hawthorn that is official in the 1998 *European Pharmacopoeia* is the dried false-fruit, which is an unapproved herb in the Commission E monographs. It must contain not less than 1.0% procyanidins, calculated as cyanidin chloride, based on the dried material (Ph.Eur.3, 1998).

HAWTHORN BERRY

Latin Name:
Crataegus monogyna

Pharmacopeial Name:
Crataegi fructus

Other Names:
haw, hawthorn tops, mayhaw, whitethorn herb

Description
Hawthorn berry consists of the dried fruit of *Crataegus monogyna* Jaquin emend. Lindman or *C. laevigata* (Poiret) de Candolle or others in a valid pharmacopeia citing *Crataegus* [Fam. Rosaceae] and preparations thereof. A recent monograph provides detailed information on the botany and chemistry of hawthorn berry (Upton, 1999a).

Chemistry and Pharmacology
There are no scientific data on which to base the pharmacology and toxicology of the herb. Spectrographic analysis of the chemical constituents of the herb distinguishes only quantitative differences between preparations from the fruit and preparations combining leaf and flower. One may assume pharmacodynamics similar to those shown for the preparation containing both leaf and flower.

Proanthocyanidins in the berry "possess a higher degree of polymerization, a characteristic that reportedly increases antioxidant activity" (Upton, 1999a).

Uses

It has been claimed that preparations of hawthorn berry have been applied to the treatment of coronary circulation, coronary complications and weak heart, heart and circulatory disturbances, hypotension, and arteriosclerosis.

Note: This monograph was published as a negative/unapproved monograph. The Commission E stated that since the effectiveness of hawthorn berry (used by itself) for its claimed applications has not been documented, therapeutic use cannot be recommended.

According to the Commission, the berry as a water extract, water-alcohol extract, wine infusion, and fresh juice has been utilized traditionally to strengthen and invigorate heart and circulatory function. These statements are based exclusively on historical record and long experience. [Ed. Note: There are no clinical studies available on hawthorn berry alone. Three clinical studies have been performed on a preparation combining extracts of hawthorn berry with leaf with flower extract (Crataegutt® novo, W. Schwabe, Germany) (Hanak and Bruckel, 1983; O'Connolly et al., 1986; O'Connolly et al., 1987; Iwamoto et al., 1981). Positive results of these studies are presumably due, at least to some significant degree, to the flavonoid content of the leaf with flower portion of the extract.]

Contraindications

No risks or contraindications are known.

Side Effects

None known (McGuffin et al., 1997; Meyer-Buchtela, 1999).

Use During Pregnancy and Lactation

No restrictions known (Anon., 1999; McGuffin et al., 1997). Not recommended during pregnancy and lactation due to potential uteroactivity (Ammon, 1981; Newall et al., 1996).

Interactions with Other Drugs

Hawthorn preparations may potentiate the actions of digitalis (McGuffin et al., 1997; Van Hellemont, 1986), though this effect has not been confirmed (Brown et al., 1999).

Dosage and Administration

See the approved monograph on hawthorn leaf with flower.

HAWTHORN FLOWER

Latin Name:
Crataegus monogyna or *C. laevigata*

Pharmacopeial Name:
Crataegi flos

Other Names:
haw, hawthorn tops, mayhaw, whitethorn herb

Description

Hawthorn flower consists of the dried flower of *Crataegus monogyna* Jaquin emend. Lindman or *C. laevigata* (Poiret) de Candolle or others in a valid pharmacopeia citing *Cratageus* [Fam. Rosaceae] and preparations thereof.

Chemistry and Pharmacology

There are no scientific data on which to base the pharmacology and toxicology of the herb. Spectrographic analysis of the chemical constituents of the herb distinguishes only quantitative differences between leaf and flower preparations. One may assume pharmacody-namics similar to those shown for preparations from the leaf.

Uses
It has been claimed that preparations of hawthorn flowers have been applied to the treatment of coronary circulation, support of the heart muscle and attendant improvement in provision for the coronary artery, autonomic heart trouble, autonomic circulatory disturbances, geriatric heart disease, enhancing activity of myocardium, preventing stress-related heart disease, cardiac boost for the elderly, strengthening the heart and circulatory system, strengthening nerves, for coronary insufficiency, angina pectoris, cardiac neurasthenia, cardiac asthma, and arrhythmia.

Note: This monograph was published as a negative/unapproved monograph. According to Commission E, since the effectiveness of hawthorn flower (by itself) for its claimed applications has not been documented, therapeutic use cannot be recommended.

The herb as a water extract, water-alcohol extract, wine infusion, and fresh juice has been used traditionally to strengthen and invigorate heart and circulatory function. These statements are based exclusively on historical record and experience.

Contraindications
No risks or contraindications are known.

Side Effects
None known (McGuffin et al., 1997; Meyer-Buchtela, 1999).

Use During Pregnancy and Lactation
No restrictions known (Anon., 1999; McGuffin et al., 1997).

Interactions with Other Drugs
Hawthorn preparations may potentiate the actions of digitalis (McGuffin et al., 1997; Van Hellemont, 1986) though this effect has not been confirmed (Brown et al., 1999).

Dosage and Administration
See the approved monograph on hawthorn leaf with flower.

HAWTHORN LEAF

Latin Name:
Crataegus monogyna or *C. laevigata*

Pharmacopeial Name:
Crataegi folium

Other Names:
haw, hawthorn tops, mayhaw, whitethorn herb

Description
Hawthorn leaf consists of the dried leaf of *Crataegus monogyna* Jaquin emend. Lindman or *C. laevigata* in a valid pharmacopeia citing *Crataeus* [Fam. Rosaceae] and preparations thereof.

Chemistry and Pharmacology
There are no scientific data on which to base the pharmacology and toxicology of the leaf alone (as of 1994, the date of publication of this monograph by the Commission E). Spectrographic analysis of the chemical constituents of the herb distinguishes only quantitative differ-

ences between leaf and flower preparations. One may assume pharmacodynamics similar to those shown for preparations from the flower.

Uses

It has been claimed that hawthorn leaf preparations may be applied prophylactically to impeded circulation in the coronary artery, for psychogenic disturbances of the heart and circulatory system, to improve the perfusion and nutrition of the myocardium, for simple circulatory disorders of the coronary artery not needing treatment with digitalis, for beginnings of diminished cardiac output due to hypertension and pulmonary disease during and after infection, for chronic disturbance of heart rhythm, to enhance treatment with cardiac glycosides, for hypotension, for heart trouble in menopause and advanced age, as well as unregulated cardiac output in children.

Note: This monograph was published as a negative/unapproved monograph. According to Commission E, since the effectiveness of hawthorn leaf (by itself) for its claimed applications has not been documented, therapeutic use cannot be recommended.

The herb as a water extract, water-alcohol extract, wine infusion, and fresh juice has been used traditionally to strengthen and invigorate heart and circulatory function. These statements are based exclusively on historical record and experience.

Contraindications

No risks or contraindications are known.

Side Effects

None known (McGuffin et al., 1997; Meyer-Buchtela, 1999).

Use During Pregnancy and Lactation

No restrictions known (Anon., 1999; McGuffin et al., 1997).

Interactions with Other Drugs

Hawthorn preparations may potentiate the actions of digitalis (McGuffin et al., 1997; Van Hellemont, 1986), though this effect has not been confirmed (Brown et al., 1999).

Dosage and Administration

See the approved monograph on hawthorn leaf with flower.

HAWTHORN LEAF WITH FLOWER

Latin Name:
Crataegus monogyna

Pharmacopeial Name:
Crataegi folium cum flore

Other Names:
haw, hawthorn tops, mayhaw, whitethorn herb

Description

Hawthorn leaf with flower, consisting of dried flowering twig tips of *Crataegus monogyna* Jaquin emend. Lindman or *C. laevigata* (Poiret) de Candolle [Fam. Rosaceae], or other members of the *Crataegus* genus cited in a valid pharmacopeia and preparations from them in an effective dosage. The preparation contains flavonoids (flavones, flavonols), including hyperoside, vitex-inrhamnose, rutin, and vitexin and oligomeric procyanidins (n=2 to n=8 catechins and/or epicatechins).

Chemistry and Pharmacology

Hawthorn leaf with flower contains 1–3% oligomeric procyanidins; 1–2% flavonoids, including flavonols and flavone derivatives such as hyperoside, vitexinrhamnose, rutin, and vitexin; amines (choline, acetylcholine, trimethylamine); catechins; phenol carboxylic acids (e.g., chlorogenic acid); purines; sterols; and approximately 0.6% triterpene acids (oleanolic, ursolic, and crataegolic acids) (Budavari, 1996; Meyer-Buchtela, 1999; Wichtl and Bisset, 1994).

The following pharmacodynamic effects have been established in isolated organs or in animal experimentation with preparations from hawthorn leaf with flower (hydroalcoholic extract with defined content of oligomeric pro-cyanidins and/or flavonoids: macerates, fresh plant extract) and with individual fractions (oligomeric procyanidins, biogenic amines): positive inotropic effect, positive dromotropic effect, negative bathmotropic effect, increased coronary and myocardial circulatory perfusion, and reduction in peripheral vascular resistance.

Pharmacological investigations have shown that the most important components in terms of improving the peripheral vascular system are flavonoids, flavonglycosides (quercetin, rutin, hyperoside, and vitexin), procyanidine derived from catechin or epicatechin (oligomeric procyanidines), pentacyclical triterpenes, and aromatic carbon dioxides (Reuter, 1994). As long as a specific effectiveness can't be assigned to a single substance, the entire *Crataegus* extract must be viewed as the effective treatment (Reuter, 1994).

In cases of cardiac insufficiency according to Stage II NYHA, an improvement of subjective findings as well as an increase in cardiac work tolerance, a decrease in pressure/heart rate product, an increase in the ejection

fraction, and a rise in the anaerobic threshold have been established in human pharmacological studies following the administration of 160 to 900 mg aqueous-alcoholic extract per day (adjusted to oligomeric procyanidins and/or flavonoids) over periods lasting up to 56 days.

The pharmacokinetics of the preparation have been investigated only in animal studies, and no scientific results are available in the context of human pharmacokinetics. Investigations of acute toxicity using a hydroalcoholic dry extract (drug/extract ratio 5:1, standardized for oligomeric procyanidins) are available, according to which no fatal events occurred after oral or peritoneal administration in mice or rats in doses of up to 3 g per kg of body weight.

Symptoms of acute toxicity in rats and mice with an intraperitoneal administration of 3 g per kg body weight include sedation, piloerection, dyspnea, and tremor. The oral administration of powdered herb at individual doses of 3 g per kg body weight in rats and 5 g per kg body weight in mice produced no fatal reactions. No toxic effects were observed after oral administration of 30, 90, and 300 mg aqueous/ethanolic dry extract per kg body weight in rats and dogs over a period of 26 weeks. For this extract, the "no effect" dose was 300 mg per kg body weight. No fatal events and no toxic effects were observed after the oral administration of 300 and 600 mg preparation powder per kg body weight over a period of four weeks. No experimental data are available concerning embryonic and fetal toxicity, fertility, and post-natal development.

Although they have indeed produced different results, more recent studies are now available in regards to testing the mutagenicity of *Crataegus* preparations. It is assumed that the mutagenic activity demonstrated on *Salmonella* is based on the quercetin content, and the induction of SCE, particularly on the presence of flavone-C-glycosides as well as of flavone aglycones. By comparison with the quantity of quercetin ingested with the food, however, the content of quercetin in the preparation is so low that a risk for humans may be practically excluded.

No experimental data are available regarding carcinogenicity. The findings regarding gene toxicity and mutagenicity give no indication of carcinogenic risk of the preparation in human use.

Animal studies have found that hawthorn shows positive inotropic and negative chronotropic effects of the alcoholic extract (IV), as well as hypotensive activity (Bruneton, 1995). Isolated human artery studies have concluded that *Crataegus* extract dilates the coronary arteries to cause a more effective flow of blood to the heart. Animal studies have proven clear hemodynamic effects along with this vasodilatatory effect (Reuter, 1994). Observations in human subjects confirm the experimental results: improvement of symptoms and of the ECG in patients with mild cardiac insufficiency (with long term treatment of aqueous extract, orally), decrease in rhythm, and improvement of systolic contraction (Bruneton, 1995).

Uses

The Commission E approved the use of hawthorn leaf with flower for decreasing cardiac output as described in functional Stage II of NYHA.

Hawthorn has been used in cases of mild bradyarrhythmia, paroxymsmal tachycardia, hypertension, arteriosclerosis, Buerger's disease, and for relief of the feeling of pressure and tightness in the cardiac region (Wichtl and Bisset, 1994). Hawthorn is often combined with conventional cardiovascular medications (such as digitalis and oubain) to speed up cardiac compensation and prevent the indigestion and nausea associated with said treatments. It is additionally used as a sedative, antispasmodic, and as a general source of flavonoids (Upton, 1999b).

Note: A physician must be consulted in cases where symptoms continue unchanged for longer than six weeks or in case of swelling of the legs. Medical diagnosis is absolutely necessary when pains occur in the region of the heart,

spreading out to the arms, upper abdomen or the area around the neck, or in cases of respiratory distress (dyspnea).

Contraindications

None known.

Side Effects

None known.

Use During Pregnancy and Lactation

No restrictions known.

Interactions with Other Drugs

None known.

Dosage and Administration

Unless otherwise prescribed:
Take orally following liquid or dry pharmaceutical forms for a minimum of six weeks: 160–900 mg native, water-ethanol extract (ethanol 45% v/v or methanol 70% v/v, drug-extract ratio = 4–7:1, with defined flavonoid or procyanidin content), corresponding to 30–168.7 mg procyanidins, calculated as epicatechin, or 3.5–19.8 mg flavonoids, calculated as hyperoside in accordance with DAB 10, in two or three individual doses.

Hawthorn fluidextract DAB 10: Equivalent individual or daily dosage must be confirmed by clinical-pharmacological experiment or clinical study.

References

Ammon, H.P.T. and M. Händel. 1981. Crataegus, toxicology and pharmacology. Parts I–III. Planta Med 43:105–120, 209–239, 313–322.

Anon. 1999. Hawthorn (Crataegus laevigata, Crataegus oxyacantha, Crataegus monogyna). Portland, OR: Healthnotes, Inc. Available at: www.healthnotes.com

Anschutz, E.P. 1900. *New, Old and Forgotten Remedies*. Philadelphia, PA: Boericke and Tafel.

Blesken, R. 1992. [*Crataegus* in cardiology] [In German]. *Fortschr Med* 110(15):290–292.

Braun, R. et al. 1997. *Standardzulassungen für Fertigarzneimittel—Text and Kommentar*. Stuttgart: Deutscher Apotheker Verlag.

British Herbal Pharmacopoeia (BHP). 1996. Exeter, U.K.: British Herbal Medicine Association. 98–101.

Brown, D. 1999. Common Drugs and Their Potential Interactions with Herbs or Nutrients. Health Notes Review of Complementary and Integrative Medicine 6(2):124–141.

Bruneton, J. 1995. *Pharmacognosy, Phytochemistry, Medicinal Plants*. Paris: Lavoisier Publishing.

Budavari, S. (ed.). 1996. *The Merck Index: An Encyclopedia of Chemicals, Drugs, and Biologicals*, 12th ed. Whitehouse Station, N.J.: Merck & Co, Inc. 435.

Deutsches Arzneibuch, 10th ed., 3rd suppl. (DAB 10). 1993. Stuttgart: Deutscher Apotheker Verlag.

Deutsches Arzneibuch (DAB 1997). 1997. Stuttgart: Deutscher Apotheker Verlag.

Europäisches Arzneibuch, 3rd ed., 1st suppl. (Ph.Eur.3). 1998. Stuttgart: Deutscher Apotheker Verlag. 667–668.

Hanack, T. and M.H. Brückel. 1983. The treatment of mild stable forms of angina pectoris using Crategutt® novo. *Therapiewoche* 33:4331–4333.

Hedrick, U.P. (ed.). 1972. *Sturtevant's Edible Plants of the World*. New York: Dover Publications [reprint of 1919 original].

Hobbs, C. and S. Foster. 1990. Hawthorn—a literature review. *HerbalGram* 22:19–33.

Iwamoto, M., I.Takashi, S.Tasuo. 1981. [Clinical actions of Crataegutt on angina pectoris of ischemic or hypertensive origin] [In German]. *Planta Med* 42:1–16.

Leuchtgens, H. 1993. [*Crataegus* special extract WS 1442 in NYHA II heart failure. A placebo controlled randomized double-blind study] [In German]. *Fortschr Med* 111(20–21):352–354.

Leung, A.Y. and S. Foster. 1996. *Encyclopedia of Common Natural Ingredients Used in Food, Drugs, and Cosmetics*, 2nd ed. New York: John Wiley & Sons, Inc. 295–297.

Loew, D., M. Albrecht, H. Podzuweit. 1996. Efficacy and tolerability of a Hawthorn preparation in patients with heart failure Stage I and II according to NYHA—a surveillance study. Munich: 2nd International Congress on Phytomedicine.

McGuffin, M., C. Hobbs, R. Upton, A. Goldberg. 1997. American Herbal Product Association's Botanical Safety Handbook. Boca Raton: CRC Press. 37.

Meyer-Buchtela, E. 1999. *Tee-Rezepturen—Ein Handbuch für Apotheker und Ärzte*. Stuttgart: Deutscher Apotheker Verlag.

New York Heart Association (NYHA). 1994. Revisions to Classification of Functional Capacity and Objective Assessment of Patients with Diseases of the Heart.

Newall, C.A., L.A. Anderson, J.D. Phillipson. 1996. Herbal Medicines: A Guide for Health-Care Professionals. London: The Pharmaceutical Press. 157–159.

O'Connolly, M., G. Bernhöft, G. Bartsch. 1987. [Treatment of stenocardia (*Angina pectoris*) pain in advanced age patients with multi-morbidity] [In German]. *Therapiewoche* 37:3587–3600.

O'Connolly, M., W. Jansen, G. Bernhöft, G. Bartsch. 1986. Behandlung der nachlassenden Herzleistung. [Treatment of decreasing cardiac performance. Therapy using standardized crataegus extract in advanced age] *Fortschr Med* 104(42):805–808.

Ph.Eur.3. See *Europäisches Arzneibuch*.

Reuter, H. 1994. *Crataegus* (Hawthorn): A Botanical Cardiac Agent. *Z Phytother* 15:73–81.

Schilcher, H. 1997. Personal communication to M. Blumenthal. Dec. 30.

Schmidt, U., U. Kuhn, M. Ploch, W.D. Hubner. 1994. Efficacy of the hawthorn (crataegus) preparation LI 132 in 78 patients with chronic congestive heart failure defined as NYHA functional class II. *Phytomedicine* 1:17–24.

Schulz, V., R. Hänsel, V.E. Tyler. 1998. *Rational Phytotherapy: A Physicians' Guide to Herbal Medicine*. New York: Springer.

These monographs, published by the Commission E in 1994, were modified based on new scientific research. They contain more extensive pharmacological and therapeutic information taken directly from the Commission E.

This material was adapted from *The Complete German Commission E Monographs—Therapeutic Guide to Herbal Medicines*. M. Blumenthal, W.R. Busse, A. Goldberg, J. Gruenwald, T. Hall, C.W. Riggins, R.S. Rister (eds.) S. Klein and R.S. Rister (trans.). 1998. Austin: American Botanical Council; Boston: Integrative Medicine Communications.

1) The Overview section is new information.

2) Description, Chemistry and Pharmacology, Uses, Contraindications, Side Effects, Interactions with Other Drugs, and Dosage sections have been drawn from the original work. Additional information has been added in some or all of these sections, as noted with references.

3) The dosage for equivalent preparations (tea infusion, fluidextract, and tincture) have been provided based on the following example:

Unless otherwise prescribed: 2 g per day of [powdered, crushed, cut or whole] [plant part]
Infusion: 2 g in 150 ml of water
Fluidextract 1:1 (g/ml): 2 ml
Tincture 1:5 (g/ml): 10 ml

4) The References and Additional Resources sections are new sections. Additional Resources are not cited in the monograph but are included for research purposes.

Steinhoff, B. 1993–1994. New developments regarding phytomedicines in Germany. *Brit J Phytother* 3(4):190–193.

———. 1997. Herbal medicines increasingly preferred. *Pharmazeutische Zeitung* 142(49):4412–4417.

Tauchert, M., M. Ploch, W.D. Hubner. 1994. Effectiveness of hawthorn extract LI 132 compared with the ACE inhibitor Captopril: Multicenter double-blind study with 132 NYHA Stage II. *Muench Med Wochenschr* 136 suppl:S27–S33.

Upton, R. (ed.) et al. 1999a. Hawthorn Berry. Santa Cruz, CA: American Herbal Pharmacopoeia.

Upton, R. (ed.) et al. 1999b. Hawthorn Leaf with Flower. Santa Cruz, CA: American Herbal Pharmacopoeia.

Van Hellemont, J. 1986. Compendium de Phytotherapie. Bruxelles, Belgique: Association Pharmaceutique Belge.

Weihmayr, T. and E. Ernst. 1996. [Therapeutic effectiveness of *Crataegus*] [In German]. *Fortschr Med* 114(1–2):27–29.

Weikl, A. et al. 1996. *Crataegus* special extract WS 1442. Assessment of objective effectiveness in patients with heart failure. *Fortschr Med* 114(24)291–296.

Wichtl, M. and N.G. Bisset (eds.). 1994. *Herbal Drugs and Phytopharmaceuticals*. Stuttgart: Medpharm Scientific Publishers. 161–166.

Zapfe, G., K.D. Assmus, H.S. Noh. 1993. Placebo-controlled multicenter study with *Crataegus* special extract WS 1442: Clinical results in the treatment of NYHA II cardiac insufficiency. Presented at the 5th Congress on Phytotherapy: Bonn, Germany; June 11.

Additional Resources

Ammon, H.P. and M. Handel. 1981. [*Crataegus*, toxicology and pharmacology, Part I: Toxicity] [In German]. *Planta Med* 43(2):105–120.

———. 1981. [*Crataegus*, toxicology and pharmacology, Part II: Pharmacodynamics] [In German]. *Planta Med* 43(3):209–239.

———. 1981. [*Crataegus*, toxicology and pharmacology, Part III: Pharmacodynamics and pharmacokinetics] [In German]. *Planta Med* 43(4):313–322.

Ammon, H.P.T. and R. Kaul. 1994. [*Crataegus*: Activity on heart and circulation of *Crataegus* extracts, flavonoids and procyanidins. Part 1: History and hormones] [In German]. *Dtsch Apoth Zeitg* 134(26):2433–2436.

———. 1994. [*Crataegus*: Activity on heart and circulation of *Crataegus* extracts, flavonoids and procyanidins. Part 2: Actions on the heart] [In German]. *Dtsch Apoth Zeitg* 134(27):2521–2527.

———. 1994. [*Crataegus*: Activity on heart and circulation of *Crataegus* extracts, flavonoids and procyanidins. Part 3: Actions on circulation] [In German]. *Dtsch Apoth Zeitg* 134(28):2631–2636.

Beretz, A., M. Haag-Berrurier, R. Anton. 1978. Choice of pharmacological methods for the study of hawthorn activities. *Plantes Med Phytothér* 12(4):305–314.

Brown, D., S. Austin, R. Reichert. 1997. Early-stage congestive heart failure. Seattle: Natural Products Research Consultants.

Gabhard, B. et al. (eds.). 1983. Wandlungen in der Therapie der Herzinsuffizienz. Wiesbaden: Friedr. Vieweg & Soyn.

Guendjev, Z. 1977. Experimental myocardial infarction of the rat and stimulation of the revascularization by the flavonoid drug crataemon. *Arnzeimforsch* 27(8):1576–1579.

McGuffin, M., C. Hobbs, R. Upton, A. Goldberg. 1997. American Herbal Product Association's *Botanical Safety Handbook*. Boca Raton: CRC Press.

Newall, C.A., L.A. Anderson, J.D. Phillipson. 1996. *Herbal Medicines: A Guide for Health-Care Professionals*. London: The Pharmaceutical Press.

Occhiuto, F., C. Circosta, R. Costa, F. Briguglio, A. Tommasini. 1986. Study comparing the cardiovascular activity of young shoots, leaves and flowers of *C. laevigata* L. II: Effects of extracts and pure isolated active principles on the isolated rabbit heart. *Plantes Med Phytothér* 20:52–63.

Rakotoarison, D.A. et al. 1997. Antioxidant activities of polyphenolic extracts from flowers, *in vitro* callus and cell suspension cultures of *Crataegus monogyna*. *Pharmazie* 52(1):60–64.

Roddewig, C., H. Hensel. 1977. [Reaction of local myocardial blood flow in non-anesthetized dogs and anesthetized cats to the oral and parenteral administration of a Crateagus fraction] [In German]. *Arnzeimforsch* 27(7):1407–1410.

Stepka, W. and A.D. Winters. 1973. A survey of the genus *Crataegus* for hypotensive activity [symposium paper]. Proceedings American Society of Pharmacognosy: Jekyll Island, Georgia; Jul 15–20. *Lloydia* 36(4):430–443.

Sticher, O. and B. Meier. Hawthorn (*Crataegus*): Biological Activity and New Strategies for Quality Control. In: Lawson, L.D. and R. Bauer (eds.) 1998. *Phytomedicines of Europe: Chemistry and Biological Activity*. Washington, DC: American Chemical Society.

Tyler, V.E. 1994. *Herbs of Choice: The Therapeutic Use of Phytomedicinals*. New York: Haworth Press.

Weng, W.L. et al. 1984. Therapeutic effect of *Crataegus* pinnatifida on 46 cases of angina pectoris—a double blind study. *J Trad Chin Med* 4(4):293–294.

HOPS

Latin Name:
Humulus lupulus

Pharmacopeial Name:
Lupuli strobulus

Other Names:
common hops, European hops,
hop strobile

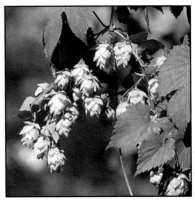

©1999 Steven Foster

Overview

Hops is a climbing perennial herb with male and female flowers on separate plants, native to Europe, Asia, and North America, extending roughly from 35 to 55 degrees north latitude, extensively cultivated in temperate zones worldwide. The material of commerce comes exclusively from female plants cultivated primarily in the United States, Germany, Great Britain, the Czech Republic, and China (BHP, 1990; Bruneton, 1995; DeLyser and Kasper, 1994; Leung and Foster, 1996; Wichtl and Bisset, 1994). The origin of hop cultivation is poorly documented, though it is first reported ca. 860 C.E. In the 1860s Germans brought hop cultivation to China and Korea, and to Japan in 1876, where German and American cultivars were used instead of the native Japanese variety (DeLyser and Kasper, 1994). Its common name is derived from the Anglo-Saxon hoppan (to climb). According to Pliny the Elder (ca. 23–79 C.E.), its species name *lupulus* is derived from Latin lupus (wolf), because when it grows among osiers (willows), it strangles them by its light, climbing embraces, as a wolf does a sheep (Grieve, 1979).

The therapeutic use of hops in Europe dates back to at least the ninth century. Before that it was used in making beers and breads, and also as a salad vegetable (DeLyser and Kasper, 1994). In North American aboriginal medicines, the Cherokee used hops as a sedative, antirheumatic, analgesic, gynecological aid for breast and womb problems, and kidney and urinary aid for "gravel" and inflamed kidneys (Hamel and Chiltoskey, 1975). In India, the *Ayurvedic Pharmacopoeia* recommends hops for restlessness associated with nervous tension, headache, and indigestion; and reports its actions as sedative, hypnotic, and antibacterial (Karnick, 1994). In traditional Chinese medicine, it is used to treat insomnia, restlessness, dyspepsia, intestinal cramps, and lack of appetite. In China, the ethanol fluidextract dosage form is the most commonly used preparation (Chang and But, 1986; Leung and Foster, 1996).

In Germany, hops is licensed as a standard medicinal tea, and about 70 prepared sedative medicines contain hops extract. In Germany and the United States, hops infusions, tinctures, and dry extracts are used in sedative preparations for anxiety and unrest (Leung and Foster, 1996; Wichtl and Bisset, 1994). Hop strobile and hops extract were listed in the United States *National Formulary* (NF) and unofficial in the *United States Pharmacopoeia* (USP) from 1831 to 1910 (Boyle, 1991).

Human studies generally investigate use of hops in combination with other herbs (e.g., valerian root). One study examined the effects of the drug Seda-Kneipp®N, which contains dry extracts of hop strobile (9.0–11.0:1) and valerian root (5.5–74:1), on patients suffering from sleep disorders. The study reported that hops lessened sleep disturbances when given in combination with valerian (Kneipp®, 1996; Müller-Limmroth and Ehrenstein, 1977; Newall et al., 1996).

However, it is not possible to determine if the action is caused by the hops, the valerian, or a possible synergy between the two.

One randomized, double-blind, controlled clinical trial in a parallel group design assessed quality of life parameters of patients with exogenous sleep disorders, such as temporary sleep onset and sleep interruption, treated with a hops-valerian preparation or a benzodiazepine drug. This trial demonstrated equivalent efficacy and tolerability according to DSM-IV criteria. The equivalence of both therapies according to sleep quality, fitness, and quality of life was demonstrated. The patients' state of health improved during therapy and then deteriorated after cessation with both preparations. The authors concluded that the investigated hop-valerian preparation in the appropriate dose is a sensible alternative to benzodiazepine for the treatment of nonchronic and non-psychiatric sleep disorders (Schmitz and Jackel, 1998).

Clinical studies conducted in China have investigated and reported positive outcomes for the use of hops preparations in the treatment of tuberculosis, leprosy, acute bacillary dysentery, silicosis, and asbestosis (Chang and But, 1986).

Though the sedative effect of hops is indisputable, its mechanism of action is not yet understood (Bradley, 1992). The approved modern therapeutic applications for hops are supportable based on its long history of use in well established systems of traditional medicine, documented pharmacological actions reported in *in vitro* and *in vivo* studies in animals, and human clinical studies.

European pharmacopeial grade hops must contain not less than 18% water soluble extractive and not less than 25% water and methanol soluble extractive. It must pass an assay that includes thin-layer chromatography (TLC) analysis of the flavonoids. Additionally, the German Standard License for hops medicinal tea requires the raw material to contain at least 0.5% flavonoids, calculated as rutin (BHP, 1996; Bradley, 1992; Braun et al., 1997; Bruneton, 1995; DAB, 1997; Wichtl and Bisset, 1994). The *Ayurvedic Pharmacopoeia* requires not less than 13% water soluble extractive (Karnick, 1994).

Description

Hops, consisting of the dried strobiles of *Humulus lupulus* L. [Fam. Cannabaceae], and their preparations in effective dosage. The preparation contains at least 0.35 % (v/w) essential oil. Other ingredients are α- and β-bitter acids and 2-methyl-3-butanol.

Chemistry and Pharmacology

Hop strobile contains resinous bitter principles (5–30%), mostly α-bitter acids (humulones 2–10%) and β-bitter acids (lupulones 2–16%) and their oxidative degradation products (2-methyl-3-buten-2-ol); polyphenolic condensed tannins (2–4%); volatile oil (0.35–1.0%), mainly monoterpenes and sesquiterpenes (β-caryophyllene, farnesene, humulene, β-myrcene); chalcones (xanthohumol); flavonoids (kaempferol, quercetin, rutin); phenolic acids; and amino acids (Bradley, 1992; Bruneton, 1995; ESCOP, 1997; Leung and Foster, 1996; Newall et al., 1996; Wichtl and Bisset, 1994). Unpublished analysis on some hops varieties by a major hops producer indicates the following ranges for some key components: resinous bitter principles (5–30%), humulones (2–18%), and volatile oil (0.5–3.0%) (Kostelecky, 1999).

The Commission E reported calming and sleep-promoting activity.

The *British Herbal Compendium* reported its actions as sedative, soporific, spasmolytic and aromatic bitter (Bradley, 1992). Hops are generally combined with other sedative herbs and have been reported to improve sleep when taken with valerian (Müller-Limmroth and Ehrenstein, 1977; Newall et al., 1996).

Uses

The Commission E approved the internal use of hops for mood disturbances such as restlessness and anxiety as well as sleep disturbances.

The *British Herbal Compendium* indicated its use for excitability, restlessness, disorders of sleep, and lack of appetite (Bradley, 1992). ESCOP indicates its use for tenseness, restlessness, and difficulty in falling asleep (ESCOP, 1997). The German Standard License for hops tea infusion indicates its use for disturbed states such as restlessness and disorders of sleep (Braun et al., 1997).

Contraindications

None known.

Side Effects

None known.

Use During Pregnancy and Lactation

No restrictions known.

Interactions with Other Drugs

None known.

Dosage and Administration

Unless otherwise prescribed: Single dosage of 0.5 g cut or powdered strobile or dry extract powder for infusions, decoctions, or other preparations. Liquid and solid preparations for internal use.

Note: Combinations with all other sedatives can be beneficial.

Infusion or decoction: 0.5 g in 150 ml water.

Fluidextract 1:1 (g/ml): 0.5 ml.

Tincture 1:5 (g/ml): 2.5 ml.

Native dry extract 6–8:1 (w/w): 0.06–0.08 g (60–80 mg).

References

Boyle, W. 1991. *Official Herbs: Botanical Substances in the United States Pharmacopoeias 1820–1990*. East Palestine, OH: Buckeye Naturopathic Press.

Bradley, P.R. (ed.). 1992. *British Herbal Compendium*, Vol. 1. Bournemouth: British Herbal Medicine Association.

Braun, R. et al. 1997. *Standardzulassungen für Fertigarzneimittel—Text and Kommentar*. Stuttgart: Deutscher Apotheker Verlag.

British Herbal Pharmacopoeia (BHP). 1990. Bournemouth, U.K.: British Herbal Medicine Association.

———. 1996. Exeter, U.K.: British Herbal Medicine Association.

Bruneton, J. 1995. *Pharmacognosy, Phytochemistry, Medicinal Plants*. Paris: Lavoisier Publishing.

Chang, H.M. and P.P.H. But. 1986. *Pharmacology and Applications of Chinese Materia Medica*. Philadelphia: World Scientific. 1077–1083.

Deutsches Arzneibuch (DAB 1997). 1997. Stuttgart: Deutscher Apotheker Verlag.

DeLyser, D.Y. and W.J. Kasper. 1994. Hopped Beer: The Case for Cultivation. *Economic Botany* 48(2):166–170.

ESCOP. 1997. "Lupuli strobulus." *Monographs on the Medicinal Uses of Plant Drugs*. Exeter, U.K.: European Scientific Cooperative on Phytotherapy.

Grieve, M. 1979. *A Modern Herbal*. New York: Dover Publications, Inc.

Hamel, P.B. and M.U. Chiltoskey. 1975. *Cherokee Plants and Their Uses—A 400-Year History*. Sylva, N.C.: Herald Publishing Co.

Karnick, C.R. 1994. *Pharmacopoeial Standards of Herbal Plants*, Vols. 1–2. Delhi: Sri Satguru Publications. Vol. 1:183–184, Vol. 2:67.

Kneipp®.1996. Wegweiser zu den Kneipp® Mitteln [Guide to Kneipp® Remedies]. Würzburg: Sebastian Kneipp Gesundheitsmittel-Verlag. 88–89.

Kostelecky, T. 1999. (John I. HAAS, Inc.). Personal communication to A. Goldberg, May 26.

Leung, A.Y. and S. Foster. 1996. *Encyclopedia of Common Natural Ingredients Used in Food, Drugs, and Cosmetics*, 2nd ed. New York: John Wiley & Sons, Inc.

Müller-Limmroth, W. and W. Ehrenstein. 1977. Untersuchungen über die Wirkung von Seda-Kneipp® auf den Schlaf schlafgestörter Menschen [Experimental studies of the effects of Seda-Kneipp® on the sleep of sleep disturbed subjects; implications for the treatment of different sleep disturbances]. *Med Klin* 72(25):1119–1125.

Newall, C.A., L.A. Anderson, J.D. Phillipson. 1996. *Herbal Medicines: A Guide for Health-Care Professionals*. London: The Pharmaceutical Press.

Schmitz, M. and M. Jackel. 1998. Vergleichsstudie zur Untersuchung der Lebensqualitat von Patienten mit exogenen Schlafstorungen (vorübergehenden Ein- und Durchschlafstorungen) unter Therapie mit einem Hopfen-Baldrian-Präparat und einem Benzodiazepin-Präparat [Comparative study for assessing quality of life of patients with exogenous sleep disorders (temporary sleep onset and sleep interruption disorders) treated with a hops-valerian preparation and a benzodiazepine drug]. *Wien Med Wochenschr* 148(13):291–298.

Wichtl, M. and N.G. Bisset (eds.). 1994. *Herbal Drugs and Phytopharmaceuticals*. Stuttgart: Medpharm Scientific Publishers.

Additional Resources

Bown, D. 1995. *Encyclopedia of Herbs and Their Uses*. New York: DK Publishing, Inc. 294.

British Pharmaceutical Codex (BPC). 1949. London: The Pharmaceutical Press.

Bravo, L., J. Cabo, A. Fraile, J. Jimenez, A. Villar. 1974. Estudio Farmacodinamico del Lupulo (*Humulus lupulus* L.). Accion Tranquilizante. *Boll Chim Farm* 113:310–315.

Caujolle, F., P.H. Chanh, P. Duch-Kan, L. Bravo-Diaz. 1969. Etude de l'action spasmolytique du houblon (*Humulus lupulus*, Cannabinacées) [Spasmolytic action of hop]. *Agressologie* 10(5):405–410.

Council of Europe. 1981. *Flavouring Substances and Natural Sources of Flavourings*, 3rd ed. Strasbourg: Maisonneuve.

Der Marderosian, A. (ed.). 1999. *The Review of Natural Products*. St. Louis: Facts and Comparisons.

Duke, J.A. 1985. *Handbook of Medicinal Herbs*. Boca Raton: CRC Press.

Hänsel, R. and H.H. Wagener. 1967. Versuche, sedativ-hypnotische Wirkstoffe im Hopfen nachzuweisen [Attempts to identify sedative-hypnotic active substances in hops.] *Arzneimforsch* 17(1):79–81.

Hänsel, R., R. Wohlfart, H. Coper. 1980. Narcotic action of 2-methyl-3-butene-2-ol contained in the exhalation of hops [in German]. *Z Naturforsch* 35(1112):1096–1097.

Hänsel, R., R. Wohlfart, H. Schmidt. 1982. The sedative-hypnotic principle of hops. 3. Communication: Contents of 2-methyl-3-butene-2-ol in hops and hop preparations. *Planta Med* 45:224–228.

Hänsel, R. and J. Schulz. 1986. Hopfen und Hopfenpräparate: Fragen zur pharmazeutischen Qualität. *Dtsch Apoth Ztg* 126:2033–2037.

———. 1986. Hopfenzapfen (*Lupuli strobulus*): Dünnschichtchromatographische Prüfung auf Identität. *Dtsch Apoth Ztg* 126:2347–2648.

Hänsel, R. 1995. Pflanzliche Beruhigungsmittel. Möglichkeiten und Grenzen in der Selbstmedikation. *Dtsch Apoth Ztg* 135:2935–2943.

Karrer, W. 1958. *Konstitution und Vorkommen der Organischen Pflanzenstoffe (exclusive Alkaloide)*. Basel: Birkhäuser Verlag.

List, P.H. and L. Hörhammer (eds.). 1973–1979. *Hagers Handbuch der Pharmazeutischen Praxis*, Vols. 1–7. New York: Springer Verlag.

McGuffin, M., C. Hobbs, R. Upton, A. Goldberg. 1997. *American Herbal Product Association's Botanical Safety Handbook*. Boca Raton: CRC Press.

Pharmacopée Française Xe Édition (Ph.Fr.X.). 1983–1990. Moulins-les-Metz: Maisonneuve S.A.

Reynolds, J.E.F. (ed.). 1982. *Martindale: The Extra Pharmacopoeia*, 28th ed. London: The Pharmaceutical Press.

Wichtl, M. 1988. In: Braun, R. (ed.). Standardzulassung für Fertigarzneimittel—Text und Kommentar. Stuttgart: Deutsche Apotheker Verlag.

Wichtl, M. 1989. In: Wichtl, M. (ed.). *Teedrogen*, 2nd ed. Stuttgart: Wissenschaftliche Verlagsgesellschaft. 242–245.

Wohlfart, R. 1993. In: Hänsel, R., K. Keller, H. Rimpler, G. Schneider (eds.). 1993. *Hagers Handbuch der Pharmazeutischen Praxis*, 5th ed. Vol. 5. Drogen E-O. Berlin-Heidelberg: Springer Verlag. 447–458.

This material was adapted from *The Complete German Commission E Monographs—Therapeutic Guide to Herbal Medicines*. M. Blumenthal, W.R. Busse, A. Goldberg, J. Gruenwald, T. Hall, C.W. Riggins, R.S. Rister (eds.) S. Klein and R.S. Rister (trans.). 1998. Austin: American Botanical Council; Boston: Integrative Medicine Communications.

1) The Overview section is new information.

2) Description, Chemistry and Pharmacology, Uses, Contraindications, Side Effects, Interactions with Other Drugs, and Dosage sections have been drawn from the original work. Additional information has been added in some or all of these sections, as noted with references.

3) The dosage for equivalent preparations (tea infusion, fluidextract, and tincture) have been provided based on the following example:

Unless otherwise prescribed: 2 g per day of [powdered, crushed, cut or whole] [plant part]
Infusion: 2 g in 150 ml of water
Fluidextract 1:1 (g/ml): 2 ml
Tincture 1:5 (g/ml): 10 ml

4) The References and Additional Resources sections are new sections. Additional Resources are not cited in the monograph but are included for research purposes.

Horehound Herb

Latin Name:
Marrubium vulgare

Pharmacopeial Name:
Marrubii herba

Other Names:
white horehound

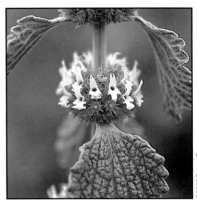

©1999 Steven Foster

Overview

White horehound is a perennial aromatic herb native to the region between the Mediterranean Sea and Central Asia, now naturalized in North America (Budavari, 1996; Knöss and Zapp, 1998; Leung and Foster, 1996). In Asia, its range includes the western temperate Himalayas, Kashmir, the N.W. Frontier Province (India) and Baluchistan (southwest Pakistan and southeast Iran) (Karnick, 1994; Nadkarni, 1976). The material of commerce comes mainly from Hungary and also from France, Italy, and Morocco (BHP, 1996; Wichtl and Bisset, 1994).

Horehound has been used as an expectorant cough remedy since ancient Egyptian times (Bown, 1995). Its name comes from the word hoary, due to the white hairs that cover horehound leaves, and hound, because it was used in ancient Greek medicine to treat bites from rabid dogs (Tyler, 1993). The sixteenth century Elizabethan herbalist John Gerard indicated its use for wheezing and tuberculosis (Tyler, 1993) as did seventeenth century English herbalist Nicholas Culpepper (Grieve, 1979). Horehound is used in Indian Ayurvedic medicine to treat acute or chronic bronchitis and whooping cough (Karnick, 1994; Nadkarni, 1976). Its uses in North American aboriginal medicines are comparable to the Asian and European uses. The Cherokee use horehound as a cold remedy, cough medicine, and throat aid and prepare a cough syrup by combining the infusion with sugar. The Navajo prepare the infusion to treat sore throat. The Kawaiisu prepared hot or cold aqueous infusions of the leaves and flowering tops to treat coughs and colds. Additionally, they prepared a syrup to treat respiratory ailments (Moerman, 1998).

In Germany, horehound is used to treat dyspeptic complaints such as feeling of repletion, flatulence, and loss of appetite. It is also used for catarrh of the respiratory tract (BAnz, 1998; Meyer-Buchtela, 1999; Wichtl and Bisset, 1994) as a component of some antitussive and expectorant drugs. It is also an ingredient in various multi-herb "liver and bile teas" such as "Species cholagogae ÖAB" (ÖAB, 1983; Wichtl and Bisset, 1994). It is a common expectorant component of Europeanmade herbal cough remedies (e.g., Ricola® lozenges) that are sold in the United States. It was formerly official in the *United States Pharmacopeia* (Boyle, 1991).

Horehound has been used traditionally as an expectorant, to treat whooping cough and non-productive coughs of bronchitis and tuberculosis (Felter and Lloyd, 1985; Grieve, 1979; Newall et al., 1996; Tyler, 1993). Since these conditions are now primarily treated with antibiotics or prevented with vaccines, horehound's use as an expectorant is not as common, despite evidence that attests to its probable efficacy (Tyler, 1993). Animal studies have shown that horehound preparations are choleretic. This activity is attributed to the marrubic acid, which, in laboratory tests, increased bile flow in rats (Krejci and Zadina, 1959). Marrubiin has also been observed to enhance bronchial mucosa secretion, and to have cardiac actions. It is anti-arrhythmic in therapeutic doses, but pro-arrhythmic in large doses (Tyler, 1993). The approved modern therapeutic applications for horehound are supportable based on its long history of use in well established systems of traditional medicine, phytochemical investigations, *in vitro* studies, and pharmacological studies in animals.

Pharmacopeial grade white horehound consists of the dried leaves and flowering tops of *Marrubium vulgare* L. Botanical identity must be carried out with thin-layer chromatography (TLC), macroscopic and microscopic examinations, and organoleptic evaluations. It must contain not less than 15% water-soluble extractive (BHP, 1996). *The Hungarian Pharmacopoeia VII* requires microscopic tests for identity, qualitative tests for other plant parts, foreign organic matter, and bitter value. Based on recent phytochemical studies, a proposal has been made to amend the monograph to include new qualitative and quantitative chemical tests for determination of the main terpenoid substances, premarubiin and marrubiin (Ph.Hg.VII, 1986; Telek et al., 1997). Marrubiin is a furanic labdane diterpene with a lactone ring system and it evolves from the genuine diterpene premarrubiin during the extraction process (Knöss and Zapp, 1998). The *Austrian Pharmacopoeia* requires a bitterness value of not less than 3,000 (ÖAB, 1983; Wichtl and Bisset, 1994).

Description

Horehound herb consists of the fresh or dried, aboveground parts of *M. vulgare* L. [Fam. Lamiaceae] and their preparations in effective dosage. The herb contains bitter principles and tannins.

Chemistry and Pharmacology

Horehound contains 0.3–1% bitter diterpene principles, mainly marrubiin, which has a bitterness index (BI) of 65,000 (Leung and Foster, 1996; Wagner et al., 1984); diterpene alcohols, including peregrinol, vulgarol, marrubiol, marrubenol, and phytol; up to 7% tannins; alkaloids including approximately 0.3% betonicine and stachydrine; 0.2% choline; 0.05%–0.06% volatile oil, mainly monoterpenes; flavonoids (apigenin, luteolin, quercetin, and their glycosides); and minerals, particularly potassium (Bradley, 1992; Hänsel et al., 1992–1994; Leung and Foster, 1996; Meyer-Buchtela, 1999).

The Commission E reported that marrubinic acid works as a choleretic. *The Merck Index* reported expectorant action (Budavari, 1996). The *British Herbal Compendium* reported expectorant and bitter tonic actions. Marrubiin and the volatile oil contribute to the expectorant action by stimulating secretion from the respiratory tract's mucous membranes (Bradley, 1992).

Uses

The Commission E approved horehound herb for loss of appetite and dyspepsia, such as bloating and flatulence.

The *British Herbal Compendium* indicates its use for acute bronchitis, nonproductive coughs and catarrh of the respiratory tract as well as for lack of appetite and dyspepsia (Bradley, 1992). In France, it is indicated for use as a cough remedy and to treat acute benign bronchial affections (Bradley, 1992; Bruneton, 1995; DPM, 1992).

Contraindications

None known.

Side Effects

None known.

Use During Pregnancy and Lactation

Not recommended during pregnancy. No restrictions known during lactation (McGuffin et al., 1997).

Interactions with Other Drugs

None known.

Dosage and Administration

Unless otherwise prescribed: 4.5 g per day of cut herb, freshly expressed plant juice and other equivalent galenical preparations for internal use.
Dried herb: 4.5 g.
Succus: 2–6 tablespoons fresh pressed juice.
Infusion: Steep 1.5 g in 150–250 ml boiling water for 5 to 10 minutes, three times daily (Meyer-Buchtela, 1999; ÖAB, 1991; Wichtl and Bisset, 1994).
Fluidextract 1:1 (g/ml): 1.5 ml, three times daily.
Syrup: 2–4 ml (BPC, 1949; Bradley, 1992).
Tincture 1:5 (g/ml): 7.5 ml, three times daily.

References

BAnz. See *Bundesanzeiger.*
Bown, D. 1995. *Encyclopedia of Herbs and Their Uses.* New York: DK Publishing, Inc. 308–309.
Boyle, W. 1991. *Official Herbs: Botanical Substances in the United States Pharmacopoeias 1820–1990.* East Palestine, OH: Buckeye Naturopathic Press.
Bradley, P.R. (ed.). 1992. *British Herbal Compendium,* Vol. 1. Bournemouth: British Herbal Medicine Association.
British Herbal Pharmacopoeia (BHP). 1996. Exeter, U.K.: British Herbal Medicine Association. 53.
British Pharmaceutical Codex (BPC). 1949. London: The Pharmaceutical Press.
Bruneton, J. 1995. *Pharmacognosy, Phytochemistry, Medicinal Plants.* Paris: Lavoisier Publishing.
Budavari, S. (ed.). 1996. *The Merck Index: An Encyclopedia of Chemicals, Drugs, and Biologicals,* 12th ed. Whitehouse Station, N.J.: Merck & Co, Inc. 812.
Bundesanzeiger (BAnz). 1998. Monographien der Kommission E (Zulassungs- und Aufbereitungskommission am BGA für den humanmed. Bereich, phytotherapeutische Therapierichtung und Stoffgruppe). Köln: Bundesgesundheitsamt (BGA).
Direction de la Pharmacie et du Médicament (DPM). 1992. Bulletin Officiel (Fascicule spécial) No. 90/22 bis. [English edition]. Paris: Ministère des Affaires Sociales et de la Solidarité.
Felter, H.W. and J.U. Lloyd. 1985. *King's American Dispensatory,* Vols. 1–2. Portland, OR: Eclectic Medical Publications [reprint of 1898 original].

Grieve, M. 1979. *A Modern Herbal.* New York: Dover Publications, Inc.
Hänsel, R., K. Keller, H. Rimpler, G. Schneider (eds.). 1992–1994. *Hagers Handbuch der Pharmazeutischen Praxis,* 5th ed. Vol. 4–6. Berlin-Heidelberg: Springer Verlag.
Karnick, C.R. 1994. *Pharmacopoeial Standards of Herbal Plants,* Vols. 1–2. Delhi: Sri Satguru Publications. Vol. 1:255–256; Vol. 2:140.
Knöss, W. and J. Zapp. 1998. Accumulation of furanic labdane diterpenes in *Marrubium vulgare* and *Leonurus cardiaca. Planta Med* 64:357–361.
Krejci, I. and R. Zadina. 1959. Die Gallentreibende Wirkung von Marrubiin und Marrabinsäure. *Planta Med* 7.
Leung, A.Y. and S. Foster. 1996. *Encyclopedia of Common Natural Ingredients Used in Food, Drugs, and Cosmetics,* 2nd ed. New York: John Wiley & Sons, Inc.
McGuffin, M., C. Hobbs, R. Upton, A. Goldberg. 1997. American Herbal Product Association's *Botanical Safety Handbook.* Boca Raton: CRC Press. 74.
Meyer-Buchtela, E. 1999. *Tee-Rezepturen—Ein Handbuch für Apotheker und Ärzte.* Stuttgart: Deutscher Apotheker Verlag.
Moerman, D.E. 1998. *Native American Ethnobotany.* Portland, OR: Timber Press.
Nadkarni, K.M. 1976. *Indian Materia Medica.* Bombay: Popular Prakashan. 771.
Newall, C.A., L.A. Anderson, J.D. Phillipson. 1996. *Herbal Medicines: A Guide for Health-Care Professionals.* London: The Pharmaceutical Press.
Österreichisches Arzneibuch, 1st and 2nd suppl. (ÖAB). 1991. Wien: Verlag der Österreichischen Staatsdruckerei.
Österreichisches Arzneibuch, Vols. 1–2, 1st suppl. (ÖAB). 1981–1983. Wien: Verlag der Österreichischen Staatsdruckerei.
Pharmacopoeia Hungarica, 7th ed (Ph.Hg.VII). 1986. Budapest: Medicina Konyvkiado.
Telek, E., L. Toth, L. Botz, I. Mathe. 1997. Marrubium fajok novenykemiai vizsgalata Adatok a VII. Magyar Gyogyszerkonyv Marrubii herba cikkelyehez [Chemical tests with *Marrubium* species. Official data on Marubii herba in *Pharmacopoeia Hungarica* VII]. *Acta Pharm Hung* 67(1):31–37.
Tyler, V. 1993. *The Honest Herbal: A Sensible Guide to the Use of Herbs and Related Remedies,* 3rd ed. New York: Pharmaceutical Products Press.
Wagner, H., S. Bladt, E.M. Zgainski. 1984. *Plant Drug Analysis–A Thin Layer Chromatography Atlas.* Berlin-Heidelberg: Springer Verlag. 128, 134.
Wichtl, M. and N.G. Bisset (eds.). 1994. *Herbal Drugs and Phytopharmaceuticals.* Stuttgart: Medpharm Scientific Publishers.

Additional Resources

Bartarelli M. 1966. *Marrubium vulgare* and its pharmaceutical uses. *Boll Chim Farm* 105(11):787–798.

Cahen R. 1970. [Pharmacologic spectrum of *Marrubium vulgare* L.] [In French]. *C R Seances Soc Biol Fil* 164(7):1467–1472.

Karryev, M.O., C.B. Bairyev, A.S. Ataeva. 1977. Some therapeutic properties of common horehound. *Chem Abstr* (86): 2355.

List, P.H. and L. Hörhammer (eds.). 1976. *Hagers Handbuch der Pharmazeutischen Praxis,* Vol. 5. New York: Springer Verlag. 703–706.

Paudler, W.W. and S. Wagner. 1963. The major alkaloid of *Marrubium vulgare*. London: Chem Ind.

Saleh, M.M. and K.W. Glombitza. 1989. Volatile oil of *Marrubium vulgare* and its anti-schistosomal activity. *Planta Med* 55:105.

This material was adapted from *The Complete German Commission E Monographs—Therapeutic Guide to Herbal Medicines.* M. Blumenthal, W.R. Busse, A. Goldberg, J. Gruenwald, T. Hall, C.W. Riggins, R.S. Rister (eds.) S. Klein and R.S. Rister (trans.). 1998. Austin: American Botanical Council; Boston: Integrative Medicine Communications.

1) The Overview section is new information.

2) Description, Chemistry and Pharmacology, Uses, Contraindications, Side Effects, Interactions with Other Drugs, and Dosage sections have been drawn from the original work. Additional information has been added in some or all of these sections, as noted with references.

3) The dosage for equivalent preparations (tea infusion, fluidextract, and tincture) have been provided based on the following example:

   Unless otherwise prescribed: 2 g per day of [powdered, crushed, cut or whole] [plant part]
   Infusion: 2 g in 150 ml of water
   Fluidextract 1:1 (g/ml): 2 ml
   Tincture 1:5 (g/ml): 10 ml

4) The References and Additional Resources sections are new sections. Additional Resources are not cited in the monograph but are included for research purposes.

HORSE CHESTNUT SEED EXTRACT

Latin Name:
Aesculus hippocastanum

Pharmacopeial Name:
Hippocastani semen

Other Names:
buckeye, Spanish chestnut

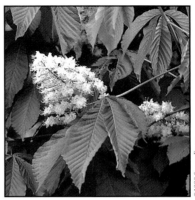

© 1999 Steven Foster

Overview

Horse chestnut seed extract (HCSE) is derived from a deciduous tree that grows up to 25 meters. It has spread throughout the northern hemisphere, but is native to the central Balkan peninsula. HCSE is relatively new on the United States botanical market. This phytomedicine is gaining in popularity due to the significant quantity of clinical evidence that documents its efficacy as a treatment for varicose veins, chronic venous insufficiency (CVI), and related vascular disorders.

In 1994, Commission E revised the previous horse chestnut monograph to include a detailed description of the pharmacokinetics (the absorption/resorption of substances in the human body) of the approved herb. The old monograph (December 5, 1984) on horse chestnut leaf and flower did not include these findings, and thus the herb was not approved. Also, the approved formulation for horse chestnut was more rigorously defined than earlier. The 1984 monograph defined the drug as horse chestnut seed with 3% triterpene glycosides calculated as escin (aescin), and indicated a daily dose corresponding to 30–150 mg escin. The 1994 monograph pertains to a defined extract only with an escin content of 16–21% in a slow-release dosage form.

Numerous studies have been performed on the defined extract. A clinical study of 22 patients with proven venous insufficiency measured by capillary filtration coefficient and intravascular volume of the lower legs showed that 1200 mg of HCSE, standardized to 50 mg escin per capsule, lowered capillary filtration by 22% in three hours (Bisler et al., 1986). In a randomized, placebo-controlled, parallel, double-blind study of 40 patients with venous edema in chronic deep vein incompetence, the edema-reducing effect of HCSE was deemed statistically significant. Measurements of leg circumference and other relevant indicators showed HCSE to be a safe and effective adjunct to compression therapy (Diehm et al., 1992). A study of 240 patients indicated that HCSE is effective as an adjunct therapy with compression stockings for the treatment of edema resulting from CVI (Diehm et al., 1996).

Other recent clinical studies have evaluated oral HCSE and topically applied gel for CVI. In a multi-center, placebo-controlled study on 60 patients (half receiving placebo), HCSE tablets (63–90 mg extract, standardized to 20 mg escin) (Aesculaforce®/Venaforce®, Bioforce, Switzerland), given in a dosage of three tablets twice daily for six weeks, were effective in reducing edema in the ankles and the venous filling rate (Shah et al., 1997). A gel (Aesculuaforce®/Venacorce® Vein Gel, Bioforce) containing 2% escin was successful in a recent non-controlled multi-center trial for six weeks on 71 patients with CVI and edema (Geissbühler and Degenring, 1999). Ankle circumference was reduced by a statistically significant 0.7 cm and the sum of the symptoms score was reduced by approximately 60% as determined by physicians and patients. In both studies, the principal author was employed by the manufacturer.

An observational study of 800 German general practitioners treating over five thousand patients concluded that the symptoms (pain, tiredness, tension and swelling in the leg, itching, and tendency towards edema) all improved significantly or disappeared completely. The authors, employees of the leading manufacturer of HCSE (Venostasin® retard, Klinge Pharma, Germany), concluded that compared to compression therapy, HCSE had the advantage of better compliance (Greeske and Pohlmann, 1996).

A recent systematic review of 13 clinical studies conducted on HCSE concluded that the superiority of the medication compared to placebo was established by the studies. HCSE was as effective as rutosides (the conventional treatment) in five studies. Adverse effects were mild and infrequent (Pittler and Ernst, 1998). In addition to studies published in 1999 on the external gel, at least 22 clinical studies of various designs have been conducted on HCSE on a total of 918 patients: 12 trials were double-blind, placebo-controlled, two were double-blind compared with a conventional drug, one was single-blind, placebo-controlled, two were open and placebo-controlled and five were open studies (Degenring, 1996; Shah et al., 1997). Clinical and pharmacological studies were evaluated in a recent literature review of HCSE (Bombardelli and Morazzoni, 1996).

German pharmacopeial grade horse chestnut seed, which is the material required for manufacture of the above specified native dry extract, consists of the dried seed of *Aesculus hippocastanum* L. It must contain not less than 3.0% triterpene glycosides, calculated as anhydrous escin, with reference to the dried drug. Botanical identity must be confirmed using thin-layer chromatography (TLC) as well as macroscopic and microscopic examinations (DAB, 1997). The typical drug-to-extract ratio for this native dry extract will fall within the range of 5.0–8.0:1 (w/w) depending on the chemical composition of the starting material and the subsequent yield of soluble extractive.

Description

A dry extract manufactured from horse chestnut seeds, *A. hippocastanum* L. [Fam. Hippocastanaceae], adjusted to a content of 16–20% triterpene glycosides calculated as anhydrous escin.

Chemistry and Pharmacology

Horse chestnut seed contains 3–6% of a complex mixture of triterpene saponins collectively referred to as escin (Morgan and Bone, 1998), including the triterpene oligoglycosides escins, Ia, Ib, IIa, IIb, and IIIa (Yoshikawa et al., 1996), the acylated polyhydroxy-oleanene triterpene oligoglycosides escins IIIb, IV, V, and VI and isoescins Ia, Ib, and V (Yoshikawa et al., 1998), and the sapogenols hippocaesculin and barringtogenol-C (Konoshima and Lee, 1986); flavonoids (e.g., flavonol glycosides); condensed tannins (Newall et al., 1996); quinones; sterols, including stig-

masterol, *alpha*-spinasterol, and *beta*-sitosterol; and fatty acids, such as linolenic, palmitic, and stearic acids (Leung and Foster, 1996).

As found in different animal experiments, the principal ingredient in HCSE is the triterpene glycoside mixture, aescin (escin), which has an anti-exudative and vascular-tightening effect. There are indications that HCSE reduces the activity of lysosomal enzymes that is increased in chronic pathological conditions of the veins, so that the breakdown of glycoacalyx (mucopolysaccharides) in the region of the capillary walls is inhibited. The filtration of low-molecular proteins, electrolytes, and water into the interstitium is inhibited through a reduction of vascular permeability. Using placebo as reference, a significant reduction of transcapillary filtration has been demonstrated in pharmacological studies involving human subjects, and a significant improvement shown in the symptoms of chronic venous insufficiency (sensation of tiredness, heaviness and tension, pruritus, pain and swelling in the legs) in randomized double-blind studies and cross-over studies.

Pilot studies are available on the toxicology of HCSE. The oral LD50 of the extract is 990 mg per kg body weight in mice, 2,150 mg per kg body weight in rats, 1,530 mg per kg body weight in rabbits, and 130 mg per kg body weight in dogs. In rats, the "no effect" dose is between 9 and 30 mg per kg body weight after intravenous administration of HCSE over a period of eight weeks. Chronic administration above 80 mg per kg body weight over a period of 34 weeks produced gastric irritation in dogs. In rats, no toxic changes were observed throughout the same period up to an oral dose of 400 mg per kg body weight.

Uses

The Commission E approved the use of horse chestnut seed for treatment of complaints found in pathological conditions of the veins of the legs (chronic venous insufficiency, CVI), for example, pain and a sensation of heaviness in the legs, cramps in the calves, pruritus, and swelling of the legs. Note: Other non-invasive treatment measures prescribed by a physician, such as leg compresses, wearing of supportive elastic stockings, or cold water applications, must be observed under all circumstances.

Horse chestnut seed preparations are indicated for treatment of CVI, varicose veins, edema of the lower limbs, and hemorrhoids. It is reported to combine well with other herbs that improve peripheral circulation such as ginkgo leaf, gotu kola leaf, and bilberry fruit (Morgan and Bone, 1998).

Contraindications

None known.

Side Effects

Pruritis, nausea, and gastric complaints may occur in isolated cases after oral intake.

Use During Pregnancy and Lactation

No restrictions known.

Interactions with Other Drugs

None known.

Dosage and Administration

Unless otherwise prescribed:
Dry extract 5.0–8.0:1 (w/w): 250–312.5 mg, two times per day in delayed release form, corresponding to 100 mg escin daily. Take one dose in the morning and the other in the evening with ample liquids during meals.

References

Bisler, H., R. Pfeifer, N. Kluken, P. Pauschinger. 1986. Wirkung von Rosskastaniensamenextrakt auf die traskapillare filtration bei chronischer venoser insuffizien [Effects of horse-chestnut seed extract on transcapillary filtration in chronic venous insufficiency]. *Dtsch Med Wochenschr* 111(35):1321–1329.

Bombardelli, E. and P. Morazzoni. 1996. *Aesculus hippocastanum* L. Fitoterapia 67(6):483–511.

Degenring, F.H. 1996. *Aesculus Hipp*. Semen for the treatment of venous blood flow disorders. Clinical Expert Report for Bioforce AG (unpublished).

Deutsches Arzneibuch (DAB 1997). 1997. Stuttgart: Deutscher Apotheker Verlag.

Diehm C., D. Vollbrecht, K Amendt, H.U. Comberg. 1992. Medical edema protection—Clinical benefit in patients with chronic deep vein incompetence. A placebo-controlled double-blind study. *Vasa* 21(2):188–192.

Diehm, C., H.J. Trampisch, S. Lange, C. Schmidt. 1996. Comparison of leg compression stocking and oral horse-chestnut seed extract therapy in patients with chronic venous insufficiency. *Lancet* 347(8997):292–294.

Geissbühler, S. and F.H. Degenring. 1999. Treatment of chronic venous insufficiency with Aesculaforce Vein Gel. *Schweiz Zschr Ganzheits Medizin* 11:82–87.

Greeske, K. and B.K. Pohlmann. 1996. [Horse chestnut seed extract—an effective therapy principle in general practice. Drug therapy of chronic venous insufficiency] [In German]. *Fortschr Med* 114(15):196–200.

Konoshima, T. and K.H. Lee. 1986. Antitumor agents, 82. Cytotoxic sapogenols from *Aesculus hippocastanum*. *J Nat Prod* 49(4):650–656.

Leung, A.Y. and S. Foster. 1996. *Encyclopedia of Common Natural Ingredients Used in Food, Drugs, and Cosmetics*, 2nd ed. New York: John Wiley & Sons, Inc. 304–306.

Morgan, M. and K. Bone. 1998. *Professional Review*: Horsechestnut. *Medi Herb* (65):1–4.

Newall, C.A., L.A. Anderson, J.D. Phillipson. 1996. *Herbal Medicines: A Guide for Health-Care Professionals*. London: The Pharmaceutical Press. 166–167.

Pittler, M.H. and E. Ernst. 1998. Horse-chestnut seed extract for chronic venous insufficiency. A criteria-based systematic review. *Arch Dermatol* 134(11):1356–1360.

Shah, D., S. Bommer, F.H. Degenring. 1997. Aesculaforce in chronic venous insufficiency. *Schweiz Zschr Ganzheits Medizin* 9(2):86–91.

Yoshikawa, M. et al. 1996. Bioactive saponins and glycosides. III. Horse chestnut. (1): The structures, inhibitory effects on ethanol absorption, and hypoglycemic activity of escins Ia, Ib, IIa, IIb, and IIIa from the seeds of *Aesculus hippocastanum* L. *Chem Pharm Bull* (Tokyo) 44(8):1454–1464.

Yoshikawa, M. et al. 1998. Bioactive saponins and glycosides. XII. Horse chestnut. (2): Structures of escins IIIb, IV, V and VI and isoescins Ia, Ib, and V, acylated polyhydroxyoleanene triterpene oligoglycosides, from the seeds of horse chestnut tree (*Aesculus hippocastanum* L., Hippocastanaceae). *Chem Pharm Bull (Tokyo)* 46(11):1764–1769.

Additional Resources

Boiadzhiev, T. et al. 1973. Experimental studies on the action of total extracts of *Aesculus hippocastanum* L. (horse chestnut) on cellular respiration. *Eksp Med Morfol* 12(1):11–14.

Chan, E.H. et al. (eds.). 1985. *Advances in Chinese Medicinal Materials Research*. Singapore: World Scientific Pub. Co.

Longiave, D., C. Omini, S. Nicosia, F. Berti. 1978. The mode of action of aescin on isolated veins, relationship with PGF2. *Pharmacol Res Commun* 10(2):145–152.

Popp, W. et al. 1992. Horse chestnut (*Aesculus hippocastanum*) pollen: a frequent cause of allergic sensitization in urban children. *Allergy* 47(4 pt. 2):380–383.

This monograph, published by the Commission E in 1994, was modified based on new scientific research. It contains more extensive pharmacological and therapeutic information taken directly from the Commission E.

This material was adapted from *The Complete German Commission E Monographs—Therapeutic Guide to Herbal Medicines*. M. Blumenthal, W.R. Busse, A. Goldberg, J. Gruenwald, T. Hall, C.W. Riggins, R.S. Rister (eds.) S. Klein and R.S. Rister (trans.). 1998. Austin: American Botanical Council; Boston: Integrative Medicine Communications.

1) The Overview section is new information.

2) Description, Chemistry and Pharmacology, Uses, Contraindications, Side Effects, Interactions with Other Drugs, and Dosage sections have been drawn from the original work. Additional information has been added in some or all of these sections, as noted with references.

3) The dosage for equivalent preparations (tea infusion, fluidextract, and tincture) have been provided based on the following example:

Unless otherwise prescribed: 2 g per day of [powdered, crushed, cut or whole] [plant part]
Infusion: 2 g in 150 ml of water
Fluidextract 1:1 (g/ml): 2 ml
Tincture 1:5 (g/ml): 10 ml

4) The References and Additional Resources sections are new sections. Additional Resources are not cited in the monograph but are included for research purposes.

HORSERADISH

Latin Name:
Armoracia rusticana

Pharmacopeial Name:
Armoraciae rusticanae radix

Other Names:
n/a

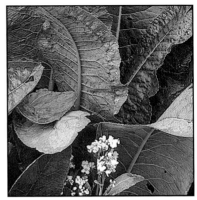

© 1999 Steven Foster

Overview

Horseradish is a perennial plant native to southeastern Europe and western Asia, now naturalized in North America (Budavari, 1996; Grieve, 1979; Lust, 1974). It was brought westward to North America by colonists (Mills, 1985). Today, horseradish is one of Germany's most important domestically cultivated medicinal plant and spice crops (Lange and Schippmann, 1997).

Horseradish has been used traditionally to treat both bronchial and urinary infections, joint and tissue inflammation, and swelling (Mills, 1985). It has been cultivated since ancient times. Roman naturalist Pliny the Elder (ca. 23–79 C.E.) described a plant by the name of *Amoracia*, which was probably horseradish (Grieve, 1979). In his book *The Herball* (1597), Elizabethan herbalist John Gerard referred to horseradish as *Raphanus rusticanus* and reported on its culinary and therapeutic uses (Bown, 1995; Grieve, 1979). Nicholas Culpepper, the seventeenth century English herbalist, reported its use as a poultice for local application to treat sciatica, gout, joint-aches, and hard swellings. In the eighteenth century, it entered the *London Pharmacopoeia* as *R. rusticanus*. Linnaeus later renamed it *Cochlearia armoracia* (Grieve, 1979).

In Germany, horseradish root is approved in the Commission E monographs for treatment of infections of the respiratory tract and as supportive treatment in urinary tract infections. In the United States, horseradish root is the active ingredient of Rasapen®, a urinary antiseptic drug (Budavari, 1996). It is listed as generally recognized as safe (GRAS) in the FDA's Code of Federal Regulations. It has also been used somewhat in North American aboriginal medicine. The Cherokee people use it as a urinary aid for gravel, as a diuretic, as a gastrointestinal aid to improve digestion, and as a respiratory aid to treat asthma (Moerman, 1998).

Although there are no recent modern human clinical studies, some older German studies investigated its effect on non-specific urinary tract infections (Schindler et al., 1960) and the antibacterial action of its essential oils (Kienholz and Kemkes, 1960). One animal study determined that its therapeutic activity was due mostly to its peroxidase enzymes, which act by triggering arachidonic acid metabolites. Intravenous administration of horseradish peroxidase to cats produced a significant hypotensive effect (Sjaastad et al., 1984). Horseradish peroxidase also serves as a catalyst of low-density lipoprotein (LDL) peroxidation (Natella et al., 1998). The approved modern therapeutic applications for horseradish are based on its long history of use in well established systems of traditional medicine, pharmacological studies in animals, and on its well documented chemical composition. A pharmacopeial grade horseradish root has not been defined at this time.

Description

Horseradish consists of the fresh or dried roots of *Armoracia rusticana* Ph. Gaertner, B. Meyer et Scherbius (syn. *Cochlearia armoracia* L.) [Fam. Brassicaceae], and their preparations in effective dosage. The root contains mustard oil and mustard oil glycosides.

Chemistry and Pharmacology

Horseradish root contains volatile oils: glucosinolates (mustard oil glycosides) gluconasturtiin and sinigrin (S-glucosides), which yield allyl isothiocyanate on hydrolysis with peroxidase or myrosinase (Budavari, 1996; Hansen, 1974; Newall et al., 1996); coumarins (aesculetin and scopoletin); phenolic acids, including caffeic acid derivatives and hydroxycinnamic acid derivatives (Newall et al., 1996; Stoehr and Herrman, 1975); ascorbic acid; asparagin; resin; and peroxidase enzymes (Budavari, 1996; Karnick, 1994; Newall et al., 1996).

The Commission E reported antimicrobial and hyperemic activity.

Uses

The Commission E approved the internal use of horseradish for catarrhs of the respiratory tract and supportive therapy for infections of the urinary tract. It was approved externally for catarrhs of the respiratory tract and hyperemic treatment for minor muscle aches.

Contraindications

Internal: Stomach and intestinal ulcers, kidney disorders. No administration to children under the age of 4.

Side Effects

Internal: Discomforts of the gastrointestinal tract.

Use During Pregnancy and Lactation

Not recommended during pregnancy and lactation.

Interactions with Other Drugs

None known.

Dosage and Administration

Unless otherwise prescribed: 20 g per day of fresh or dried, cut or ground root, freshly pressed juice as well as other equivalent galenical preparations for internal use.

External: Preparations with a maximum of 2% mustard oil.

Internal: Fresh root: 2–4 g before meals (Mills, 1985; Newall et al., 1996).

Infusion: Steep 2 g in 150 ml boiled water for 5 minutes, several times daily (Hoffmann, 1992).

Succus: Fresh pressed juice from 20 g.

Syrup: First prepare a concentrated infusion by steeping 2 g root in 150 ml boiled water in a covered cup for two hours. Strain and add an equal amount of sugar (150 g) to liquid (150 ml) to thicken (Cowper, 1996; Lust, 1974).

External: Poultice: Grate the fresh root and spread it onto a linen cloth or thin gauze. Apply locally with cloth against the skin, until a burning sensation is experienced (Hoffmann, 1992; Lust, 1974).

References

Bown, D. 1995. *Encyclopedia of Herbs and Their Uses.* New York: DK Publishing, Inc. 242.

Budavari, S. (ed.). 1996. *The Merck Index: An Encyclopedia of Chemicals, Drugs, and Biologicals,* 12th ed. Whitehouse Station, N.J.: Merck & Co, Inc. 812.

Cowper, A.B. 1996. *Manufacturing Handbook for Herbal Medicines.* Morisset, Australia: Anne B. Cowper. 21.

Grieve, M. 1979. *A Modern Herbal.* New York: Dover Publications, Inc.

Hansen, H. 1974. Content of glucosinolates in horseradish (*Armoracia rusticana*). *Tidsskr Planteavl* 73:408–410.

Hoffmann, D. 1992. *The New Holistic Herbal.* Rockport, MA: Element Books Limited. 163, 207.

Karnick, C.R. 1994. *Pharmacopoeial Standards of Herbal Plants,* Vol. 2. Delhi: Sri Satguru Publications. 69.

Kienholz, N. and B. Kemkes. 1960. [The antibacterial action of ethereal oils from horseradish root (*Cochlearia armoracia* L.)] [In German]. *Arzeneimforsch* 10:917–918.

Lange, D. and U. Schippmann. 1997. *Trade Survey of Medicinal Plants in Germany—A Contribution to International Plant Species Conservation.* Bonn: Bundesamt für Naturschutz. 32–34.

Lust, J.B. 1974. *The Herb Book.* New York: Bantam Books. 40–41, 233.

Mills, S.Y. 1985. *The Dictionary of Modern Herbalism.* Wellingborough: Thorsons.

Moerman, D.E. 1998. *Native American Ethnobotany.* Portland, OR: Timber Press. 92.

Natella, F. et al. 1998. Oxidative modification of human low-density lipoprotein by horseradish peroxidase in the absence of hydrogen peroxide. *Free Radic Res* 29(5):427–434.

Newall, C.A., L.A. Anderson, J.D. Phillipson. 1996. *Herbal Medicines: A Guide for Health-Care Professionals.* London: The Pharmaceutical Press.

Schindler, E.H. Zipp, I. Marth. 1960. [Comparative clinical studies on non-specific urinary tract infections with an enzyme-glycoside mixture obtained from horseradish roots (*Cochlearia armoracia* L.)] [In German]. *Arzeneimforsch* 10:919-921.

Sjaastad, O.V., A.K. Blom, R. Haye. 1984. Hypotensive effects in cats caused by horseradish peroxidase mediated by metabolites of arachidonic acid. *J Histochem Cytochem* 32(12):1328–1330.

Stoehr, H. and K. Herrman. 1975. Phenolic acids of vegetables. III. Hydroxycinnamic acids and hydroxybenzoic acids of root vegetables. *Z Lebensm-Unters Forsh* 159:219–224.

Additional Resources

Flocco, C.G., M.A. Alvarez, A.M. Giulietti. 1998. Peroxidase production *in vitro* by *Armoracia lapathifolia* (horseradish)-transformed root cultures: effect of elicitation on level and profile of isoenzymes. *Biotechnol Appl Biochem* 28(1):33–38.

Foster, S. 1993. *Herbal Renaissance: Growing, Using and Understanding Herbs in the Modern World.* Salt Lake City: Gibbs-Smith.

Mabey, R. (ed.). 1988. *The Complete New Herbal.* London: Elm Tree Books.

Tisserand, R. and T. Balacs. 1995. *Essential Oil Safety.* Edinburgh: Churchill Livingstone.

van der Want, J.J. et al. 1997. Tract-tracing in the nervous system of vertebrates using horseradish peroxidase and its conjugates: tracers, chromogens and stabilization for light and electron microscopy. *Brain Res Brain Res Protoc* 1(3):269–279.

Wren, R.C. 1988. *Potter's New Cyclopaedia of Botanical Drugs and Preparations.* Essex: The C.W. Daniel Company Ltd.

This material was adapted from *The Complete German Commission E Monographs—Therapeutic Guide to Herbal Medicines.* M. Blumenthal, W.R. Busse, A. Goldberg, J. Gruenwald, T. Hall, C.W. Riggins, R.S. Rister (eds.) S. Klein and R.S. Rister (trans.). 1998. Austin: American Botanical Council; Boston: Integrative Medicine Communications.

1) The Overview section is new information.

2) Description, Chemistry and Pharmacology, Uses, Contraindications, Side Effects, Interactions with Other Drugs, and Dosage sections have been drawn from the original work. Additional information has been added in some or all of these sections, as noted with references.

3) The dosage for equivalent preparations (tea infusion, fluidextract, and tincture) have been provided based on the following example:
   Unless otherwise prescribed: 2 g per day of [powdered, crushed, cut or whole] [plant part]
   Infusion: 2 g in 150 ml of water
   Fluidextract 1:1 (g/ml): 2 ml
   Tincture 1:5 (g/ml): 10 ml

4) The References and Additional Resources sections are new sections. Additional Resources are not cited in the monograph but are included for research purposes.

HORSETAIL HERB

Latin Name:
Equisetum arvense

Pharmacopeial Name:
Equiseti herba

Other Names:
bottlebrush, common horsetail, field
horsetail, shave grass, shavetail grass

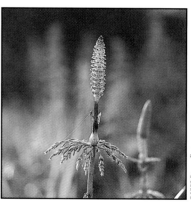

©1999 Steven Foster

Overview

Horsetail is a dimorphic perennial plant common throughout the temperate northern hemisphere in Asia, Europe, and North America. Two distinct chemotypes have
been identified, one from Europe and the other from Asia and North America,
which can be differentiated chemically by the detection of certain characteristic
flavonoids unique to each chemotype (Leung and Foster, 1996). The material of
commerce comes from Albania, Hungary, Poland, the former Yugoslavia, the
United Kingdom, and the former USSR (BHP, 1996; Wichtl and Bisset, 1994). A
relative to ferns, horsetails reproduce through spore transport, not by seeds (Tyler,
1993).

Horsetail's therapeutic use in Europe dates back to at least ancient Roman and
Greek medicine; it was recorded by Greek physician Claudius Galenus (130–200
C.E.). The genus name *Equisetum* is derived from the Latin *equus* meaning horse
and *seta* meaning bristle (Grieve, 1979). Nicholas Culpepper, the seventeenth century English herbalist, indicated horsetail juice or decoction as a remedy to stop
bleeding, to treat ulcers, wounds, ruptures and inflammations in the skin, as well as
for kidney stones and strangury (painful and interrupted urination in drops)
(Grieve, 1979). In Indian Ayurvedic medicine, horsetail is used as a treatment for
inflammation or benign enlargement of the prostate gland, for urinary inconti-
nence, and for enuresis (involuntary discharge of urine) of children (Karnick,
1994). In the nineteenth century, American Eclectic physicians used it to treat gon-
orrhea, prostatitis, and enuresis (Ellingwood, 1983). Some of its uses in North
American aboriginal medicine are comparable to the Asian and European uses. The
Cherokee people prepared the infusion as a kidney aid. The Chippewa Ojibwe
people prepared a decoction of the stems as a urinary aid to treat dysuria (painful
or difficult urination). The Okanagan-Colville people prepared an infusion of the
stems as a diuretic drug to stimulate the kidneys. The Potawatomi people prepared
an infusion as a urinary aid for bladder trouble (Moerman, 1998).

The approved modern therapeutic applications for horsetail herb are supportable
based on its long history of clinical use in well established systems of traditional
medicine, phytochemical investigations, and pharmacological studies. Its diuretic
actions are mild, according to studies, and are attributed to horsetail's flavonoid
and saponin constituents (Bradley, 1992; Tyler, 1993). The plant's actions in healing bones and strengthening connective tissue are thought to be due to silicic acid.
The mineral content is significant: silica and silicic acid concentrations in the stems
are usually from five to eight percent, which is probably why the hollow weeds
were used to scour pots, and why horsetail is also called scouring rush (Tyler,
1993).

In Germany, horsetail is official in the *German Pharmacopoeia*, approved in the
Commission E monographs, and the tea form is official in the German Standard

License monographs (BAnz, 1998; Braun et al., 1997; DAB, 1998). It is used as a monopreparation and also as a component of various prepared diuretic drugs (Wichtl and Bisset, 1994). For example, it is a component in Kneipp® "Blasen- und Nieren-Tee" (Kidney and Bladder Tea) composed of 30% horsetail herb, 25% giant goldenrod herb (*S. gigantea*), 20% birch leaf (*Betula alba*), 10% spiny restharrow root (*Ononis spinosa*), 5% rose hip shells (*Rosa canina*), 5% peppermint leaf (*Mentha x piperita*), and 5% marigold blossoms (*Calendula officinalis*) (Kneipp®, 1996). In the United States, horsetail is commonly found as a component of dietary supplement products in fluid (infusion or tincture) or solid (capsules and tablets) dosage forms for its mineral nutrient content and/or for its diuretic action.

Pharmacopeial grade horsetail herb consists of the dried, green, sterile stems of *Equisetum arvense* L. in whole, cut or powdered forms. Botanical identity must be carried out by thin-layer chromatography (TLC), macroscopic and microscopic examinations, and organoleptic evaluations. It must contain no more than 3% blackish rhizome fragments and maximum 5% stems or branches from hybrids and/or from other *Equisetum* species. The fertile cambium may not be present (DAB, 1998; Wichtl and Bisset, 1994). It must contain not less than 15% water-soluble extractive (BHP, 1996; Karnick, 1994).

Description

Horsetail consists of the fresh or dried, green, sterile stems of *E. arvense* L. [Fam. Equisetaceae] and its preparations in effective dosage. The herb contains silicic acid and flavonoids.

Chemistry and Pharmacology

Constituents include 10–20% minerals, of which over 66% are silicic acids and silicates, plus potassium, aluminum, and manganese; 0.3–1% flavonoids, mainly quercetin glycosides (quercetin 3-glucoside and its malonyl esters); phenolic acids, including up to 0.008% di-*E*-caffeoyl-*meso*-tartaric acid, plus methyl esters of protocatechuic and caffeic acids; alkaloids (traces of nicotine); polyenic acids and rare dicarboxylic acids; and phytosterols (Bradley, 1992; Hänsel et al., 1992–1994; Leung and Foster, 1996; Meyer-Buchtela, 1999; Wichtl and Bisset, 1994).

The Commission E reported mild diuretic properties.

The *British Herbal Compendium* reported weak diuretic, hemostyptic (an astringent that stops bleeding), vulnerary (wound healing) and mild leukocytosis causing (increases leukocyte count in the blood) actions (Bradley, 1992).

Uses

The Commission E approved internal use of horsetail herb in irrigation therapy for post-traumatic and static edema and for bacterial infections and inflammation of the lower urinary tract and renal gravel. Externally, horsetail is indicated as supportive to poorly healing wounds.

The German Standard License horsetail tea monograph allows the same indications for use as those reported in the Commission E monograph (Braun et al., 1997). In France, it is indicated for use to promote renal and digestive elimination functions and as an adjuvant in slimming diets (Bradley, 1992; Bruneton, 1995; DPM, 1992). The *British Herbal Compendium* indicates its internal use for inflammation or mild infections of the genito-urinary tract and external use for poorly healing wounds (Bradley, 1992).

Contraindications

None known.
Note: No irrigation therapy in the case of edema due to impaired heart and kidney function.

Side Effects

None known.

Use During Pregnancy and Lactation

No restrictions known.

Interactions with Other Drugs

None known.

Dosage and Administration

Unless otherwise prescribed: 6 g per day of cut herb for infusions and other equivalent galenical preparations for oral administration. For irrigation therapy, ensure an abundant fluid intake.
External: Cut herb for decoctions and other equivalent galenical preparations.
Internal: Decoction: Pour 150 ml boiling water over 2 g and continue boiling for 5 minutes, then allow to steep for another 10 to 15 minutes before straining; take three times daily (Wichtl and Bisset, 1994).
Infusion: Steep 2 g of herb in 150 ml boiled water for 10 to15 minutes; take three times daily (Braun et al., 1997). [Note: 34% of the potentially available flavonoids are yielded into the tea after 5 minutes of steeping and 40% are released after 10 minutes (Meyer-Buchtela, 1999).]
Cold Macerate: Soak 2 g of herb in 150 ml cold water for 10 to 12 hours; take three times daily (Meyer-Buchtela, 1999; Wichtl and Bisset, 1994).
Fluidextract 1:1 (g/ml): 2 ml, three times daily.
Tincture 1:5 (g/ml): 10 ml, three times daily.
External: Bath additive: Add 2 g herb per 1 liter hot bathwater and allow to steep one hour before bathing (Hänsel et al., 1992–1994; Meyer-Buchtela, 1999).
Decoction: To prepare a decoction for use in making a cataplasm or compress, boil 10 g herb in 1 liter water for 10 to 15 minutes (Braun et al., 1997; Meyer-Buchtela, 1999).
Cataplasm: Semi-solid paste prepared from horsetail aqueous decoction for a moist-heat direct application to the skin; used like a poultice to remove deep-seated inflammation.
Compress: Saturate a stupe with hot semi-solid preparation containing horsetail aqueous decoction; fold and apply firmly for a moist-heat direct application to the skin to relieve pain or inflammation.
Note: The herb in powdered form is not recommended for children or for prolonged use due to the inorganic silica content. Toxicity of the herb was found to be similar to nicotine poisoning in children who chewed the stem (McGuffin et al., 1997).

References

BAnz. See *Bundesanzeiger.*
Bradley, P.R. (ed.). 1992. *British Herbal Compendium,* Vol. 1. Bournemouth: British Herbal Medicine Association.
Braun, R. et al. 1997. *Standardzulassungen für Fertigarzneimittel—Text and Kommentar.* Stuttgart: Deutscher Apotheker Verlag.
British Herbal Pharmacopoeia (BHP). 1996. Exeter, U.K.: British Herbal Medicine Association. 76.
Bruneton, J. 1995. *Pharmacognosy, Phytochemistry, Medicinal Plants.* Paris: Lavoisier Publishing.
Bundesanzeiger (BAnz). 1998. Monographien der Kommission E (Zulassungs- und Aufbereitungskommission am BGA für den humanmed. Bereich, phytotherapeutische Therapierichtung und Stoffgruppe). Köln: Bundesgesundheitsamt (BGA).
Deutsches Arzneibuch, Ergänzungslieferung 1998 (DAB). 1998. Stuttgart: Deutscher Apotheker Verlag.
Direction de la Pharmacie et du Médicament (DPM). 1992. Bulletin Officiel (Fascicule spécial) No. 90/22 bis. [English edition]. Paris: Ministère des Affaires Sociales et de la Solidarité.
Ellingwood, F. 1983. *American Materia Medica, Therapeutics and Pharmacognosy.* Portland, OR: Eclectic Medical Publications [reprint of 1919 original].
Grieve, M. 1979. *A Modern Herbal.* New York: Dover Publications, Inc.
Hänsel, R., K. Keller, H. Rimpler, G. Schneider (eds.). 1992–1994. *Hagers Handbuch der Pharmazeutischen Praxis,* 5th ed. Vol. 4–6. Berlin-Heidelberg: Springer Verlag.
Karnick, C.R. 1994. *Pharmacopoeial Standards of Herbal Plants,* Vol. 1. Delhi: Sri Satguru Publications. Vol. 1:129–130.
Kneipp®, 1996. *Wegweiser zu den Kneipp® Mitteln* [Guide to Kneipp® Remedies]. Würzburg: Sebastian Kneipp Gesundheitsmittel-Verlag. 124–125.
Leung, A.Y. and S. Foster. 1996. *Encyclopedia of Common Natural Ingredients Used in Food, Drugs, and Cosmetics,* 2nd ed. New York: John Wiley & Sons, Inc.
McGuffin, M., C. Hobbs, R. Upton, A. Goldberg. 1997. American Herbal Product Association's *Botanical Safety Handbook.* Boca Raton: CRC Press.

Meyer-Buchtela, E. 1999. *Tee-Rezepturen—Ein Handbuch für Apotheker und Ärzte.* Stuttgart: Deutscher Apotheker Verlag.

Moerman, D.E. 1998. *Native American Ethnobotany.* Portland, OR: Timber Press. 213–214.

Tyler, V. 1993. *The Honest Herbal*, 3rd ed. New York: Pharmaceutical Products Press.

Wichtl, M. and N.G. Bisset (eds.). 1994. *Herbal Drugs and Phytopharmaceuticals.* Stuttgart: Medpharm Scientific Publishers.

Additional Resources

Harnischfeger, G. and H. Stolze. 1983. *Bewährte Pflanzendrogen in Wissenschaft und Medizin.* Bad Homburg/Melsungen, Germany: Notamed Verlag.

Newall, C.A., L.A. Anderson, J.D. Phillipson. 1996. *Herbal Medicines: A Guide for Health-Care Professionals.* London: The Pharmaceutical Press.

Piekos, R. and S. Paslawska. 1975. Studies on the optimum conditions of extraction of silicon species from plants with water. I. *Equisetum arvense* L. Herb. *Planta Med* 27(2):145–150.

Piekos, R., S. Paslawska, W. Grinczelis. 1976. Studies on the optimum conditions of extraction of silicon species from plants with water. III. On the stability of silicon species in extracts from *Equisetum arvense* herb. *Planta Med* 29(4):351–356.

Sudan, B.J. 1985. Seborrhoeic dermatitis induced by nicotine of horsetails (*Equisetum arvense* L.). *Contact Dermatitis* 13(3):201–202.

Veit, M. 1987. Die Schachtelhalme (Equisetaceae) Objekte der Forschung und der Praxis. *Dtsch Apoth Ztg* (127): 2049–2056.

This material was adapted from *The Complete German Commission E Monographs—Therapeutic Guide to Herbal Medicines.* M. Blumenthal, W.R. Busse, A. Goldberg, J. Gruenwald, T. Hall, C.W. Riggins, R.S. Rister (eds.) S. Klein and R.S. Rister (trans.). 1998. Austin: American Botanical Council; Boston: Integrative Medicine Communications.

1) The Overview section is new information.

2) Description, Chemistry and Pharmacology, Uses, Contraindications, Side Effects, Interactions with Other Drugs, and Dosage sections have been drawn from the original work. Additional information has been added in some or all of these sections, as noted with references.

3) The dosage for equivalent preparations (tea infusion, fluidextract, and tincture) have been provided based on the following example:
   Unless otherwise prescribed: 2 g per day of [powdered, crushed, cut or whole] [plant part]
   Infusion: 2 g in 150 ml of water
   Fluidextract 1:1 (g/ml): 2 ml
   Tincture 1:5 (g/ml): 10 ml

4) The References and Additional Resources sections are new sections. Additional Resources are not cited in the monograph but are included for research purposes.

ICELAND MOSS

Latin Name:
Cetraria islandica

Pharmacopeial Name:
Lichen islandicus

Other Names:
fucus, muscus

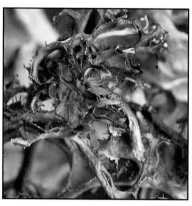

© 1999 Steven Foster

Overview

Iceland moss is a lichen harvested and prepared in Scandinavia and Europe as a medicinal agent to stimulate the appetite and relieve dry cough and inflamed oral tissues (Schulz et al., 1998; Tyler, 1994). The therapeutic actions of Iceland moss are attributed to its mucilaginous polysaccharides (Tyler, 1994). Contemporary and traditional use of Iceland moss for the relief of upper respiratory catarrh is supported by results from recent clinical studies. In a randomized trial, Iceland moss was found to prevent both dryness and inflammation of the oral cavity in patients who had undergone surgery of the nasal septum and were subjected to prolonged mouth breathing following surgery. Emollient effects were noticeable with the daily use of 0.48 mg Iceland moss lozenges (Kempe et al., 1997).

Iceland moss polysaccharides have been the focus of a number of experimental studies. One in particular, protolichesterinic acid, may prove to be valuable in the treatment of ulcers and cancers, and in AIDS prevention. *In vitro* activity against *Helicobacter pylori* (Ingolfsdottir et al., 1997) and DNA polymerase activity of human immunodeficiency virus-1 reverse transcriptase (Pengsuparp et al., 1995) have been documented. Protolichesterinic acid is also antiproliferative and cytotoxic to T-47D and ZR-75-1 cell lines cultured from breast carcinomas, and to K-562 from erythro-leukemia. Significant inhibition of 5-lipoxygenase may stimulate these activities and contribute to protolichesterinic acid's reported anti-inflammatory actions (Ogmundsdottir et al., 1998).

Historically, Iceland moss has provided both medicine and food for the people of Iceland, Norway, Finland, Russia, and Sweden. It has been made into flour for bread (Schneider, 1904), and gelled and mixed with lemon, sugar, chocolate, or almonds to make confections (Dannfelt, 1917). During the 1807–1814 famine in Norway, it was used as food (Richardson, 1988). During World War II, Iceland moss was prepared into a type of molasses in Russia (Llano, 1956). Always, powdered material must be soaked in lye for 24 hours or filtered through ash in order to properly extricate lichen acids. Studies demonstrate that poorly prepared Iceland moss contains probably toxic levels of lead (Airaksinen et al., 1986).

Medicinal uses include as a tonic during convalescence, gastrointestinal demulcent, and treatment for upper respiratory catarrh (Lindley, 1849). Iceland moss decoctions, infusions, and gargles have been used to treat colds, whooping cough, asthma, diabetes, and nephritis (Ahmadjian and Nilsson, 1963), and for post-tuberulosis convalescence (Lokar and Poldini, 1988). Cough drops for sore throats and laxative and tonic formulations are available in European pharmacies (Richardson, 1991).

Description

Iceland moss consists of the dried thallus of *Cetraria islandica* (L.) Acharius *s.l.* [Fam. Parmeliaceae] and its preparations in effective dosage. The herb contains mucilage and bitter principles.

Chemistry and Pharmacology

Constituents include about 50% water-soluble polysaccharides, including lichenin, a linear cellulose-like polymer of β-D-glucose, and isolichenin, a linear starch-like polymer of α-D-glucose (Wichtl and Bisset, 1994). Iceland moss also contains galactomannans and an acidic, branched polysaccharide containing D-glucose and D-glucuronic acid units. Other constituents include bitter-tasting lichen acids, including the depsidones fumarprotocetraric acid and protocetraric acid, and the aliphatic lactone protolichesterinic acid (ESCOP, 1997).

The Commission E reported soothing and mildly antimicrobial acitivities. The polysaccharides are thought to form a soothing, protective, mucilaginous layer on the mucosa of the upper respiratory tract. Significant immunostimulating activity was shown in an *in vitro* study on an alkali-soluble galactomannan isolated from Iceland moss (ESCOP, 1997).

Uses

The Commission E approved Iceland moss to treat irritation of the oral and pharyngeal mucous membranes and accompanying dry cough, and loss of appetite. In an open clinical trial, 100 patients with pharyngitis, laryngitis, or bronchial ailments were treated with lozenges containing 160 mg of an aqueous extract of Iceland moss. The results were determined to be positive in 86 cases with good gastric tolerance and lack of side effects (ESCOP, 1997).

Contraindications

Iceland moss is contraindicated in gastro-duodenal ulcers due to its mucosa-irritating properties (McGuffin et al., 1997).

Side Effects

None known.

Use During Pregnancy and Lactation

No restrictions known.

Interactions with Other Drugs

None known.

Dosage and Administration

Unless otherwise prescribed: 4–6 g per day of cut herb.
Infusion: 4–6 g of herb in 150 ml water.
Fluidextract 1:1 (g/ml): 4–6 ml.
Tincture 1:5 (g/ml): 20–30 ml.

References

Ahmadjian, V. and S. Nilsson. 1963. *Swedish lichens.* Yearbook (American Swedish Historical Foundation).

Airaksinen, M.M. et al. 1986. Toxicity of plant material used as emergency food during famines in Finland. *J Ethnopharmacol* 18(3):273–296.

Dannfelt, H.J. 1917. *Kungl Lantbrukssakad Tidskr* 6:483–498.

ESCOP. 1997. "Lichen islandicus." *Monographs on the Medicinal Uses of Plant Drugs.* Exeter, U.K.: European Scientific Cooperative on Phytotherapy.

Ingolfsdottir, K. et al. 1997. *In vitro* susceptibility of *Helicobacter pylori* to protolichesterinic acid from the lichen *Cetraria islandica. Antimicrob Agents Chemother* 41(1):215–217.

Kempe, C., H. Gruning, N. Stasche, K. Hormann. 1997. [Icelandic moss lozenges in the prevention or treatment of oral mucosa irritation and dried out throat mucosal] [In German]. *Laryngorhinootologie* 76(3):186–188.

Lindley, J. 1849. *Medical and Economical Botany.* London: Bradbury and Evans.

Llano, G.A. 1956. Utilization of lichens in the arctic and subarctic. *Econ Bot* 10(4):367–392.

Lokar, L.C. and L. Poldini. 1988. Herbal remedies in the traditional medicine of the Venezia Giulia region (north east Italy). *J Ethnopharmacol* 22(3):231–279.

McGuffin, M., C. Hobbs, R. Upton, A. Goldberg. 1997. American Herbal Product Association's *Botanical Safety Handbook.* Boca Raton: CRC Press.

Ogmundsdottir, H.M., G.M. Zoega, S.R. Gissurarson, K. Ingolfsdottir. 1998. Anti-proliferative
effects of lichen-derived inhibitors of 5-lipoxyge-
nase on malignant cell-lines and mitogen-stimu-
lated lymphocytes. *J Pharm Pharmacol*
50(1):107–115.

Pengsuparp, T. et al. 1995. Mechanistic evaluation
of new plant-derived compounds that inhibit
HIV-1 reverse transcriptase. *J Nat Prod*
58(7):1024–1031.

Richardson, D.H.S. 1988. *Handbook of Lichenol-
ogy*, Vol. 3. Boca Raton: CRC Press.

———. 1991. *Frontiers in Mycology*. Honorary
and General Lectures from the Fourth International Mycological Congress, Rengensburg, Germany, 1990.

Schneider, A. 1904. *A Guide to the Study of
Lichens*. Boston: Knight and Miller.

Schulz, V., R. Hänsel, V.E. Tyler. 1998. *Rational
Phytotherapy: A Physicians' Guide to Herbal
Medicine*. New York: Springer.

Tyler, V.E. 1994. *Herbs of Choice: The Therapeutic
Use of Phytomedicinals*. New York: Pharmaceutical Products Press.

Wichtl, M. and N.G. Bisset (eds.). 1994. *Herbal
Drugs and Phytopharmaceuticals*. Stuttgart:
Medpharm Scientific Publishers.

Additional Resources

Braun, R. et al. 1997. *Standardzulassungen für Fertigarzneimittel—Text and Kommentar.* Stuttgart:
Deutscher Apotheker Verlag.

British Herbal Pharmacopoeia (BHP). 1983. Keighley, U.K.: British Herbal Medicine Association.

Deutsches Arzneibuch, 10th ed. Vol. 1–6. (DAB 10).
1991. Kommentar. (4 Lfg. 1994) Stuttgart: Wissenschaftliche Verlagsgesellschaft mbH. M84.

Ingolfsdottir, K., K. Jurcic, B. Fischer, H. Wagner.
1994. Immunologically active polysaccharide
from *Cetraria islandica. Planta Med*
60(6):527–531.

Ingolfsdottir, K., G.A. Chung, V.G. Skulason, S.R.
Gissurarson, M. Vilhelmsdottir. 1998. Antimy-
cobacterial activity of lichen metabolites *in vitro*.
Eur J Pharm Sci 6(2):141–144.

Kartnig, T. 1987. *Cetraria islandica*—Islandisches
Moos. *Z Phytother* (8):127–130.

Stecher, P.G. (ed.). 1968. *The Merck Index: An
Encyclopedia of Chemicals and Drugs*, 8th ed.
Rahway, N.J.: Merck & Co., Inc.

Vorberg, G. 1981. Flechtenwirkstoffe lindern Reiz-
zustande der Atemwege. Neben den entzundung-
shemmenden Eigenschaften wirkt sich der
Schleimhautschutz besonders gunstig aus. *Arztl
Praxis* (33):3068.

Weiss, R.F. 1988. *Herbal Medicine*. Beaconsfield,
England: Beaconsfield Publishers.

This material was adapted from *The Complete German Commission E Monographs—Therapeutic Guide to
Herbal Medicines*. M. Blumenthal, W.R. Busse, A. Goldberg, J. Gruenwald, T. Hall, C.W. Riggins, R.S. Ris-
ter (eds.) S. Klein and R.S. Rister (trans.). 1998. Austin: American Botanical Council; Boston: Integrative
Medicine Communications.

1) The Overview section is new information.

2) Description, Chemistry and Pharmacology, Uses, Contraindications, Side Effects, Interactions with
Other Drugs, and Dosage sections have been drawn from the original work. Additional information has
been added in some or all of these sections, as noted with references.

3) The dosage for equivalent preparations (tea infusion, fluidextract, and tincture) have been provided
based on the following example:
Unless otherwise prescribed: 2 g per day of [powdered, crushed, cut or whole] [plant part]
Infusion: 2 g in 150 ml of water
Fluidextract 1:1 (g/ml): 2 ml
Tincture 1:5 (g/ml): 10 ml

4) The References and Additional Resources sections are new sections. Additional Resources are not cited
in the monograph but are included for research purposes.

IVY LEAF

Latin Name:
Hedera helix

Pharmacopeial Name:
Hederae helicis folium

Other Names:
English ivy, woodbine

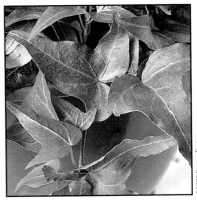

©1999 Steven Foster

Overview

Ivy grows across Europe and into northern and central Asia, and has been naturalized to the United States. It has been cultivated to climb along trellises, and to provide ornamental covering to stone and brickwork buildings. Commission E approves the use of ivy for the symptomatic relief of acute and chronic respiratory inflammation. An *in vitro* study recently confirmed the antispasmodic action of ivy, showing significant activity for both the saponial and phenolic compounds (Trute et al., 1997). Not much clinical research is available on the medicinal use of ivy; however, traditional healers in Europe had more uses for the plant than contemporary herbalists. They described ivy leaves as cathartic, anthelmintic, and useful for lowering fever, and inducing perspiration. As far back as classical Greece, ivy leaves were bruised and simmered in wine, and drunk as a deterrent to intoxication. It has been proposed that this is why Bacchus is depicted wearing an ivy wreath around his head in old paintings and statues. Greek priests gave newlyweds ivy wreaths to signify fidelity (Grieve, 1979).

Early experimental tests isolated glycosidic saponins in ivy leaf, and demonstrated that they were antifungal and molluscicidal *in vitro*, and able to kill liver flukes both *in vitro* and *in vivo* (Wren, 1988). More recently, biochemists have postulated that these saponins are responsible for the plant's expectorant actions: Saponins trigger responses in gastric mucosa, which in turn activate mucous glands in the bronchi through parasympathetic signaling, to aid in the removal of mucous. Ivy leaves contain up to 6% saponin (Schulz et al., 1998).

Saponins are a common focus in plant research. Bitter tasting, saponins foam when shaken with water, and their irritant nature can cause nausea and vomiting. Because they have been shown to be effective in the treatment of chronic venous insufficiency (CVI), saponins occuring in significant levels in plants target those plants for further circulatory research. Recently, however, ivy's purported use as an alternative treatment for CVI was disproved, and its saponins were found to be ineffective for this indication (Facino et al., 1995). Ivy saponins do demonstrate significant antileishmanial activity. Specifically, the monodesmosides are as effective as pentamidine against the flagellate promastigote, and hederagenin is as effective as N-methylglucamine against amastigote (Majester-Savornin et al., 1991). Leishmaniasis is an infection caused by the flagellate protozoans of sand flies, such as promastigote and amastigote. Because ulcers that form with the infection can lead to blindness, further study of ivy's saponin effects may one day be useful to the people of Africa, India, and Asia, where sand flies are prevalent.

In addition, in ongoing experimental anticancer testing, ivy's saponins were found to be cytotoxic to cultured B16-melanoma cells (Danloy et al., 1994).

Description

Ivy leaf consists of the dried leaf of *Hedera helix* L. [Fam. Araliaceae] and its preparations in effective dosage. The preparation contains saponins.

Chemistry and Pharmacology

The main constituents include saponins, comprising the hederagenin glycosides hederacoside C and α-hederin and the oleanolic-acid glycosides hederacoside B and β-hederin (Wichtl and Bisset, 1994). The saponins range in concentration from 5–8%. Ivy leaves contain sterols, flavonoids, polyalkynes: falcarinol, falcarinone, 11-dehydrofalcarinol (Bruneton, 1995). Other constituents include the polyacetylenes falcarinone and falcarinol; the sterols stigmasterol, sitosterol, cholesterol, campesterol, α-spinasterol, and 5α-stigma-7-en-3β-ol; scopolin; chlorogenic acid; caffeic acid; the sesquiterpene hydrocarbons germacrene; β-elemene; and elixin (Wichtl and Bisset, 1994).

The Commission E reported that skin and mucosa are sensitive to ivy leaf and it performs correspondingly expectorant and antispasmodic activity. There are also apparent antiparasitic properties in the leaf extract (Bruneton, 1995). Experiments have found that the extract is cytotoxic and antibacterial (Bruneton, 1995). Specifically, the constituent falcarinol has been confirmed as having antibacterial, analgesic, and sedative effects. Both falcarinone and falcarinol are considered antimycotic (Wichtl and Bisset, 1994). *In vitro* studies conclude that the sodium salts of the monodesmosides create a toxicity toward *Amoeba*, *Trichomonas*, and *Leishmania* (Bruneton, 1995).

Uses

The Commission E confirms ivy leaf as treatment for catarrhs of the respiratory passages and for symptoms of chronic inflammatory bronchial conditions. Ivy is suggested as an expectorant, secretolytic, and antispasmodic in response to, specifically, whooping cough, spastic bronchitis, and chronic catarrh (Wichtl and Bisset, 1994). Topical applications of ivy-based products are suggested for their anti-cellulite and weight loss properties. Emollient and itch-relieving preparations, including creams, lotions, and shampoos, are used cosmetically and in the treatment of skin disorders (Bruneton, 1995). The ivy leaf is additionally indicated for arthritis, rheumatism, and scrofula (Wichtl and Bisset, 1994).

Contraindications

None known.

Side Effects

Contact dermatitis (Bruneton, 1995).

Use During Pregnancy and Lactation

No restrictions known.

Interactions with Other Drugs

None known.

Dosage and Administration

Unless otherwise prescribed: 0.3 g per day of cut herb.
Infusion: 0.3 g of herb in 150 ml water.
Fuidextract 1:1 (g/ml): 0.3 ml.
Tincture 1:5 (g/ml): 1.5 ml.
Note: Repeated contact with ivy leaves may cause erythematous or vesicular reactions of the face, hands, and arms up to 48 hours after contact (Bruneton, 1995).

References

Bruneton, J. 1995. *Pharmacognosy, Phytochemistry, Medicinal Plants*. Paris: Lavoisier Publishing.

Danloy, S. et al. 1994. Effects of alpha-hederin, a saponin extracted from *Hedera helix*, on cells cultured *in vitro*. *Planta Med* 60(1):45–49.

Facino, R.M., M. Carini, R. Stefani, G. Aldini, L. Saibene. 1995. Anti-elastase and anti-hyaluronidase activities of saponins and sapogenins from *Hedera helix*, *Aesculus hippocastanum*, and *Ruscus aculeatus*: factors contributing to their efficacy in the treatment of venous insufficiency. *Arch Pharm (Weinheim)* 328(10):720–724.

Grieve, M. 1979. *A Modern Herbal*. New York: Dover Publications, Inc.

Majester-Savornin, B. et al. 1991. Saponins of the ivy plant, *Hedera helix*, and their leishmanicidic activity. *Planta Med* 57(3):260–262.

Schulz, V., R. Hänsel, V.E. Tyler. 1998. *Rational Phytotherapy: A Physicians' Guide to Herbal Medicine*. New York: Springer.

Trute, A. et al. 1997. *In vitro* antispasmodic compounds of the dry extract obtained from *Hedera helix*. *Planta Med* 63(2):125–129.

Wichtl, M. and N.G. Bisset (eds.). 1994. *Herbal Drugs and Phytopharmaceuticals*. Stuttgart: Medpharm Scientific Publishers.

Wren, R.C. 1988. *Potter's New Cyclopaedia of Botanical Drugs and Preparations*. Essex: The C.W. Daniel Company Ltd.

Additional Resources

Garcia, M., E. Fernandez, J.A. Navarro, M.D. del Pozo, L. Fernandez de Corres. 1995. Allergic contact dermatitis from *Hedera helix* L. *Contact Dermatitis* 33(2):133–134.

Johnke, H. et al. 1994. [Contact dermatitis allergy to common ivy] [In Danish]. *Ugeskr Laeger* 156(25):3778–3779.

This material was adapted from *The Complete German Commission E Monographs—Therapeutic Guide to Herbal Medicines*. M. Blumenthal, W.R. Busse, A. Goldberg, J. Gruenwald, T. Hall, C.W. Riggins, R.S. Rister (eds.) S. Klein and R.S. Rister (trans.). 1998. Austin: American Botanical Council; Boston: Integrative Medicine Communications.

1) The Overview section is new information.
2) Description, Chemistry and Pharmacology, Uses, Contraindications, Side Effects, Interactions with Other Drugs, and Dosage sections have been drawn from the original work. Additional information has been added in some or all of these sections, as noted with references.
3) The dosage for equivalent preparations (tea infusion, fluidextract, and tincture) have been provided based on the following example:
   Unless otherwise prescribed: 2 g per day of [powdered, crushed, cut or whole] [plant part]
   Infusion: 2 g in 150 ml of water
   Fluidextract 1:1 (g/ml): 2 ml
   Tincture 1:5 (g/ml): 10 ml
4) The References and Additional Resources sections are new sections. Additional Resources are not cited in the monograph but are included for research purposes.

JUNIPER BERRY

Latin Name:
Juniperus communis

Pharmacopeial Name:
Juniperi fructus

Other Names:
common juniper

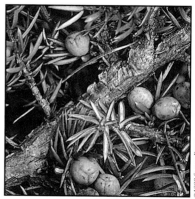

©1999 Steven Foster

Overview

Juniper grows in the temperate regions of Europe, Asia, and North America. Its berries, female cones more closely related to pine cones than to fruit, are used commercially for the preparation of gin and essential oil. Gin has been drunk in the Western world for at least three hundred years. The oil is diuretic and has gastrointestinal irritant and antiseptic properties (Leung and Foster, 1996). Commission E approves the use of juniper dried fruit preparations or oil to relieve dyspepsia.

In traditional medicine, preparations made from juniper berries were used to relieve flatulence and indigestion and to stimulate the appetite. Berries themselves were eaten to relieve rheumatism (Tyler, 1993) or were made into topical ointments and rubbed into joints and aching muscles (Newall et al., 1996). Spirit of juniper, made by extracting the oil with 70% alcohol, has been used to treat dropsy, intestinal pain (Grieve, 1979), and lack of appetite (Tyler, 1993). Steam inhalations were used for bronchitis, extracts were made to treat snakebites and intestinal worms, and some types of cancers were treated with juniper (Leung and Foster, 1996). It was also used for cystitis (Newall et al., 1996). In veterinary medicine, juniper oil was mixed with lard and used to heal wounds; the concoction also protected open wounds from fly infestation (Grieve, 1979).

Juniper's therapeutic actions are due primarily to its volatile oil, which contains the constituent terpinen-4-ol. Diuretic actions stimulated by terpinen-4-ol are reportedly aquaretic, meaning that glomerular filtration rates increase, but electrolyte secretion does not. Excessive use may cause kidney irritation and damage because terpinen-4-ol has demonstrated irritant activities (Newall et al., 1996). Other constituents that may have applications in the future are juniper berries' lignan, desoxypodophyllotoxin, and flavonoid, amentoflavone. Desoxypodophyllotoxin may stimulate juniper extract inhibition of cytopathogenesis caused by herpes simplex virus type 1 in primary human amnion cell cultures (Markkanen et al., 1981). Amentoflavone appears to have some antiviral potential (Chandler, 1986).

Laboratory tests provide support for the use of juniper oil and berry to relieve inflammation. Oral administration to rats was 60% effective in preventing paw edema, compared to a 45% efficacy rate for indomethacin. Extracts were also fungicidal against *Penicillium notatum*. The scientific studies available on the therapeutic actions of juniper berry and berry oil have been performed mostly on laboratory animals, and human studies are needed. Because the oil has been found to stimulate uterine contractions, use is not advised during pregnancy (Tyler, 1993).

Description

Juniper berry is the ripe, fresh or dried spherical ovulate cone ("berry") of *Juniperus communis* L. [Fam. Cupressaceae] and its preparations in effective dosage. Juniper berry contains at least 1% (v/w) volatile oil in reference to the dried preparation. Main ingredients of the volatile oil are terpene hydrocarbons such as α-pinene, β-pinene, myrcene, sabinene, thujone, and limonene. Also contained are sesquiterpene hydrocarbons such as caryophyllene, cadinene, and elemene, and terpene alcohols such as 4-terpineol. Furthermore, juniper berries contain flavonoid glycosides, tannins, sugar, and resin- and wax-containing compounds.

Chemistry and Pharmacology

Constituents include volatile oil, sugars, glucuronic acid, L-ascorbic acid, resin, catechins, proanthocyanidins, fatty acids, sterols, gallotannins, geijerone, diterpene acids, and flavonoid glycosides (Leung and Foster, 1996). The volatile oils consist of about 58% monoterpenes, including α-pinene, myrcene and sabinene, and camphene, camphor, 1,4-cineole, p-cymene, α- and γ-cadinene, limonene, β-pinene, γ-terpinene, terpinen-4-ol, terpinyl acetate, α-thujene, and borneol (ESCOP, 1997; Newall et al., 1996). The sesquiterpenes include caryophyllene, eposydihydrocaryophyllene, and β-elemem-7α-ol (Newall et al., 1996). Factors that influence the concentrations of constituents include geographic location, altitude, degree of ripeness, and other environmental factors (Leung and Foster, 1996).

The Commission E reported an increase in urine excretion and a direct effect on smooth muscle contraction in animal experiments.

The berry has diuretic, digestive, antiseptic, carminative, stomachic, and antirheumatic properties (Leung and Foster, 1996).

Uses

The Commission E approved the use of juniper berry for dyspepsia. It has also been used in combination with other botanicals for bladder and kidney conditions (Bruneton, 1995; Leung and Foster, 1996; Newall et al., 1996).

Contraindications

Pregnancy and inflammation of the kidneys.

Note: Juniper berry may increase glucose levels in diabetics (ESCOP, 1997).

Side Effects

Prolonged usage or overdosing may cause kidney damage.

Use During Pregnancy and Lactation

Not recommended during pregnancy and lactation (ESCOP, 1997).

Interactions with Other Drugs

None known.

Dosage and Administration

Unless otherwise prescribed: 2 g to a maximum of 10 g per day of whole, crushed, or powdered fruit, corresponding to 20–100 mg of the essential oil, for infusions and decoctions, alcohol extracts, and in wine.

Essential oil: Liquid and solid medicinal forms only for oral application.

Infusion: Steep 2–3 g in 150 ml boiled water for 20 minutes, take three times daily.

Fluidextract 1:1 (g/ml): 2–3 ml, three times daily.

Essential oil: 0.02–0.1 ml, three times daily.

Spirit of juniper: A mixture of oil of juniper and alcohol corresponding to 20–100 ml oil.

Note: Combinations with other plant preparations in teas and similar preparations for treating bladder and kidney diseases may be helpful.

References

Bruneton, J. 1995. *Pharmacognosy, Phytochemistry, Medicinal Plants.* Paris: Lavoisier Publishing.

Chandler, R.F. 1986. An inconspicuous but insidious drug. *Rev Pharm Can* 563–566.

ESCOP. 1997. "Juniperi fructus." *Monographs on the Medicinal Uses of Plant Drugs.* Exeter, U.K.: European Scientific Cooperative on Phytotherapy.

Grieve, M. 1979. *A Modern Herbal.* New York: Dover Publications, Inc.

Leung, A.Y. and S. Foster. 1996. *Encyclopedia of Common Natural Ingredients Used in Food, Drugs, and Cosmetics,* 2nd ed. New York: John Wiley & Sons, Inc.

Newall, C.A., L.A. Anderson, J.D. Phillipson. 1996. *Herbal Medicines: A Guide for Health-Care Professionals.* London: The Pharmaceutical Press.

Markkanen, T. et al. 1981. Antiherpetic agent from juniper tree (*Juniperus communis*), its purification, identification, and testing in primary human amnion cell cultures. *Drugs Exp Clin Res* 7:691–697.

Tyler, V. 1993. *The Honest Herbal,* 3rd ed. New York: Pharmaceutical Products Press.

Additional Resources

Agrawal, O.P., B. Santosh., R. Mathur. 1980. Antifertility effects of fruits of *Juniperus communis. Planta Med* (Suppl):98–101.

British Herbal Pharmacopoeia (BHP). 1983. Keighley, U.K.: British Herbal Medicine Association.

Czygan, F.C. 1987. Warnung vor unkritischem Gebrauch von Wacholderbeeren. *Z Phytotherapie* (8):10.

Deutsches Arzneibuch, 10th ed., 1st–2nd suppl. (DAB 10). 1991–1993. Stuttgart: Deutscher Apotheker Verlag.

Hänsel, R. and H. Haas. 1984. *Therapie mit Phytopharmaka.* Berlin: Springer Verlag.

Harnischfeger, G. and H. Stolze. 1983. *Bewahrte Pflanzendrogen in Wissenschaft und Medizin.* Bad Homburg/Melsungen, Germany: Notamed Verlag.

Markkanen, T. 1981. Antiherpetic agent(s) from juniper tree (*Juniperus communis*) preliminary communication. *Drugs Exp Clin Res* (7):69–73.

McGuffin, M., C. Hobbs, R. Upton, A. Goldberg. 1997. American Herbal Product Association's *Botanical Safety Handbook.* Boca Raton: CRC Press.

Prakash, A.O. 1986. Potentialities of some indigenous plants for antifertility activity. *Int J Crude Drug Res* (24):19–24.

Sanchez de Medina, F. et al. 1994. Hypoglycemic activity of Juniper "Berries." *Planta Med* 60(3):197–200.

Schilcher, H. 1992. *Phyotherapie in der Urologie.* Stuttgart: Hippokrates Verlag.

———. 1995. Juniper berry oil in diseases of the efferent urinary tract. *Med Monatsschr Pharm* 18(7):198–199.

Schilcher, H. and B.M. Heil. 1993. Nierentoxizitat von Wacholderbeerzubereitungen. Eine kritische Literaturauswertung von 1844 bis 1993. *Z Phytotherapie* (15):205–213.

Van der Weijden, G.A., et al. 1998. The effect of herbal extracts in an experimental mouthrinse on established plaque and gingivitis. *J Clin Periodontol* 25(5):399–403.

Wichtl, M. and N.G. Bisset (eds.). 1994. *Herbal Drugs and Phytopharmaceuticals.* Stuttgart: Medpharm Scientific Publishers.

Wichtl, M. (ed.). 1989. *Teedrogen,* 2nd ed. Stuttgart: Wissenschaftliche Verlagsgesellschaft.

This material was adapted from *The Complete German Commission E Monographs—Therapeutic Guide to Herbal Medicines.* M. Blumenthal, W.R. Busse, A. Goldberg, J. Gruenwald, T. Hall, C.W. Riggins, R.S. Rister (eds.) S. Klein and R.S. Rister (trans.). 1998. Austin: American Botanical Council; Boston: Integrative Medicine Communications.

1) The Overview section is new information.

2) Description, Chemistry and Pharmacology, Uses, Contraindications, Side Effects, Interactions with Other Drugs, and Dosage sections have been drawn from the original work. Additional information has been added in some or all of these sections, as noted with references.

3) The dosage for equivalent preparations (tea infusion, fluidextract, and tincture) have been provided based on the following example:
Unless otherwise prescribed: 2 g per day of [powdered, crushed, cut or whole] [plant part]
Infusion: 2 g in 150 ml of water
Fluidextract 1:1 (g/ml): 2 ml
Tincture 1:5 (g/ml): 10 ml

4) The References and Additional Resources sections are new sections. Additional Resources are not cited in the monograph but are included for research purposes.

KAVA KAVA RHIZOME (ROOT)

Latin Name:
Piper methysticum

Pharmacopeial Name:
Piperis methystici rhizoma

Other Names:
kava, awa

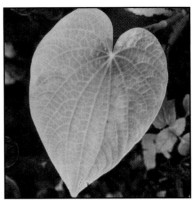
©1999 Steven Foster

Overview

Kava (also known as kava kava) is the most respected herb in the islands of the South Pacific. It is used as a ritual beverage for ceremonial purposes, including the welcoming of important guests. Pope John Paul II, Queen Elizabeth, President Lyndon B. Johnson, Lady Bird Johnson, and Hillary Rodham Clinton are all known to have drunk kava upon being welcomed to Fiji (the Pope) and Samoa (others) (Singh and Blumenthal, 1997).

Kava has been used in native medicine for its relaxing qualities, for urinary tract infections, asthma (Hope et al., 1993), as a topical anesthetic, and other applications. The primary interest in the West has been its well documented anxiolytic effects.

Numerous clinical studies, including laboratory testing, conducted in Germany reveal the relative safety and efficacy of kava extracts for reduction of symptoms in patients with anxiety disorders (Kinzler et al., 1991; Volz and Kieser, 1997). The results of the clinical studies and the experiences of German patients using kava phytomedicines have shown that kava is an appropriate treatment compared to tricyclic antidepressants and benzodiazepines in anxiety disorders. Kava has also been shown effective for long-term use without the tolerance problems associated with the use of tricyclics and benzodiazepines (Volz and Kieser, 1997).

There is some documentation to support the increased popularity of kava with menopausal women. An eight-week study on a special kava extract (Laitan®, W. Schwabe, Germany) resulted in reduction of neurovegetative and psychosomatic dysfunctions (hot flashes, depressive moods, irritability) after only one week of treatment (Warnecke, 1991).

Although usually contraindicated with alcohol, a recent study designed to determine any adverse synergies between the two substances concluded that no negative "multiplicative" (i.e., synergistic) effects of a special proprietary kava extract (WS 1490) were observed with persons ingesting alcohol (0.05% blood alcohol concentration) (Herberg, 1993).

Other safety concerns with kava deal with the observed yellowing and scaling of the skin in persons using kava beverages heavily for an extended period, a condition known as "kava dermopathy." A study (Ruze, 1990) of male kava drinkers in the Tongan Islands concluded that the observed pellagroid dermopathy was not due to niacin deficiency as had previously been suggested.

The general safety of kava was assessed in an industry-sponsored review of the historical and scientific literature, and it was concluded that, "When used in normal therapeutic doses, kava appears to offer safe and effective anti-anxiety and muscle relaxant actions without depressing centers of higher thought. The safe use of kava as a dietary supplement in cultures that do not have historical experience with its use depends on responsible manufacturing, marketing, individual consumer patterns, and education (Dentali, 1997).

Due to concerns about the relative safety of kava, in September 1997 the American Herbal Products Association recommended the following label warning to all its members: "Caution: Not for use by persons under the age of 18. If pregnant, nursing, or taking a prescription drug, consult healthcare practitioner prior to use. Do not exceed recommended dosage. Excessive consumption may impair ability to drive or operate heavy equipment" (Anon, 1999). This warning is consistent with cautions published by the Commission E.

German pharmacopeial grade kava kava consists of the peeled and cut dried rhizome of *Piper methysticum* G. Forster, mostly removed from the root. It must contain not less than 3.5% total kavalactones, calculated as kavain. Botanical identification is confirmed by thin-layer chromatography (TLC), macroscopic and microscopic examinations, as well as organoleptic evaluations including taste, smell, and chewing the rhizome to stimulate salivation and a long lasting anesthetic effect on the tongue (DAC, 1986–1989).

Description

Kava kava rhizome consists of the dried rhizomes of *P. methysticum* G. Forster [Fam. Piperaceae], as well as their preparations in effective dosage. The rhizome contains kava pyrones (kawain).

Chemistry and Pharmacology

Kava kava rhizome contains >3.5% kavalactones, a.k.a. kavapyrones, mainly methysticin, dihydromethysticin, kavain, 7,8-dihydrokavain, 5,6-dehydrokavain, 5-6,dehydromethysticin, and yangonin; chalcones, including flavokavains A, B, and C (He et al., 1997). The major kavalactones can be classified into enolides (e.g., 5,6-dihydro-α-pyrones with an asymmetric carbon atom) and dienolides (e.g., achiral α-pyrones) (Häberlein et al., 1997); approximately 3.2% minerals, including potassium (approximately 2.2%), calcium, magnesium, sodium, aluminum, iron; approximately 3.5% amino acids (Leung and Foster, 1996; Mack, 1994).

The Commission E reported anti-anxiety activity for kava kava. In animal experiments a potentiation of narcosis (sedation), as well as anticonvulsive, antispasmodic, and central muscular relaxant effects were described.

The neuropharmacologic effects of kava include analgesia, anesthesia, sedation, and hyporeflexia (Holm et al., 1991; Jamieson et al., 1989; Singh, 1983). Kava affects motor and muscular function (Holm et al., 1991; Jamieson et al., 1989; Meyer, 1962; Singh, 1983), while mental function appears to remain clear (Pfeiffer et al., 1967). Kava pyrones have been shown to protect mice from strychnine-induced convulsions (Klohs et al., 1959). Kava has also been shown to improve seizure control in epileptic patients but with unacceptable skin-yellowing side effects (Pfeiffer et al., 1967).

The mechanism of action by kava on the central nervous system is not clear. *In vitro* and *in vivo* studies have produced differing conclusions regarding whether kava binds at GABA receptors. A possible noradrenaline uptake effect has been shown in 3 kavalactones. Anticonvulsant activity may be a result of mediation of Na+ channel receptor sites, common targets of anti-epileptic drugs (Anon, 1998). One of the more interesting features about kava is its ability to relax skeletal muscles, yet it does not act as a central nervous system depressant. Studies show that kava actually helps to retain or increase mental processes (Emser, 1993; Heinze et al., 1994; Münte et al., 1993; Pfeiffer et al., 1967; Saletu et al., 1989).

Uses

Commission E approved kava for use in conditions of nervous anxiety, stress, and restlessness.

Clinical trials have also studied the use of kava for cognitive enhancement (Emser, 1993; Heinze et al., 1994; Münte et al., 1993; Saletu et al., 1989) and climacteric symptom reduction (Warnecke, 1991).

Contraindications
Endogenous depression.

Side Effects
None known.
Note: Extended continuous intake can cause a temporary yellow discoloration of skin, hair, and nails. In this case, application of this preparation must be discontinued. In rare cases, allergic skin reactions can occur. Also, accommodative disturbances, such as enlargement of the pupils and disturbances of the oculomotor equilibrium, have been described.

Use During Pregnancy and Lactation
Not recommended.

Interactions with Other Drugs
Potentiation of effectiveness is possible for substances acting on the central nervous system, such as alcohol, barbiturates, and psychopharmacological agents.

Dosage and Administration
Unless otherwise prescribed: 1.7–3.4 g per day of cut rhizome and other galenical preparations for oral use, equivalent to 60–120 mg kava pyrones. Do not exceed recommended dose.
Note: The equivalency of 1.7–3.4 g dry rhizome to 60–120 mg kava pyrones is based on the drug codex requirement of minimum 3.5% (35 mg/g) kava pyrones content in the raw material.
Cold macerate: Soak 1.7–3.4 g of ground rhizome in 150 ml cold water for several hours, then strain.
Dried rhizome: 1.5–3 g, in divided doses throughout the day (Bone,

1993–1994; Burgess, 1998); 2–4 g (Karnick, 1994).
Note: The rhizome needs to be chewed well and suffiently mixed with saliva while ingesting (Alschuler, 1998).
Fluidextract 1:2 (g/ml): 3–6 ml, in divided doses (Alschuler, 1998; Bone, 1993–1994; Burgess, 1998).
Dry normalized extract containing 30% (300 mg/g) kava pyrones: 0.2–0.4 g (200–400 mg).
Soft native extract containing approximately 55% (550 mg/g) kava pyrones: 0.1–0.2 g (100–200 mg).
Note: The traditional kava preparation in a single dose is reported to deliver approximately 250–300 mg of active α-pyrones (Dentali, 1997).
Duration of administration: Not more than 3 months without medical advice.
Note: Even when administered within its prescribed dosages, this herb may adversely affect motor reflexes and judgment for driving and/or operating heavy machinery.

References
Alschuler, L. 1998. Kava: an herb for our hectic times. *Nature's Impact™* by Impact Communications, Inc.

Anon. 1999. AHPA's Recommended Label Language for Kava Products. *HerbalGram* 45.

Anon. 1998. Monograph: *Piper methysticum* (kava kava). *Alt Med Rev* 3(6):458–460.

Bone, K. 1993–1994. Kava—a safe herbal treatment for anxiety. *Brit J Phytother* 3(4):147–153.

Burgess, N. 1998. Regulatory issues on *Piper methysticum* (kava). *Aust J Med Herbalism* 10(1):2–3.

Dentali, S.J. 1997. *Herb Safety Review: Kava, Piper methysticum Forster f. (Piperaceae).* Bethesda, MD: American Herbal Products Association.

Deutscher Arzneimittel-Codex, 1st suppl. (DAC). 1986–1989. Stuttgart: Deutscher Apotheker Verlag. K-155:1–6.

Emser, W. 1993. Phytotherapy of insomnia—a critical overview. *Pharmacopsychiatry* 26:150.

Häberlein, H., G. Boonen, M.A. Beck. 1997. *Piper methysticum*: enantiomeric separation of kavapyrones by high performance liquid chromatography. *Planta Med* 63:63–65.

He, X., L. Lin, L. Lian. 1997. Electrospray high performance liquid chromatography-mass spectrometry in phytochemical analysis of kava (*Piper methysticum*) extract. *Planta Med* 63:70–74.

Heinze, H.J., T.F. Munthe, J. Steitz, M. Matzke. 1994. Pharmacopsychological effects of oxazepam and kava-extract in a visual search paradigm assessed with event-related potentials. *Pharmacopsychiatry* 27(6):224–230.

Herberg, K.W. 1993. [Effect of kava-special extract WS 1490 combined with ethyl alcohol on safety-relevant performance parameters] [In German]. *Blutalkohol* 30(2):96–105.

Holm, E. et al. 1991. Untersuchungen zum Wirkungsprofil von D, L-Kavain. *Arzneimforsch/Drug Res* 41(7):673–683.

Hope, B.E., D.B. Massey, G. Fournier-Massey. 1993. Hawaiian materia medica for asthma. *Hawaii Med J* 52(6):160–166.

Jamieson, D.D., P.H. Duffield, D. Cheng, A.M. Duffield. 1989. Comparison of the central nervous system activity of the aqueous and lipid extract of kava (*Piper methysticum*). *Arch Int Pharmacodyn Ther* 301:66–80.

Karnick, C.R. 1994. *Pharmacopoeial Standards of Herbal Plants,* Vol. 2. Delhi: Sri Satguru Publications. 79.

Kinzler, E., J. Kromer, E. Lehmann. 1991. [Effect of a special kava extract in patients with anxiety-, tension-, and excitation states of non-psychotic genesis. Double blind study with placebos over four weeks] [In German]. *Arzneimforsch* 41(6):584–588.

Klohs, M.W.F. et al. 1959. A chemical and pharmacological investigation of *Piper methysticum* Forst. *J Med Pharm Chem* 1:95–99.

Leung, A.Y. and S. Foster. 1996. *Encyclopedia of Common Natural Ingredients Used in Food, Drugs, and Cosmetics*, 2nd ed. New York: John Wiley & Sons, Inc. 330–331.

Mack, R. 1994. Kava kava. *Piper methysticum*—a unique economic plant of the Pacific Islands. *J Health Sci* 1(1):43–48.

Meyer, H.J. 1962. Pharmakologie der Wirksamen Prinzipien de Kawa-rhizoms (*Piper methysticum* Forst.) *Arch Int Pharmacodyn Ther* 138:505–536.

Münte, T.F. et al. 1993. Effects of oxazepam and an extract of kava roots (*Piper methysticum*) on event-related potentials in a word recognition task. *Neuropsychobiology* 27(1):46–53.

Pfeiffer, C.C., H.G. Murphree, L. Goldstein. 1967. Effects of kava in normal subjects and patients. Ethnopharmacologic search for psychoactive drugs: Proceedings of a symposium held in San Francisco, California. January 28–30. *Public Health Service Publication* No. 1645:155–161.

Ruze, P. 1990. Kava-induced dermopathy: a niacin deficiency? *Lancet* 335(8703):1442–1445.

Saletu, B. et al. 1989. EEG-brain mapping, psychometric and psychophysiological studies on central effects of kavain—a kava plant derivative. *Hum Psychopharmacol* 4:169–190.

Singh, Y.N. 1983. Effects of kava on neuromuscular transmission and muscle contractility. *J Ethnopharmacol* 7(3):267–276.

Singh, Y.N. and M. Blumenthal. 1997. Kava—An Overview. *HerbalGram* 39:33–56.

Volz, H.P. and M. Kieser. 1997. Kava-kava extract WS 1490 versus placebo in anxiety disorders—A randomized placebo controlled 25-week outpatient trial. *Pharmacopsychiatry* 30(1):1–5.

Warnecke, G. 1991. [Psychosomatic dysfunction in the female climacteric. Clinical effectiveness and tolerance of Kava Extract WS 1490] [In German]. *Fortschr Med* 109(4):119–122.

Additional Resources

Frater, A.S. 1976. Medical aspects of yaqona. *Fiji Med J* 4:526–530.

Lebot, V., M. Merlin, L. Lindstrom. 1992. *Kava: the Pacific Drug*. New Haven: Yale University Press.

Lebot, V. and P. Cabalion. 1988. *Kavas of Vanuatu: Cultivars of Piper Methysticum* Forst. Technical Paper No. 1955. Noumea, New Caledonia: South Pacific Commission. 3–53.

Lebot, V. and J. Levesque. 1989. The origin and distribution of kava (*Piper methysticum* Forst. f., Piperaceae): a phytochemical approach. *Allertonia* 5:223–281.

Lehmann, E. et al. 1996. [Effects of a special Kava extract (*Piper methysticum*) in patients with states of anxiety, tension and excitedness of non-mental origin—A double blind placebo controlled study of four weeks treatment] [In German]. *Phytomedicine* 3(2):113–119.

This material was adapted from *The Complete German Commission E Monographs—Therapeutic Guide to Herbal Medicines.* M. Blumenthal, W.R. Busse, A. Goldberg, J. Gruenwald, T. Hall, C.W. Riggins, R.S. Rister (eds.) S. Klein and R.S. Rister (trans.). 1998. Austin: American Botanical Council; Boston: Integrative Medicine Communications.

1) The Overview section is new information.

2) Description, Chemistry and Pharmacology, Uses, Contraindications, Side Effects, Interactions with Other Drugs, and Dosage sections have been drawn from the original work. Additional information has been added in some or all of these sections, as noted with references.

3) The dosage for equivalent preparations (tea infusion, fluidextract, and tincture) have been provided based on the following example:
   Unless otherwise prescribed: 2 g per day of [powdered, crushed, cut or whole] [plant part]
   Infusion: 2 g in 150 ml of water
   Fluidextract 1:1 (g/ml): 2 ml
   Tincture 1:5 (g/ml): 10 ml

4) The References and Additional Resources sections are new sections. Additional Resources are not cited in the monograph but are included for research purposes.

Lindenberg, Von D. and H. Pitule-Schodel. 1990. D,L-Kavain in comparison with oxazepam in anxiety states. Double-blind clinical trial. *Forschr Med* 108(2):49–50; 53–54.

McGuffin, M., C. Hobbs, R. Upton, A. Goldberg. 1997. American Herbal Product Association's *Botanical Safety Handbook*. Boca Raton: CRC Press.

Russell, P.N., D. Bakker, N.N. Singh. 1987. The effects of kava on alerting and speed of access of information from long-term memory. *Bull Psychonomic Society* 25:236–237.

Shulgin, A.T. 1973. The narcotic pepper: the chemistry and pharmacology of *Piper methysticum* and related species. *Bulletin on Narcotics* 25:59–74.

Singh, Y.N. 1992. Kava—An Overview. *J Ethnopharmacol* 37(1):13–45.

Smith, RM. 1979. Pipermethystine: a novel pyridone alkaloid from *Piper methysticum*. *Tetrahedron Lett* 35:437–439.

Titcomb, M. 1948. Kava in Hawaii. *J Polynesian Society* 57:105–171.

LAVENDER FLOWER

Latin Name:
Lavandula angustifolia

Pharmacopeial Name:
Lavandulae flos

Other Names:
English lavender,
garden lavender, true lavender

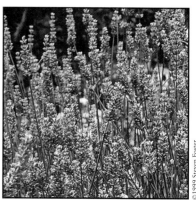
©1999 Steven Foster

Overview

Lavender is an aromatic subshrub native to the low mountains (800–1,800 meters) of the Mediterranean basin, cultivated in France, Bulgaria, Italy, Spain, the former Yugoslavia, the Netherlands, the United Kingdom, the United States, and Australia. The material of commerce comes mainly from France (Bruneton, 1995; Grieve, 1979; Leung and Foster, 1996; Wichtl and Bisset, 1994).

Lavender was used as an antiseptic in ancient Arabian, Greek, and Roman medicines. Its genus name comes from the Latin *lavare*, to wash, probably referring to its use as a bath additive for the purification of body and spirit. It was also used as a bactericide to disinfect hospitals and sick rooms in ancient Persia, Greece, and Rome. The ancient Greeks called the plant *nardus* and later the Romans called it *asarum*. In the time of Pliny the Elder (ca. 23–79 B.C.E.), the blossoms sold for 100 Roman denarii per pound (Bown, 1995; Grieve, 1979; Savinelli, 1993). Knowledge of its healing abilities spread to India and then to Tibet. In the book *Makhzan-El-Adwiya*, it is called the broom of the brain, because it is reputed to sweep away all kafa impurities (Nadkarni, 1976). The *Gyu-zhi*, or *Four Tantras*, by Chandranandana is the earliest Indian medical text to be translated into Tibetan (eighth century B.C.E.). In it, lavender (*Pri-yangku* in Tibetan) is included in psychiatric formulas, still used today in Tibetan Buddhist medicine, for treating insanity and psychoses, in an edible ointment or medicine butter dosage form. (Clifford, 1984). The *Ayurvedic Pharmacopoeia* (AP) lists *Lavandula officinalis*, along with a related Indian species, L. burmani, and specifically indicates its use for depressive states associated with digestive dysfunction. The AP reports its actions as carminative, antispasmodic, antidepressant, sedative, and antirheumatic; oil is a rubefacient (Karnick, 1994).

In Germany, lavender is licensed as a standard medicinal tea for sleep disorders and nervous stomach. Lavender flower and extract are also used in sedative and cholagogue medical preparations. In Germany and the United States, the aqueous infusion is used in balneotherapy and the essential oil is used in aromatherapy. Additionally, lavender flower is often used in the United States as a component of dietary supplement products, mainly in aqueous infusions. Lavender oil is also official in the *United States National Formulary* (Leung and Foster, 1996; NF, 1985; Wichtl and Bisset, 1994).

Modern clinical studies have investigated the neurophysical effects of its essential oil (Tasev et al, 1969), its choleretic and cholagogic actions (Gruncharov, 1973), its use as a bath additive for perineal discomfort and repair following childbirth (Dale and Cornwell, 1994; Cornwell and Dale, 1995), and its use as an alternative to tamoxifen (Ziegler, 1996).

The approved modern therapeutic applications for lavender are supportable based on its use in well established systems of traditional medicine, on phytochemical investigations, and on its documented pharmacological actions reported in *in vitro* studies and *in vivo* experiments in animals.

German pharmacopeial grade lavender flower must contain not less than 1.3% volatile oil and pass a botanical identity test determined by thin-layer chromatography (TLC). French pharmacopeial grade lavender flower must contain not less than 0.8% volatile oil. German pharmacopeial grade lavender oil must contain not less than 35.0% ester, calculated as linalyl acetate, and must also pass a number of purity tests including detection of foreign esters. French pharmacopeial grade lavender oil must contain 25–38% linalool, 25–45% linalyl acetate, 0.1–0.5% limonene, 0.3–1.5% 1,8-cineole, 0.2–0.5% camphor, and 0.3–1.0% α-terpineol (DAB 1997; DAC, 1986; Ph.Fr.X., 1990; Wichtl and Bisset, 1994).

Description

Lavender flower consists of the dried flower of *Lavandula angustifolia* Miller [Fam. Lamiaceae], gathered shortly before fully unfolding, and its preparations in effective dosage. The preparation contains at least 1.5% (v/w) essential oil with linalyl acetate, linalool, camphor, β-ocimene, and 1,8-cineole as its main components. Furthermore, the preparation contains about 12% tannins unique to the Lamiaceae.

Note: In U.S. commerce, lavandin (*L. xintermedia*) is often interchanged with *L. angustifolia* (Tucker, 1999). However, the official species approved for medicinal use by the Commission E is *L. angustifolia*.

Chemistry and Pharmacology

Lavender flower contains 1.5–3% volatile oil, of which 25–55% is linalyl acetate, 20–38% linalool, 4–10% cis-β-ocimene, 2–6% trans-β-ocimene, 2–6% 1-terpinen-4-ol, <2% 3-octanone, 0.3–1.5% 1,8-cineole, 0.3–1% α-terpineol, 0.2–0.5% camphor, and 0.1–0.5% limonene; tannins (5–10%); coumarins; flavonoids (luteolin); phytosterols; and triterpenes (Bruneton, 1995; Leung and Foster, 1996; Wichtl and Bisset, 1994).

The Commission E reported sedative and antiflatulent activity.

Lavender oil exhibited central nervous system-depressive activities on experimental animals (Leung and Foster, 1996).

Uses

The Commission E approved the internal use of lavender for restlessness or insomnia and nervous stomach irritations, Roehmheld's syndrome, meteorism, and nervous intestinal discomfort. For balneotherapy: Treatment of functional circulatory disorders.

The German Standard License for lavender tea lists it for restlessness, sleeplessness, lack of appetite, nervous irritable stomach, meteorism, and nervous disorders of the intestines (Wichtl and Bisset, 1994). Lavender preparations are traditionally used to treat symptoms of neurotonic disorders, especially minor sleeplessness (Bruneton, 1995).

Contraindications

None known.

Side Effects

None known.

Use During Pregnancy and Lactation

No restrictions known.

Interactions with Other Drugs

None known.

Dosage and Administration

Unless otherwise prescribed: Tea extract, and bath additive.

Internal: Infusion: 1–2 teaspoons (approximately 0.8–1.6 g) in 150 ml water (Note: 1 teaspoon flower = 0.8 g).
Essential oil: 1–4 drops (approximately 20–80 mg), e.g., on a sugar cube.
Note: Combinations with other sedative or carminative herbs may be beneficial.
External: Bath additive: 20–100 g for a 20 liter bath.

References

Bown, D. 1995. *Encyclopedia of Herbs and Their Uses.* New York: DK Publishing, Inc. 301–302.

Bruneton, J. 1995. *Pharmacognosy, Phytochemistry, Medicinal Plants.* Paris: Lavoisier Publishing.

Clifford, T. 1984. *Tibetan Buddhist Medicine and Psychiatry.* York Beach, ME: Samuel Weiser, Inc. 171–186.

Cornwell, S. and A. Dale. 1995. Lavender oil and perineal repair. *Mod Midwife* 5(3):31–33.

Dale, A. and S. Cornwell. 1994. The role of lavender oil in relieving perineal discomfort following childbirth: a blind randomized clinical trial. *J Adv Nurs* 19(1):89–96.

Deutsches Arzneibuch (DAB 1997). 1997. Stuttgart: Deutscher Apotheker Verlag.

Deutscher Arzneimittel-Codex (DAC). 1986. Stuttgart: Deutscher Apotheker Verlag.

Grieve, M. 1979. *A Modern Herbal.* New York: Dover Publications, Inc.

Gruncharov, V. 1973. [Clinico-experimental study on the choleretic and cholagogic action of Bulgarian lavender oil] [In Bulgarian]. *Vutr Boles* 12(3):90–96.

Karnick, C.R., 1994. *Pharmacopoeial Standards of Herbal Plants,* Vols. 1–2. Delhi: Sri Satguru Publications. Vol. 1:213–214; Vol. 2:82.

Leung, A.Y. and S. Foster. 1996. *Encyclopedia of Common Natural Ingredients Used in Food, Drugs, and Cosmetics,* 2nd ed. New York: John Wiley & Sons, Inc.

Nadkarni, K.M. 1976. *Indian Materia Medica.* Bombay: Popular Prakashan. 730.

National Formulary (NF), 16th ed. 1985. Washington, D.C.: American Pharmaceutical Association.

Pharmacopée Française Xe Édition (Ph.Fr.X.). 1983–1990. Moulins-les-Metz: Maisonneuve S.A.

Savinelli, A. 1993. *Plants of Power.* Taos, NM: Alfred Savinelli. 26–29.

Tasev, T., P. Toleva, V. Balabanova. 1969. Effet neuro-physique des huiles essentielles bulgares de rose, de lavande et de geranium [Neurophysical effect of Bulgarian essential oils from rose, lavender and geranium]. *Folia Med (Plovdiv)* 11(5):307–317.

Tucker, A. 1999. Personal communication to A. Goldberg. July 13.

Wichtl, M. and N.G. Bisset (eds.). 1994. *Herbal Drugs and Phytopharmaceuticals.* Stuttgart: Medpharm Scientific Publishers.

Ziegler, J. 1996. Raloxifene, retinoids, and lavender: "me too" tamoxifen alternatives under study [news]. *J Natl Cancer Inst* 88(16):1100–1102.

Additional Resources

Atanasova-Shopova, S. and K.S. Rusinov. 1970. [On certain central neurotropic effects of lavender essential oil]. *Izv Inst Fiziol Bulg Akad Nauk* 13:69–76.

Braun, R. et al. 1997. *Standardzulassungen für Fertigarzneimittel—Text and Kommentar.* Stuttgart: Deutscher Apotheker Verlag.

British Herbal Pharmacopoeia (BHP). 1983. Keighley, U.K.: British Herbal Medicine Association.

Buchbauer, G., L. Jirovetz, W. Jager, H. Dietrich, C. Plank. 1991. Aromatherapy: evidence for sedative effects of the essential oil of lavender after inhalation. *Z Naturforsch* 46(11–12):1067–1072.

Delaveau, P., J. Guillemain, G. Narcisse, A. Rousseau. 1989. [Neuro-depressive properties of essential oil of lavender] [In French]. *C R Seances Soc Biol Fil* 183(4):342–348.

Deutsches Arzneibuch (DAB 1998). 1998. Stuttgart: Deutscher Apotheker Verlag.

Food Chemicals Codex, 2nd ed. (FCC II). 1972. Washington, D.C.: National Academy of Sciences.

Frohlich, E. 1968. [Lavender oil, review of clinical, pharmacological and bacteriological studies. Contribution to clarification of the mechanism of action] [In German]. *Wien Med Wochenschr* 118(15):345–350.

Guillemain, J., A. Rousseau, P. Delaveau. 1989. Effets neurodepresseurs de l'huile essentielle de *Lavandula angustifolia* Mill [Neurodepressive effects of the essential oil of *Lavandula angustifolia* Mill]. *Ann Pharm Fr* 47(6):337–343.

Hänsel, R., K. Keller, H. Rimpler, G. Schneider (eds.). 1992–1994. *Hagers Handbuch der Pharmazeutischen Praxis,* 5th ed. Vol. 4–6. Berlin-Heidelberg: Springer Verlag.

Karrer, W. 1958. *Konstitution und Vorkommen der Organischen Pflanzenstoffe (exclusive Alkaloide).* Basel: Birkhäuser Verlag.

Kustrak, D. and J. Besic. 1975. Aetheroleum Lavandulae und Aetheroleum Lavandulae hybridae in Ph. Jug. III. [In German]. *Pharm Acta Helv* 50(11):373–378.

List, P.H. and L. Hörhammer (eds.). 1973–1979. *Hagers Handbuch der Pharmazeutischen Praxis,* Vols. 1–7. New York: Springer Verlag.

McGuffin, M., C. Hobbs, R. Upton, A. Goldberg. 1997. American Herbal Product Association's *Botanical Safety Handbook.* Boca Raton: CRC Press.

Reynolds, J.E.F. (ed.). 1982. *Martindale: The Extra Pharmacopoeia,* 28th ed. London: The Pharmaceutical Press.

Steinegger, E. and R. Hänsel. 1992. *Pharmakog-nosie*, 5th ed. Berlin-Heidelberg: Springer Verlag.

Wichtl, M. (ed.). 1997. *Teedrogen,* 4th ed. Stuttgart: Wissenschaftliche Verlagsgesellschaft.

This material was adapted from *The Complete German Commission E Monographs—Therapeutic Guide to Herbal Medicines.* M. Blumenthal, W.R. Busse, A. Goldberg, J. Gruenwald, T. Hall, C.W. Riggins, R.S. Rister (eds.) S. Klein and R.S. Rister (trans.). 1998. Austin: American Botanical Council; Boston: Integrative Medicine Communications.

1) The Overview section is new information.

2) Description, Chemistry and Pharmacology, Uses, Contraindications, Side Effects, Interactions with Other Drugs, and Dosage sections have been drawn from the original work. Additional information has been added in some or all of these sections, as noted with references.

3) The dosage for equivalent preparations (tea infusion, fluidextract, and tincture) have been provided based on the following example:
Unless otherwise prescribed: 2 g per day of [powdered, crushed, cut or whole] [plant part]
Infusion: 2 g in 150 ml of water
Fluidextract 1:1 (g/ml): 2 ml
Tincture 1:5 (g/ml): 10 ml

4) The References and Additional Resources sections are new sections. Additional Resources are not cited in the monograph but are included for research purposes.

LEMON BALM

Latin Name:
Melissa officinalis

Pharmacopeial Name:
Melissae folium

Other Names:
balm, common balm, melissa,
sweet balm

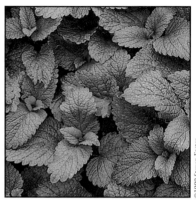

©1999 Steven Foster

Overview

Lemon balm is an aromatic perennial subshrub native to the eastern Mediterranean region and western Asia, widely cultivated throughout much of Europe. The material of commerce comes from Bulgaria, Romania, and Spain (BHP, 1996; Bruneton, 1995; Leung and Foster, 1996; Wichtl and Bisset, 1994). Lemon balm is one of Germany's more important medicinal crops (Lange and Schippmann, 1997). Its genus name *Melissa* is from the Greek word for "bee," referring to the bee's attraction to its flower and the quality of the honey produced from it (Grieve, 1979).

Lemon balm steeped in wine was used orally and topically in ancient Greek and Roman medicines, as surgical dressing for wounds, and to treat venomous bites and stings, as mentioned in the writings of Dioscorides and Pliny the Elder. These same uses and medicinal wine dosage form, stemming from traditional Greek medicine, are also used in the *Indian Materia Medica* (Nadkarni, 1976). Old European medical herbals also report its memory-improving properties, recently corroborated as cholinergic activities identified in extracts of lemon balm (Perry et al., 1998). The *Ayurvedic Pharmacopoeia* (AP) lists *Melissa officinalis*, along with the related Indian species *M. parviflora*, for dyspepsia associated with anxiety or depressive states, in a dried herb or alcoholic fluidextract dosage form. The AP reports its actions as carminative, antispasmodic, diaphoretic, and sedative (Karnick, 1994).

In Germany, lemon balm is licensed as a standard medicinal tea for sleep disorders and gastrointestinal tract disorders (Braun et al., 1997; Meyer-Buchtela, 1999; Wichtl and Bisset, 1994). Aqueous and alcoholic extract of balm are also used as components of various sedative and hypnotic drug preparations (Wichtl and Bisset, 1994). It is often combined with other sedative and/or carminative herbs (BAnz, 1998; Wichtl and Bisset, 1994). In the United States, lemon balm is often used as a component of mild sleep aid and/or stomachic dietary supplement products, mainly in aqueous infusion and hydroalcoholic fluidextract and tincture dosage forms (Leung and Foster, 1996). Lemon balm was formerly official in the *United States Pharmacopoeia* (Leung and Foster, 1996).

No significant human studies in English relate to its Commission E-approved *internal* uses. Some modern studies have investigated its external use to treat cutaneous herpes simplex lesions (ESCOP, 1997). In one study on 115 patients, a proprietary preparation of lemon balm extract in a lip balm showed efficacy in treating lip sores associated with the herpes simplex virus (Wöbling and Leonhardt, 1994). The approved modern therapeutic applications for lemon balm are supportable based on its long history of use in well established systems of traditional medicine, on phytochemical investigations, and on its documented pharmacological actions reported in *in vitro* studies and *in vivo* experiments in animals.

Pharmacopeial grade lemon balm must contain not less than 0.05% volatile oil with citral, and pass a botanical identity test determined by thin-layer chromatography (TLC) (Bruneton, 1995; DAB, 1997; ÖAB, 1981; Ph.Fr.X, 1990; Wichtl and Bisset, 1994). Its water-soluble extractive content must be not less than 15% (BHP, 1996; Karnick, 1994). A technical note to the *French Pharmacopoeia* 10th edition recommends that pharmacopeial grade lemon balm be defined by at least of 6% total hydroxycinnamic derivatives, calculated as rosmarinic acid, as opposed to the current minimum volatile oil content requirement (Bruneton, 1995). Manufacturers of lemon balm extracts are already guaranteeing minimum content levels for both rosmarinic acid and total volatile oils.

Description

Lemon balm contains the fresh or dried leaf of *M. officinalis* L. [Lamiaceae], and its preparations in effective dosage. The leaf contains at least 0.05% (v/w) essential oil based on the dried herb. Main components are citronellal, citral a, and citral b, as well as other monoterpenes and sesquiterpenes. Other ingredients are tannins unique to the Lamiaceae, such as triterpenylic acid, bitter principles, and flavonoids.

Chemistry and Pharmacology

Lemon balm contains the flavonoids quercitrin, rhamnocitrin, and the 7-glucosides of apigenin, kaempferol, quercetin, and luteolin; phenolic acids and tannins, chiefly rosmarinic acid (up to 4%), and glycosidically bound caffeic and chlorogenic acids; triterpenes (ursolic, oleanolic acids); volatile oil (0.05–0.375%), of which the monoterpenoid citronellal is 30–40%, geranial (citral a) and neral (citral b) are 10–30%; and sesquiterpenes (β-caryophyllene, germacrene D). (Bruneton, 1995; ESCOP, 1997; Leung and Foster, 1996; Wichtl and Bisset, 1994).

The Commission E reported sedative and carminative activity.

The *British Herbal Pharmacopoeia* reported it is internally a sedative and externally a topical antiviral (BHP, 1996). The hydroalcoholic lemon balm extract is a central nervous system sedative in animal studies; its essential oil content does not appear to play a role in this activity (Bruneton, 1995). Preparations of lemon balm have sedative, spasmolytic, and antibacterial actions (Wichtl and Bisset, 1994).

Uses

The Commission E approved the internal use of lemon balm for nervous sleeping disorders and functional gastrointestinal complaints.

ESCOP lists its internal use for tenseness, restlessness, irritability, and symptomatic treatment of digestive disorders, such as minor spasms; externally, for herpes labialis (cold sores) (ESCOP, 1997). The German Standard License for lemon balm tea approves it for nervous disorders of slccp and of the gastrointestinal tract, and to stimulate the appetite (Wichtl and Bisset, 1994).

Contraindications

None known.

Side Effects

None known.

Use During Pregnancy and Lactation

No restrictions known.

Interactions with Other Drugs

None known.

Dosage and Administration

Unless otherwise prescribed: 1.5–4.5 g cut herb several times daily, as needed. Note: Combinations with other sedative and/or carminative herbs may be beneficial.
Infusion: 1.5–4.5 g in 150 ml water.
Fluidextract 1:1 (g/ml): 1.5–4.5 ml.
Native dry extract 5.0–6.0:1 (w/w): 0.3–0.9 g.

References

BAnz. See *Bundesanzeiger*.

Braun, R. et al. 1997. *Standardzulassungen für Fertigarzneimittel—Text and Kommentar*. Stuttgart: Deutscher Apotheker Verlag.

British Herbal Pharmacopoeia (BHP). 1996. Exeter, U.K.: British Herbal Medicine Association. 29–30.

Bruneton, J. 1995. *Pharmacognosy, Phytochemistry, Medicinal Plants*. Paris: Lavoisier Publishing.

Bundesanzeiger (BAnz). 1998. Monographien der Kommission E (Zulassungs- und Aufbereitungskommission am BGA für den humanmed. Bereich, phytotherapeutische Therapierichtung und Stoffgruppe). Köln: Bundesgesundheitsamt (BGA).

Deutsches Arzneibuch (DAB 1997). 1997. Stuttgart: Deutscher Apotheker Verlag.

ESCOP. 1997. "Melissae folium." *Monographs on the Medicinal Uses of Plant Drugs*. Exeter, U.K.: European Scientific Cooperative on Phytotherapy.

Grieve, M. 1979. *A Modern Herbal*. New York: Dover Publications, Inc.

Karnick, C.R. 1994. *Pharmacopoeial Standards of Herbal Plants,* Vols. 1–2. Delhi: Sri Satguru Publications. Vol. 1:259–260; Vol. 2: 83.

Lange D. and U. Schippmann. 1997. *Trade Survey of Medicinal Plants in Germany—A Contribution to International Plant Species Conservation*. Bonn: Bundesamt für Naturschutz. 32–33.

Leung, A.Y. and S. Foster. 1996. *Encyclopedia of Common Natural Ingredients Used in Food, Drugs, and Cosmetics*, 2nd ed. New York: John Wiley & Sons, Inc.

Meyer-Buchtela, E. 1999. *Tee-Rezepturen—Ein Handbuch für Apotheker und Ärzte*. Stuttgart: Deutscher Apotheker Verlag.

Nadkarni, K.M. 1976. *Indian Materia Medica*. Bombay: Popular Prakashan. 786.

*Österreichisches Arzneibuch,*1st suppl. (ÖAB). 1981–1983. Wien: Verlag der Österreichischen Staatsdruckerei.

Perry, E.K., A.T. Pickering, W.W. Wang, P. Houghton, N.S. Perry. 1998. Medicinal plants and Alzheimer's disease: Integrating ethnobotanical and contemporary scientific evidence. *J Altern Complement Med* 4(4):419–428.

Pharmacopée Française Xe Édition (Ph.Fr.X.). 1983–1990. Moulins-les-Metz: Maisonneuve S.A.

Wichtl, M. and N.G. Bisset (eds.). 1994. *Herbal Drugs and Phytopharmaceuticals*. Stuttgart: Medpharm Scientific Publishers.

Wöbling, R.H. and K. Leonhardt. 1994. Local therapy of herpes simplex with dried extract from *Melissa officinalis*. *Phytomedicine* 1:25–31.

Additional Resources

Enjalbert, F., J.M. Bessière, J. Pellecuer, G. Privat, G. Doucet. 1983. Analyse des essences de Mélisse. *Fitoterapia* 2:59–65.

Glowatzki, G. 1970. [*Melissa*, a drug for 2000 years] [In German]. *Med Klin* 65(16):800–803.

Karrer, W. 1958. *Konstitution und Vorkommen der Organischen Pflanzenstoffe (exclusive Alkaloide)*. Basel: Birkhäuser Verlag.

Morelli, I. 1977. Costituenti e usi della "*Melissa officinalis*" [Constituents and uses of *Melissa officinalis*]. *Boll Chim Farm* 116(6):334–340.

Mulkens, A. and I. Kapetanidis. 1987. [Flavonoids of the leaves of *Melissa officinalis* L. (Lamiaceae)] [In French]. *Pharm Acta Helv* 62(1):19–22.

Soulimani, R. et al. 1991. Neurotropic action of the hydroalcoholic extract of *Melissa officinalis* in the mouse. *Planta Med* 57(2):105–109.

Tagashira, M. and Y. Ohtake. 1998. A new antioxidative 1,3-benzodioxole from *Melissa officinalis*. *Planta Med* 64:555–558.

Vogt, H.J., I. Tausch, R.H. Wöbling, P.M. Kaiser. 1991. Melissenextrakt bei Herpes simplex. *Der Allgemeinarzt* 13:832–841.

Wöbling, R.H. and R. Milbradt. 1984. Klinik und Therapie des Herpes simplex. Vorstellung eines neuen phytotherapeutischen Wirkstoffes. *Therapiewoche* 34:1193–1200.

This material was adapted from *The Complete German Commission E Monographs—Therapeutic Guide to Herbal Medicines*. M. Blumenthal, W.R. Busse, A. Goldberg, J. Gruenwald, T. Hall, C.W. Riggins, R.S. Rister (eds.) S. Klein and R.S. Rister (trans.). 1998. Austin: American Botanical Council; Boston: Integrative Medicine Communications.

1) The Overview section is new information.

2) Description, Chemistry and Pharmacology, Uses, Contraindications, Side Effects, Interactions with Other Drugs, and Dosage sections have been drawn from the original work. Additional information has been added in some or all of these sections, as noted with references.

3) The dosage for equivalent preparations (tea infusion, fluidextract, and tincture) have been provided based on the following example:
   Unless otherwise prescribed: 2 g per day of [powdered, crushed, cut or whole] [plant part]
   Infusion: 2 g in 150 ml of water
   Fluidextract 1:1 (g/ml): 2 ml
   Tincture 1:5 (g/ml): 10 ml

4) The References and Additional Resources sections are new sections. Additional Resources are not cited in the monograph but are included for research purposes.

LICORICE ROOT

Latin Name:
Glycyrrhiza glabra

Pharmacopeial Name:
Liquiritiae radix

Other Names:
Liquorice, Gancao, Glycyrrhiza,
sweet root, Yasti-madhu

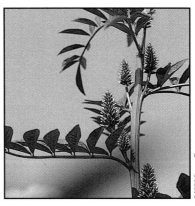

©1999 Steven Foster

Overview

Licorice is a perennial herb native to the Mediterranean region, central to southern Russia, and Asia Minor to Iran, now widely cultivated throughout Europe, the Middle East, and Asia. The material of commerce comes from wild plants and "semiwild" plants cultivated in the former U.S.S.R., Turkey, Greece, Iran, China, India, Pakistan, Afghanistan, Syria, Italy, and Spain (Bruneton, 1995; Karnick, 1994; Leung and Foster, 1996; Wichtl and Bisset, 1994). In the Chinese pharmacopeia, *Glycyrrhiza glabra*, *G. uralensis*, and *G. inflata* are officially recognized and are the species usually employed in commerce (Tu, 1992). Licorice is one of the most widely used medicinal herbs and is found in numerous traditional formulas (Leung and Foster, 1996). Until about 1000 C.E., licorice was collected in the wild. Its cultivation was first recorded by Piero de Cresenzi of Bologna in the thirteenth century. Cultivated roots are harvested after three to four years of growth. Its genus name, *Glycyrrhiza*, given by first century Greek physician Dioscorides, comes from *glukos* (sweet) and *riza* (root) (Foster and Yue, 1992; Grieve, 1979).

Licorice is one of the most extensively researched medicinal and food plants (Chandler, 1997). The roots and stolons contain glycyrrhizin (also knows as glycyrrhizic or glycyrrhizinic acid, about 5–9% by weight), a compound that is about 50 times sweeter than sucrose. Commercial extracts usually contain gycyrrhizin in its ammonium salt form. The sweet taste is reduced or lost in an acidic medium (Leung and Foster, 1996; Foster and Tyler, 1999). Licorice extracts are widely used to flavor food and liqueurs. Millions of pounds of licorice are imported into the United States each year, about 90% for use in flavoring tobacco products (Foster and Tyler, 1999).

Licorice root has been used therapeutically for several thousand years in both Western and Eastern systems of medicine (Bradley, 1992; Leung and Foster, 1996). A chronological, documented summary of its medical uses since 2100 B.C.E. to the present, with correlations to modern pharmacological research, has been published (Gibson, 1978). Its use is first documented in Assyrian clay tablets (ca. 2500 B.C.E.) and Egyptian papyri. It was used in ancient Arabia to treat coughs and to relieve the unwanted effects of laxatives (Bruneton, 1995). Its use in ancient Scythia spread to Greece. Greek natural scientist Theophrastus (ca. 372–287 B.C.E.) reported its use for dry cough, asthma, and all pectoral diseases (Grieve, 1979). Pliny the Elder (ca. 23–79 C.E.) reported licorice cleared the voice and had expectorant and carminative actions (Der Marderosian, 1999). In China, licorice is first mentioned in the *Shen Nong Ben Cao Jing* (ca. 25 C.E.), reconstructed "materia medica" from lost text attributed to Shen Nong Shi (ca. 3000 B.C.E.) (Foster and Yue, 1992). According to the Chinese pharmacopeia, licorice, either aqueous dry extract or hydroalcoholic fluidextract, is an abirritant, often used in combination with expectorants and antitussives to diminish irritation of the mucous membrane of the pharynx. It also relieves spasms of the gastrointestinal smooth muscle and shows desoxycorticosterone-like action (Tu, 1992). In India, licorice is used in traditional Ayurvedic, Siddha, and Unani medicines (Nadkarni, 1976). The present-day *Ayurvedic Pharmacopoeia* reports it is expectorant, demulcent, spasmolytic, antinflammatory, an adrenal agent, and a mild laxative (Karnick, 1994). It is also official in the *Indian Pharmacopoeia* as a demulcent (IP, 1996).

In Germany, licorice root is licensed as a standard medicinal tea for bronchitis and for chronic gastritis. It is also used in bronchial teas, stomach teas, and laxative teas available only in the pharmacy. Aqueous and alcoholic extracts of licorice root are used in many bronchial, gastrointestinal, liver and bile, and urological preparations. In the United States, licorice root is often a component of demulcent, expectorant, or laxative preparations (dietary supplement and OTC drug) in aqueous infusion, hydroalcoholic fluidextract and tincture, and solid dosage forms. Licorice root and extracts, fluid and solid, are official in the U.S. *National Formulary* (NF, 1985).

Many of the modern therapeutic uses of licorice were known in earlier times. Early claims for a broad spectrum of uses for licorice appear to be borne out by modern research (Gibson, 1978). Human studies have investigated efficacy in subacute hepatic failure (Acharya et al., 1993), chronic hepatitis C (Arase et al., 1997), infectious hepatitis (Chang and But, 1986), hemophilia with HIV-1 infection (Mori et al., 1990), and inhibition of HIV replication in patients with AIDS (Hattori et al., 1989). Studies have investigated its effects, in its traditional context as a component of multi-herb formulas, on testosterone secretion in patients with polycystic ovary syndrome (Takahashi et al., 1988), on treating anxiety (Chen et al., 1985), and on gastric and duodenal ulcer (Chang and But, 1986), among others. However, its use in combination formulas cannot determine definitively that the outcome of studies might not also be the result of the effects of other herbs in the formulas, and not attributable to the presence of the licorice alone.

Licorice preparations have been studied for possible benefits in treating digestive tract ulcers. In one clinical study, licorice root fluidextract was used to treat 100 patients with early peptic ulcer, of which 86 cases had been unresponsive to conventional treatment, at a dose of 15 ml four times daily for six weeks. Positive effects were reported in 90% of the cases, in 22 of which ulcer craters disappeared by X-ray examination and 28 others showed improvement. In subsequent studies, researchers reported that licorice powder at a dosage of 2.5–5.0 g three times daily was more effective than the fluidextract (Chang and But, 1986).

Reports in the literature of adverse effects of the consumption of excessive amounts of licorice (more than 20 g per day) have raised concerns about the potential for glycyrrhizin in licorice to produce pseudoaldesteronism (excessive levels of aldesterone, a hormone produced by the adrenalcortex) and resulting risks (headache, lethargy, sodium and water retention, hypertension, potassium loss that upsets the sodium-potassium balance, possibly resulting in cardiac problems, including cardiac arrest). The therapeutic uses and risks of licorice has been reviewed by Chandler (1997) and Stormer et al. (1993).

A deglycyrrhizinated licorice (DGL) preparation has been developed to provide some of the therapeutic benefits of licorice while reducing risk. A DGL preparation efficacy in treating duodenal and gastric ulcers in clinical trials (D'Imperio et al., 1978; Morgan et al., 1982). DGL may be useful in maintenance therapy for patients with gastric ulcers, although its superiority compared to conventional drugs has been questioned. In a two-year comparison study of a DGL product (Caved –S® tablets; two twice per day) and cimetidine, 400 mg at night, 12% (4 of 34) of the DGL subjects had ulcer recurrence compared with 10% (4 of 41) of the drug group in the first year of treatment; in the second year, 29% (9 of 31) for DGL and 25% (8 of 32) for cimetidine (Morgan et al., 1982). After termination of treatment in two years, ulcers recurred rapidly: 2 of 22 DGL patients and 7 of 23 cimetidine patients. The study concluded that long-term maintenance therapy was safe and reasonably effective.

DGL has shown success in treating duodenal gastric ulcers in clinical trials (D'Imperio et al., 1978; Morgan et al., 1982) although its superiority, compared to conventional drugs like cimetidine, has not been confirmed.

Glycyrrhizin itself, in a controlled dosage form with other natural products, has been investigated as a therapy for patients with human immuno-deficiency virus (HIV). One clinical study investigated the effects of glycyrrhizin (SNMC: stronger neo-minophagen C) in 42 hemophilia patients with HIV-1 infection. SNMC is made of 0.2% glycyrrhizin, 0.1% cysteine, and 2.0% glycine dissolved in a saline solution. Patients showed improvement in their clinical symptoms (oral candidiasis, lymph node swelling, rash), immunological functions, and liver functions (Mori et al., 1990). A subsequent study investigated the long-term efficacy of SNMC in 84 patients with chronic hepatitis C. Patients received 100 ml intravenously daily for eight weeks and then two to seven times a week for 2 to 16 years. A reduction in serum alanine aminotransferase (ALT) levels was reported in 34 of the 84 patients (35.7%). This trend toward stabilization of ALT levels was statistically significant. Hepatocellular carcinoma (HCC) in 30 patients with normal ALT levels was slightly lower than the 54 remaining patients with higher ALT scores (p=0.08). An increase in blood pressure was noted in 3 of the 84 patients. The authors concluded that the long-term administration of SNMC for chronic HCC is effective in reducing the risk of liver carcinogenesis (Arase et al., 1997).

The modern therapeutic applications for licorice root are supportable based on its use in well established systems of traditional medicine, on well documented phytochemical investigations, on pharmacological actions reported from *in vitro* and *in vivo* studies in animals, and on human clinical studies.

Pharmacopeial grade licorice root must contain not less than 4% glycyrrhizic acid, calculated on the dried root, and must pass a thin-layer chromatography (TLC) assay to show the presence of glycyrrhetic acid. Its water-soluble extractive content must be not less than 20% (Bruneton, 1995; IP, 1996; Ph.Eur.3, 1998; Ph.Fr.X., 1990; Wichtl and Bisset, 1994). The *Japanese Pharmacopoeia* also requires not less than 25% dilute ethanol-soluble extractive (JPXII, 1993).

Description

Licorice root consists of unpeeled, dried roots and stolons of *Glycyrrhiza glabra* L. [Fam. Fabaceae], and their preparations in effective dosage. The unpeeled roots contain at least 4% glycyrrhizic acid and 25% water-soluble matter. Licorice root also consists of the peeled, dried roots and stolons of G. glabra and their preparations in effective dosage. The peeled roots contain at least 20% water-soluble matter. The root contains flavanone and isoflavanone derivatives, potassium and calcium salts of glycyrrhizic acid, phytosterols, and coumarins.

Chemistry and Pharmacology

Licorice root contains triterpenoid saponins (4–24%), mostly glycyrrhizin,

a mixture of the potassium and calcium salts of glycyrrhizic acid; flavonoids (1%), mainly the flavanones liquiritin and liquiritigenin, chalcones isoliquiritin, isoliquiritigenin and isoflavonoids (formononetin); amines (1–2%) asparagine, betaine, and choline; amino acids; 3–15% glucose and sucrose; starch (2–30%); polysaccharides (arabinogalactans); sterols (β-sitosterol); coumarins (glycerin); resin; and volatile oils (0.047%) (Bruneton, 1995; Bradley, 1992; Budavari, 1996; Leung and Foster, 1996; List and Hörhammer, 1973–1979; Newall et al., 1996; Wichtl and Bisset, 1994). An extensive review of licorice chemistry has been published recently (Tang and Eisenbrand, 1992).

The Commission E reported that, according to controlled clinical studies, glycyrrhizic acid and the aglycone of glycyrrhizic acid accelerate the healing of gastric ulcers. Secretolytic and expectorant effects have been confirmed in tests on rabbits. In the isolated rabbit ileum, an antispasmodic action has been observed at concentrations of 1:2500–1:5000.

The *British Herbal Compendium* reported its actions as anti-inflammatory, expectorant, demulcent, and adrenocorticotropic (Bradley, 1992).

The pseudo-aldosterone-like effects are generally attributed to the glycyrrhizic acid. New research suggests that the glycyrrhetenic acid, the hydrolytic metabolite of glycyrrhizic acid, is the primary active component that causes inhibition of peripheral metabolism of corticol, which binds to mineralocorticoid receptors in the same way as aldosterone (Heikens et al., 1995).

Research suggests two hypotheses for licorice's mechanism of action: binding of glycyrretinic acid to mineralocorticoid receptors and blocking the action of 11-beta-hydroxysteroid dehydrogenase. Recent publications suggest that both may be involved, especially with the confirmation that the blocking of the 11-beta-hydroxysteroid dehydrogenase is temporary and that after this occurs, the pseudoaldesteronism is directly related to increased plasma concentration of licorice metabolites and their binding to mineralocorticoid receptors. Glucocorticoids are usually rapidly metabolized into inactive compounds by 11-beta-hydroxysteroid dehydrogenase, thus controlling glucocorticoid access to mineralocorticoid and glucocorticoid receptors. When licorice prevents the inactivation of hydrocortisone, the result is increased glucocorticoid concentration in mineralocorticoid-responsive tissues, thus resulting in glucocorticoids' occupying mineralocorticoid receptors and producing a mineralocorticoid response, as shown by increased sodium retention and hypertension (Chandler, 1997).

Uses

The Commission E approved the internal use of licorice root for catarrhs of the upper respiratory tract and gastric or duodenal ulcers.

The *British Herbal Compendium* indicates its use for bronchitis, peptic ulcer, chronic gastritis, rheumatism and arthritis, and adrenocorticoid insufficiency (Bradley, 1992). The German Standard License approves licorice root infusions for loosening mucus, alleviating discharge in bronchitis, and as an adjuvant in treating spasmodic pains of chronic gastritis (Bradley, 1992; Braun et al., 1997; Wichtl and Bisset, 1994). In France, licorice preparations may be used to treat epigastric bloating, impaired digestion, and flatulence (Bruneton, 1995).

The World Health Organization recognizes no uses for licorice as being supported by clinical data; WHO recognizes the following uses as being described in pharmacopeias and in traditional systems of medicine: demulcent for sore throats; expectorant in treatment of coughs and bronchial catarrh; prophylaxis and treatment of gastric and duodenal ulcers; used in dyspepsia; anti-inflammatory in treating allergic reactions, rheumatism, and arthritis; to prevent liver toxicity; and to treat tuberculosis and adrenocorticoid insufficiency (WHO, 1999).

Contraindications

Cholestatic liver disorders, liver cirrhosis, hypertonia, hypokalemia, severe kidney insufficiency.

Side Effects

On prolonged use and with higher doses, sodium and water retention and potassium loss may occur, accompanied by hypertension, edema, hypokalemia, and, in rare cases, myoglobinuria. [Ed. Note: Within several weeks of discontinuing use, any symptoms of hyperaldosteronism disappear (Mantero, 1981).]

Use During Pregnancy and Lactation

Not recommended during pregnancy (McGuffin et al., 1997). No restrictions known during lactation.

Interactions with Other Drugs

Potassium loss due to other drugs, e.g., thiazide diuretics, can be increased. With potassium loss, sensitivity to digitalis glycosides increases.

Dosage and Administration

Unless otherwise prescribed: About 5–15 g per day of cut or powdered root, or dry extracts equivalent to 200–600 mg of glycyrrhizin.

Succus liquiritiae: 0.5–1.0 ml for catarrhs of the upper respiratory tract, 1.5–3.0 ml for gastric or duodenal ulcers.

Infusion or decoction: 2–4 g in 150 ml water, after meals three times daily.

Fluidextract 1:1 (g/ml): 2–4 ml, after meals three times daily.

Native dry extract 5–6:1 (w/w): 0.33–0.8 g, after meals three times daily.

DGL tablets (380 mg DGL 4:1): acute cases (gastric or duodenal ulcers): chew 2–4 tablet before each meal; chronic cases: chew 1–2 tablets before meals (Murray and Pizzorno, 1998).

Duration of administration: Not longer than four to six weeks without medical advice. There is no objection to using licorice root as a flavoring agent up to a maximum daily dosage equivalent to 100 mg glycyrrhizin.

References

Acharya, S.K., S. Dasarathy, A. Tandon, Y.K. Joshi, B.N. Tandon. 1993. A preliminary open trial on interferon stimulator (SNMC) derived from *Glycyrrhiza glabra* in the treatment of subacute hepatic failure. *Indian J Med Res* 98:69–74.

Arase, Y. et al. 1997. The long term efficacy of glycyrrhizin in chronic hepatitis C patients. *Cancer* 79(8):1494–1500.

Bradley, P.R. (ed.). 1992. *British Herbal Compendium*, Vol. 1. Bournemouth: British Herbal Medicine Association.

Braun, R. et al. 1997. *Standardzulassungen für Fertigarzneimittel—Text und Kommentar*. Stuttgart: Deutscher Apotheker Verlag.

Bruneton, J. 1995. *Pharmacognosy, Phytochemistry, Medicinal Plants*. Paris: Lavoisier Publishing.

Budavari, S. (ed.). 1996. *The Merck Index: An Encyclopedia of Chemicals, Drugs, and Biologicals,* 12th ed. Whitehouse Station, N.J.: Merck & Co, Inc.

Chandler, R.F. *Glycyrrhiza Glabra*. De Smet, P.A., K. Keller, Hänsel R., Chandler, R.F. (eds.). 1997. *Adverse Effects of Herbal Drugs*, Vol. 3. New York: Springer Verlag.

Chang, H.M. and P.P.H. But (eds.). 1986. *Pharmacology and Applications of Chinese Materia Medica*, Vol. 1. Philadelphia: World Scientific. 304–316.

Chen, H.C., M.T. Hsieh, E. Lai. 1985. Studies on the Suanzaorentang in the treatment of anxiety. *Psychopharm* (Berl) 85(4):486–487.

Der Marderosian, A. (ed.). 1999. *The Review of Natural Products*. St. Louis: Facts and Comparisons.

D'Imperio, N. G.G. Piccari, F. Sarti, et al. 1978. Double-blind trial in duodenal and gastric ulcers. *Acta Gastro-Enterologica Belgica* 41:427–434.

Europäisches Arzneibuch, 3rd ed., 1st suppl. (Ph.Eur.3). 1998. Stuttgart: Deutscher Apotheker Verlag. 622–623.

Foster, S. and V.E. Tyler. 1999. *Tyler's Honest Herbal: A Sensible Guide to the Use of Herbs and Related Remedies*. New York: Haworth Herbal Press. 241–243.

Foster, S. and C. Yue. 1992. *Herbal Emissaries Bringing Chinese Herbs to the West*. Rochester, VT: Healing Arts Press. 112–121.

Gibson, M.R. 1978. Glycyrrhiza in old and new perspectives. *Lloydia* 41(4):348–354.

Grieve, M. 1979. *A Modern Herbal*. New York: Dover Publications, Inc.

Hattori, T. et al. 1989. Preliminary evidence for inhibitory effect of glycyrrhizin on HIV replication in patients with AIDS. *Antiviral Res* 11(5–6):255–262.

Heikens, J., E. Fliers, E. Endert, M. Ackermans, G. van Montfrans. 1995. Liquorice-induced hypertension—a new understanding of an old disease: case report and brief review. *Neth J Med* 47(5):230–234.

Indian Pharmacopoeia, Vol. 1. (IP). 1996. Delhi: Government of India Ministry of Health and Family Welfare—Controller of Publications. 440–442.

Japanese Pharmacopoeia, 12th ed. (JP XII). 1993. Tokyo: Government of Japan Ministry of Health and Welfare—Yakuji Nippo, Ltd. 130–133.

Karnick, C.R. 1994. *Pharmacopoeial Standards of Herbal Plants*, Vols. 1–2. Delhi: Sri Satguru Publications. Vol. 1:158–159; Vol. 2:86.

Leung, A.Y. and S. Foster. 1996. *Encyclopedia of Common Natural Ingredients Used in Food, Drugs, and Cosmetics*, 2nd ed. New York: John Wiley & Sons, Inc.

List, P.H. and L. Hörhammer (eds.). 1973–1979. *Hagers Handbuch der Pharmazeutischen Praxis*, Vols. 1–7. New York: Springer Verlag.

Mantero, F. 1981. Exogenous mineralocorticoid-like disorders. *Clin Endocrinol Metab* 10(3): 465–478.

McGuffin, M., C. Hobbs, R. Upton, A. Goldberg. 1997. American Herbal Product Association's *Botanical Safety Handbook*. Boca Raton: CRC Press.

Morgan, A.G., W.A. McAdam, C. Pacsoo, A. Darnborough. 1982. Comparison between cimetidine and Caved-S® in the treatment of gastric ulceration, and subsequent maintenance therapy. *Gut* 23(6):545–551.

Murray, M. and J. Pizzorno. 1998. *Encyclopedia of Natural Medicine*. Rocklin, CA: Prima Publishing. 817.

Mori, K. et al. 1990. Effects of glycyrrhizin (SNMC: stronger neo-minophagen C) in hemophilia patients with HIV-1 infection. *Tohoku J Exp Med* 162(2):183–193.

Nadkarni, K.M. 1976. *Indian Materia Medica*. Bombay: Popular Prakashan. 582–584.

National Formulary (NF), 16th ed. 1985. Washington, D.C.: American Pharmaceutical Association.

Newall, C.A., L.A. Anderson, J.D. Phillipson. 1996. *Herbal Medicines: A Guide for Health-Care Professionals*. London: The Pharmaceutical Press.

Pharmacopée Française Xe Édition (Ph.Fr.X.). 1983–1990. Moulins-les-Metz: Maisonneuve S.A.

Ph.Eur.3. See *Européisches Arzneibuch*.

Stormer, F.C., R. Reistad, J. Alexander. 1993. Glycyrrhizic acid in liquorice—evaluation of health hazard. *Food and Chemical Toxicology* 31(4):303–312.

Takahashi, K. et al. 1988. Effect of a traditional herbal medicine (shakuyaku-kanzo-to) on testosterone secretion in patients with polycystic ovary syndrome detected by ultrasound. *Nippon Sanka Fujinka Gakkai Zasshi* 40(6):789–792.

Tang, W. and G. Eisenbrand. 1992. *Chinese Drugs of Plant Origin: Chemistry, Pharmacology, and Use in Traditional and Modern Medicine*. New York: Springer Verlag.

Tu, G. (ed.). 1992. *Pharmacopoeia of the People's Republic of China* (English Edition 1992). Beijing: Guangdong Science and Technology Press. 118–119.

WHO. See World Health Organization.

Wichtl, M. and N.G. Bisset (eds.). 1994. *Herbal Drugs and Phytopharmaceuticals*. Stuttgart: Medpharm Scientific Publishers.

World Health Organization. 1999. "Radix Glycyrrhizae." *WHO Monographs on Selected Medicinal Plants*, Vol. 1. Geneva: World Health Organization. 183–194.

Additional Resources

Bardhan, K.D., D.C. Cumberland, R.A. Dixon, C.D. Holdsworth. 1976. Deglycyrrhizinated liquorice in gastric ulcer: a double blind controlled study. *Gut* 17(5):397.

Bensky, D. and A. Gamble.1993. *Chinese Herbal Medicine*. Seattle: Eastland Press, Inc. 323–325.

British Pharmaceutical Codex (BPC). 1973. London: The Pharmaceutical Press.

British Pharmacopoeia (BP). 1988. (With subsequent Addenda up to 1992.) London: Her Majesty's Stationery Office.

Deutsches Arzneibuch, 9th ed. (DAB 9). 1986. Stuttgart: Deutscher Apotheker Verlag.

Deutscher Arzneimittel-Codex (DAC). 1986. Stuttgart: Deutscher Apotheker Verlag.

Engqvist, A., F. von Feilitzen, E. Pyke, H. Reichard. 1973. Double-blind trial of deglycyrrhizinated liquorice in gastric ulcer. *Gut* 14(9):711–715.

Hartke, K. and E. Mutschler (eds.). 1988. DAB 9—*Kommentar: Deutsches Arzneibuch* 9, Vol. 3. Stuttgart: Wissenschaftliche Verlagsgesellschaft. 3187–3192.

Ming, O. (ed.). 1989. *Chinese-English Manual of Common-Used in Traditional Chinese Medicine*. Hong Kong: Joint Publishing (H.K.) Co., Ltd. 127–129.

Morton, J.F. 1977. *Major Medicinal Plants: Botany, Culture and Uses*. Springfield, IL: Charles C. Thomas. 155–158.

This material was adapted from *The Complete German Commission E Monographs—Therapeutic Guide to Herbal Medicines*. M. Blumenthal, W.R. Busse, A. Goldberg, J. Gruenwald, T. Hall, C.W. Riggins, R.S. Rister (eds.) S. Klein and R.S. Rister (trans.). 1998. Austin: American Botanical Council; Boston: Integrative Medicine Communications.

1) The Overview section is new information.

2) Description, Chemistry and Pharmacology, Uses, Contraindications, Side Effects, Interactions with Other Drugs, and Dosage sections have been drawn from the original work. Additional information has been added in some or all of these sections, as noted with references.

3) The dosage for equivalent preparations (tea infusion, fluidextract, and tincture) have been provided based on the following example:
   Unless otherwise prescribed: 2 g per day of [powdered, crushed, cut or whole] [plant part]
   Infusion: 2 g in 150 ml of water
   Fluidextract 1:1 (g/ml): 2 ml
   Tincture 1:5 (g/ml): 10 ml

4) The References and Additional Resources sections are new sections. Additional Resources are not cited in the monograph but are included for research purposes.

Pharmacopoeia Helvetica, 7th ed. Vol. 1–4. (Ph.Helv.VII). 1987. Bern: Office Central Fédéral des Imprimés et du Matériel.

Rees, W.D., J. Rhodes, J.E. Wright, L.F. Stamford, A. Bennett. 1979. Effect of deglycyrrhizinated liquorice on gastric mucosal damage by aspirin. Scand J *Gastroenterol* 14(5):605–607.

Reynolds, J.E.F. (ed.). 1989. *Martindale: The Extra Pharmacopoeia,* 29th ed. London: The Pharmaceutical Press.

Trease, G.E. and W.C. Evans. 1989. *Trease and Evans' Pharmacognosy,* 13th ed. London; Philadelphia: Baillière Tindall.

Yen, K.Y. 1992. *The Illustrated Chinese Materia Medica—Crude and Prepared.* Taipei: SMC Publishing, Inc. 42.

LINDEN FLOWER

Latin Name:
Tilia cordata

Pharmacopeial Name:
Tiliae flos

Other Names:
large leafed linden, lime tree flower

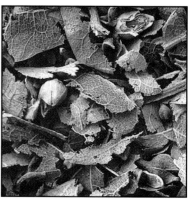

©1999 Steven Foster

Overview

Linden is a tall deciduous tree native throughout Europe as far north as 65° in latitude. It is also cultivated in Europe and North America (List and Hörhammer,
1979; Wichtl and Bisset, 1994). The material of commerce comes mainly from Bulgaria, Romania, Turkey, the former Yugoslavia, and in part from China (BHP, 1996;
Wichtl and Bisset, 1994). The trees can grow to be as tall as one hundred feet. The
two species from which the flower is primarily harvested, *Tilia cordata* and *T.
platypus,* are referred to as small-leaved linden and large-leaved linden, respectively. These species are preferred because the tannin and mucilage content in their
flowers produce more flavorful teas and extracts (Tyler, 1993). Traditionally, linden
flowers were used to soothe nerves and to treat conditions associated with anxiety.
Flowers were added to baths to quell hysteria, and steeped as a tea to relieve anxi-
ety-related indigestion, heart palpitation, and vomiting (Grieve, 1979). Linden's
primary use since the Middle Ages, however, has been as a diaphoretic to promote
perspiration (Tyler, 1993).

In Germany, linden flower is official in the *German Pharmacopoeia,* approved
in the Commission E monographs, and the tea form is official in the German
Standard License monographs (BAnz, 1998; Bradley, 1992; Braun, et al. 1997;
DAB 10, 1991; Wichtl and Bisset, 1994). It was also official in the pharmacopeia
of the former German Democratic Republic (DAB 7–DDR, 1972; List and
Hörhammer, 1979; Wagner et al., 1984). It is used as a component of common
cold and antitussive preparations and also used in urological and sedative drugs
(Wichtl and Bisset, 1994). In German pediatric medicine, it is used as a
diaphoretic component of an influenza tea for children comprised of linden
flower, willow bark, meadow-sweet flower, chamomile flower, and bitter orange
peel. It is also a primary component of "Schweisstreibender Tee" (diaphoretic tea)
composed of linden flower, peppermint leaf, meadowsweet flower, and bitter
orange (Schilcher, 1997). The pharmacopeia of Switzerland lists a comparable
diaphoretic tea composed of linden, elder flower, mint leaves, and jaborandi leaf
(List and Hörhammer, 1979; Ph.Helv.VI, 1971).

The approved modern therapeutic applications for linden flower are based on
its long history of use in well established systems of traditional and conventional
medicine, *in vitro* pharmacological studies and on its well documented chemical
composition.

Pharmacopeial grade linden flower consists of the whole, dried inflorescence of
T. cordata Mill., of *T. platyphyllos* Scop., of *T. x vulgaris* Hayne, or a mixture of
these species. It must have a swelling index of not less than 32. Botanical identity is
confirmed by thin-layer chromatography (TLC), macroscopic and microscopic
examinations, organoleptic assessment, as well as a UV spectrophotometry test for
total flavonoids. Microscopic and organoleptic tests are also used for detection of

adulteration by other species (e.g., *T. argentea*), which is common (DAB 10, 1991; List and Hörhammer, 1979; Ph.Eur.3., 1997; Wichtl and Bisset, 1994). Linden should contain not less than 15% water-soluble extractive (BHP, 1990; Wichtl and Bisset, 1994). The pharmacopeia of Hungary requires not less than 18% water-soluble extractive (List and Hörhammer, 1979).

Description

Linden flower consists of the dried flower of *T. cordata* Miller and/or *T. platyphyllos* Scopoli [Fam. Tiliaceae] and its preparations in effective dosage. The flower contains flavonoids, tannins, and mucilage.

Chemistry and Pharmacology

Linden flower contains 3–10% mucilage polysaccharides, mainly arabinogalactans and uronic acids; approximately 2% condensed tannins (procyanidin dimers B-2 and B-2); approximately 1% flavonoids, mainly quercetin glycosides (rutin, hyperoside, quercitrin, isoquercitrin) and also kaempferol glycosides (astragalin); phenolic acids (caffeic, p-coumaric, and chlorogenic acids); and 0.02–0.1% essential oil containing alkanes and monoterpenes (Bradley, 1992; List and Hörhammer, 1979; Newall et al., 1996; Wichtl and Bisset, 1994).

The Commission E reported diaphoretic activity.

The *British Herbal Compendium* reported antispasmodic, diaphoretic, sedative, hypotensive, emollient, and mildly astringent actions (Bradley, 1992). The flavonoids and phenols in the flowers are reportedly diaphoretic *in vitro*. A substance occurring in linden flower volatile oil, farnesol, demonstrates some sedative and antispasmodic activity on rat duodenum *in vitro* (Lanza and Steinmetz, 1986). Although it is present only in small amounts in linden extracts, it may be therapeutically active (Taddei et al., 1988). In initial, experimental tests, both hypotensive and vasodilative actions were noted in animals receiving linden flower extract intravenously. Their heart rate increased and cardiac muscle tone relaxed (Bradley, 1992). This effect on the heart has been a matter of some concern. In excess amounts, linden flower is known to be cardiotoxic (Pahlow, 1979; Newall et al., 1996; Tyler, 1993).

Uses

The Commission E approved linden flower for colds and cold-related coughs.

The *British Herbal Compendium* indicates its use for upper respiratory catarrh, common colds, irritable coughs, hypertension, and restlessness (Bradley, 1992). The German Standard License for linden flower infusion indicates its use for alleviation of cough irritation due to catarrh of the respiratory tract and for feverish colds for which a sweat treatment is desired (Bradley, 1992; Braun et al., 1997; Wichtl and Bisset, 1994).

Contraindications

None known.

Side Effects

None known.

Use During Pregnancy and Lactation

No restrictions known.

Interactions with Other Drugs

None known.

Dosage and Administration

Unless otherwise prescribed: 2–4 g per day of cut herb for teas and other galenical preparations for internal use. Infusion: Steep 1.8–2.0 g flower in 150 ml boiled water for 10 to 15 minutes, once or twice daily (Braun et al., 1997;

Meyer-Buchtela, 1999). [Note: After 2.5 minutes of steeping, 17% of the available flavonoids are yielded into the tea; after 10 minutes, 19% are released (Meyer-Buchtela, 1999)].
Cold infusion: Soak 1.8–2.0 g flower in 150 ml cold water for 10 to 15 minutes, then bring to a boil before drinking, once or twice daily.
Fluidextract 1:1 (g/ml): 2 ml, once or twice daily.
Tincture 1:5 (g/ml): 10 ml, once or twice daily.

References

BAnz. See *Bundesanzeiger*.

Bradley, P.R. (ed.). 1992. *British Herbal Compendium*, Vol. 1. Bournemouth: British Herbal Medicine Association.

Braun, R. et al. 1997. *Standardzulassungen für Fertigarzneimittel—Text and Kommentar*. Stuttgart: Deutscher Apotheker Verlag.

British Herbal Pharmacopoeia (BHP). 1996. Exeter, U.K.: British Herbal Medicine Association. 122.

———. 1990. Bournemouth, U.K.: British Herbal Medicine Association.

Bundesanzeiger (BAnz). 1998. Monographien der Kommission E (Zulassungs- und Aufbereitungskommission am BGA für den humanmed. Bereich, phytotherapeutische Therapierichtung und Stoffgruppe). Köln: Bundesgesundheitsamt (BGA).

Deutsches Arzneibuch, 10th ed. (DAB 10). 1991. Stuttgart: Deutscher Apotheker Verlag.

Deutsches Arzneibuch der Deutsche Demokratische Republik, 7th ed. (DAB-DDR). 1972. Berlin: Akademie Verlag.

Europäisches Arzneibuch, 3rd ed. (Ph.Eur.3). 1997. Stuttgart: Deutscher Apotheker Verlag. 1197-1198.

Grieve, M. 1979. *A Modern Herbal*. New York: Dover Publications, Inc.

Lanza, J.P. and M. Steinmetz. 1986. Actions comparees des exraits aqueux de graines de *Tilia platyphylla* et de *Tilia vulgaris* sur l'intestin isole de rat. *Fitoterapia* (57):185.

List, P.H. and L. Hörhammer (eds.). 1979. *Hagers Handbuch der Pharmazeutischen Praxis*, 4th ed., Vol. 6, Part C:T–Z. Berlin-Heidelberg: Springer Verlag. 180–184.

Meyer-Buchtela, E. 1999. *Tee-Rezepturen—Ein Handbuch für Apotheker und Ärzte*. Stuttgart: Deutscher Apotheker Verlag.

Newall, C.A., L.A. Anderson, J.D. Phillipson. 1996. *Herbal Medicines: A Guide for Health-Care Professionals*. London: The Pharmaceutical Press.

Pahlow, M. 1979. *Das Grosse Buch der Heilpflanzen*. Munich: Grafe und Unzer.

Pharmacopoeia Helvetica, 6th ed. (Ph.Helv.VI). 1971. Bern: Office Central Fédéral des Imprimés et du Matériel.

Ph.Eur.3. See *Europäisches Arzneibuch*.

Schilcher, H. 1997. *Phytotherapy in Paediatrics: Handbook for Physicians and Pharmacists*. Stuttgart: Medpharm Scientific Publishers. 41–42.

Taddei, I. et al. 1988. Spasmolytic activity of peppermint, sage, and rosemary essences and their major constituents. *Fitoterapia* (59):463–468.

Tyler, V.E. 1993. *The Honest Herbal*, 3rd ed. New York: Pharmaceutical Products Press.

Wagner, H., S. Bladt, E.M. Zgainski. 1984. *Plant Drug Analysis—A Thin Layer Chromatography Atlas*. Berlin-Heidelberg: Springer Verlag. 167.

Wichtl, M. and N.G. Bisset (eds.). 1994. *Herbal Drugs and Phytopharmaceuticals*. Stuttgart: Medpharm Scientific Publishers.

Additional Resources

Benigni, R., C. Capra, P.E. Cattorini. 1964. *Piante Medicinali—Cemica, farmacologia e Terapia*, Vol. 2. Milan: Inverni & Della Beffa.

Bezanger-Beauquesne, L. et al. 1980. *Plantes Medicinales des Regions Temperees*. Paris: Maloine S.A.

This material was adapted from *The Complete German Commission E Monographs—Therapeutic Guide to Herbal Medicines*. M. Blumenthal, W.R. Busse, A. Goldberg, J. Gruenwald, T. Hall, C.W. Riggins, R.S. Rister (eds.) S. Klein and R.S. Rister (trans.). 1998. Austin: American Botanical Council; Boston: Integrative Medicine Communications.

1) The Overview section is new information.
2) Description, Chemistry and Pharmacology, Uses, Contraindications, Side Effects, Interactions with Other Drugs, and Dosage sections have been drawn from the original work. Additional information has been added in some or all of these sections, as noted with references.
3) The dosage for equivalent preparations (tea infusion, fluidextract, and tincture) have been provided based on the following example:
   Unless otherwise prescribed: 2 g per day of [powdered, crushed, cut or whole] [plant part]
   Infusion: 2 g in 150 ml of water
   Fluidextract 1:1 (g/ml): 2 ml
   Tincture 1:5 (g/ml): 10 ml
4) The References and Additional Resources sections are new sections. Additional Resources are not cited in the monograph but are included for research purposes.

British Herbal Pharmacopoeia (BHP). 1983. Keighley, U.K.: British Herbal Medicine Association.

British Pharmaceutical Codex (BPC). 1949. London: The Pharmaceutical Press.

Bruneton, J. 1995. *Pharmacognosy, Phytochemistry, Medicinal Plants.* Paris: Lavoisier Publishing.

Deutsches Arzneibuch, 10th ed. Vol. 1–6. (DAB 10). 1991. Kommentar. Stuttgart: Wissenschaftliche Verlagsgesellschaft.

Duquenois, P.A. 1977. Retrospective sur les Hydrolats de Tilleul, Narcisse, Bourrache et Primevere. [French/English summary]. *Quart J Crude Drug Res* (15):203–211.

Guerin, J-C. and H-P. Reveillere. 1984. [Antifungal activity of plant extracts used therapeutically. Study of 41 plant extracts against 9 fungi species] [In French]. *Ann Pharm Fr* 42(6):553–559.

Österreichisches Arzneibuch, Vols. 1–2, 1st suppl. (ÖAB). 1981–1983. Wien: Verlag der Österreichischen Staatsdruckerei.

Pharmacopoeia Helvetica, 7th ed. Vol. 1–4. (Ph.Helv.VII). 1987. Bern: Office Central Fédéral des Imprimés et du Matériel.

Pharmacopoeia Hungarica, 7th ed. 1986. Budapest: Medicina Konyvkiado.

Reynolds, J.E.F. (ed.). 1989. *Martindale: The Extra Pharmacopoeia*, 29th ed. London: The Pharmaceutical Press.

Schmersahl, K.J. 1964. Über die Wirkstoffe der Diaphoretischen Drogen des DAB 6. *Naturwissenschaften* (51):361.

State Pharmacopoeia of the Union of Soviet Socialist Republics, 10th ed. 1973. [English Version]. Moscow: Ministry of Health of the U.S.S.R.

Sticher, O. 1977. *New Natural Products with Pharmacological, Biological or Therapeutical Activity*. Berlin: Springer Verlag.

Svendsen, A.B. and J.J.C. Scheffer. 1984. *Essential oils and aromatic plants*. Proceedings of the 15th international symposium on essential oils. Dordrecht: Martinus Nijhoff.

MARSHMALLOW:

MARSHMALLOW LEAF
(page 245)

MARSHMALLOW ROOT
(page 246)

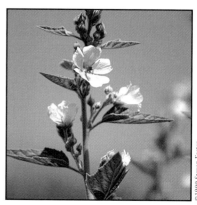

© 1999 Steven Foster

Overview

Marshmallow is a perennial herb native throughout damp areas of Europe and western Asia, naturalized in North America in salt marshes from Massachusetts to Virginia, now cultivated from western Europe to Russia (Karnick, 1994; Leung and Foster, 1996; Wichtl and Bisset, 1994). The material of commerce is harvested from cultivated plants mainly from Belgium, Bulgaria, Hungary, the former Yugoslavia, and the former U.S.S.R. (BHP, 1996; Wichtl and Bisset, 1994). The plant must be at least two years old before harvesting the roots (Bradley, 1992). In Germany, marshmallow is listed in Annex 1 of the German Federal Ordinance on the Conservation of Species (BArtSchV) and a permit is necessary for import or export of any wild-collected material (Lange and Schippmann, 1997).

Marshmallow has been used in traditional European medicines for more than two thousand years (Leung and Foster, 1996). Its therapeutic use was first recorded in the ninth century B.C.E.; it was widely used in Greek medicine (Bown, 1995). Its genus name *Althaea* comes from the Greek *altho*, to cure, and its order name, *Malvaceae*, is derived from the Greek *malake*, soft (Grieve, 1979). Its use in traditional Greek medicine spread to Arabian medicine and to traditional Indian Ayurvedic and Unani medicines. Early Arab physicians prepared a poultice with the leaves to suppress inflammation. The present day *Ayurvedic Pharmacopoeia* reports its actions as demulcent, diuretic, emollient, and vulnerary (Karnick, 1994).

In Germany, marshmallow root and leaf are both licensed as standard medicinal teas. The root is also used as a component of a few prepared cough tea and cough syrup medicines. In the United States, marshmallow is used as a component of dietary supplement antitussive and demulcent preparations. Marshmallow root and extract were formerly official in the *United States Pharmacopeia* and the *National Formulary*.

The approved modern therapeutic applications for marshmallow are supportable based on its history of use in well established systems of traditional medicine, on phytochemical investigations, and *in vitro* studies and *in vivo* experiments in animals.

Pharmacopeial grade marshmallow leaf must have a swelling index of not less than 12 and pass botanical identification by macroscopic and microscopic authentication (DAC, 1986; ÖAB, 1981). The *British Herbal Pharmacopoeia* requires marshmallow leaf to be harvested before the flowering period, pass identification by thin-layer chromatography (TLC), and conform with additional quantitative standards, including water-soluble extractive not less than 15% (BHP, 1996).

Pharmacopeial grade marshmallow root, peeled or unpeeled, must have a swelling index of not less than 10, with the pulverized root, and pass macroscopic and microscopic authentication tests (DAB, 1997; ÖAB, 1981; Ph.Eur.3, 1998; Wichtl and Bisset, 1994). The *British Herbal Pharmacopoeia* requires peeled marshmallow root to pass botanical identification by a TLC method, plus additional quantitative standards, including not less than 22% water-soluble extractive, calculated with reference to the oven-dried material (BHP, 1996). The *Swiss Pharmacopoeia* requires a swelling index of not less than 15 (Ph.Helv.VII, 1987; Wichtl and Bisset, 1994).

MARSHMALLOW LEAF

Latin Name:
Althaea officinalis

Pharmacopeial Name:
Althaeae folium

Other Names:
Althaea leaf, Althea leaf

Description
Marshmallow leaf consists of the dried leaf of *Althaea officinalis* L. [Fam. Malvaceae], and its preparations in effective dosage. The preparation contains mucilage.

Chemistry and Pharmacology
Marshmallow leaf contains mucilage polysaccharides (6–9%) composed of arabinogalactans and galacturonorhamnans; flavonoids 8-hydroxyluteolin and 8-β-gentiobioside; phenolic acids; tannins; and volatile oil (List and Hörhammer, 1973–1979; Newall et al., 1996; Wichtl and Bisset, 1994).

The Commission E reported that it acts to alleviate local irritation.

The *British Herbal Pharmacopoeia* reported that it acts as a demulcent (BHP, 1996). Its major constituent is mucilage, which supports the reputed demulcent action (Newall et al., 1996).

Uses
The Commission E approved the internal use of marshmallow leaf for irritation of the oral and pharyngeal mucosa and associated dry cough.

The German Standard License for marshmallow leaf tea indicates its use to alleviate irritation of the mucous membranes of the mouth and throat and the gastrointestinal tract; and to ease irritation of the throat in bronchial catarrh (Wichtl and Bisset, 1994). It is used traditionally to treat respiratory catarrh and cough, and inflammation of the mouth and pharynx (Newall et al., 1996).

Contraindications
None known.

Side Effects
None known.

Use During Pregnancy and Lactation
No restrictions known.

Interactions with Other Drugs
Absorption of other drugs taken simultaneously may be delayed.

Dosage and Administration
Unless otherwise prescribed: 5 g per day of cut leaf.
Infusion: 1–2 g in 150 ml boiled water, two to three times daily.
Cold maceration: 1–2 g in 150 ml cold water for 60 minutes stirring occasion-

ally; strain and warm before drinking, two to three times daily.
Fluidextract 1:1 (g/ml): 1–2 ml, two to three times daily.

Tincture 1:5 (g/ml): 5–10 ml, two to three times daily.

MARSHMALLOW ROOT

Latin Name:
Althaea officinalis

Pharmacopeial Name:
Althaeae radix

Other Names:
Althaea root, Althea root

Description
Marshmallow root consists of the dried root, unpeeled or peeled, of *Althaea officinalis* L. [Fam. Malvaceae], and its preparations in effective dosage.

Chemistry and Pharmacology
Marshmallow root contains mucilage polysaccharides (6.2–11.6%) composed of galacturonorhamnans, arabinans, glucans, and arabinogalactans; carbohydrates (25–35% starch, 11% pectin); the flavonoid glycosides kaempferol and quercetin; caffeic, chlorogenic, ferulic, and syringic phenolic acids; tannins; sugars (10% sucrose); amines (up to 2% asparagine); fat (1.7%); calcium oxalate; coumarins; and sterols (Bradley, 1992; ESCOP, 1997; Leung and Foster, 1996; List and Hörhammer, 1973–1979; Newall et al., 1996; Wichtl and Bisset, 1994).

The Commission E reported that it alleviates local irritation, inhibits mucociliary activity, and stimulates phagocytosis.

The *British Herbal Compendium* reported its actions internally as demulcent and topically as emollient and vulnerary (Bradley, 1992). The mucilage from marshmallow root coats the mucosa, protecting them from local irritations (ESCOP, 1997).

Uses
The Commission E approved the internal use of marshmallow root for irritation of the oral and pharyngeal mucosa and associated dry cough, and for mild inflammation of the gastric mucosa.

The *British Herbal Compendium* indicates its use internally for gastroenteritis, peptic and duodenal ulceration, common and ulcerative colitis, and enteritis. Topically: as a mouthwash or gargle for inflammation of the mouth and pharynx; as a poultice or ointment/cream in furunculosis, eczema and dermatitis (Bradley, 1992). ESCOP lists its use for dry cough and irritations of the oral, pharyngeal, or gastric mucosa (ESCOP, 1997). The German Standard License for marshmallow root tea approves its use for soothing of irritation from mucosal inflammations in the mouth and pharynx, upper respiratory tract, and gastrointestinal tract (Bradley, 1992; Wichtl and Bisset, 1994).

Contraindications
None known.

Side Effects
None known.

Use During Pregnancy and Lactation

No restrictions known.

Interactions with Other Drugs

The absorption of other drugs taken simultaneously may be delayed.

Dosage and Administration

Unless otherwise prescribed: 6 g per day of cut or ground root.

Cold maceration: 2–5 g in 150 ml cold water for 30 minutes stirring frequently; strain and warm before drinking, up to three times daily.

Dried root: 2–5 g, up to three times daily.

Fluidextract 1:1 (g/ml): 2–5 ml, up to three times daily.

Tincture 1:5 (g/ml): 10–25 ml, up to three times daily.

Native dry extract 3.5–5.0:1 (w/w): 0.4–0.6 g, up to three times daily.

Native soft extract 2.3–3.2:1 (w/w): 0.6–0.9 g, up to three times daily.

Syrupus Althaeae: Single dose: 10 ml, to be used only in treating throat irritation.

Note: Marshmallow syrup: diabetics need to allow for sugar concentration.

References

Bown, D. 1995. *Encyclopedia of Herbs and Their Uses.* New York: DK Publishing, Inc. 236.

Bradley, P.R. (ed.). 1992. *British Herbal Compendium*, Vol. 1. Bournemouth: British Herbal Medicine Association.

British Herbal Pharmacopoeia (BHP). 1996. Exeter, U.K.: British Herbal Medicine Association. 63–64.

Deutsches Arzneibuch (DAB 1997). 1997. Stuttgart: Deutscher Apotheker Verlag.

Deutscher Arzneimittel-Codex (DAC). 1986. Stuttgart: Deutscher Apotheker Verlag.

ESCOP. 1997. "Althaeae folium" and "Althaeae radix." *Monographs on the Medicinal Uses of Plant Drugs.* Exeter, U.K.: European Scientific Cooperative on Phytotherapy.

Europäisches Arzneibuch, 3rd ed., 1st suppl. (Ph.Eur.3). 1998. Stuttgart: Deutscher Apotheker Verlag.

Grieve, M. 1979. *A Modern Herbal.* New York: Dover Publications, Inc.

Karnick, C.R. 1994. *Pharmacopoeial Standards of Herbal Plants*, Vols. 1–2. Delhi: Sri Satguru Publications. Vol. 1:30–31; Vol. 2:90.

Lange, D. and U. Schippmann. 1997. *Trade Survey of Medicinal Plants in Germany—A Contribution to International Plant Species Conservation.* Bonn: Bundesamt für Naturschutz. 32–33, 114–121.

Leung, A.Y. and S. Foster. 1996. *Encyclopedia of Common Natural Ingredients Used in Food, Drugs, and Cosmetics*, 2nd ed. New York: John Wiley & Sons, Inc.

List, P.H. and L. Hörhammer (eds.). 1973–1979. *Hagers Handbuch der Pharmazeutischen Praxis*, Vols. 1–7. New York: Springer Verlag.

Newall, C.A., L.A. Anderson, J.D. Phillipson. 1996. *Herbal Medicines: A Guide for Health-Care Professionals.* London: The Pharmaceutical Press.

Österreichisches Arzneibuch, Vols. 1–2, 1st suppl. (ÖAB). 1981–1983. Wien: Verlag der Österreichischen Staatsdruckerei.

Ph.Eur.3. See *Europäisches Arzneibuch.*

Pharmacopoeia Helvetica, 7th ed. Vol. 1–4. (Ph.Helv.VII). 1987. Bern: Office Central Fédéral des Imprimés et du Matériel.

Wichtl, M. and N.G. Bisset (eds.). 1994. *Herbal Drugs and Phytopharmaceuticals.* Stuttgart: Medpharm Scientific Publishers.

This material was adapted from *The Complete German Commission E Monographs—Therapeutic Guide to Herbal Medicines.* M. Blumenthal, W.R. Busse, A. Goldberg, J. Gruenwald, T. Hall, C.W. Riggins, R.S. Rister (eds.) S. Klein and R.S. Rister (trans.). 1998. Austin: American Botanical Council; Boston: Integrative Medicine Communications.

1) The Overview section is new information.

2) Description, Chemistry and Pharmacology, Uses, Contraindications, Side Effects, Interactions with Other Drugs, and Dosage sections have been drawn from the original work. Additional information has been added in some or all of these sections, as noted with references.

3) The dosage for equivalent preparations (tea infusion, fluidextract, and tincture) have been provided based on the following example:
Unless otherwise prescribed: 2 g per day of [powdered, crushed, cut or whole] [plant part]
Infusion: 2 g in 150 ml of water
Fluidextract 1:1 (g/ml): 2 ml
Tincture 1:5 (g/ml): 10 ml

4) The References and Additional Resources sections are new sections. Additional Resources are not cited in the monograph but are included for research purposes.

Additional Resources

Braun H. and D. Frohne. 1987. *Heilpflanzen-lexikon für Ärzte und Apotheker*, 5th ed. Stuttgart-New York: Gustav Fischer Verlag. 14–15.

Braun, R. et al. 1997. *Standardzulassungen für Fertigarzneimittel—Text and Kommentar*. Stuttgart: Deutscher Apotheker Verlag.

British Herbal Pharmacopoeia (BHP). 1990. Bournemouth, U.K.: British Herbal Medicine Association.

———. 1983. Keighley, U.K.: British Herbal Medicine Association.

Council of Europe. 1981. *Flavouring Substances and Natural Sources of Flavourings*, 3rd ed. Strasbourg: Maisonneuve.

Franz, G. 1966. Die Schleimpolysaccharide vom *Althaea officinalis* und *Malva sylvestris*. *Planta Med* 14:90–110.

———. 1989. Polysaccharides in pharmacy: current applications and future concepts. *Planta Med* 55(6):493–497.

Franz, G. and M. Chladek. 1973. Vergleichende Untersuchungen über die Zusammensetzung von Rohschleimen aus Kreuzungsnachkommen von *Althaea officinalis* L. x *Althaea armeniaca* Ten [Comparative studies on the composition of crude mucus from crossbred descendants of *Althaea officinalis* L. and *Althaea armeniaca* Ten]. *Pharmazie* 28(2):128–129.

Franz, G. and A. Madaus. 1990. Stabilität von Polysacchariden. Untersuchungen am Beispiel des Eibischschleims. *Dtsch Apoth Ztg* 130:2194–2199.

Hänsel, R., K. Keller, H. Rimpler, G. Schneider (eds.). 1992. *Hagers Handbuch der Pharmazeutischen Praxis*, 5th ed. Vol. 4. Berlin-Heidelberg: Springer Verlag. 233–239.

Kantee, H. 1973. *Althaea*, ipecacuanha, senega ja thymus yskanlaakkeissa [*Althaea*, ipecac, senega and thyme as cough medicines]. *Sairaanhoitaja* 49(5):32.

Kapoor, L.D. 1990. *Handbook of Ayurvedic Medicinal Plants*. Boca Raton: CRC Press. 32.

McGuffin, M., C. Hobbs, R. Upton, A. Goldberg. 1997. American Herbal Product Association's *Botanical Safety Handbook*. Boca Raton: CRC Press.

Nadkarni, K.M. 1976. *Indian Materia Medica*. Bombay: Popular Prakashan. 84–85.

Pharmacopée Française Xe Édition (Ph.Fr.X.). 1983–1990. Moulins-les-Metz: Maisonneuve S.A.

Reynolds, J.E.F. (ed.). 1993. *Martindale: The Extra Pharmacopoeia*, 30th ed. London: The Pharmaceutical Press.

Trease, G.E. and W.C. Evans. 1989. *Trease and Evans' Pharmacognosy*, 13th ed. London; Philadelphia: Baillière Tindall. 375.

Wagner, H., S. Bladt, E.M. Zgainski. 1984. *Plant Drug Analysis*. Berlin-Heidelberg: Springer Verlag. 163 et seq.

Weiss, R.F. 1991. *Lehrbuch der Phytotherapie*, 7th ed. Stuttgart: Hippokrates Verlag. 258–259.

Wichtl, M. (ed.). 1997. *Teedrogen*, 4th ed. Stuttgart: Wissenschaftliche Verlagsgesellschaft.

MATÉ

Latin Name:
Ilex paraguariensis

Pharmacopeial Name:
Maté folium

Other Names:
yerba maté, kali chaye, Paraguay tea

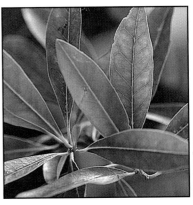

Overview

Maté is an evergreen tree growing wild near streams in South America between latitudes 30° and 20° South, now cultivated and maintained as a bush in Argentina, Brazil, and Paraguay (Bruneton, 1995; Goldberg et al., 1997; Wichtl and Bisset, 1994) from whence the material of commerce is produced (BHP, 1996; Wichtl and Bisset, 1994).

Wild-collected maté has been used by Native Americans in Brazil and Paraguay since ancient times. It was first brought under cultivation by Jesuit missionaries (Hagemann, 1997). Like green and black tea (*Camellia sinensis*), maté is processed into both green and fermented forms. In much of South America it is used more commonly than coffee or tea as a daily stimulant. Its name *maté* derives from the name of the traditional vessel in which the tea is prepared with boiling water, lemon juice, and sweetener (Goldberg et al., 1997; Grieve, 1979; Hagemann, 1997; Wichtl and Bisset, 1994). In Paraguay, the ethnomedical uses of maté infusion (*ka'a* in Paraguayan) are as a stimulant, diuretic, and eupeptic tonic (Gupta, 1996). Commercial maté farming has caused the disappearance of rainforest understory, and middle strata flora and fauna. Few canopy birds remain where maté is cropped. Experiments with sustainable yerba maté production are being conducted to identify methods less destructive to local fauna, for example, inside the forest, without removing middle strata, sub-canopy, or canopy vegetation (Lowen et al., 1995).

Its traditional uses in South American aboriginal medicines have spread to North America, Europe, and India. In northern India, maté grows in Lucknow. The *Ayurvedic Pharmacopoeia* lists maté for psychogenic headache, fatigue, nervous depression, and rheumatic pains (Karnick, 1994). In Germany, maté leaf is used as a monopreparation in an aqueous infusion dosage form and also as a component of prepared bladder and kidney teas, headache teas, and laxative teas. Maté dry extract is found as a component of instant teas and the alcoholic tincture is used in compound fluid preparations. In the United States, maté is used in monopreparations and as a component of central nervous system stimulant dietary supplements for mental and physical fatigue, aqueous infusion, alcoholic tincture, and aqueous dry extract. Ethnic South Americans living in the United States prepare and use maté in its traditional manner as an aqueous infusion in a gourd (*cuja*) through a straw or tube with a sieve-like bottom (*bombilla*).

The approved modern therapeutic applications for maté are supportable based on its long history of use in well-established systems of traditional medicine, on phytochemical investigations, and *in vitro* studies and *in vivo* pharmacological experiments in animals.

Pharmacopeial grade maté leaf is briefly cured by strong heating, then more gently dried. It must pass identification by macroscopic and microscopic authentication and by thin-layer chromatography (TLC). Quantitative standards include not less than 20% water-soluble extractive content (BHP, 1996; Erg.B.6, 1926; Wichtl and Bisset, 1994).

Description
Maté consists of the dried leaf and leaf stem of *Ilex paraguariensis* A. Saint-Hilaire [Fam. Aquifoliaceae], and their preparations in effective dosage. The herb contains caffeine.

Chemistry and Pharmacology
Maté leaf contains xanthene alkaloids (1–2% caffeine, 0.45–0.9% theobromine, 0.05% theophylline); tannin-like substances (4–16% caffeic and chlorogenic acids); the amines choline and trigonelline; amino acids; the flavonoids kaempferol, quercetin, and rutin; ursolic acid; vitamins B_2, B_6, C, niacin, and pantothenic acid; and volatile oil (Bruneton, 1995; Budavari et al., 1989; List and Hörhammer, 1973–1979; Newall et al., 1996; Wichtl and Bisset, 1994).

The Commission E reported analeptic, diuretic, positively inotropic, positively chronotropic, glycogenolytic, and lipolytic properties.

Maté is reported to have central nervous system stimulant, thymoleptic, diuretic, antirheumatic, and mild analgesic activities. The pharmaceutical use of maté can be attributed to caffeine (BHP, 1983 and 1990; Bruneton, 1995; Newall et al., 1996).

Uses
The Commission E approved the internal use of maté leaf for mental and physical fatigue. In France, maté leaf preparations are permitted for the treatment of asthenia, as an adjunctive treatment in weight loss programs orally and topically, and to increase the renal excretion of water (Bruneton, 1995). Maté is used for fatigue, nervous depression, rheumatic pains, psychogenic headache, and is specifically indicated for headache from fatigue (BHP, 1983 and 1990; Newall et al., 1996; Wichtl and Bisset, 1994).

Contraindications
None known.

Side Effects
None known.

Use During Pregnancy and Lactation
No restrictions known.

Interactions with Other Drugs
None known.

Dosage and Administration
Unless otherwise prescribed: 3 g per day of cut herb.
Infusion: 2 g in 150 ml water, one to two times daily.
Fluidextract 1:1 (g/ml): 2 ml, one to two times daily.
Tincture 1:5 (g/ml): 10 ml, one to two times daily.
Native dry extract 4.5–5.5:1 (w/w): 0.36–0.44 g, one to two times daily.

References
British Herbal Pharmacopoeia (BHP). 1996. Exeter, U.K.: British Herbal Medicine Association. 130–131.

———. 1990. Bournemouth, U.K.: British Herbal Medicine Association.

———. 1983. Keighley, U.K.: British Herbal Medicine Association.

Bruneton, J. 1995. *Pharmacognosy, Phytochemistry, Medicinal Plants*. Paris: Lavoisier Publishing.

Budavari, S., M.J. O'Neil, A. Smith, P.E. Heckelman (eds.). 1989. *The Merck Index: An Encyclopedia of Chemicals, Drugs, and Biologicals*, 11th ed. Rahway, N.J.: Merck & Co., Inc.

Ergänzungsbuch zum Deutschen Arzneibuch, 6th ed. (Erg.B.6). 1953. Stuttgart: Deutscher Apotheker Verlag.

Goldberg, A., P. Altaffer, M. Altaffer (eds.). 1997. *Brazilian Botanical Monographs*, 1st ed. Oakland: New World Enterprises, Inc.

Grieve, M. 1979. *A Modern Herbal*. New York: Dover Publications, Inc.

Gupta, M.P. (ed.). 1996. *270 Plantas Medicinales Iberoamericanas*. CYTED Programa Iberoamericano de ciencia y tecnologia para el desarrollo. Subprograma de quimica fina farmaceutica: Convenio Andres Bello. 46–47.

Hagemann, R.C. (ed.). 1997. *The Review of Natural Products*. St. Louis: Facts and Comparisons.

Karnick, C.R. 1994. *Pharmacopoeial Standards of Herbal Plants*, Vol. 1. Delhi: Sri Satguru Publications. 197–198.

List, P.H. and L. Hörhammer (eds.). 1973–1979. *Hagers Handbuch der Pharmazeutischen Praxis*, Vols. 1–7. New York: Springer Verlag.

Lowen, J.C., L. Bartrina, R.P. Clay, J.A. Tobias. 1995. *Biological Surveys and Conservation Priorities in Eastern Paraguay*. Itabó, Paraguay: CSB Conservation Publications. 55–61.

Newall, C.A., L.A. Anderson, J.D. Phillipson. 1996. *Herbal Medicines: A Guide for Health-Care Professionals*. London: The Pharmaceutical Press.

Wichtl, M. and N.G. Bisset (eds.). 1994. *Herbal Drugs and Phytopharmaceuticals*. Stuttgart: Medpharm Scientific Publishers.

Additional Resources

Barreto, R.C.R. 1956. Microbiological determination of choline in herba maté. *Rev Quim Ind (Rio de Janeiro)* 25(28):12.

Bertoni, M.S. Medicina Guarani: CAP. XXI: Accion de la Yerba Maté. Civilizacion Guarani. Etnografia 462–490.

British Pharmaceutical Codex (BPC). 1934. London: The Pharmaceutical Press.

Council of Europe. 1981. *Flavouring Substances and Natural Sources of Flavourings*, 3rd ed. Strasbourg: Maisonneuve.

Der Marderosian, A. (ed.). 1999. *The Review of Natural Products*. St. Louis: Facts and Comparisons.

Duke, J.A. 1985. *Handbook of Medicinal Herbs*. Boca Raton: CRC Press.

———. 1992. *Handbook of Phytochemical Constituents of GRAS Herbs and Other Economic Plants*. Boca Raton: CRC Press. 305–306.

Fossati, C. 1976. Sulle virtu e sulle proprieta terapeutiche della "yerba-maté" [On the virtue and therapeutic properties of "yerba-maté"]. *(Ilex paraguayensis o paraguariensis*, St. Hilaire 1838). *Clin Ter* 78(3):265–272.

Gosmann, G. and E.P. Schenkel. 1989. A new saponin from maté (*Ilex paraguariensis*) leaf and beverage. *Food Chem* 35(1):13–21.

Gosmann, G., D. Guillaume, A.T. Taketa, E.P. Schenkel. 1995. Triterpenoid saponins from *Ilex paraguariensis*. *J Nat Prod* 58(3):438–441.

Gugliucci, A. and A.J. Stahl. 1995. Low density lipoprotein oxidation is inhibited by extracts of *Ilex paraguariensis*. *Biochem Mol Biol Int* 35(1):47–56.

Gugliucci, A. 1996. Antioxidant effects of *Ilex paraguariensis*: induction of decreased oxidability of human LDL *in vivo*. *Biochem Biophys Res Commun* 224(2):338–344.

Lust, J.B. 1974. *The Herb Book*. Simi Valley, CA: Benedict Lust Publications. 229.

May, G. and G. Willuhn. 1978. [Antiviral activity of aqueous extracts from medicinal plants in tissues cultures] [In German]. *Arzneimforsch* 28(1):1–7.

McGuffin, M., C. Hobbs, R. Upton, A. Goldberg. 1997. American Herbal Product Association's *Botanical Safety Handbook*. Boca Raton: CRC Press.

Muccillo Baisch, A.L., K.B. Johnston, F.L. Paganini Stein. 1998. Endothelium-dependent vasorelaxing activity of aqueous extracts of *Ilex paraguariensis* on mesenteric arterial bed of rats. *J Ethnopharmacol* 60(2):133–139.

No Borders Net Services. 1997. Yerba Maté: Chemical Features and Therapeutic Properties. Available at: www.noborders.net/mate/ingredients.html

Ohem, N. and J. Holzl. 1988. Some new investigations on *Ilex paraguariensis*—Flavonoids and triterpenes. *Planta Med* 54:576.

Pharmacopée Française Xe Édition (Ph.Fr.X.). 1983–1990. Moulins-les-Metz: Maisonneuve S.A.

This material was adapted from *The Complete German Commission E Monographs—Therapeutic Guide to Herbal Medicines*. M. Blumenthal, W.R. Busse, A. Goldberg, J. Gruenwald, T. Hall, C.W. Riggins, R.S. Rister (eds.) S. Klein and R.S. Rister (trans.). 1998. Austin: American Botanical Council; Boston: Integrative Medicine Communications.

1) The Overview section is new information.

2) Description, Chemistry and Pharmacology, Uses, Contraindications, Side Effects, Interactions with Other Drugs, and Dosage sections have been drawn from the original work. Additional information has been added in some or all of these sections, as noted with references.

3) The dosage for equivalent preparations (tea infusion, fluidextract, and tincture) have been provided based on the following example:
   Unless otherwise prescribed: 2 g per day of [powdered, crushed, cut or whole] [plant part]
   Infusion: 2 g in 150 ml of water
   Fluidextract 1:1 (g/ml): 2 ml
   Tincture 1:5 (g/ml): 10 ml

4) The References and Additional Resources sections are new sections. Additional Resources are not cited in the monograph but are included for research purposes.

Reynolds, J.E.F. (ed.). 1993. *Martindale: The Extra Pharmacopoeia,* 30th ed. London: The Pharmaceutical Press.

Schenkel, E.P., J.A. Montanha, G. Gosmann. 1996. Triterpene saponins from maté, *Ilex paraguariensis. Adv Exp Med Biol* 405:47–56.

Tenorio Sanz, M.D. and M.E. Torija Isasa. 1991. Elementos minerales en la yerba maté [Mineral elements in maté herb] (*Ilex paraguariensis* St. H.). *Arch Latinoam Nutr* 41(3):441–454.

Valduga, E. 1995. Chemical and anatomic characterization of *Ilex paraguariensis* Saint Hilaire leaf and some species used in adulterating Yerba Maté. [Post-graduation thesis presented at the University of Paraná, Curitiba.]

Vasquez, A. and P. Moyna. 1986. Studies on maté drinking. *J Ethnopharmacol* 18(3):267–272.

Vera Garcia, R., I. Basualdo, I. Peralta, M. de Herebia, S. Caballero. 1997. Minerals content of Paraguayan yerba maté (*Ilex paraguariensis,* S.H.). *Arch Latinoam Nutr* 47(1):77–80.

Wagner, H., S. Bladt, E.M. Zgainski. 1984. *Plant Drug Analysis.* Berlin-Heidelberg: Springer Verlag. 86.

MEADOWSWEET

Latin Name:
Filipendula ulmaria; syn. *Spiraea ulmaria*

Pharmacopeial Name:
Spiraeae flos, Spiraeae herba

Other Names:
bridewort, queen of the meadow

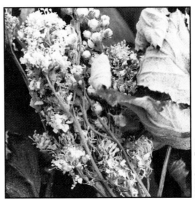

©1999 Steven Foster

Overview

Meadowsweet is a tall, stout, fragrant, perennial herb, native to Europe and Asia, found in damp meadows and moist banks, naturalized in North America as an escape from cultivation, now found wild from Newfoundland and eastern Quebec to Nova Scotia, New England, New Jersey, New York, West Virginia, and as far west as Ohio (Grieve, 1979; HPUS, 1992; Lust, 1974). The material of commerce is obtained from Poland, Bulgaria, the former Yugoslavia, and the United Kingdom (BHP, 1996; Wichtl and Bisset, 1994).

Meadowsweet was one of the three most sacred herbs used by ancient Celtic Druid priests. It is mentioned in the *Knight's Tale* by Geoffrey Chaucer (fourteenth century C.E.), and described in old European herbals, including those of John Gerard (*The Herball*, 1597) and Nicholas Culpepper (*The English Physitian*, 1652). The analgesic substance *salicin* was first isolated from meadowsweet leaves in 1827. Salicylic acid was made in 1838, and synthesized in 1859, which provided the basis for acetylsalicylic acid, first produced in 1899. The word *aspirin* owes its origin to meadowsweet's former genus name *Spiraea*, having been coined from "a" (for acetyl) and "spirin" (from *Spiraea*) (Bown, 1995; Duke, 1985; Grieve, 1979). Meadowsweet's traditional use in Britain eventually spread to India where it is now used somewhat in Ayurvedic medicine. Meadowsweet is official in the *French Pharmacopoeia* and also monographed in the Ayurvedic pharmacopoeia, the *British Herbal Pharmacopoeia* and *British Herbal Compendium*, the Commission E monographs, and the German Standard Licenses (BAnz, 1998; Bradley, 1992; Braun et al., 1997; Karnick, 1994; Ph.Fr.X, 1990; Wichtl and Bisset, 1994). The Ayurvedic pharmacopoeia specifically indicates its use for prophylaxis and treatment of peptic ulcer and for rheumatic muscle and joint pains (Karnick, 1994).

In Germany, meadowsweet is licensed as a standard medicinal tea, approved in the Commission E monographs, and used for feverish common colds for which a sweat treatment is desired. The Commission E specifies a tea infusion dosage form and it appears as a component of some influenza, rheumatism, and kidney-bladder compound herbal tea drugs (BAnz, 1998; Braun et al., 1997; Meyer-Buchtela, 1999; Wichtl and Bisset, 1994). In German pediatric medicine, meadowsweet is an antipyretic and diaphoretic component of an effective influenza tea combined with willow bark, tilia flower, chamomile flower, and orange peel (Schilcher, 1997). The American Herbal Products Association gives it a Class 1 rating (herbs that can be safely consumed when used appropriately) (McGuffin et al., 1997). It is not commonly found in consumer products in the U.S. market, though medical herbalists and naturopaths include it in some prescribed formulas.

The approved modern therapeutic applications for meadowsweet are supportable based on its history of use in well established systems of traditional medicine, phytochemical investigations, and pharmacological studies in animals.

Pharmacopeial grade meadowsweet must be composed of the dried aerial (above-ground) parts (flower, leaf, and stem), collected when the plant is in bloom. Botanical identity must be confirmed by thin-layer chromatography (TLC) as well as by macroscopic and microscopic examinations and organoleptic evaluation. It must contain not less than 12% water-soluble extractive, among other quantitative standards (BHP, 1996). The German Standard License monograph requires the dried flower as opposed to the dried aerial parts. A test for absence of known adulterants (e.g., elder flower) is also required among other purity tests. The Standard License includes specific packaging requirements for shelf-life stability and indications for use, dosage, and mode of administration (Braun et al., 1997).

Description

Meadowsweet flower consists of the dried flower of *Filipendula ulmaria* (L.) Maximowicz (syn. *Spiraea ulmaria* L.) [Fam. Rosaceae] and its preparations in effective dosage. Meadowsweet herb consists of the dried, above-ground parts of *F. ulmaria* (L.) Maximowicz, harvested during flowering season, and its preparations in effective dosage. The preparation contains flavonoids, essential oil, and, mainly in the flowers, phenol glycosides.

Chemistry and Pharmacology

Meadowsweet contains 10–15% polyphenolic tannins, especially rugosin-D; 0.5–1.0% flavonoids (up to 6% in the fresh flowers), mostly spireoside (quercetin-4'-glucoside) and other quercetin and kaempferol derivatives; 0.3–0.5% phenolic glycosides, mostly spiraein and monotropitin, the primeverosides of salicylaldehyde and methyl salicylate, also isosalicin, a glucoside of salicyl alcohol; about 0.2% volatile oil, mainly salicylaldehyde (up to 75%); mucilage; and ascorbic acid (Bradley, 1992; Braun et al., 1997; Wichtl and Bisset, 1994).

The Commission E did not report pharmacological actions for meadowsweet.

The *British Herbal Compendium* reported anti-inflammatory, diuretic, stomachic, and astringent actions (Bradley, 1992).

Uses

The Commission E approved the internal use of meadowsweet as supportive therapy for colds.

The *British Herbal Compendium* indicates its use for atonic and acid dyspepsia, gastritis, peptic ulceration, and rheumatic and arthritic pains (Bradley, 1992). In France, traditional indications for use are allowed, including for fever and influenza (Bradley, 1992; DPM, 1990). The German Standard License for meadowsweet tea indicates its use for feverish common colds for which a sweat treatment is desired and also to increase the amount of urine (Bradley, 1992; Braun et al., 1997; Wichtl and Bisset, 1994).

Contraindications

Meadowsweet flowers contain salicylate. They should not be used where a salicylate sensitivity exists.

Side Effects

None known.

Use During Pregnancy and Lactation

No restrictions known (McGuffin et al., 1997).

Interactions with Other Drugs

None known.

Dosage and Administration

Unless otherwise prescribed: 2.5–3.5 g
per day of cut meadowsweet flower or
4–5 g per day of cut meadowsweet
herb, and other galenical preparations
for infusions; a cup of the infusion
drunk as hot as tolerable several times
daily.
Infusion: Steep 2–3 g in 150 ml boiled
water for about 10 minutes.
Fluidextract 1:1 (g/ml): 2–3 ml.

References

BAnz. See *Bundesanzeiger.*
Bown, D. 1995. *Encyclopedia of Herbs and Their Uses.* New York: DK Publishing, Inc. 17, 283.
Bradley, P.R. (ed.). 1992. *British Herbal Compendium,* Vol. 1. Bournemouth: British Herbal Medicine Association.
Braun, R. et al. 1997. *Standardzulassungen für Fertigarzneimittel—Text and Kommentar.* Stuttgart: Deutscher Apotheker Verlag.
British Herbal Pharmacopoeia (BHP). 1996. Exeter, U.K.: British Herbal Medicine Association. 131–132.
Bundesanzeiger (BAnz). 1998. Monographien der Kommission E (Zulassungs- und Aufbereitungskommission am BGA für den humanmed. Bereich, phytotherapeutische Therapierichtung und Stoffgruppe). Köln: Bundesgesundheitsamt (BGA).
Direction de la Pharmacie et du Médicament (DPM). 1992. Bulletin Officiel (Fascicule spécial) No. 90/22 bis. [English edition]. Paris: Ministère des Affaires Sociales et de la Solidarité.
Duke, J.A. 1985. *Handbook of Medicinal Herbs.* Boca Raton: CRC Press. 196–197.
Grieve, M. 1979. *A Modern Herbal.* New York: Dover Publications, Inc.
The Homeopathic Pharmacopoeia of the United States (HPUS). 1992. Arlington, VA: Pharmacopoeia Convention of the American Institute of Homeopathy.
Karnick, C.R. 1994. *Pharmacopoeial Standards of Herbal Plants,* Vols. 1–2. Delhi: Sri Satguru Publications. Vol. 1:144–145; Vol. 2:91.
Lust, J.B. 1974. *The Herb Book.* New York: Bantam Books. 269–270.
McGuffin, M., C. Hobbs, R. Upton, A. Goldberg. 1997. *American Herbal Product Association's Botanical Safety Handbook.* Boca Raton: CRC Press.
Meyer-Buchtela, E. 1999. *Tee-Rezepturen—Ein Handbuch für Apotheker und Ärzte.* Stuttgart: Deutscher Apotheker Verlag.
Pharmacopée Française Xe Édition (Ph.Fr.X.). 1983–1990. Moulins-les-Metz: Maisonneuve S.A.
Schilcher, H. 1997. *Phytotherapy in Paediatrics—Handbook for Physicians and Pharmacists.* Stuttgart: Medpharm Scientific Publishers. 41, 63–64, 113.
Wichtl, M. and N.G. Bisset (eds.). 1994. *Herbal Drugs and Phytopharmaceuticals.* Stuttgart: Medpharm Scientific Publishers.

Additional Resources

Barnaulov, O.D. and P.P. Denisenko. 1980. [Antiulcerogenic action of a decoction from flowers of *Filipendula ulmaria* (L.) Maxim] [In Russian]. *Farmakol Toksikol* (Moscow) 43(6):700–705.
Csedö, K. et al. 1993. The antibiotic activity of *Filipendula ulmaria. Planta Med* 59(7):A675.
Hänsel, R., K. Keller, H. Rimpler, G. Schneider (eds.). 1992–1994. *Hagers Handbuch der Pharmazeutischen Praxis,* 5th ed. Vol. 4–6. Berlin-Heidelberg: Springer Verlag.
Hörhammer, L., R. Hänsel, W. Endres. 1956. Über die Flavonglykoside der Gattungen Filipendula und Spiraea. *Arch Pharm (Weinheim)* 289(61):133–140.
Malhotra, S.C. 1990. *Phytochemical Investigations of Certain Medicinal Plants Used in Ayurveda.* New Delhi, India: CCRA & S, Government of India.
Newall, C.A., L.A. Anderson, J.D. Phillipson. 1996. *Herbal Medicines: A Guide for Health-Care Professionals.* London: The Pharmaceutical Press.

This material was adapted from *The Complete German Commission E Monographs—Therapeutic Guide to Herbal Medicines.* M. Blumenthal, W.R. Busse, A. Goldberg, J. Gruenwald, T. Hall, C.W. Riggins, R.S. Rister (eds.) S. Klein and R.S. Rister (trans.). 1998. Austin: American Botanical Council; Boston: Integrative Medicine Communications.

1) The Overview section is new information.
2) Description, Chemistry and Pharmacology, Uses, Contraindications, Side Effects, Interactions with Other Drugs, and Dosage sections have been drawn from the original work. Additional information has been added in some or all of these sections, as noted with references.
3) The dosage for equivalent preparations (tea infusion, fluidextract, and tincture) have been provided based on the following example:
Unless otherwise prescribed: 2 g per day of [powdered, crushed, cut or whole] [plant part]
Infusion: 2 g in 150 ml of water
Fluidextract 1:1 (g/ml): 2 ml
Tincture 1:5 (g/ml): 10 ml
4) The References and Additional Resources sections are new sections. Additional Resources are not cited in the monograph but are included for research purposes.

Novikova, N.N. 1969. Use of *Filipendula ulmaria* in medicine. Tr Perm Farm Inst 267–270.

Wichtl, M. (ed.). 1997. *Teedrogen*, 4th ed. Stuttgart: Wissenschaftliche Verlagsgesellschaft.

Yanutsh, A.Y. et al. 1982. A study of the antiulcerative action of the extracts from the supernatant part and roots of *Filipendula ulmaria*. *Farm Zh* (Kiev) 37:53–56.

Milk Thistle Fruit

Latin Name:
Silybum marianum (L.) Gaertner

Pharmacopeial Name:
Cardui mariae fructus

Other Names:
blessed milk thistle, St. Mary thistle

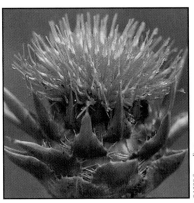

©1999 Steven Foster

Overview

The milk thistle of commerce is a standardized preparation extracted from the fruits (seeds) of *Silybum marianum* (L.) Gaertn., Asteraceae (syn. *Carduus marianus* L.), a plant native to the Mediterranean. The leaves have been used since Greco-Roman times as an herbal remedy for a variety of ailments, particularly liver problems. Eclectic physicians in the United States in the latter nineteenth and early twentieth centuries acknowledged the clinical benefits of preparations from the milk thistle seeds (technically the fruits) for "Congestion of the liver, spleen, and kidneys ..." (Felter and Lloyd, 1983). It is widely used in German phytotherapy for "chronic hepatitis of all types," and especially for fatty liver (cirrhosis) associated with alcoholics (Weiss, 1988).

Milk thistle is an example of a preparation that is required to be in the standardized, concentrated form in order to fully convey the desired, in this case, hepatoprotectant, effects. Milk thistle preparations are usually standardized to a concentration of 70 to 80% of three flavonolignans (silibinin, silychristin, and silydianin), collectively known as silymarin. According to research conducted by the original manufacturer and primary researcher of milk thistle extract, Madaus AG of Cologne, Germany, this level of concentration of silymarin is required to survive degradation by gastric fluids and in order to enter into the bloodstream via the intestinal wall. Silymarin is poorly absorbed (20–50%) from the gastrointestinal tract; thus, the concentrated extract is recommended (Foster and Tyler, 1999; Robbers and Tyler, 1999).

The original product in Germany contains 70 mg silymarin. The Commission E approved uses and the subsequent use of milk thistle standardized extracts in the United States are based on a significant amount of chemical, pharmacological, and clinical research. There have been an estimated 120 clinical studies carried out on the proprietary milk thistle preparation from Madaus, known in Germany as Legalon®. A comprehensive and detailed review of the pharmacokinetics and clinical pharmacology of Legalon® has been published in English by the manufacturer (Anon., 1989).

Clinical studies suggest or confirm the efficacy of milk thistle extract for various hepatic disorders, including hepatitis A, alcoholic cirrhosis, and exposure to hazardous chemicals. Another relatively esoteric use is as a preventive and/or antidote to poisoning by the deathcap mushroom, *Amanita phalloides*. A preparation of the silibinin fraction is available in Germany as an intravenous (i.v.) drip for such acute cases.

A primary use for silymarin is in the treatment of liver damage due to ingestion of alcohol. An early double-blind study examined 66 patients, most with alcohol-induced toxic liver disease (Fintelmann and Albert, 1980). The 31 patients who received 420 mg/day of Legalon® showed a significant influence on serum levels of glutamic-oxalacetic transaminase (GOT), glutamic-pyruvic transaminase (GPT), and Gamma-GT over those 35 patients receiving placebo, with levels returning to normal more quickly in the treated group than placebo. Another double-blind study with 36 patients suffering from alcohol-induced liver disease found that pathological liver parameters (GOT, GPT, Gamma-GT, and bilirubin) were significantly reduced in the patients receiving silymarin (Legalon®) after six months of treatment compared to the placebo group (Feher et al., 1990). However, a multi-center study conducted in Spain from 1986 to 1989 found no effect for silymarin on the survival of patients or the clinical course of alcohol-induced cirrhosis (Pares et al., 1998). In another study, a randomized, controlled trial was performed to determine the effect of silymarin in the treatment of patients with alcohol- and non-alcohol-induced cirrhosis (Ferenci et al., 1989). Of the 170 patients, 87 received 420 mg of silymarin daily, compared with 83 placebo patients. The mean observation period was 41 months, with 10 dropouts in the placebo group and 14 in the treatment group. The four-year survival rate was $58\pm9\%$ in the silymarin-treated patients, and $39\pm9\%$ in the placebo group (p=0.036). No adverse side effects of drug treatment were observed.

In another double-blind, controlled study, the effects of silymarin on chemical, functional, and morphological alterations of the liver were examined (Salmi and Sarna, 1982). The 106 patients with liver disease in the study were selected on the basis of elevated serum transaminase levels. A total of 97 patients completed the four-week trial (47 treated and 50 placebo). A dose of 420 mg a day of silymarin produced a statistically significant greater decrease of GPT and GOT liver enzymes in the treated group than in the control. Serum total and bilirubin decreased more in the treated than in the control group, but the differences were not statistically significant.

Some forms of hepatitis have responded to silymarin treatment. A study reported on 67 subjects treated as outpatients for toxic metabolic liver damage, chronic hepatitis, and bile duct inflammation (Poser, 1971). After three months of treatment (525 mg/day of silymarin), chronic hepatitis was found to be significantly improved bioptically. Conditions associated with bile duct inflammation also responded particularly well. Another double-blind study looked at the effect of silymarin in the treatment of acute viral hepatitis (Magliulo et al., 1978). A daily dose of 420 mg therapeutically influenced the increased serum levels of bilirubin, GOT, and GPT characteristically associated with acute viral hepatitis. After five days of treatment, the laboratory parameters regressed more in the treated group than for the placebo group. After three weeks, more patients in the treated group had attained normal values than in the placebo group. A statistical analysis showed a difference between GOT and bilirubin values in the silymarin and placebo groups, with a regression of GPT values in favor of silymarin. A recent case report of chronic infection by hepatitis B virus and hepatitis C virus demonstrated potential efficacy of treatment with milk thistle (10 g ground-up seeds in oatmeal with standardized (70%) milk thistle extract capsules three times daily) in combination with another herb known for its hepatoprotectant activity, *Phyllanthus amarus* (200 mg, three times daily) (McPartland, 1996).

In a review of important European clinical studies ranging from 1971 to 1988 (including those summarized above), the authors found the data suggests the effectiveness of silymarin not only in toxic and metabolic liver damage, but also in acute and chronic hepatitis (Hikino and Kiso, 1988). Silymarin's ability to stabilize the cell membrane and stimulate protein synthesis, while accelerating the process of regeneration in damaged liver tissue, was found to be important in its therapeutic efficacy.

The hepatoprotectant effect of milk thistle fractions (silymarin) is documented in other studies: these compounds can produce both a protective and curative effect on liver damage resulting from the highly toxic compounds phalloidin and alpha-amanitin (from the deathcap mushroom, *A. phalloides*). A multicenter trial conducted from 1979 to 1982 involved 220 cases of Amanita poisoning treated in German, Swiss, and Austrian hospitals (Hruby, 1984). Silibinin (administered i.v.) in supportive treatment was used. The mortality rate was 12.8%, compared to a mortality rate of 22.4% in a study where only 16 of the 205 patients were treated with 20 to 50 mg/kg/day of silibinin (Floersheim et al., 1982). Hruby concluded that the use of silibinin in addition to current methods of treating Amanita poisoning could lower mortality rates below any previously achieved.

A literature review noted that Legalon® is the best documented agent for the treatment of toxic liver impairment (Morazzani and Bombardelli, 1995). These authors also reviewed studies which suggest future use in dermatological and cosmetic products, based on a number of activities including promoting healing at wound sites, improved burn healing, and counteracting skin degeneration and aging via anti-inflammatory and free radical scavenging mechanisms. A more recent review concluded that despite some flaws in methodology of some of the clinical studies, Legalon® has not demonstrated adverse side effects and it "may be effective in improving the clinical courses of both acute and chronic viral, drug- and toxin-induced and alcoholic hepatitis" (Flora et al., 1998).

Because the well-documented antioxidant activity of silymarin has been shown to prevent lipoperoxidative hepatic damage by xenobiotic compounds (e.g., alcohol and certain pharmaceutical drugs), researchers attempted to determine whether milk thistle would be helpful for patients being administered psychotropic drugs. In a double-blind, placebo-controlled study, the efficacy of silymarin was evaluated in patients receiving psychotropic drugs as long-term therapy (Palasciano et al., 1994). Sixty women in the psychiatric ward of an Italian hospital were selected for the trial, all having been treated with either phenothiazines and/or butyrophenones for at least five years. They were randomly divided into four groups, with the silymarin patients receiving 800 mg a day for 90 days. Results showed that 800 mg/day of silymarin may be useful in the treatment of some instances of lipoperoxidative hepatic damage, such as the damage that may occur during long-term treatment with the psychotropic drugs.

Milk thistle extract has become increasingly popular in the United States as a dietary supplement for people with livers compromised by alcohol or exposure to toxic chemicals. Based on the increasing number of clinical studies indicating its safety and suggesting efficacy, consumers are also using this preparation as a means to ensure proper liver function and to assist in "detoxification" measures. Given this phytomedicine's well established safety and its reasonable documentation of efficacy, future clinical use of milk thistle extract should be explored as an adjunct therapy in chemotherapy to help offset the effects of powerful and potentially hepatotoxic conventional drugs.

U.S. pharmacopeial grade milk thistle consists of the dried ripe fruit of *S. marianum* with its pappus removed. It must contain not less than 2% of silymarin, calculated as silybin, as determined by a USP spectrophotometric assay method. Botanical identification must be confirmed by thin-layer chromatography (TLC) and macroscopic and microscopic examinations (USP 24–NF 19, 1999). German pharmacopeial grade milk thistle also consists of the ripe fruit with the pappus removed. However, it must contain not less than 1.5% silymarin, calculated as silybin with reference to the dried drug. Total silymarin must be determined by a liquid chromatagraphic method (DAB method V.6.20.4). Botanical identity must be confirmed by TLC, macroscopic and microscopic examinations, and organoleptic evaluations. For example, the seed husk should have a bitter taste while the seed has an oleaginous taste, and it may not smell or taste rancid (DAB, 1997). The *German Homeopathic Pharmacopoeia* monograph requires that it contain not less than 1% of silymarin, calculated as silybin (GHP, 1993).

Description

Milk thistle fruit consists of ripe seed of *S. marianum* (L.) Gaertner [Fam. Asteraceae], freed from the pappus, and its preparations in effective dosage. The preparation contains silibinin, silydianin, and silychristin.

Chemistry and Pharmacology

Milk thistle seed contains 1.5–3% flavone lignans, collectively referred to as silymarin (Bruneton, 1995; Wichtl and Bisset, 1994); 20–30% fixed oil, of which approximately 60% is linoleic acid, approximately 30% is oleic acid, and approximately 9% is palmitic acid; 25–30% protein; 0.038% tocopherol; 0.63% sterols, including cholesterol, campesterol, stigmasterol, and sitosterol; and some mucilage (Meyer-Buchtela, 1999; Wichtl and Bisset, 1994). The three principle components of silymarin are the flavanolignans silybin, silychristin, and silidianin (Bruneton, 1995; Leung and Foster, 1996; Wichtl and Bisset, 1994).

The Commission E reported that silymarin acts as an antagonist in many experimental liver-damage models: phalloidin and amanitin (deathcap toxins), lanthanides, carbon tetrachloride, galactosamine, thioacetamide, and the hepatotoxic virus FV3 of cold-blooded vertebrates.

The therapeutic activity of silymarin is based on two sites or mechanisms of action:

(a) It alters the structure of the outer cell membrane of the hepatocytes in such a way as to prevent penetration of the liver toxin into the interior of the cell.

(b) It stimulates the action of nucleolar polymerase A, resulting in an increase in ribosomal protein synthesis, and thus stimulates the regenerative ability of the liver and the formation of new hepatocytes.

Milk thistle extract provides hepatocellular protection by stabilizing hepatic cell membranes (McPartland, 1996). Other actions include interruption of enterohepatic recirculation of toxins, stimulation of protein synthesis and regeneration of damaged hepatocytes, as well as antioxidant activity (McPartland, 1996).

Recent research on silibinin and silichristin to promote faster regeneration of diseased liver tissue has focused on the ability of silibinin to stimulate the activity of the DNA-dependent RNA-polymerase I, causing an increase in rRNA synthesis and an accelerated formation of intact ribosomes. This results in a general increase in the rate of synthesis of all cellular proteins. *In vivo* and *in vitro* molecular modeling experiments indicate that silibinin may imitate a steroid hormone by binding specifically to polymerase I, thus stimulating enzyme activity (Sonnenbichler et al., 1998).

Uses

The Commission E approved the internal use of crude milk thistle fruit preparations for dyspeptic complaints. Formulations* are approved for toxic liver damage and for supportive treatment in chronic inflammatory liver disease and hepatic cirrhosis.

*[Ed. note: A "formulation" refers to an extract standardized to at least 70–80% silymarin, the collective name for the three compounds listed in the Description section.]

The German Standard License for milk thistle seed tea infusion indicates its use for digestive disorders, particularly for functional disturbances of the biliary systems (Braun et al., 1997).

Contraindications

None known.

Side Effects

Crude preparation: None known. Formulations: A mild laxative effect has been observed in occasional instances.

Use During Pregnancy and Lactation

No restrictions known.

Interactions with Other Drugs
None known.

Dosage and Administration
Unless otherwise prescribed: 12–15 g
per day of powdered seed for making
infusions and other galenical formulations to be taken by mouth. Formulations (e.g., dry extract noted below)
equivalent to 200–400 mg per day of
silymarin, calculated as silibinin.
For liver diseases:
Dry extract 40–70:1 (w/w), 70–80%
silymarin: Swallow one capsule containing 100–200 mg of silymarin, twice
daily in the morning and evening. Swallow with sufficient amounts of fluid; or,
take one capsule containing approximately 140 mg of silymarin, two to
three times daily (Brown, 1996).
For digestive disorders:
Decoction: Place approximately 3.0 g
seed in 150 ml cold water, bring to a
boil and simmer for 20 to 30 minutes,
three to four times daily (Wichtl and
Bisset, 1994).
Infusion: Steep approximately 3.5 g
seed in 150 ml boiled water for 10 to
15 minutes, three to four times daily
one half-hour before meals (Braun et
al., 1997; Meyer-Buchtela, 1999;
Wichtl and Bisset, 1994).
[Note: Silymarin is poorly soluble in
water; teas have been analyzed with
only about 10% of the original levels of
silymarin from the fruits. Thus, for
hepatic benefits, the concentrated
extract is recommended (Foster and
Tyler, 1999).]
Tincture: 15–25 drops, four to five
times daily (Lust, 1974); 1–2 ml, three
times daily (Hoffmann, 1992).

References
Anon. 1989. Legalon®. Cologne, Germany: Madaus AG.

Braun, R. et al. 1997. *Standardzulassungen für Fertigarzneimittel—Text and Kommentar.* Stuttgart: Deutscher Apotheker Verlag.

Brown, D.J. 1996. *Herbal Prescriptions for Better Health.* Rocklin, CA: Prima Publishing. 151–158.

Bruneton, J. 1995. *Pharmacognosy, Phytochemistry, Medicinal Plants.* Paris: Lavoisier Publishing.

Deutsches Arzneibuch (DAB 1997). 1997. Stuttgart: Deutscher Apotheker Verlag.

Feher, J. et al. 1990. Hepatoprotective activity of silymarin therapy in patients with chronic alcoholic liver disease. *Orv Hetil* 130:51.

Felter, H.W. and J.U. Lloyd. 1983. *King's American Dispensatory,* 18th ed., 3rd rev. Portland, OR: Eclectic Medical Publications [reprint of 1898 original].

Ferenci, P. et al. 1989. Randomized controlled trial of silymarin treatment in patients with cirrhosis of the liver. *J Hepatol* 9(1):105–113.

Fintelmann, V. and A. Albert. 1980. The therapeutic activity of Legalon® in toxic hepatic disorders demonstrated in a double-blind trial. *Therapiewoche* 30:5589–5594.

Floersheim, G.L., O. Weber, P. Tschumi, M. Ulbrich. 1982. [Poisoning by the deathcap fungus (*Amanita phalloides*): Prognostic factors and therapeutic measures] [In German]. *Schweiz Med Wochenschr* 112(34):1164–1177.

Flora, K., M. Hahn, H. Rosen, K. Benner. 1998. Milk thistle (*Silybum marianum*) for the therapy of liver disease. *Am J Gastroenterol* 93(2):139–143.

Foster, S. and V.E. Tyler. 1999. *Tyler's Honest Herbal: A Sensible Guide to the Use of Herbs and Related Remedies,* 4th ed. New York: Haworth Herbal Press.

The German Homeopathic Pharmacopoeia (GHP). 1993. Translation of the *Deutsches Homöopathisches Arzneibuch* (HAB 1), 5th suppl. 1991 to the 1st ed. 1978. Stuttgart: Deutscher Apotheker Verlag. 821–827.

Hikino, H. and Y. Kiso. 1988. Natural Products for Liver Disease. In: Wagner, H., H. Hikino, N.R. Farnsworth. *Economic and Medicinal Plant Research,* Vol. 2. New York: Academic Press. 39–72.

Hoffmann, D. 1992. *The New Holistic Herbal.* Rockport, MA: Element Books Ltd. 215.

Hruby, C. 1984. Silibinin in the treatment of deathcap fungus poisoning. *Forum* 6:23–26.

Leung, A.Y. and S. Foster. 1996. *Encyclopedia of Common Natural Ingredients Used in Food, Drugs, and Cosmetics,* 2nd ed. New York: John Wiley & Sons, Inc. 366–368.

Lust, J.B. 1974. *The Herb Book.* New York: Bantam Books. 272–273.

Magliulo, E., B. Gagliardi, G.P. Fiori. 1978. [Results of a double blind study on the effect of silymarin in the treatment of acute viral hepatitis, carried out at two medical centers] [In German]. *Med Klin* 73(28–29):1060–1065.

McPartland, J.M. 1996. Viral hepatitis treated with *Phyllanthus amarus* and milk thistle (*Silybum marianum*): a case report. *Complementary Medicine International* 3(2):40–42.

Meyer-Buchtela, E. 1999. *Tee-Rezepturen—Ein Handbuch für Apotheker und Ärzte.* Stuttgart: Deutscher Apotheker Verlag.

Morazzani, P. and E. Bombardelli. 1995. *Silybum marianum* (*Carduus marianus*). Fitoterapia 66:3–42.

Palasciano, G. et al. 1994. The effect of Silymarin on plasma levels of Malon-Dialdehyde in patients receiving long-term treatment with psychotropic drugs. *Curr Therapeut Res* 55(5):537–545.

Pares, A. et al. 1998. Effects of silymarin in alcoholic patients with cirrhosis of the liver: results of a controlled, double-blind, randomized and multicenter trial. *J Hepatol* 28(4):615–621.

Poser, G. 1971. [Experience in the treatment of chronic hepatitis with silymarin] [In German]. *Arzneimforsch* 21(8):1209–1212.

Robbers, J.E. and V.E. Tyler. 1999. *Tyler's Herbs of Choice: The Therapeutic Use of Phytomedicinals.* New York: Haworth Herbal Press.

Salmi, H.A. and S. Sarna. 1982. Effect of silymarin on chemical, functional, and morphological alterations of the liver. A double-blind controlled study. *Scand J Gastroenterol* 17(4):517–521.

Sonnenbichler, J., I. Sonnenbichler, F. Scalera. 1998. Influence of the Flavonolignan Silibinin of Milk Thistle on Hepatocytes and Kidney Cells. In: L.D. Lawson and R. Bauer (eds.) *Phytomedicines of Europe: Chemistry and Biological Activity.* Washington, DC: American Chemical Society, 263–277.

United States Pharmacopeia, 24th rev. and *National Formulary*, 19th ed. (USP24–NF19). 1999. Rockville, MD: United States Pharmacopeial Convention, Inc. 2481–2482.

Weiss, R.F. 1988. *Herbal Medicine.* Beaconsfield, England: Beaconsfield Publishers.

Wichtl, M. and N.G. Bisset (eds.). 1994. *Herbal Drugs and Phytopharmaceuticals.* Stuttgart: Medpharm Scientific Publishers. 121–123.

Additional Resources

Albrecht, M. et al. 1992. Therapy of toxic liver pathologies with Legalon®. *Z Klin Med* 47:87–92.

Bindoli, A., L. Cavallini, N. Siliprandi. 1977. Inhibitory action of silymarin of lipid peroxide formation in the rat liver mitochondria and microsomes. *Biochem Pharmacol* 26(24):2405–2409.

Campos, R., A. Garrido, R. Guerra, A. Valenzuela. 1989. Silybin dihemisuccinate protects against glutathione depletion and lipid peroxidation induced by acetaminophen on rat liver. *Planta Med* 55(5):417–419.

Foster, S. 1995. *Milk Thistle Bibliography and Abstracts.* Austin, TX: American Botanical Council.

Hikino, H., Y. Kiso, H. Wagner, M. Fiebig. 1984. Antihepatotoxic actions of flavonolignans from *Silybum marianum* fruits. *Planta Med* 50(3):248–250.

Kiesewetter, E., I. Leodolter, H. Thaler. 1977. [Results of two double-blind studies on the effect of silymarin in chronic hepatitis] [In German]. *Leber Magen Darm* 7(5):318–323.

Krecman, V., N. Skottova, D. Walterova, J. Ulrichova, V. Simanek. 1998. Silymarin inhibits the development of diet-induced hypercholesterolemia in rats. *Planta Med* 64(2):138–142.

McGuffin, M., C. Hobbs, R. Upton, A. Goldberg. 1997. American Herbal Product Association's *Botanical Safety Handbook.* Boca Raton: CRC Press.

Mourelle, M., P. Muriel, L. Favari, T. Franco. 1989. Prevention of CC14-induced liver cirrhosis by silymarin. *Fundam Clin Pharm* 3(3):183–191.

Plomteux, G. et al. 1977. Hepatoprotector action of silymarin in human acute viral hepatitis. *Int Res Commun Syst* 5.

Saba, P. et al. 1976. Effetti terapeutica della silimarina nelle epatopatie croniche indotte da psicofarmaci. *Gaz Med Ital* 135:236–251.

Schulz, V., R. Hänsel, V.E. Tyler. 1998. *Rational Phytotherapy: A Physicians' Guide to Herbal Medicine.* New York: Springer.

Skottova, N. and V. Krecman. 1998. Silymarin as a potential hypocholesterolaemic drug. *Physiol Res* 47(1):1–7.

Valenzuela, A., C. Lagos, K. Schmidt, L. Videla. 1985. Silymarin protection against hepatic lipid peroxidation induced by acute ethanol intoxication in the rat. *Biochem Pharmacol* 34(12):2209–2212.

Wagner, H. 1981. *Natural Products as Medicinal Agents.* Stuttgart: Hippokrates.

This material was adapted from *The Complete German Commission E Monographs—Therapeutic Guide to Herbal Medicines.* M. Blumenthal, W.R. Busse, A. Goldberg, J. Gruenwald, T. Hall, C.W. Riggins, R.S. Rister (eds.) S. Klein and R.S. Rister (trans.). 1998. Austin: American Botanical Council; Boston: Integrative Medicine Communications.

1) The Overview section is new information.
2) Description, Chemistry and Pharmacology, Uses, Contraindications, Side Effects, Interactions with Other Drugs, and Dosage sections have been drawn from the original work. Additional information has been added in some or all of these sections, as noted with references.
3) The dosage for equivalent preparations (tea infusion, fluidextract, and tincture) have been provided based on the following example:
   Unless otherwise prescribed: 2 g per day of [powdered, crushed, cut or whole] [plant part]
   Infusion: 2 g in 150 ml of water
   Fluidextract 1:1 (g/ml): 2 ml
   Tincture 1:5 (g/ml): 10 ml
4) The References and Additional Resources sections are new sections. Additional Resources are not cited in the monograph but are included for research purposes.

Wagner, H. et al. 1984. *Plant Drug Analysis*. Berlin-Heidelberg; New York; Tokyo: Springer Verlag.

Wang, M. et al. 1996. Hepatoprotective properties of *Silybum marianum* herbal preparation on ethanol-induced liver damage. *Fitoterapia* 67(2):166–171.

MINT OIL

Latin Name:
Mentha arvensis

Pharmacopeial Name:
Menthae arvensis aetheroleum

Other Names:
cornmint oil, field mint oil, Japanese
mint oil, marsh mint oil

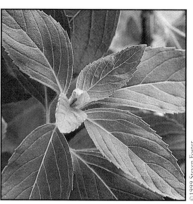

©1999 Steven Foster

Overview

Mint oil is steam distilled from the flowering tops of Japanese mint, a perennial
aromatic herb native to Japan, now cultivated in subtropical climates around the
world (Bruneton, 1995; Leung and Foster, 1996; Tyler et al., 1988). The material
of commerce comes from China, Japan, Taiwan, Brazil, India, and Paraguay
(Bruneton, 1995; Leung and Foster, 1996). Mint oil is used to produce menthol,
isolated and purified from the essential oil (Tyler et al., 1988). The partially
dementholated essential oil is official in the pharmacopeias of India, France, and
China (IP, 1996; Ph.Fr.X., 1990; Tu, 1992) and approved in the Commission E
monographs.

Mint oil is official in the *Indian Pharmacopoeia* as a carminative at dosage
60μl–200μl (IP, 1996). It is official in the Chinese pharmacopeia as an aromatic,
flavoring agent, and carminative, for application to the skin or mucous membrane,
and to relieve pain or discomfort, at single dosage of 0.02–0.2 ml and daily dosage
of 0.06–0.6 ml (Tu, 1992). In Germany, it is taken internally as a carminative or
cholagogue, inhaled as a secretolytic, and applied externally for its cooling property. In the United States, the essential oils of other mints (e.g., peppermint and
spearmint) are more commonly used in dietary supplement, health food, and OTC
drug products than Japanese mint oil (Leung and Foster, 1996). However, menthol, derived from mint oil, is widely used as an antipruritic component of OTC
preparations to treat burns and sunburn, poison ivy rash, athlete's foot, and as a
counterirritant in external analgesic preparations (Tyler et al., 1988).

The approved modern therapeutic applications for mint oil are supportable
based on its history of clinical use in well established systems of traditional medicine, on phytochemical investigations, and *in vitro* studies and *in vivo* pharmacological experiments in animals.

French pharmacopeial grade mint oil is the essential oil of Japanese mint, partially dementholated by freezing and crystallization processes, composed of
30–45% menthol, 17–35% menthone, 5–13% isomenthone, 2–7% menthyl
acetate, 1.5–7% limonene, <1% menthofuran, <1.5% cineole and pulegone, and
<2% carvone (Bruneton, 1995; Ph.Fr.X., 1990). The Commission E monograph
requires 3–17% esters, calculated as menthyl acetate, at least 42% free alcohols,
calculated as menthol, and 25–40% ketones, calculated as menthone. The *Indian
Pharmacopoeia* requires not less than 50% w/w of total menthol, and other standards, including tests for acidity or alkalinity, optical rotation, and solubility in
ethanol (IP, 1996). The Chinese pharmacopeia requires not less than 50% (g/g)
total alcohols, calculated as menthol, 2.0–6.5% (g/g) ester, calculated as menthyl
acetate, and other standards, including tests for relative density, optical rotation,
refractive index, identification, and insoluble matter in ethanol (Tu, 1992). The
Japanese Pharmacopoeia specifies a simple colormetric test for positive identification of the essential oil (JP XII, 1993).

Description

Mint oil consists of volatile oil obtained from *Mentha arvensis* L. var. *piperascens* Malinv. [Fam. Lamiaceae], and its preparations in effective dosage. The oil is obtained by steam distillation of the fresh, flowering herb, followed by partial removal of menthol and rectification.

Chemistry and Pharmacology

Mint oil contains at least 42% free alcohols (30–45% menthol); 25–40% ketones (17–35% menthone, 5–13% isomenthone); 3–17% esters (2–7% menthyl acetate); 1.5–7% limonene; <1% menthofuran, cineole and pulegone <1.5%, and <2% carvone (Bruneton, J., 1995; Leung and Foster, 1996; List and Hörhammer, 1973–1979).

The Commission E reported carminative, cholagogic, antibacterial, secretolytic, and cooling properties.

Mint oil has antimicrobial activities *in vitro* (Leung and Foster, 1996).

Uses

The Commission E approved internal use of mint oil for flatulence, functional gastrointestinal and gallbladder disorders, catarrhs of the upper respiratory tract, and external use for myalgia and neuralgic ailments.

Mint and its oil are used in China for treating indigestion, nausea, sore throat, diarrhea, colds, and headaches (Leung and Foster, 1996).

Contraindications

Internal: Obstruction of the bile ducts, inflammation of the gallbladder, severe liver damage. To be used only after consulting a physician.

External: For infants and young children, mint oil-containing preparations should not be used on areas of the face, especially the nose.

Side Effects

Sensitive people may experience stomach disorders.

Use During Pregnancy and Lactation

No restrictions known.

Interactions with Other Drugs

None known.

Dosage and Administration

Unless otherwise prescribed: 3–6 drops per day essential oil.

Internal: Inhalant: Inhale deeply the steam vapor by adding 3–4 drops of essential oil in hot water.

External: Essential oil: Several drops rubbed into the skin (may be diluted with lukewarm water or vegetable oil). Ointment: Semi-solid preparation containing 5–20% essential oil in a base of paraffin and petroleum jelly for local application.

Nasal ointment: Semi-solid preparation containing 1–5% essential oil.

Tincture: Aqueous-alcoholic preparation containing 5–10% essential oil for local application.

References

Bruneton, J. 1995. *Pharmacognosy, Phytochemistry, Medicinal Plants.* Paris: Lavoisier Publishing.

Indian Pharmacopoeia, Vol. 1. (IP 1996). 1996. Delhi: Government of India Ministry of Health and Family Welfare—Controller of Publications. 454–466.

Japanese Pharmacopoeia, 12th ed. (JP XII). 1993. Tokyo: Government of Japan Ministry of Health and Welfare—Yakuji Nippo, Ltd. 174.

Leung, A.Y. and S. Foster. 1996. *Encyclopedia of Common Natural Ingredients Used in Food, Drugs, and Cosmetics*, 2nd ed. New York: John Wiley & Sons, Inc.

List, P.H. and L. Hörhammer (eds.). 1973–1979. *Hagers Handbuch der Pharmazeutischen Praxis*, Vols. 1–7. New York: Springer Verlag.

Pharmacopée Française Xe Édition (Ph.Fr.X.). 1983–1990. Moulins-les-Metz: Maisonneuve S.A.

Tu, G. (ed.). 1992. *Pharmacopoeia of the People's Republic of China* (English Edition 1992). Beijing: Guangdong Science and Technology Press. 129–130.

Tyler, V.E., L.R. Brady, J.E. Robbers. 1988. *Pharmacognosy*, 9th ed. Philadelphia: Lea & Febiger. 118–119.

Additional Resources

Bown, D. 1995. *Encyclopedia of Herbs and Their Uses*. New York: DK Publishing, Inc. 311.

Bradu, B.L., S.G. Agarval, V.N. Vashist, C.K. Atal. 1971. Comparative performance of diploid and tetraploid *Mentha arvensis* and evaluation of their oils. *Planta Med* 20(3):219–222.

Dost, F.H. and B. Leiber (eds.). 1967. *Menthol and Menthol-containing External Remedies. Use, Mode of Effect and Tolerance in Children.* Stuttgart: George Thieme Verlag.

Ellis, B.E. and G.H. Towers. 1970. Biogenesis of rosmarinic acid in *Mentha*. *Biochem J* 118(2):291–297.

Food Chemicals Codex, 2nd ed. (FCC II). 1972. Washington, D.C.: National Academy of Sciences.

Grieve, M. 1979. *A Modern Herbal*. New York: Dover Publications, Inc.

Jiangsu Institute of Modern Medicine. 1977. *Zhong Yao Da Ci Dian* (Encyclopedia of Chinese Materia Medica), Vols. 1–3. Shanghai: Shanghai Scientific and Technical Publications.

Lombard, A., M.L. Tourn, M. Buffa. 1977. In situ reactions on silica gel thin layers in studies on plant oligosaccharides. *J Chromatogr* 134(1):242–245.

Morton, J.F. 1977. *Major Medicinal Plants: Botany, Culture and Uses*. Springfield, IL: Charles C. Thomas.

Nadkarni, K.M. 1976. *Indian Materia Medica*. Bombay: Popular Prakashan. 788–789.

NF T 75-306. Dec. 1985. [The French standard for cornmint oil].

Nigam, I.C. and L. Levi. 1964. Essential oils and their constituents. XX. Detection and estimation of menthofuran in *Mentha arvensis* and other mint species by coupled gas-liquid-thin-layer chromatography. *J Pharm Sci* 53:1008–1013.

van Os, F.H. and D. Smith. 1970. De vluchtige olie van *Mentha arvensis* L. subsp. *austriaca* (Jacquin) Briquet [The essential oil of *Mentha arvensis* L. subsp. austriaca (Jaquin) Briquet]. *Pharm Weekbl* 105(44):1273–1276.

Panadero, M. 1959. [Study of Japanese mint cultivated in Spain] *Farmacognosia* 19:225–253.

Poetsch, C.E. 1967. Brief history of topical rub therapy. In: Dost, F.H. and B. Leiber (eds.). *Menthol and Menthol-containing External Remedies*. Stuttgart: George Thieme Verlag.

This material was adapted from *The Complete German Commission E Monographs—Therapeutic Guide to Herbal Medicines.* M. Blumenthal, W.R. Busse, A. Goldberg, J. Gruenwald, T. Hall, C.W. Riggins, R.S. Rister (eds.) S. Klein and R.S. Rister (trans.). 1998. Austin: American Botanical Council; Boston: Integrative Medicine Communications.

1) The Overview section is new information.

2) Description, Chemistry and Pharmacology, Uses, Contraindications, Side Effects, Interactions with Other Drugs, and Dosage sections have been drawn from the original work. Additional information has been added in some or all of these sections, as noted with references.

3) The dosage for equivalent preparations (tea infusion, fluidextract, and tincture) have been provided based on the following example:

Unless otherwise prescribed: 2 g per day of [powdered, crushed, cut or whole] [plant part]
Infusion: 2 g in 150 ml of water
Fluidextract 1:1 (g/ml): 2 ml
Tincture 1:5 (g/ml): 10 ml

4) The References and Additional Resources sections are new sections. Additional Resources are not cited in the monograph but are included for research purposes.

MOTHERWORT HERB

Latin Name:
Leonurus cardiaca

Pharmacopeial Name:
Leonuri cardiacae herba

Other Names:
common motherwort

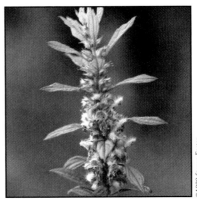

© 1999 Steven Foster

Overview

Motherwort's several species are native to temperate regions of Europe and Asia and grow wild in Canada and the United States (Foster, 1993). For therapeutic purposes, the species are generally interchangeable (Newall et al., 1996). As its name implies, motherwort was used by the people in these geographical regions as a folk remedy for female reproductive disorders. It was also used for certain types of heart conditions, as the Latin word *cardiaca* indicates. Today, it is recommended by herbalists and Commission E for heart palpitations occurring with anxiety attacks or other nervous disorders (Foster, 1993).

Although current clinical research is lacking, earlier studies demonstrated hypotensive and negatively chronotropic effects on laboratory animals. Sedative actions and protective effects during cerebral ischemia were reported (Bradley, 1992), and alcohol extracts of motherwort were noted to have direct myocardial actions, inhibiting the effects of calcium chloride and stimulating alpha and beta adrenoceptors (Newall et al., 1996). Alkaloids in the plant depress the central nervous system and lower blood pressure in preliminary testing, and are considered responsible for these effects (Bradley, 1992). However, these studies are exploratory. Further research may determine the usefulness of motherwort, or its possible detrimental effects. Of concern are its uterine-stimulant and myocardial effects, and how it will interact with concurrent cardiac medications.

Motherwort's uterine stimulant effects were recognized by native Americans. The Delaware, Micmac, Modheman, and Shinnecock tribes used motherwort to treat gynecological disorders (Moerman, 1998), as did the nineteenth century Eclectic physicians. Indications included difficult, painful, or absent menstruation, and especially for anxiety occurring along with it (Ellingwood, 1983). One alkaloid in particular, leonurine, is uterotonic *in vitro*, and another, stacydrine, may stimulate the release of oxytocin (Newall et al., 1996); both actions support the use of motherwort for menstrual disorders. The herb was also a noted antispasmodic and laxative (Hutchens, 1991). Native Americans, herbalists, and the Eclectic physicians used motherwort for delirium tremens, typhoid fever, disturbed sleep, minor gastrointestinal distress, heart palpitations (Ellingwood, 1983), rheumatism, goiter, epilepsy, and high blood pressure (Hutchens, 1991).

In the Middle Ages, motherwort was a remedy for fainting and other symptoms of nervousness or weakness due to emotional excitement or illness. It was also used to protect individuals from evil spirits. In the late sixteenth century, the English herbalist John Gerard noted its effectiveness in treating cardiac weakness, and while his successor, Nicholas Culpepper, recommended it for chest colds, intestinal worms, and aches and pains, he emphasized motherwort's ability to make the mind cheerful (Grieve, 1979).

Description

Motherwort herb consists of the above-ground parts of *Leonurus cardiaca* L. [Fam. Lamiaceae], gathered during flowering season, and their preparations in effective dosage. The preparation contains alkaloids (stachydrine), glycosides of bitter principles, and bufenolide.

Chemistry and Pharmacology

Constituents include alkaloids (stachydrine, betonicine, turicin, leonurine, leonuridin, and leonurinine), flavonoids (glycosides of apigenin, kaempferol, and quercetin), iridoids (ajugol, ajugoside, galiridoside, and leonurid), tannins (pseudotannins: pyrogallol and catechins), terpenoids (volatile oil, resin, wax, ursolic acid, leocardin, and a diterpene lactone similar to marrubiin), and triterpenes (ursolic acid) (Bradley, 1992; Newall et al., 1996). Other constituents include citric acid, malic acid, oleic acid, bitter principles, carbohydrates, choline, and a phenolic glycoside (caffeic acid 4-rutinoside) (Brieskorn, 1972; Tschesche et al., 1980).

Studies have found that ursolic acid has demonstrated tumor-inhibiting, antiviral, cardioactive, and cytotoxic properties (Kuo-Hsiung et al., 1988; Tokuda et al., 1986; Yanxing, 1983). An *in vitro* study found that ursolic acid acted similarly to retinoic acid, a known tumor inhibitor. In mice, it inhibited the Epstein-Barr virus and tumor production (Tokuda et al., 1986). Motherwort demonstrated cytotoxicity during an *in vitro* study on lymphocytic leukemia, KB cells, human lung carcinoma, mammary tumors and human colon (Kuo-Hsiung et al., 1988). The alkaloids in motherwort may contribute to the activity of the herb: leonurine produces central nervous depressant and hypotensive effects in animals and stachydrine may be involved (Bradley, 1992).

Uses

The Commission E approved motherwort herb for nervous cardiac disorders and as an adjuvant for thyroid hyperfunction. It has been used as a sedative, hypotensive, cardiotonic, and antispasmodic (Bradley, 1992; Newall et al., 1996). The herb has been given to patients who have neuropathic cardiac disorders and cardiac complaints of nervous origin (Bradley, 1992). Traditionally it has been used for cardiac debility, simple tachycardia, effort syndrome, amenorrhea, and cardiac symptoms associated with neurosis.

Contraindications

None known.

Side Effects

None known.

Use During Pregnancy and Lactation

Not recommended during pregnancy. No restrictions known during lactation.

Interactions with Other Drugs

None known.

Dosage and Administration

Unless otherwise prescribed: 4.5 g per day of cut herb.
Infusion: 4.5 g of herb in 150 ml water.
Fluidextract 1:1 (g/ml): 4.5 ml.
Tincture 1:5 (g/ml): 22.5 ml.
Note: The *Botanical Safety Handbook* states, "A dose in excess of 3.0 grams of a powdered extract may cause diarrhea, uterine bleeding, and stomach irritation" (McGuffin et al., 1997).

$4.5/150 = 0.03 \times 20 = 0.6 \, g$

$600 \, mg$

References

Bradley, P.R. (ed.). 1992. *British Herbal Compendium*, Vol. 1. Bournemouth: British Herbal Medicine Association.

Brieskorn, C.H. and W. Broschek. 1972. Analysis of bitter principles and furanoid compounds of *Leonurus cardiaca* L. *Pharm Acta Helv* 47(2):123–132.

Ellingwood, F. 1983. *American Materia Medica, Therapeutics and Pharmacognosy.* Portland, OR: Eclectic Medical Publications [reprint of 1919 original].

Foster, S. 1993. *Herbal Renaissance: Growing, Using and Understanding Herbs in the Modern World.* Salt Lake City: Gibbs-Smith.

Grieve, M. 1979. *A Modern Herbal.* New York: Dover Publications, Inc.

Hutchens, A. 1991. *Indian Herbology of North America.* Boston: Shambala.

Kuo-Hsiung, L. et al. 1988. The cytotoxic principles of *Prunella vulgaris, Psychotria serpens,* and *Hyptis capitata:* Ursolic acid and related derivatives. *Planta Med* (54):308.

McGuffin, M., C. Hobbs, R. Upton, A. Goldberg. 1997. American Herbal Product Association's *Botanical Safety Handbook.* Boca Raton: CRC Press.

Moerman, D.E. 1998 *Native American Ethnobotany.* Portland, OR: Timber Press.

Newall, C.A., L.A. Anderson, J.D. Phillipson. 1996. *Herbal Medicines: A Guide for Health-Care Professionals.* London: The Pharmaceutical Press.

Tokuda, H., H. Ohigashi, K. Koshimizu, Y. Ito. 1986. Inhibitory effects of ursolic and oleanolic acid on skin tumor promotion by 12Otetrade canoylphor bol13acetate. *Cancer Lett* 33(3):279–285.

Tschesche, R. et al. 1980. Caffeic acid 4-rutinoside-from *Leonurus cardiaca. Phytochemistry* 19: 2783.

Yanxing, X. 1983. The inhibitory effect of motherwort extract on pulsating myocardial cells *in vitro. J Tradit Chin Med* 3(3):185–188.

Additional Resources

Benigni, R., C. Capra, P.E. Cattorini. 1964. *Piante Medicinali—Chimica, Farmacologia e Terapia,* Vol. 2. Milan: Inverni & Della Beffa.

British Herbal Pharmacopoeia (BHP). 1983. Keighley, U.K.: British Herbal Medicine Association.

———. 1990. Bournemouth, U.K.: British Herbal Medicine Association.

Kong, Y.C. et al. 1976. Isolation of the uterotonic principle from *Leonurus cardiaca,* the Chinese motherwort. *Am J Chin Med* 4(4):373–382.

Kuang, P.G., X.F. Zhou, F.Y. Zhang, S.Y. Lang. 1988. Motherwort and cerebral ischemia. *J Tradit Chin Med* 8(1):37–40.

Nahrstedt, A. 1985. Drogen und Phytopharmaka mit sedierender Wirkung. *Z Phytotherapie* (6):101–109.

Reuter, G. and H.J. Diehl. 1970. Arzneipflanzen der gattung *Leonurus* und ihre wirkstoffe [Medicinal plants of species *Leonurus* and their active substances]. *Pharmazie* 25(10):586–589.

Schultz, O.E. and M. Alhyane. 1973. Inhaltsstoffe von *Leonurus cardiaca* L. *Sci Pharm* (41):149–155.

State Pharmacopoeia of the Union of Soviet Socialist Republics, 10th ed. 1973. [English edition]. Moscow: Ministry of Health of the U.S.S.R.

Yeung, H.W. et al. 1977. The structure and biological effect of leonurine. A uterotonic principle from the Chinese drug, I-mu Ts'ao. *Planta Med* 31(1):51–56.

This material was adapted from *The Complete German Commission E Monographs—Therapeutic Guide to Herbal Medicines.* M. Blumenthal, W.R. Busse, A. Goldberg, J. Gruenwald, T. Hall, C.W. Riggins, R.S. Rister (eds.) S. Klein and R.S. Rister (trans.). 1998. Austin: American Botanical Council; Boston: Integrative Medicine Communications.

1) The Overview section is new information.

2) Description, Chemistry and Pharmacology, Uses, Contraindications, Side Effects, Interactions with Other Drugs, and Dosage sections have been drawn from the original work. Additional information has been added in some or all of these sections, as noted with references.

3) The dosage for equivalent preparations (tea infusion, fluidextract, and tincture) have been provided based on the following example:
   Unless otherwise prescribed: 2 g per day of [powdered, crushed, cut or whole] [plant part]
   Infusion: 2 g in 150 ml of water
   Fluidextract 1:1 (g/ml): 2 ml
   Tincture 1:5 (g/ml): 10 ml

4) The References and Additional Resources sections are new sections. Additional Resources are not cited in the monograph but are included for research purposes.

MULLEIN FLOWER

Latin Name:
Verbascum densiflorum

Pharmacopeial Name:
Verbasci flos

Other Names:
large-flowered mullein

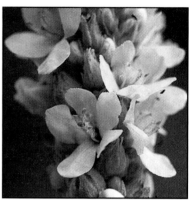

©1999 Steven Foster

Overview

Great mullein (*Verbascum thapsus* L.), orange mullein (*V. phlomoides* L.) and large-flowered mullein (*V. densiflorum* Bertol., syn. *V. thapsiforme* Schrad.) are biennial plants native throughout Europe, northern Africa (Egypt) and Ethiopia, and temperate Asia as far as the Himalayas (Grieve, 1979; Wichtl and Bisset, 1994). In India, it grows wild in the temperate Himalayas from Kashmir to Bhutan (Nadkarni, 1976). The material of commerce comes mainly from cultivated sources in Bulgaria, the Czech Republic, and Egypt (BHP, 1996; Wichtl and Bisset, 1994).

Both the leaves and the flower of mullein have been used as medicine since ancient times. Mullein preparations were used during the Middle Ages as a remedy for skin and lung disease in cattle and humans. By the end of the nineteenth century, mullein was given in Europe, the United Kingdom, and the United States to tuberculosis patients. Its actions on the lungs are demulcent and emollient (Grieve, 1979). Nineteenth century Eclectic physicians used mullein for inflammatory diseases of the respiratory and genitourinary tracts and the ear canal (Ellingwood, 1983). It is still prescribed today by naturopathic physicians and medical herbalists as a treatment for chronic otitis media and eczema of the ear (Caradonna, 1997; Winston, 1997).

In Germany, mullein flower is approved in the Commission E monographs, listed in the *German Drug Codex*, and it is also used as a component of various cough and bronchial tea medicines (BAnz, 1998; DAC, 1986; Schilcher, 1997; Wichtl and Bisset, 1994). For example, it is a component of Kneipp® Husten-Tee (cough tea) and Salus® Bronchial-Tee (bronchial tea) (Wichtl and Bisset, 1994). In German pediatric medicine, mullein flower is used as a component of various herbal tea mixtures indicated to treat cough with viscid expectoration (productive cough). For example, the cough tea mixture *Species pectorales* DAB 6 is composed of 40% althea root (*Althaea officinalis*), 20% licorice root (*Glycyrrhiza glabra*), 20% coltsfoot leaf (*Tussilago farfara*), 10% mullein flower, and 10% anise seed (*Pimpinella anisum*) (DAB 6, 1951; Schilcher, 1997). In the United States, mullein flower became official in the fourth edition of the U.S. *National Formulary*, as a component in pectoral remedies, but has been removed from its official status due to a lack of therapeutic validation (Tyler, 1993).

The approved modern therapeutic applications for mullein flower in Europe are supportable based on its long history of use in well established systems of traditional and conventional medicine, phytochemical investigations, *in vitro* studies, and pharmacological studies in animals. Mullein flowers have demonstrated antiviral action, *in vitro*, against fowl plague virus, several strains of influenza A and B, and herpes simplex virus (Slagowska et al., 1987; Zgorniak-Nowosielska et al., 1991), and both flowers and leaves possess mildly demulcent, expectorant, and astringent properties. Expectorant actions may be due to the plant's saponin content (Tyler, 1993), its actual mucilage content is a sparse 3% (Schulz et al., 1998).

German pharmacopeial grade mullein flower must have a swelling index of not less than 9 and it must contain not more than 5% calices and discolored flowers (brown corollas). Botanical identity must be confirmed by macroscopic and microscopic examinations as well as analysis of flavonoids (DAC, 1986; Wichtl and Bisset, 1994). The Swiss pharmacopeia requires a swelling index of not less than 12 (Ph.Helv.VII, 1987; Wichtl and Bisset, 1994).

Description
Mullein flower consists of the dried petals of V. *densiflorum* Bertoloni and V. *phlomoides* L. (syn. V. thapsus L.) [Fam. Scrophulariaceae], and their preparations in effective dosage. The preparation contains saponins and mucopolysaccharides.

Chemistry and Pharmacology
Mullein flower contains approximately 3% water-soluble mucilage polysaccharides, which after hydrolysis yields 47% D-galactose, 25% arabinose, 14% D-glucose, 6% D-xylose, 4% L-rhamnose, 2% D-mannose, 1% L-fucose, and 12.5% uronic acids (arabinogalactans) (Kraus and Franz, 1987; Meyer-Buchtela, 1999; Wichtl and Bisset, 1994); approximately 1.5–4% flavonoids (apignein, luteolin and their 7-O-glucosides, plus kaempferol and rutin); caffeic acid derivatives including caffeic, ferulic, protocatechuic acids, and verbascoside; iridoid monoterpenes (aucubin, 6-β-xylosylaucubin, methylcatalpol, isocatalpol); triterpene saponins (verbascosaponin) (Klimek, 1996a; Klimek, 1996b; Meyer-Buchtela, 1999; Wichtl and Bisset, 1994); sterols; and 11% invert sugar (fructose + glucose) (Meyer-Buchtela, 1999; Wichtl and Bisset, 1994).

The Commission E reported expectorant activity and alleviation of irritation. *In vitro*, mullein flower infusion has demonstrated antiviral action against herpes simplex type I virus and influenza A and B strains (Slagowska et al., 1987; Zgorniak-Nowosielska et al., 1991).

Uses
The Commission E approved mullein flower for catarrhs of the respiratory tract.

Mullein is useful as a component of preparations indicated for symptomatic treatment of sore throat and cough (Der Marderosian, 1999). Other uses of the flower are for chills, dry coughs, and phlegm congestion due to the mild expectorant action of the saponins (Schulz et al., 1998; Wichtl and Bisset, 1994).

Contraindications
None known.

Side Effects
None known.

Use During Pregnancy and Lactation
No restrictions known.

Interactions with Other Drugs
None known.

Dosage and Administration
Unless otherwise prescribed: 3–4 g of cut herb for teas and other equivalent galenical preparations for internal use. [Note: According to the *Pharmacopeia of Austria*, the usual single dose for mullein flower decoction or infusion is 1.5 g dried herb per cup (Meyer-Buchtela, 1999; ÖAB, 1991).]
Decoction: Place 1.5–2 g of herb in 150–250 ml cold water and bring to a boil for 10 minutes, twice daily (Meyer-

Buchtela, 1999; Wichtl and Bisset, 1994).
Infusion: Steep 1.5–2 g of herb in 150–250 ml boiled water for 10 to 15 minutes, twice daily (Meyer-Buchtela, 1999; Wichtl and Bisset, 1994).
Note: 18% of the potentially available flavonoids are yielded into the tea after 10 minutes of steeping time. However, a 10 minute decoction will result in a more exhaustive extraction of the flavonoids than a 10 minute infusion (Meyer-Buchtela, 1999).
Fluidextract 1:1 (g/ml): 1.5–2 ml, twice daily.
Tincture 1:5 (g/ml): 7.5–10 ml, twice daily (dilute in warm water if desired).

References

BAnz. See *Bundesanzeiger*.
British Herbal Pharmacopoeia (BHP). 1996. Exeter, U.K.: British Herbal Medicine Association. 140–141.
Bundesanzeiger (BAnz). 1998. Monographien der Kommission E (Zulassungs- und Aufbereitungskommission am BGA für den humanmed. Bereich, phytotherapeutische Therapierichtung und Stoffgruppe). Köln: Bundesgesundheitsamt (BGA).
Caradonna, W. 1997. Naturopathic Condition Review: Otitis media. *Protocol J Botanical Med* 2(2):100.
Der Marderosian, A. (ed.). 1999. *The Review of Natural Products*. St. Louis: Facts and Comparisons.
Deutscher Arzneimittel-Codex (DAC). 1986. Stuttgart: Deutscher Apotheker Verlag.
Deutsches Arzneibuch, 6th ed. (DAB 6). 1951. Hamburg: R.V. Decker's Verlag.
Ellingwood, F. 1983. *American Materia Medica, Therapeutics and Pharmacognosy*. Portland, OR: Eclectic Medical Publications [reprint of 1919 original].

Grieve, M. 1979. *A Modern Herbal*. New York: Dover Publications, Inc.
Klimek, B. 1996a. 6'-O-apiosyl-verbascoside in the flowers of mullein (*Verbascum* species). *Acta Pol Pharm* 53(2):137–140.
———. 1996b. Hydroxycinnamoyl ester glycosides and saponins from flowers of *Verbascum phlomoides*. *Phytochemistry* 43(6):1281–1284.
Kraus, K. and G. Franz. 1987. *Dtsch Apoth Ztg* 127:665–669.
Meyer-Buchtela, E. 1999. *Tee-Rezepturen—Ein Handbuch für Apotheker und Ärzte*. Stuttgart: Deutscher Apotheker Verlag.
Nadkarni, K.M. 1976. *Indian Materia Medica*. Bombay: Popular Prakashan. 1266–1267.
Österreichisches Arzneibuch (ÖAB). 1991. Wien: Verlag der Österreichischen Staatsdruckerei.
Pharmacopoeia Helvetica, 7th ed. Vol. 1–4. (Ph.Helv.VII). 1987. Bern: Office Central Fédéral des Imprimés et du Matériel.
Schilcher, H. 1997. *Phytotherapy in Paediatrics—Handbook for Physicians and Pharmacists*. Stuttgart: Medpharm Scientific Publishers. 36.
Schulz, V., R. Hänsel, V.E. Tyler. 1998. *Rational Phytotherapy: A Physicians' Guide to Herbal Medicine*. New York: Springer.
Slagowska, A., I. Zgorniak-Nowosielska, J. Grzybek. 1987. Inhibition of herpes simplex virus replication by Flos verbasci infusion. *Pol J Pharmacol Pharm* 39(1):55–61.
Tyler, V.E. 1993. *The Honest Herbal*, 3rd ed. New York: Pharmaceutical Products Press.
Wichtl, M. and N.G. Bisset (eds.). 1994. *Herbal Drugs and Phytopharmaceuticals*. Stuttgart: Medpharm Scientific Publishers.
Winston, D. 1997. *Protocol J Bot Med* 2(2):106.
Zgorniak-Nowosielska, I., J. Grzybek, N. Manolova, J. Serkedjieva, B. Zawilinska. 1991. Antiviral activity of Flos verbasci infusion against influenza and Herpes simplex viruses. *Arch Immunol Ther Exp (Warsz)* 39(1–2):103–108.

Additional Resources

Bruneton, J. 1995. *Pharmacognosy, Phytochemistry, Medicinal Plants*. Paris: Lavoisier Publishing.

This material was adapted from *The Complete German Commission E Monographs—Therapeutic Guide to Herbal Medicines*. M. Blumenthal, W.R. Busse, A. Goldberg, J. Gruenwald, T. Hall, C.W. Riggins, R.S. Rister (eds.) S. Klein and R.S. Rister (trans.). 1998. Austin: American Botanical Council; Boston: Integrative Medicine Communications.
1) The Overview section is new information.
2) Description, Chemistry and Pharmacology, Uses, Contraindications, Side Effects, Interactions with Other Drugs, and Dosage sections have been drawn from the original work. Additional information has been added in some or all of these sections, as noted with references.
3) The dosage for equivalent preparations (tea infusion, fluidextract, and tincture) have been provided based on the following example:
   Unless otherwise prescribed: 2 g per day of [powdered, crushed, cut or whole] [plant part]
   Infusion: 2 g in 150 ml of water
   Fluidextract 1:1 (g/ml): 2 ml
   Tincture 1:5 (g/ml): 10 ml
4) The References and Additional Resources sections are new sections. Additional Resources are not cited in the monograph but are included for research purposes.

MYRRH

Latin Name:
Commiphora molmol
Pharmacopeial Name:
Myrrha
Other Names:
common myrrh, gum myrrh, hirabol
myrrh, heerabol myrrh, gummi
myrrh

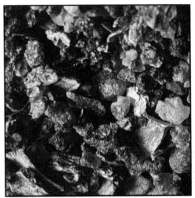

©1999 Steven Foster

Overview

Gum-resin myrrh is a product of several species of *Commiphora*, a perennial tree or shrub native to Nubia (Egypt and Sudan), Somaliland (northeast Somalia, Djibouti, and east Ethiopia) and the Arabian Peninsula of southwest Asia (Yemen) (Budavari, 1996; Leung and Foster, 1996; Tyler, 1993; Wichtl and Bisset, 1994). The material of commerce is collected mainly from wild trees in the Horn of Africa (Erythrea, Ethiopia, Somalia), Sudan, and Yemen (BHP, 1996; Iwu, 1990; Wichtl and Bisset, 1994; Yen, 1992). It is also under cultivation in Kenya, Tanzania, Ethiopia and other north African countries (Iwu, 1990). The material used in traditional Chinese medicine, *Commiphora molmol* Engl. = *C. myrrha* Engl., is imported from Africa and Arabia and is wrapped in dogskin (Yen, 1992). The species used in Ayurvedic medicine (*C. mukul* Engl.) grows in the rocky tracts of the northwestern Indian state of Rajasthan and in the west Indian state of Gujarat (API, 1989). It is also found in the northeast Indian state of Assam, in Bangladesh, and in the province of Sind, Pakistan (Kapoor, 1990). When the bark is cut, myrrh seeps out in yellow to reddish brown agglutinated (stuck together), tear-shaped, irregular masses that are sometimes as big as walnuts (BHP, 1996; Grieve, 1979; Karnick, 1994; Tyler, 1993).

Myrrh has been used in Middle Eastern medicine for treatment of infected wounds and bronchial complaints for thousands of years (Bown, 1995). It was also used as an embalming agent by the ancient Egyptians. It is familiar to many cultures as incense used in religious rituals. Myrrh is a Jewish holy oil, and is mentioned in the first books of the Jewish, Muslim, and Christian holy texts (Grieve, 1979). In the time of Christ, the gum-resin of both frankincense (*Boswellia* spp.) and myrrh were some of the most highly valued commodities in trade (Wilford, 1997). Today, crude myrrh is dispensed throughout eastern Africa and Saudi Arabia as an anti-inflammatory and anti-rheumatism drug (Iwu, 1990).

Myrrh has a long history of therapeutic use in the Indian Ayurvedic system of medicine (Bown, 1995), where it is used to treat mouth ulcers, gingivitis and pharyngitis, as well as respiratory catarrh (Karnick, 1994). As a treatment for stomatitis (inflammation of the mouth), it is combined with honey and rectified spirit, then dissolved in rose petal infusion, and taken as a mouthwash. Externally, it is used as an astringent topical application to ulcers and as a gargle for spongy gums (Nadkarni, 1976). Myrrh tincture is also used to treat many disorders associated with the female reproductive cycle, particularly dysmenorrhea and amenorrhea, and to help relieve some of the uncomfortable symptoms of menopause (Frawley and Lad, 1986; Nadkarni, 1976). These uses have not been corroborated by clinical studies. Its use was later introduced into both the Chinese and Tibetan systems of medicine sometime during the seventh century C.E. (Bown, 1995; Clifford,

1984; Leung and Foster, 1996). The *Gyu-zhi, or Four Tantras*, by Chandranandana is the earliest Indian medical text to be translated into Tibetan (eighth century C.E.). In it, Indian myrrh (*C. mukul*) is included as a component of various psychiatric incenses, still used in Tibetan Buddhist medicine (Clifford, 1984). It is available today, for example, as a component of the Tibetan drug "Agar 31" in an incense-stick dosage form for inhaling, produced in India and Nepal (Tsarong, 1986). In Chinese medicine, Somalian myrrh (*C. myrrha*) is used to treat impact injury, incised wounds, sinew and bone pain, menstrual block, and hemorrhoids, among other conditions. It is used as a component in many patent medicines, including *bu-gu-zhi-wan* (Psoralea Pills) and *zhi-wan* (Hemorrhoid Pills), as well as various topical plaster-adhesives and lotions, including *die-da-yao-jing* (Traumatic Injury Medicine Essence) (Fratkin, 1986; Yen, 1992).

In Germany, myrrh gum-resin and myrrh tincture are both official in the *German Pharmacopeia*, approved in the Commission E monographs, and the tincture dosage form is official in the German Standard License monographs (Braun et al., 1997; DAB, 1997; Wichtl and Bisset, 1994). The tincture is used as a mono-preparation and also as a component of various dental remedies and mouthwashes, ointments, paints, and coated tablets. Application by paint, gargle, and/or rinse are used in dentistry (Wichtl and Bisset, 1994). For example, the product Merfluan® is an effervescent dentifrice salt with myrrh (Mielck, 1970). In German pediatric medicine, tincture of myrrh is used to treat oral candidiasis (thrush), which is common in infants. It is applied undiluted with a cotton-wool tip to small areas of affection, or diluted 1:1 with chamomile flower tea for larger areas (Schilcher, 1997). In the United States, myrrh was formerly official in the *United States Pharmacopeia* and *National Formulary* (Leung and Foster, 1996; Taber, 1962). It was used as an aromatic, astringent mouthwash (Taber, 1962). Myrrh's constituents include aldehydes and phenols, which stimulate drying and cleansing actions through topical administration. As a salve, myrrh is used to treat hemorrhoids, wounds, and bed sores. In tincture form, gargles and mouthwashes are considered useful in treating sore throats or other oral mucosal or gingival irritations (Tyler, 1993). The approved modern therapeutic applications for myrrh are based on its long history of use in well established systems of traditional and conventional medicine, case studies, *in vitro* studies, pharmacological studies in animals, and on phytochemical studies of its volatile oil, gum, and resin fractions.

German pharmacopeial grade myrrh consists of the air-dried oleo-gum resin exuded from the bark of *C. molmol* Engler and/or other chemically similar species. It may contain no more than 65% ethanol-insoluble extractive. Botanical identity is confirmed by thin-layer chromatography (TLC), macroscopic and microscopic examinations, and organoleptic evaluations. Myrrh tincture is also official in the *German Pharmacopeia*. It must be manufactured according to the DAB tincture monograph, macerating 1 part pulverized myrrh with 5 parts ethanol 90% (v/v) (DAB, 1997; Wichtl and Bisset, 1994). The *Pharmacopeia of Austria* requires myrrh to have an acid value of 19.5–22.0 and also includes color reaction tests for the presence of characteristic sesquiterpenes (ÖAB, 1981–1983; Wichtl and Bisset, 1994). The *British Herbal Pharmacopoeia* defines myrrh as the oleo-gum resin obtained from the stems of *C. molmol* Engler and/or other related species. It must contain not less than 6% volatile oil and not more than 70% ethanol (90%)-insoluble residue. Botanical identity is confirmed by TLC and macroscopic and organoleptic evaluations (BHP, 1996). Indian pharmacopeial grade myrrh, referred to as *guggulu*, consists of the exudate of *C. wightii* (Arn.) Bhand [syn. Balsamodendron mukul Hook. ex Stocks (*C. mukul* Engl.)] collected by making incisions in the bark during winter. It must contain not less than 1% (v/w) volatile oil, not less than 53% water-soluble extractive and not less than 27% alcohol-soluble extractive. Botanical identity is confirmed by macroscopic and organoleptic evaluations as well as by chemical tests (API, 1989). [Note: Some European references refer to the official species used in India as false myrrh and consider it to be an adulterant to genuine myrrh (Wichtl and Bisset, 1994).]

Description

Myrrh consists of oleo-gum resin extruded from the stems of *C. molmol* Engler [Fam. Burseraceae], then air-dried, and its preparations in effective dosage. Myrrh can also originate from other *Commiphora* species, if the chemical composition is comparable to the official preparation.

Chemistry and Pharmacology

Myrrh contains approximately 30–60% water-soluble gum; 20–40% alcohol-soluble resins consisting of commiphoric acids, commiphorinic acid and heerabomyrrhols; approximately 8% volatile oil (Bradley, 1992; Leung and Foster, 1996; Newall et al., 1996). The volatile oil fraction contains myrcene and α-camphorene; steroids including Z-guggulsterol, and I, II, III guggulsterol (Huang, 1999; Kapoor, 1990). The water-soluble gum or mucilage fraction is composed mainly of acidic polysaccharide with galactose, 4-O-methyl-glucuronic acid and arabinose in a ratio of 8:7:2 with approximately 18–20% proteins (Bradley, 1992; Jones and Nunn, 1955; Wichtl and Bisset, 1994). Characteristic constituents are mainly terpenoids, including furanosesquiterpenoids with eudesmane, germacrane, elemane, or guaiane structures (Bradley, 1992; Wichtl and Bisset, 1994). Its characteristic odor is due to the furanosesquiterpenes (Bruneton, 1995), which may also be the characteristic components of pharmaceutical myrrh (Wichtl and Bisset, 1994).

The Commission E reported astringent activity.

The *British Herbal Pharmacopoeia* reported antiseptic action (BHP, 1996). *The Merck Index* reported its therapeutic action as carminative and astringent (Budavari, 1996). It has also been shown to have disinfecting, deodorizing, and granulation-promoting properties (Wichtl and Bisset, 1994).

Uses

The Commission E approved myrrh for topical treatment of mild inflammations of the oral and pharyngeal mucosa.

The *British Herbal Compendium* indicates the use of myrrh tincture as a gargle to treat pharyngitis and tonsillitis, as a mouthwash for gingivitis and ulcers, and external application to treat sinusitis and minor skin inflammations (Bradley, 1992). In France, its topical use is approved for the treatment of small wounds, for nasal congestion from the common cold, and for local application as an anodyne to treat affections of the buccal cavity and/or the oropharynx (Bradley, 1992; Bruneton, 1995). The German Standard License for myrrh tincture indicates its use for inflammations of the gums and mouth mucosa such as gingivitis and stomatitis, and also for prosthesis pressure marks (Braun et al., 1997).

Contraindications

None known.

Side Effects

None known.

Use During Pregnancy and Lactation

Not recommended during pregnancy. No restrictions known for lactation.

Interactions with Other Drugs

None known.

Dosage and Administration

Unless otherwise prescribed: Powdered resin, myrrh tincture, and other galenical preparations for topical use.
Tincture of myrrh 1:5 (g/ml), 90% ethanol (DAB 10): For use in gargles, mouthwashes, rinses, and paints.

Gargle or rinse: Add 5–10 drops of tincture to a glass of warm water (Commission E).

Mouthwash or gargle solution: Add 30–60 drops of tincture to a glass of warm water (Braun et al., 1997).

Paint: Apply the undiluted tincture to the affected areas on the gums or the mucous membranes of the mouth and paint with a brush or swab, two to three times daily (Commission E; Braun et al., 1997).

Undiluted tincture 1:5 (g/ml): Apply locally to affected areas of the gums or mucous membranes of the mouth, two to three times daily (Braun et al., 1997).

Dental powders: Containing 10% powdered resin (Commission E).

References

The *Ayurvedic Pharmacopoeia* of India, Part 1, Vol. 1, 1st ed. (API). 1989. Delhi: Government of India—Ministry of Health and Family Welfare, Department of Health. 43.

Bown, D. 1995. *Encyclopedia of Herbs and Their Uses.* New York: DK Publishing, Inc. 265.

Bradley, P.R. (ed.). 1992. *British Herbal Compendium*, Vol. 1. Bournemouth: British Herbal Medicine Association.

Braun, R. et al. 1997. *Standardzulassungen für Fertigarzneimittel—Text and Kommentar.* Stuttgart: Deutscher Apotheker Verlag.

British Herbal Pharmacopoeia (BHP). 1996. Exeter, U.K.: British Herbal Medicine Association. 141.

Bruneton, J. 1995. *Pharmacognosy, Phytochemistry, Medicinal Plants.* Paris: Lavoisier Publishing.

Budavari, S. (ed.). 1996. *The Merck Index: An Encyclopedia of Chemicals, Drugs, and Biologicals*, 12th ed. Whitehouse Station, N.J.: Merck & Co, Inc. 1086.

Clifford, T. 1984. *Tibetan Buddhist Medicine and Psychiatry.* York Beach, ME: Samuel Weiser, Inc.

Deutsches Arzneibuch, 10th ed. Vol. 1–6. (DAB 10). 1991. Kommentar. Stuttgart: Wissenschaftliche Verlagsgesellschaft.

Deutsches Arzneibuch (DAB 1997). 1997. Stuttgart: Deutscher Apotheker Verlag.

Fratkin, J. 1986. *Chinese Herbal Patent Formulas—A Practical Guide.* Boulder, CO: Shya Publications. 125–134, 142–148.

Frawley, D. and V. Lad. 1986. *The Yoga of Herbs: An Ayurvedic Guide to Herbal Medicine.* Twin Lakes: Lotus Press.

Grieve, M. 1979. *A Modern Herbal.* New York: Dover Publications, Inc.

Huang, K.C. 1999. *The Pharmacology of Chinese Herbs*, 2nd ed. Boca Raton: CRC Press. 183.

Iwu, M.M. 1990. *Handbook of African Medicinal Plants.* Boca Raton: CRC Press. 160–161.

Jones, J.K. and J.R. Nunn. 1955. The constitution of gum myrrh. *J Chem Soc* 3001–3004.

Kapoor, L.D. 1990. *Handbook of Ayurvedic Medicinal Plants.* Boca Raton: CRC Press. 131–132.

Karnick, C.R. 1994. *Pharmacopoeial Standards of Herbal Plants,* Vol. 1. Delhi: Sri Satguru Publications. 103–104.

Leung, A.Y. and S. Foster. 1996. *Encyclopedia of Common Natural Ingredients Used in Food, Drugs, and Cosmetics*, 2nd ed. New York: John Wiley & Sons, Inc.

Mielck, W. 1970. Merfluan—ein brausendes zahnsalz mit myrrhe [Merfluan—an effervescent dentifrice salt with myrrh]. *Dent Dienst* 22(11):21.

Nadkarni, K.M. 1976. *Indian Materia Medica.* Bombay: Popular Prakashan. 170–171.

Newall, C.A., L.A. Anderson, J.D. Phillipson. 1996. *Herbal Medicines: A Guide for Health-Care Professionals.* London: The Pharmaceutical Press.

Österreichisches Arzneibuch, Vols. 1–2, 1st suppl. (ÖAB). 1981–1983. Wien: Verlag der Österreichischen Staatsdruckerei.

Schilcher, H. 1997. *Phytotherapy in Paediatrics—Handbook for Physicians and Pharmacists.* Stuttgart: Medpharm Scientific Publishers. 29.

Taber, C.W. 1962. *Taber's Cyclopedic Medical Dictionary.* Philadelphia, PA: F.A. Davis Company. M–65.

This material was adapted from *The Complete German Commission E Monographs—Therapeutic Guide to Herbal Medicines.* M. Blumenthal, W.R. Busse, A. Goldberg, J. Gruenwald, T. Hall, C.W. Riggins, R.S. Rister (eds.) S. Klein and R.S. Rister (trans.). 1998. Austin: American Botanical Council; Boston: Integrative Medicine Communications.

1) The Overview section is new information.

2) Description, Chemistry and Pharmacology, Uses, Contraindications, Side Effects, Interactions with Other Drugs, and Dosage sections have been drawn from the original work. Additional information has been added in some or all of these sections, as noted with references.

3) The dosage for equivalent preparations (tea infusion, fluidextract, and tincture) have been provided based on the following example:
Unless otherwise prescribed: 2 g per day of [powdered, crushed, cut or whole] [plant part]
Infusion: 2 g in 150 ml of water
Fluidextract 1:1 (g/ml): 2 ml
Tincture 1:5 (g/ml): 10 ml

4) The References and Additional Resources sections are new sections. Additional Resources are not cited in the monograph but are included for research purposes.

Tsarong, T.J. 1986. *Handbook of Traditional Tibet Drugs—Their Nomenclature, Composition, Use, and Dosage.* Kalimpong, India: Tibetan Medical Publications. 4–5.

Tyler, V.E. 1993. *The Honest Herbal*, 3rd ed. New York: Pharmaceutical Products Press.

Wichtl, M. and N.G. Bisset (eds.). 1994. *Herbal Drugs and Phytopharmaceuticals.* Stuttgart: Medpharm Scientific Publishers.

Wilford, J.N. 1997. *Ruins in Yemeni Desert Mark Route of Frankincense Trade.* New York Times. Jan. 28:B1, B10.

Yen, K.Y. 1992. *The Illustrated Chinese Materia Medica—Crude and Prepared.* Taipei: SMC Publishing, Inc. 202.

Additional Resources

Felter, H.W. and J.U. Lloyd. 1985. *King's American Dispensatory*, Vols. 1–2. Portland, OR: Eclectic Medical Publications [reprint of 1898 original].

McGuffin, M., C. Hobbs, R. Upton, A. Goldberg. 1997. American Herbal Product Association's *Botanical Safety Handbook.* Boca Raton: CRC Press.

Pharmacopoeia Helvetica, 7th ed. Vol. 1–4. (Ph.Helv.VII). 1987. Bern: Office Central Fédéral des Imprimés et du Matériel.

OAK BARK

Latin Name:
Quercus robur and/or *Q. petraea,*
Q. alba

Pharmacopeial Name:
Quercus cortex

Other Names:
white oak bark (*Q. alba*)

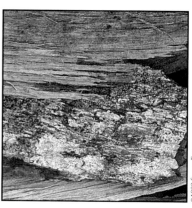

©1999 Steven Foster

Overview

The name *quercus* comes from the Celtic words *quer* (fine) and *cuez* (tree) (Grieve, 1979). Oak was so respected that a branch of the tree was stamped onto British coins for centuries. Oaks, being both pliable and extremely strong, were used for British ship building, and also for train cars and knife handles. Historically, oak bark decoctions or tinctures have been used for lung, throat, and gastrointestinal disorders, particularly in England, although the Greeks and Romans were also well acquainted with oak's astringent actions (Grieve, 1979). It has been used to treat hemorrhaging, intermittent fevers, chronic diarrhea, and dysentery. As a gargle, oak bark has been used to relieve chronic sore throats; it has also been prepared as a vaginal wash to treat leucorrhea (Hutchins, 1991). *Quercus alba* was listed in the *United States Pharmacopoeia* from 1820 until 1910 (Boyle, 1991).

Future uses for oak bark require examination. Oak bark may also prove to be useful in the treatment of ureteral and kidney lithiasis. One study found that a proprietary medicine inhibited not only the formation of stones, but also the growth of bacteria surrounding them. Litiax® was also shown to be diuretic and significantly reduced inflammation and pain (Mandana-Rodriguez and Gausa-Rull, 1980). Oak bark may also be useful in treating patients with pyoinflammatory skin diseases. A water alcohol glycerol extract has shown antistaphylococcal activity (Molochko et al., 1990).

Description

Oak bark consists of the dried bark of young branches and saplings of *Quercus robur* L. and *Q. petraea* (Mattuschka) Lieblein [Fam. Fagaceae], harvested in the spring, and their preparations in effective dosage. The preparation contains tannins.

Chemistry and Pharmacology

Constituents include about 10% saponins, 10–15% tannins, calcium oxalate, starch, and a mixture of different triterpene glycosides with quillaic acid as the main sapogenin (Wichtl and Bisset, 1994). Other constituents include tannic acid, oak-red, resin,

pectin, levulin, and quercitol (Stecher, 1968).

The Commission E reported astringent and virustatic activity.

Recent animal experiments have found that through oral administration, the saponins of the bark are able to reduce serum cholesterol levels. This activity is thought to be due to a reaction between the saponins and the bile acids, resulting in micelle formation and leading to inhibition of cholesterol uptake. The saponins are also thought to raise antibody production in the mouse; the experiments found that the immune response after viral infections was accelerated (Wichtl and Bisset, 1994).

Uses

The Commission E approved the internal use of oak bark for nonspecific, acute diarrhea, and local treatment of mild inflammation of the oral cavity and pharyngeal region, and genital and anal area. It was also approved externally for inflammatory skin diseases. The bark's saponin content is thought to possess expectorant activity in respiratory complaints (Wichtl and Bisset, 1994). Oak bark can be used topically for its astringent properties in cases of dermatitis without risk of irritation (Weiss, 1988).

Contraindications

Internal: None known.
External: Skin damage over a large area.
Baths: Full baths should not be taken.

Side Effects

None known.

Use During Pregnancy and Lactation

No restrictions known.

Interactions with Other Drugs

External: None known.
Internal: The absorption of alkaloids and other alkaline drugs may be reduced or inhibited.

Dosage and Administration

Unless otherwise prescribed: 3 g per day of cut herb.
Infusion: 3 g of herb in 150 ml water.
Fluidextract 1:1 (g/ml): 3 ml.
Tincture 1:5 (g/ml): 15 ml.
For rinses, compresses and gargles: 20 g preparation per 1 liter of water; equivalent preparations.
For full and partial baths: 5 g preparation per 1 liter of water; equivalent preparations.
If diarrhea persists longer than three to four days, consult a physician.

Other areas of application: Not more than two to three weeks.

References

Boyle, W. 1991. *Official Herbs: Botanical Substances in the United States Pharmacopoeias 1820–1990.* East Palestine, OH: Buckeye Naturopathic Press.

Grieve, M. 1979. *A Modern Herbal.* New York: Dover Publications, Inc.

Hutchins, A. 1991. *Indian Herbology of North America.* Boston: Shambala.

Mandana-Rodriguez, A. and P. Gausa-Rull. 1980. [Therapeutic effects of *Quercus* extract in urolithiasis] [In Spanish]. *Arch Esp Urol* 33(2):205–226.

Molochko, V.A., T.M. Lastochkina, I.A. Krylov, K.A. Brangulis. 1990. [The antistaphylococcal properties of plant extracts in relation to their prospective use as therapeutic and prophylactic formulations for the skin] [In Russian]. *Vestn Dermatol Venerol* (8):54–56.

Stecher, P.G. (ed.). 1968. *The Merck Index: An Encyclopedia of Chemicals and Drugs,* 8th ed. Rahway, N.J.: Merck & Co., Inc.

Weiss, R.F. 1988. *Herbal Medicine.* Beaconsfield, England: Beaconsfield Publishers.

Wichtl, M. and N.G. Bisset (eds.). 1994. *Herbal Drugs and Phytopharmaceuticals.* Stuttgart: Medpharm Scientific Publishers.

Additional Resources

Deutscher Arzneimittel-Codex (DAC). 1986. Stuttgart: Deutscher Apotheker Verlag.

Maharaj, I., K.J. Froh, J.B. Campbell. 1986. Immune responses of mice to inactivated rabies vaccine administered orally: potentiation by Quillaja saponin. *Can J Microbiol* 32(5):414–420.

McGuffin, M., C. Hobbs, R. Upton, A. Goldberg. 1997. American Herbal Product Association's *Botanical Safety Handbook.* Boca Raton: CRC Press.

Oakenfull, D. 1986. Aggregation of saponins and bile acids in aqueous solution. *Aust J Chem* 39(10):1671–1683.

Österreichisches Arzneibuch, Vols. 1–2, 1st suppl. (ÖAB). 1981–1983. Wien: Verlag der Österreichischen Staatsdruckerei.

Pharmacopoeia Helvetica, 7th ed. Vol. 1–4. (Ph.Helv.VII). 1987. Bern: Office Central Fédéral des Imprimés et du Matériel.

Rao, A.V. and C.W. Kendall. 1986. Dietary saponins and serum lipids. *Food Chem Toxicol* 24(5):441.

Scott, M.T., M. Goss-Sampson, R. Bomford. 1985. Adjuvant activity of saponin: antigen localization studies. *Int Arch Allergy Appl Immunol* 77(4):409–412.

Sidhu, G.S. and D.G. Oakenfull. 1986. A mechanism for the hypocholesterolemic activity of saponins. *Br J Nutr* 55(3):643–649.

Tyler, V.E. 1994. *Herbs of Choice: The Therapeutic Use of Phytomedicinals.* New York: Pharmaceutical Products Press.

This material was adapted from *The Complete German Commission E Monographs—Therapeutic Guide to Herbal Medicines.* M. Blumenthal, W.R. Busse, A. Goldberg, J. Gruenwald, T. Hall, C.W. Riggins, R.S. Rister (eds.) S. Klein and R.S. Rister (trans.). 1998. Austin: American Botanical Council; Boston: Integrative Medicine Communications.

1) The Overview section is new information.

2) Description, Chemistry and Pharmacology, Uses, Contraindications, Side Effects, Interactions with Other Drugs, and Dosage sections have been drawn from the original work. Additional information has been added in some or all of these sections, as noted with references.

3) The dosage for equivalent preparations (tea infusion, fluidextract, and tincture) have been provided based on the following example:
Unless otherwise prescribed: 2 g per day of [powdered, crushed, cut or whole] [plant part]
Infusion: 2 g in 150 ml of water
Fluidextract 1:1 (g/ml): 2 ml
Tincture 1:5 (g/ml): 10 ml

4) The References and Additional Resources sections are new sections. Additional Resources are not cited in the monograph but are included for research purposes.

Oat Straw

Latin Name:
Avena sativa

Pharmacopeial Name:
Avenae stramentum

Other Names:
oats, green oats, green tops

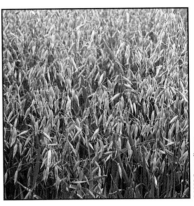

© 1999 Steven Foster

Overview

Oat straw is the aboveground part of a plant more often associated with the commercial product milled from its seed. The cultivation of oatmeal dates back to at least 2000 B.C.E. Oats are native to warm Mediterranean regions of the world. In Europe, the oat plant is used for much more than its yield of grain. Extracts and tinctures prepared from the oat straw and the plant's immature, milky seed are readily available. These formulas are used as a nervous system restorative, to assist convalescence, and to strengthen a weakened constitution. Neurasthenia, shingles, herpes zoster, and herpes simplex are also treated with oat straw. It is sometimes recommended by European alternative practitioners as a phytomedicine for multiple sclerosis patients (Mills, 1988), but the efficacy of this application is not well documented.

Commission E limits its approval to topical applications, allowing the administration of oat straw through baths to reduce inflammation and pruritis.

In the 1970s, much research was conducted to determine if oat straw extracts helped cigarette smokers to quit. The results of these tests were negative, but led to research on oat straw's potential influence on reproductive hormones (Connor et al., 1975; Schmidt and Geckeler, 1976). In an experimental study, oat straw stimulated the release of luteinizing hormone from the adenohypophysis (a gland in the brain) of rats (Fukushima et al., 1976).

Description

Oat straw consists of the dried, threshed leaf and stem of *Avena sativa* L. [Fam. Poaceae] and its preparations in effective dosage. The preparation contains silicic acid.

Chemistry and Pharmacology

Two percent silicon dioxide occurs in the leaves and in the straw in soluble form as esters of silicic acid with polyphenols and monosaccharides and oligosaccharides. Oat straw contains a high content of iron (39 mg/kg dry weight), manganese (8.5 mg), and zinc (19.2 mg) (Wichtl and Bisset, 1994).

The leaves contain triterpenoid saponins of the furostanol type (avenacosides) with strong *in vitro* fungicidal activity (Wichtl and Bisset, 1994). In vitro and *in vivo*, beta-glucan from oats has been shown to stimulate immune functions (Estrada et al., 1997).

Uses

The Commission E approved the topical use of oat straw in baths for inflammatory and seborrheic skin diseases, especially those with itching.

Contraindications
None known.

Side Effects
None known.

Use During Pregnancy and Lactation
No restrictions known.

Interactions with Other Drugs
None known.

Dosage and Administration
Unless otherwise prescribed: 100 g of cut herb for one full bath; equivalent preparations.

References

Connor, J., T. Connor, P.B. Marshall, A. Reid, M.J. Turnbull. 1975. The pharmacology of *Avena sativa*. *J Pharm Pharmacol* 27(2):92–98.

Estrada, A. et al. 1997. Immunomodulatory activities of oat beta-glucan *in vitro* and *in vivo*. *Microbiol Immunol* 41(12):991–998.

Fukushima, M., S. Watanabe, K. Kushima. 1976. Extraction and purification of a substance with luteinizing hormone releasing activity from the leaves of *Avena sativa*. *Tohoku J Exp Med* 119(2):115–122.

Mills, S.Y. 1988. *The Dictionary of Modern Herbalism*. New York: MJF Books.

Schmidt, K. and K. Geckeler. 1976. Pharmacotherapy with *Avena sativa*—a double blind study. Int *J Clin Pharmacol* Biopharm 14(3):214–216.

Wichtl, M. and N.G. Bisset (eds.). 1994. *Herbal Drugs and Phytopharmaceuticals*. Stuttgart: Medpharm Scientific Publishers.

Additional Resources

Anand, C.L. 1971. Effect of *Avena sativa* on cigarette smoking. *Nature* 233(5320):496.

Grieve, M. 1979. *A Modern Herbal*. New York: Dover Publications, Inc.

This material was adapted from *The Complete German Commission E Monographs—Therapeutic Guide to Herbal Medicines*. M. Blumenthal, W.R. Busse, A. Goldberg, J. Gruenwald, T. Hall, C.W. Riggins, R.S. Rister (eds.) S. Klein and R.S. Rister (trans.). 1998. Austin: American Botanical Council; Boston: Integrative Medicine Communications.

1) The Overview section is new information.

2) Description, Chemistry and Pharmacology, Uses, Contraindications, Side Effects, Interactions with Other Drugs, and Dosage sections have been drawn from the original work. Additional information has been added in some or all of these sections, as noted with references.

3) The dosage for equivalent preparations (tea infusion, fluidextract, and tincture) have been provided based on the following example:
Unless otherwise prescribed: 2 g per day of [powdered, crushed, cut or whole] [plant part]
Infusion: 2 g in 150 ml of water
Fluidextract 1:1 (g/ml): 2 ml
Tincture 1:5 (g/ml): 10 ml

4) The References and Additional Resources sections are new sections. Additional Resources are not cited in the monograph but are included for research purposes.

ONION

Latin Name:
Allium cepa

Pharmacopeial Name:
Allii cepae bulbus

Other Names:
n/a

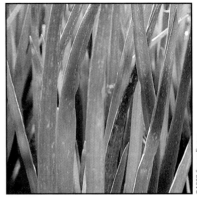

© 1999 Steven Foster

Overview

Onion is a bulbous perennial or biennial herb believed to be native to western Asia. Numerous varieties are cultivated worldwide (Leung and Foster, 1996). It is cultivated throughout India (Kapoor, 1990). Some sources state that it is native to Hungary (Felter and Lloyd, 1985; HPUS, 1992).

Onion bulb has been used as a food for thousands of years. It has also been used medicinally. According to traditional European herbalists, onions are antiseptic and diuretic in action (Grieve, 1979). They are used therapeutically in the Ayurvedic, Siddha, and Unani systems of Indian medicine, in various dosage forms including the decoction, infusion, and fresh juice, as well as raw, cooked, and/or roasted bulb. The juice form is usually combined with honey, ginger rhizome juice, and ghee (liquid clarified butter) (Nadkarni, 1976). Its introduction into traditional Chinese medicine is fairly recent and its use limited (Leung and Foster, 1996). The official onion bulb of the *Pharmacopoeia of the People's Republic of China* is a different species (*Allium macrostemon* Bge.) than that of the Commission E monographs (*A. cepa*). The Chinese pharmacopeia indicates its use for treatment of angina pectoris, cough, and dyspnea (painful, difficult breathing), and also tenesmus (painful spasmodic contraction of anal or vesical sphincter) in dysentery (Tu, 1992).

In Germany, onion bulb is approved in the Commission E monographs for loss of appetite and prevention of atherosclerosis. The World Health Organization supports Commission E, noting that the following use is supported by clinical data: "treatment of age-dependent changes in the blood vessels, and loss of appetite" (WHO, 1999). Onions are also cooked in milk and eaten in order to clear congestion in the lungs (Shultz et al., 1998). In the United States, onion bulb was used somewhat in the Eclectic system of medicine during the nineteenth century and early twentieth century. Its actions were considered to be comparable to those of garlic, though milder. It was dispensed as a syrup, made from the fresh juice with sugar, for treatment of cough and bronchial conditions. It was also given as a tincture, made with gin, for kidney gravel and/or dropsy (Felter and Lloyd, 1985). Onion is presently classified in the *Homeopathic Pharmacopoeia of the United States* as an OTC Class C drug prepared as a 1:10 (w/v) alcoholic tincture of the mature bulb (preferably the red variety), in 45% v/v alcohol (HPUS, 1992).

Several clinical studies have been found in the literature. Recent investigations suggest that therapies aimed toward the prevention of atherosclerosis should include a diet rich with onions. Contemporary studies have shown that onions, like garlic, may inhibit platelet aggregation and interfere with fibrinolyis (Leung and Foster, 1996; Reynolds, 1989). The antiplatelet activity is genotype dependent and correlates directly with bulb sulfur content (Goldman et al., 1996). Antihypercholesterolemic and hypoglycemic uses for onions have also been supported by research. Clinical studies have reported that onions lowered lipid levels and inhibited the formation of blood clots in study subjects (Schulz et al., 1998). Other studies have investigated the effect of butter fat and onion on coagulability of blood (Jain, 1971), its effects on serum triglyceride, betalipoprotein-cholesterol, and phospholipids in alimentary lipemia (Jain et al., 1973), the fibrinolytic activator action of steam-distilled and ether extract of onion (Augusti et al., 1975), the effects of an oily chloroform extract of onion on platelet aggregation and thromboxane synthesis (Makheja et al., 1979), the effects of an aqueous extract of onion on the inhibition of platelet aggregation (Srivastava, 1984), the use of crude onion oil in the treatment of hypertension and hyperlipidemia (Louria et al., 1985), and the relationship between consumption of onions with a reduced risk of stomach carcinoma (Dorant et al., 1996; You, 1988; You et al., 1989).

A pharmacopeial grade onion bulb has not been defined at present.

Description

Onion consists of the fresh or dried, thick and fleshy leaf sheaths and stipules of *Allium cepa* L. [Fam. Alliaceae] and their preparations in effective dosage. It contains alliin and similar sulfur compounds, essential oil, peptides, and flavonoids.

Chemistry and Pharmacology

Onion bulb contains numerous organic sulfur compounds, including *trans-S*-(1-propenyl) cysteine sulfoxide, *S*-methylcysteine sulfoxide, *S*-propylcysteine sulfoxide, and cycloalliin; flavonoids; phenolic acids; sterols including cholesterol, stigmasterol, β-sitosterol; saponins; sugars; and a trace of volatile oil composed mainly of sulfur compounds, including dipropyl disulfide (Kapoor, 1990; Leung and Foster, 1996). A fresh onion bulb contains fructans with a low degree of polymerization, flavonoids, and sulfur-containing compounds. When an onion bulb is bruised, the sulfoxides are degraded by alliinase and release pyruvic acid and alkylthiosulfinates, which rapidly form into disulfides (Bruneton, 1995).

The Commission E reported antibacterial, lipid, and blood pressure-lowering properties and inhibition of thrombocyte aggregation.

Onions have appetizer and gastric tract stimulant actions (Taber, 1962). An animal study concluded that serum, liver, and aorta triglyceride levels were decreased after use of an aqueous extract of onion (Sebastian et al.,

1979). *In vitro* studies have shown antimicrobial activity and animal studies have demonstrated hypoglycemic activity (Bruneton, 1995). The antibacterial activity of onion was determined by a study that researched the activity of oral bacteria, including *Streptococcus mutans* and *Porphyromonas gingivalis* (Kim, 1997).

Uses

The Commission E approved onion for loss of appetite and prevention of atherosclerosis.

Supporting the Commission E uses, the World Health Organization notes the following uses are supported by clinical data: age related change in blood vessels and loss of appetite (WHO, 1999).

A preliminary epidemiological study suggests that increased consumption of onion, as well as other *Allium* vegetables, may reduce the risk of gastric cancer (You et al., 1989).

Contraindications

None known.

Side Effects

None known.

Use During Pregnancy and Lactation

No restrictions known.

Interactions with Other Drugs
None known.

Dosage and Administration
Unless otherwise prescribed: 50 g per day of fresh bulb or 20 g per day of cut dried bulb, pressed juice from fresh onions and other oral galenical preparations.
Dried bulb: 20 g (Commission E).
Fresh bulb: 50 g (Commission E).
Infusion: Steep 1–2 teaspoons in 120 ml water (Lust, 1974).
Succus: 5 ml (1 teaspoon) pressed juice of fresh bulb, three to four times daily (Lust, 1974).
Tincture: 5 ml (1 teaspoon), three to four times daily (Fleming et al., 1998).
Duration of administration: Note: If onion preparations are used over several months, the daily maximum amount for diphenylamine is 0.035 g.

References
Augusti, K.T., M.E. Benaim, H.A. Dewar, R. Virden. 1975. Partial identification of the fibrinolytic activators in onion. *Atherosclerosis* 21(3):409–416.

Bruneton, J. 1995. *Pharmacognosy, Phytochemistry, Medicinal Plants*. Paris: Lavoisier Publishing.

Dorant, E., P.A. van den Brandt, R.A. Goldbohm, F. Sturmans. 1996. Consumption of onions and a reduced risk of stomach carcinoma. *Gastroenterology* 110(1):12–20.

Felter, H.W. and J.U. Lloyd. 1985. *King's American Dispensatory*, Vols. 1–2. Portland, OR: Eclectic Medical Publications [reprint of 1898 original]. 146.

Fleming, T. (ed.). 1998. *PDR® for Herbal Medicines*. Montvale, N.J.: Medical Economics Company, Inc.

Goldman, I.L. M. Kopelberg, J.E. Debaene, B.S. Schwartz. 1996. Antiplatelet activity in onion (*Allium cepa*) is sulfur dependent. *Thromb Haemost* 76(3):450–452.

Grieve, M. 1979. *A Modern Herbal*. New York: Dover Publications, Inc.

The Homeopathic Pharmacopoeia of the United States (HPUS) *Revision Service Official Compendium*. 1992. Fairfax, VA: Pharmacopoeia Convention of the American Institute of Homeopathy.

Jain, R.C. 1971. Effect of butter fat and onion on coagulability of blood. *Indian J Med Sci* 25(9):598–600.

Jain, R.C., K.N. Sachdev, S.S. Kaushal. 1973. Effect of onion ingestion on serum triglyceride, betalipoprotein-cholesterol and phospholipids in alimentary lipaemia. *J Assoc Physicians India* 21(4):357–360.

Kapoor, L.D. 1990. *Handbook of Ayurvedic Medicinal Plants*. Boca Raton: CRC Press. 25.

Kim, J.H. 1997. Anti-bacterial action of onion (*Allium cepa* L.) extracts against oral pathogenic bacteria. *J Nihon Univ Sch Dent* 39(3):136–141.

Leung, A.Y. and S. Foster. 1996. *Encyclopedia of Common Natural Ingredients Used in Food, Drugs, and Cosmetics*, 2nd ed. New York: John Wiley & Sons, Inc.

Louria, D.B. et al. 1985. Onion extract in treatment of hypertension and hyperlipidemia: A preliminary communication. *Curr Ther Res* 37(1):127–131.

Lust, J. 1974. *The Herb Book*. New York: Bantam Books. 298.

Makheja, A.N., J.Y. Vanderhoek, J.M. Bailey. 1979. Effects of onion (*Allium cepa*) extract on platelet aggregation and thromboxane synthesis. *Prostaglandins Med* 2(6):413–424.

Nadkarni, K.M. 1976. *Indian Materia Medica*. Bombay: Popular Prakashan. 63–64.

Reynolds, J.E.F. (ed.). 1989. *Martindale: The Extra Pharmacopoeia*, 29th ed. London: The Pharmaceutical Press. 1597.

Schulz, V., R. Hänsel, V.E. Tyler. 1998. *Rational Phytotherapy: A Physicians' Guide to Herbal Medicine*. New York: Springer.

Sebastian, K.L., N.T. Zacharias, B. Philip, K.T. Augusti. 1979. The hypolipidemic effect of onion (*Allium cepa* Linn) in sucrose fed rabbits. *Indian J Physiol Pharmacol* 23(1):27–30.

Srivastava, K.C. 1984. Aqueous extracts of onion, garlic and ginger inhibit platelet aggregation and alter arachidonic acid metabolism. *Biomed Biochim Acta* 43(8-9):S335–S346.

Taber, C.W. 1962. *Taber's Cyclopedic Medical Dictionary*, 9th ed. Philadelphia: F.A. Davis Company. O–9.

Tu, G. (ed.). 1992. *Pharmacopoeia of the People's Republic of China* (English Edition 1992). Beijing: Guangdong Science and Technology Press. 8.

World Health Organization (WHO). 1999. "Allii cepae bulbus." *WHO Monographs on Selected Medicinal Plants*, Vol. 1. Geneva: World Health Organization. 5–15.

You, W.C. et al. 1989. *Allium* vegetables and reduced risk of stomach cancer. *J Natl Cancer Inst* 81(2):162–164.

You, W.C. 1988. [A study on the relationship between consumption of Allium vegetables and gastric cancer] [In Chinese]. *Chung Hua Yu Fang I Hsueh Tsa Chih* 22(6):321–323.

Additional Resources
Augusti, K.T. 1996. Therapeutic values of onion (*Allium cepa* L.) and garlic (*Allium sativum* L.). *Indian J Exp Biol* 34(7):634–640.

Duke, J.A. 1997. *The Green Pharmacy*. Emmaus, PA: Rodale Press. 243, 245, 254–255, 259.

Navarro, J.A. et al. 1995. *Allium cepa* seeds: a new occupational allergen. *J Allergy Clin Immunol* 96(5 Pt 1):690–693.

Zohri, A.N., K. Abdel-Gawad, S. Saber. 1995. Antibacterial, antidermatophytic and antitoxigenic activities of onion (*Allium cepa* L.) oil. *Microbiol Res* 150(2):167–172.

This material was adapted from *The Complete German Commission E Monographs—Therapeutic Guide to Herbal Medicines*. M. Blumenthal, W.R. Busse, A. Goldberg, J. Gruenwald, T. Hall, C.W. Riggins, R.S. Rister (eds.) S. Klein and R.S. Rister (trans.). 1998. Austin: American Botanical Council; Boston: Integrative Medicine Communications.

1) The Overview section is new information.
2) Description, Chemistry and Pharmacology, Uses, Contraindications, Side Effects, Interactions with Other Drugs, and Dosage sections have been drawn from the original work. Additional information has been added in some or all of these sections, as noted with references.
3) The dosage for equivalent preparations (tea infusion, fluidextract, and tincture) have been provided based on the following example:
   Unless otherwise prescribed: 2 g per day of [powdered, crushed, cut or whole] [plant part]
   Infusion: 2 g in 150 ml of water
   Fluidextract 1:1 (g/ml): 2 ml
   Tincture 1:5 (g/ml): 10 ml
4) The References and Additional Resources sections are new sections. Additional Resources are not cited in the monograph but are included for research purposes.

ORANGE PEEL, BITTER

Latin Name:
Citrus aurantium

Pharmacopeial Name:
Aurantii pericarpium

Other Names:
Seville orange, sour orange

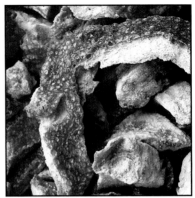

©1999 Steven Foster

Overview

Bitter orange is an aromatic variety of citrus that produces highly bitter, acidic fruits. The tree, indigenous to eastern Africa, Arabia, and Syria, was cultivated in India and in Europe by 1200 C.E. Sometimes called Seville orange, bitter orange is produced in Spain, Sicily, Tripoli, California, and Florida (Trease and Evans, 1989). Unripe dried fruits and fruit peels provide ingredients for numerous products. In China, two medicinal preparations are made from bitter orange. In Europe and North America, essential oils distilled from bitter orange flowers (neroli oil) and leaves (petitgrain oil) are commonly used by perfume, cosmetic, and aromatherapy industries (Leung and Foster, 1996). These, and bitter orange oil, flavor many foods, and mask unpleasant tastes in pharmaceuticals.

In traditional Chinese medicine, *Zhi qiao*, prepared from the dried peel of immature, green fruit, and *Zhi shi*, prepared from dried fruit, have specific applications, added to formulas that treat mild indigestion, nausea, constipation, and organ prolapse (Huang, 1993).

Like *Zhi qiao, Zhi shi* is a traditional Chinese treatment for indigestion and anal or uterine prolapse. In its contemporary use in China, it is injected for the treatment of shock syndromes, toxic and anaphylactic shock in particular (Huang, 1993). The herb's positive inotropic effects, observed improvements to circulation of blood through the heart and cerebral tissue, and its amine content, synephrine and N-methyltyramine, validate this use.

The primary indication for bitter orange tincture or extract is heartburn. Dried peel is official in the *British Pharmacopoeia* as a bitter tonic (Trease and Evans, 1989). Traditional herbalism correlates bitter substances to the digestive tract, and empirical evidence suggests that bitter orange is carminative (Leung and Foster, 1996), mostly likely due to mild spasmolysis. It may also have applications as a topical antifungal agent; oil of bitter orange was effective in curing patients with treatment-resistant fungal skin diseases in recent studies (Ramadan et al., 1996). *In vitro* tests show that limonene from citrus peels may have relevant anticancer, antitumor, and cell-differentiation promoting activities (Boik, 1995).

Bitter orange extract has been added to herbal weight loss formulas as a replacement for epinephrine. Bitter orange is believed to increase metabolism or thermogenesis due to its synephrine content, and, because of this constituent, it is used in herbal nasal decongestants as an alternative to ephedrine (Sabinsa, 1997). However, the effects of bitter orange in weight reduction, nasal decongestion, and patient safety is still controversial, and awaits clinical assessment. Synephrine, an α_1-adrenergic agonist, stimulates a rise in blood pressure through vasoconstriction. N-methyltyramine also raises blood pressure, through norepinephrine depletion (Huang, 1993).

Description

Bitter orange peel is the dried outer peel of ripe fruits of *Citrus aurantium* L. subspecies *aurantium* (synonym C. *aurantium* L. subspecies amara Engler) [Fam. Rutaceae], freed from the white pulp layer, as well as its preparations in effective dosage. The preparation contains essential oil and bitter principles.

Chemistry and Pharmacology

The main constituents include approximately 0.2–0.5% essential oil; the monoterpenes linalyl acetate, α-pinene, limonene, linalool, nerol, and geraniol; methyl anthranilate; bitter substances; and flavonoids (Wichtl and Bisset, 1994). The flavones present include: tangeretin, tetra-o-methylscutellarin, 3,5,6,7,8,3',4' –heptametoxyflavone, nobiletin, sinensetin, auranetin, and 5-hydroxyauranetin (Tang and Eisenbrand, 1992). Active principles in the peel include the alkaloid synephrine and N-methyltyramine (Tang and Eisenbrand, 1992). The carotene pigments found in *Citrus* species are derived from cryptoxanthin (major), luteoxanthin, mutatochrome, auroxanthin, and zeaxanthin (Tang and Eisenbrand, 1992).

Bitter orange peel contains choleretic, anti-inflammatory, antibacterial, and antifungal activity. Antihypercholesterolemic activity (prevents elevation of serum cholesterol level) in humans and animals is attributed to the constituent pectin (Leung and Foster, 1996).

Uses

The Commission E approved the cut peel for loss of appetite and dyspeptic ailments. Bitter orange peel is thought to facilitate weight gain by stimulating the appetite (Bruneton, 1995). The leaf and flower of bitter orange are used, by infusion, for symptoms of neurotonic disorders in both children and adults in cases of minor sleeplessness (Bruneton, 1995; Wichtl and Bisset, 1994). The German Standard License states that the peel is useful "as a supportive measure in treating stomach complaints, e.g.,

insufficient formation of gastric juice; to stimulate the appetite" (Wichtl and Bisset, 1994).

Contraindications

None known.

Side Effects

Photosensitization is possible, especially in fair-skinned individuals.

Use During Pregnancy and Lactation

Not recommended.

Interactions with Other Drugs

None known.

Dosage and Administration

Unless otherwise prescribed: 4–6 g per day of cut peel for teas, other bitter-tasting galenical preparations for oral application.
Infusion: 2 g in 150 ml boiled water, three times daily.
Cold macerate: 2 g in 150 ml cold water for 6 to 8 hours stirring occasionally, strain then heat before drinking, three times daily.
Syrupus Aurantii Amarii: 6 g diluted with water or tea infusion.
Fluidextract: 1–2 g (Erg.B.6).
Tincture: 2–3 g (DAB 7).

References

Boik, J. 1995. *Cancer and Natural Medicine: A Textbook of Basic Science and Clinical Research.* Princeton, Minnesota: Oregon Medical Press.

Bruneton, J. 1995. *Pharmacognosy, Phytochemistry, Medicinal Plants.* Paris: Lavoisier Publishing.

Deutsches Arzneibuch, 7th ed. (DAB 7). 1968. Stuttgart: Deutscher Apotheker Verlag.

Ergänzungsbuch zum Deutschen Arzneibuch, 6th ed. (Erg.B.6). 1953. Stuttgart: Deutscher Apotheker Verlag.

Huang, K.C. 1993. *The Pharmacology of Chinese Herbs.* Boca Raton: CRC Press.

The Japanese Standards for Herbal Medicines (JSHM). 1993. Tokyo: Yakuji Nippo, Ltd. 52–53.

Leung, A.Y. and S. Foster. 1996. *Encyclopedia of Common Natural Ingredients Used in Food, Drugs, and Cosmetics*, 2nd ed. New York: John Wiley & Sons, Inc.

Ramadan, W., B. Mourad, S. Ibrahim, F. Sonbol. 1996. Oil of bitter orange: new topical antifungal agent. *Int J Dermatol* 35(6):448–449.

Sabinsa Corporation. 1997. Current Issues: Newsletter of Sabinsa Corporation, October. Available at: www.sabinsa.com/news/nlr1097.htm.

Tang, W. and G. Eisenbrand. 1992. *Chinese Drugs of Plant Origin: Chemistry, Pharmacology, and Use in Traditional and Modern Medicine*. New York: Springer Verlag.

Trease, G.E. and W.C. Evans. 1989. *Trease and Evans' Pharmacognosy*, 13th ed. London; Philadelphia: Baillière Tindall.

Wichtl, M. and N.G. Bisset (eds.). 1994. *Herbal Drugs and Phytopharmaceuticals*. Stuttgart: Medpharm Scientific Publishers.

Additional Resources

BAnz. See *Bundesanzeiger*.

Bown, D. 1995. *Encyclopedia of Herbs and Their Uses*. New York: DK Publishing, Inc. 262–263.

Braun, R. et al. 1997. *Standardzulassungen für Fertigarzneimittel—Text und Kommentar*. Stuttgart: Deutscher Apotheker Verlag.

British Pharmacopoeia (BP). 1980. London: Her Majesty's Stationery Office. Vol. 1:317; Vol 2: 376, 837.

Bundesanzeiger (BAnz). 1998. Monographien der Kommission E (Zulassungs- und Aufbereitungskommission am BGA für den humanmed. Bereich, phytotherapeutische Therapierichtung und Stoffgruppe). Köln: Bundesgesundheitsamt (BGA).

Deutsches Arzneibuch (DAB 1997). 1997. Stuttgart: Deutscher Apotheker Verlag.

Grieve, M. 1979. *A Modern Herbal*. New York: Dover Publications, Inc.

Hartke, K. et al. 1991. *Deutsches Arzneibuch—Kommentar. Wissenschaftliche Erlauterungen zum Deutschen Arzneibuch*, 10. Ausgabe. [*German Pharmacopoeia*, 10th ed.—Commentary]. Vols. 1–6. Stuttgart: Wissenschaftliche Verlagsgesellschaft.

Hernández, L. et al. Use of medicinal plants by ambulatory patients in Puerto Rico. *Am J Hosp Pharm* 41(10):2060–2064.

Meyer-Buchtela, E. 1999. *Tee-Rezepturen—Ein Handbuch für Apotheker und Ärzte*. Stuttgart: Deutscher Apotheker Verlag.

Österreichisches Arzneibuch, Vols. 1–2, 1st suppl. (ÖAB). 1981–1983. Wien: Verlag der Österreichischen Staatsdruckerei.

Pei, D.K. 1985. [Dissolution of retained biliary stones with a compound prescription of orange-peel emulsion—a clinical analysis of 134 cases] [In Chinese]. *Chung Hsi I Chieh Ho Tsa Chih* 5(10):591–594, 578.

Pharmacopoeia Helvetica, 7th ed. Vol. 1–4. (Ph.Helv.VII). 1987. Bern: Office Central Fédéral des Imprimés et du Matériel.

Reynolds, J.E.F. (ed.). 1989. *Martindale: The Extra Pharmacopoeia*, 29th ed. London: The Pharmaceutical Press. 1065.

Schilcher, H. 1997. *Phytotherapy in Paediatrics: Handbook for Physicians and Pharmacists*. Stuttgart: Medpharm Scientific Publishers. 42–46.

This material was adapted from *The Complete German Commission E Monographs—Therapeutic Guide to Herbal Medicines*. M. Blumenthal, W.R. Busse, A. Goldberg, J. Gruenwald, T. Hall, C.W. Riggins, R.S. Rister (eds.) S. Klein and R.S. Rister (trans.). 1998. Austin: American Botanical Council; Boston: Integrative Medicine Communications.

1) The Overview section is new information.

2) Description, Chemistry and Pharmacology, Uses, Contraindications, Side Effects, Interactions with Other Drugs, and Dosage sections have been drawn from the original work. Additional information has been added in some or all of these sections, as noted with references.

3) The dosage for equivalent preparations (tea infusion, fluidextract, and tincture) have been provided based on the following example:

Unless otherwise prescribed: 2 g per day of [powdered, crushed, cut or whole] [plant part]
Infusion: 2 g in 150 ml of water
Fluidextract 1:1 (g/ml): 2 ml
Tincture 1:5 (g/ml): 10 ml

4) The References and Additional Resources sections are new sections. Additional Resources are not cited in the monograph but are included for research purposes.

PARSLEY HERB AND ROOT

Latin Name:
Petroselinum crispum

Pharmacopeial Name:
Petroselini herba/radix

Other Names:
common parsley, garden parsley

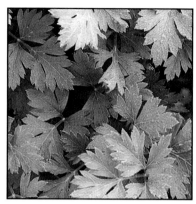

©1999 Steven Foster

Overview

Parsley is a biennial or short-lived perennial, native to the Mediterranean region, now cultivated in California, Germany, France, Belgium, former Czechoslovakia, and Hungary (BHP, 1996; Leung and Foster, 1996; Wichtl and Bisset, 1994). English botanist George Bentham (ca. 1800–1884), senior author with Joseph Palton Hooker of *Genera Plantarum*, believed it to be a native of Turkey, Algeria, and Lebanon. Its controlled cultivation dates back to ancient Rome; Pliny the Elder (ca. 23–79 C.E.) mentioned cultivation of the variety *crispum* (Grieve, 1979). Medicinal grade material is usually obtained from the plain-leafed rather than the curly-leafed varieties (BHP, 1996). The herb is harvested in the second year before flowering and the root is harvested in the late autumn of the first year, or spring of the second year (BHP, 1996; Bown, 1995; Grieve, 1979). Parsley is one of Germany's most important medicinal plants, under cultivation in seven regions (Lange and Schippmann, 1997).

The current genus name, *Petroselinum*, from the Greek, *selinon*, is believed to have been assigned by Greek physician Dioscorides in the first century C.E. The Greeks made distinctions between two related *Selinon* plants, celery (*Apium graveolens*), called *Heleioselinon*, and parsley, called *Oreoselinon*. The name *Petroselinum* became corrupted during the Middle Ages into Petrocilium, then anglicized into *petersylinge, persele, persely,* and finally *parsley* (Grieve, 1979). Its use in traditional Greek medicine spread to India where the dried root, essential oil, and fluidextract are used in traditional Indian Ayurvedic medicine. In Ayurvedic medicine celery root is substituted or used interchangeably with parsley root, reported to act as a carminative, diuretic, emmenagogue, and expectorant (Karnick, 1994; Nadkarni, 1976).

In Germany, parsley herb and root is taken for systemic irrigation for ailments of the lower urinary tract and as irrigation therapy for the prevention of renal gravel, in aqueous infusion dosage form or other equivalent galenical preparations. The dry extract is also used as a component in tablets (Leung and Foster, 1996; Wichtl and Bisset, 1994). In the United States, the herb or root is often used as a carminative or diuretic component of dietary supplements, in aqueous infusion, juice, or alcoholic tincture dosage forms.

The approved modern therapeutic applications for parsley are supportable based on its history of clinical use in well established systems of traditional medicine, on phytochemical investigations, and pharmacological studies in animals.

Pharmacopeial grade parsley herb is collected in the second year of growth before flowering. It must pass identification by macroscopic and microscopic examination and thin-layer chromatography (TLC) method. Quantitative standards include not less than 25% water-soluble extractive content. Pharmacopeial grade parsley root must pass comparable identification tests (BHP, 1996). The pharmacopeia of the former German Democratic Republic specified an essential oil content of not less than 0.3% in the root (DAB-DDR, 1985; Wichtl and Bisset, 1994).

Description

Parsley herb is the fresh or dried plant section of *Petroselinum crispum* (Miller) Nyman ex A.W. Hill [Fam. Apiaceae] and its pharmaceutical preparations. Parsley root is the dried root of *P. crispum* (Miller) Nyman ex A.W. Hill and its pharmaceutical preparations.

Chemistry and Pharmacology

Parsley contains the flavonoids apiin and luteolin; volatile oils myristicin, apiole, and β-phellandrene; fats; the furocoumarin bergapten; polyynes; protein; sugars; and vitamins A and C (Bradley, 1992; Leung and Foster, 1996; List and Hörhammer, 1973–1979; Newall et al., 1996; Wichtl and Bisset, 1994).

The Commission E did not report pharmacological actions for parsley.

The *British Herbal Compendium* reported the actions of parsley herb as diuretic, carminative, and spasmolytic (BHP, 1996; Bradley, 1992). The diuretic effect of parsley is probably due to the actions of its volatile oils myristicin and apiole (Newall et al., 1996).

Uses

The Commission E approved the use of parsley herb and root preparations for flushing out the urinary tract and for preventing and treating kidney gravel.

The *British Herbal Compendium* approves the internal use of parsley herb for flatulent dyspepsia, dysuria, and rheumatic conditions (Bradley, 1992). Parsley root is indicated for use as a mild diuretic (Wichtl and Bisset, 1994).

Contraindications

Pregnancy; inflammatory kidney conditions.

Precautions: Irrigation therapy (flush-ing out treatment) should not be carried out in the case of edema caused by impaired heart or kidney function.

Side Effects

Occasional allergic skin or mucous membrane reactions have been reported.

Use During Pregnancy and Lactation

Not recommended during pregnancy (McGuffin et al., 1997). No known restrictions during lactation.

Interactions with Other Drugs

None known.

Dosage and Administration

Unless otherwise prescribed: 6 g per day of crushed herb and root.
Infusion: 2 g in 150 ml water, three times daily.
Fluidextract 1:1 (g/ml): 2 ml, three times daily.
Irrigation therapy: Large amounts of fluids must be taken.
Warning: The essential oil should not be used in isolation because of its toxicity.

References

Bown, D. 1995. *Encyclopedia of Herbs and Their Uses.* New York: DK Publishing, Inc. 325.

Bradley, P.R. (ed.). 1992. *British Herbal Compendium*, Vol. 1. Bournemouth: British Herbal Medicine Association.

British Herbal Pharmacopoeia (BHP). 1996. Exeter, U.K.: British Herbal Medicine Association. 146–147.

Deutsches Arzneibuch der Deutsche Demokratische Republik (DAB-DDR). 1985. Berlin: Akademie Verlag.

Grieve, M. 1979. *A Modern Herbal.* New York: Dover Publications, Inc.

Karnick, C.R. 1994. *Pharmacopoeial Standards of Herbal Plants*, Vol. 1. Delhi: Sri Satguru Publications. 291–292.

Lange, D. and U. Schippmann. 1997. *Trade Survey of Medicinal Plants in Germany—A Contribution to International Plant Species Conservation.* Bonn: Bundesamt für Naturschutz. 32–33.

Leung, A.Y. and S. Foster. 1996. *Encyclopedia of Common Natural Ingredients Used in Food, Drugs, and Cosmetics,* 2nd ed. New York: John Wiley & Sons, Inc.

List, P.H. and L. Hörhammer (eds.). 1973–1979. *Hagers Handbuch der Pharmazeutischen Praxis,* Vols. 1–7. New York: Springer Verlag.

McGuffin, M., C. Hobbs, R. Upton, A. Goldberg. 1997. *American Herbal Product Association's Botanical Safety Handbook.* Boca Raton: CRC Press.

Nadkarni, K.M. 1976. *Indian Materia Medica.* Bombay: Popular Prakashan. 934–935.

Newall, C.A., L.A. Anderson, J.D. Phillipson. 1996. *Herbal Medicines: A Guide for Health-Care Professionals.* London: The Pharmaceutical Press.

Wichtl, M. and N.G. Bisset (eds.). 1994. *Herbal Drugs and Phytopharmaceuticals.* Stuttgart: Medpharm Scientific Publishers.

Additional Resources

British Herbal Pharmacopoeia (BHP). 1990. Bournemouth, U.K.: British Herbal Medicine Association.

———. 1983. Keighley, U.K.: British Herbal Medicine Association.

Chadha, Y.R. et al. (eds.). 1952–1988. *The Wealth of India (Raw Materials),* Vols. 1–11. New Delhi: Publications and Information Directorate, CSIR.

Duke, J.A. 1985. *Handbook of Medicinal Herbs.* Boca Raton: CRC Press.

———. 1992. *Handbook of Phytochemical Constituents of GRAS Herbs and Other Economic Plants.* Boca Raton: CRC Press. 438–441.

Ergänzungsbuch zum Deutschen Arzneibuch, 6th ed. (Erg.B.6). 1953. Stuttgart: Deutscher Apotheker Verlag.

Fejes, S. et al. 1998. A *Petroselinum crispum* (Mill.) Nym. ex A.W. Hill. *in vitro* antioxidans hatasanak vizsgalata [Investigation of the *in vitro* antioxidant effect of *Petroselinum crispum* (Mill.) Nym. ex A.W. Hill] *Acta Pharm Hung* 68(3):150–156.

Hänsel, R., K. Keller, H. Rimpler, G. Schneider (eds.). 1992–1994. *Hagers Handbuch der Pharmazeutischen Praxis,* 5th ed. Vol. 4–6. Berlin-Heidelberg: Springer Verlag.

Innocenti, G., F. Dall'Acqua, G. Caporale. 1976. Investigations of the content of furocoumarins in *Apium graveolens* and in *Petroselinum sativum.* *Planta Med* 29(2):165–170.

MacLeod, A.J., C.H. Snyder, G. Subramanian. 1985. Volatile aroma constituents of parsley leaves. *Phytochem* 24(11):2623–2627.

Marsh, A.C. et al. 1977. *Composition of Foods, Spices, and Herbs: Raw, Processed, Prepared.* Agriculture Handbook No. 8–2. Washington, D.C.: Agricultural Research Service, U.S. Department of Agriculture.

Reynolds, J.E.F. (ed.). 1982. *Martindale: The Extra Pharmacopoeia,* 28th ed. London: The Pharmaceutical Press.

Warncke, D. 1994. *Petroselinum crispum*—Die Gartenpetersilie. *ZPT* 15(1):50–58.

Watt, J.M. and M.G. Breyer-Brandwijk. 1962. *The Medicinal and Poisonous Plants of Southern and Eastern Africa.* Edinburgh-London: E. & S. Livingstone Ltd.

Wichtl, M. (ed.). 1997. *Teedrogen,* 4th ed. Stuttgart: Wissenschaftliche Verlagsgesellschaft.

This material was adapted from *The Complete German Commission E Monographs—Therapeutic Guide to Herbal Medicines.* M. Blumenthal, W.R. Busse, A. Goldberg, J. Gruenwald, T. Hall, C.W. Riggins, R.S. Rister (eds.) S. Klein and R.S. Rister (trans.). 1998. Austin: American Botanical Council; Boston: Integrative Medicine Communications.
1) The Overview section is new information.
2) Description, Chemistry and Pharmacology, Uses, Contraindications, Side Effects, Interactions with Other Drugs, and Dosage sections have been drawn from the original work. Additional information has been added in some or all of these sections, as noted with references.
3) The dosage for equivalent preparations (tea infusion, fluidextract, and tincture) have been provided based on the following example:
   Unless otherwise prescribed: 2 g per day of [powdered, crushed, cut or whole] [plant part]
   Infusion: 2 g in 150 ml of water
   Fluidextract 1:1 (g/ml): 2 ml
   Tincture 1:5 (g/ml): 10 ml
4) The References and Additional Resources sections are new sections. Additional Resources are not cited in the monograph but are included for research purposes.

PASSIONFLOWER HERB

Latin Name:
Passiflora incarnata

Pharmacopeial Name:
Passiflorae herba

Other Names:
Maypop passion flower, Passiflora, passion vine

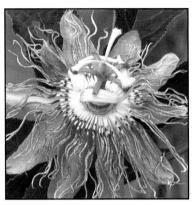

©1999 Steven Foster

Overview

Passionflower is a perennial creeping vine, native to the tropical and semi-tropical southern United States (ranging from Virginia to Florida and as far west as Missouri and Texas), Mexico, and Central and South America, now cultivated in tropical and subtropical regions, including Florida, Guatemala, and India. The material of commerce is obtained from wild and cultivated plants, mainly from the United States, India, and the West Indies (Bergner, 1995; Bruneton, 1995; Leung and Foster, 1996; Der Marderosian, 1999; Wichtl and Bisset, 1994).

Passionflower was first cultivated by native Americans for its edible fruit (Hedrick, 1972; Uphof, 1968). Spanish conquerors first learned of passionflower from the Aztecs of Mexico who used it as a sedative to treat insomnia and nervousness. The plant was taken back to Europe where it became widely cultivated and introduced into European medicine. The unusual construction of its whitish violet flowers caused Spanish missionaries to name this plant with reference to elements of the *passion* of Christ: Its coronal threads were seen as a symbol for the crown of thorns, the curling tendrils for the cords of the whips, the five stamens for the wounds, the three stigmas for the nails on the cross, the ovary for the hammer, and the five petals and five sepals of the flower for the ten "true" apostles (Brill and Dean, 1994; Der Marderosian, 1999; Tyler, 1987; Wichtl and Bisset, 1994).

Its traditional uses, in American aboriginal medicine, by the Cherokees of the southern Allegheny mountains, the Houmas of Louisiana, and the Aztecs of Mexico, are well documented and predate its entry into conventional American and European medicine. It was introduced into conventional North American medicine in the mid-1800s, from Europe, or through Native or slave use in the South, and possibly through all of these avenues (Bergner, 1995; Bown, 1995; Ellingwood, 1983; Hamel and Chiltoskey, 1975; Perry, 1975; Speck, 1941). Today, passionflower is official in the national pharmacopeias of Egypt, France, Germany, and Switzerland, and also monographed in the *British Herbal Pharmacopoeia* and the *British Herbal Compendium*, the ESCOP monographs, the Commission E, the German Standard Licenses, the *German Homeopathic Pharmacopoeia*, and the *Homeopathic Pharmacopoeia of the United States* (BAnz, 1998; BHP, 1996; Bradley, 1992; Braun et al., 1997; Bruneton, 1995; DAB, 1997; ESCOP, 1997; DHAB 1, 1978; HPUS, 1992; Newall et al., 1996; Ph.Fr.X, 1990; Ph.Helv.VII, 1987; Wichtl and Bisset, 1994).

In Germany, passionflower is used as a component of prepared sedative (in combination with lemon balm and valerian root) and cardiotonic (in combination with hawthorn) nonprescription drugs in various dosage forms including coated tablets, tinctures, and infusions (BAnz, 1998; Bradley, 1992; Braun et al., 1997; Leung and Foster, 1996; Wichtl and Bisset, 1994). It is also used in German homeopathic medicine to treat pain, insomnia related to neurasthenia, and nervous exhaustion

(DHAB 1, 1978; Der Marderosian, 1999). In German pediatric medicine, it is used as a component of *Species nervinae pro infantibus* (sedative tea for children), which contains 30% lemon balm leaf, 30% lavender flower, 30% passionflower herb, and 10% St. John's wort herb. It is also a component of a standard Commission E fixed formula "Sedative Tea," which contains 40% valerian root, 30% passionflower herb, and 30% lemon balm leaf (BAnz, 1998; Schilcher, 1997). In the United States, passionflower is used as a sedative component of dietary supplement sleep aid formulations. It was official in the fourth (1916) and fifth (1926) United States *National Formulary* and removed in 1936. It was also an approved OTC sedative and sleep aid up until 1978 (Bown, 1995; Leung and Foster, 1996; NF, 1926).

Very few pharmacological studies have been undertaken, though its central nervous system sedative properties have been documented, supporting its traditional indications for use (Newall et al., 1996). The approved modern therapeutic applications for passionflower are supportable based on its history of use in well established systems of traditional and conventional medicine, pharmacodynamic studies supporting its empirically acknowledged sedative and anxiolytic effects, and phytochemical investigations.

German pharmacopeial grade passionflower must be composed of the whole or cut dried aerial parts, collected during the flowering and fruiting period, containing not less than 0.4% flavonoids calculated as hyperoside. Botanical identity must be confirmed by thin-layer chromatography (TLC) as well as by macroscopic and microscopic examinations and organoleptic evaluation. Purity tests are required for the absence of pith-containing stem fragments greater than 3 mm in diameter and also for the absence of other species (e.g., *P. coerulea* L.) (DAB 1997; Wichtl and Bisset, 1994). The *British Herbal Pharmacopoeia* requires not less than 15% water-soluble extractive, among other quantitative standards (BHP, 1996). The *French Pharmacopoeia* requires not less than 0.8% total flavonoids calculated as vitexin by measuring the absorbence after reaction (Bradley, 1992; Bruneton, 1995; ESCOP, 1997; Ph.Fr.X, 1990). The ESCOP monograph requires that the material comply with the French, German, or Swiss pharmacopeias (ESCOP, 1997).

Description

Passionflower herb consists of fresh or dried, aboveground parts of *Passiflora incarnata* L. [Fam. Passifloraceae] and their preparations in effective dosage. The preparation contains flavonoids (vitexin), maltol, coumarin derivatives, and small amounts of essential oil. The content of harman alkaloids varies; it must not exceed 0.01%.

Chemistry and Pharmacology

Passionflower contains 0.8–2.5% apigenin and luteolin glycosides, vitexin, isovitexin and their C-glycosides, kaempferol, quercetin, and rutin; indole alkaloids (0.01–0.09%), mainly harman, harmaline, harmine; coumarin derivatives; cyanogenic glycosides (gynocardin); fatty acids (linoleic and linolenic); gum; maltol; phytosterols (stigmasterol); sugars (sucrose); and a trace of volatile oil (Bradley, 1992; Bruneton, 1995; ESCOP, 1997; Leung and Foster, 1996; Newall et al., 1996; Wichtl and Bisset, 1994).

The Commission E reported that a motility-inhibiting effect has been observed in animal experiments.

The *British Herbal Compendium* reported its actions as sedative, anxiolytic, and antispasmodic (Bradley, 1992). The available pharmacodynamic studies generally support the empirically accepted central nervous system sedative and anxiolytic effects (ESCOP, 1997; Newall et al., 1996). The specific constituents responsible for these actions remain unclear and it is possibly a synergy of multiple constituents instead (Bradley, 1992; Bruneton, 1995; ESCOP, 1997; Newall et al., 1996).

Uses

The Commission E approved the internal use of passionflower for nervous restlessness.

The *British Herbal Compendium* indicates its use for sleep disorders, restlessness, nervous stress, and anxiety. Other uses include neuralgia and nervous tachycardia (Bradley, 1992). The German Standard License for passionflower tea indicates its use for nervous restlessness, mild disorders of sleeplessness, and gastrointestinal disorders of nervous origin (Bradley, 1992; Wichtl and Bisset, 1994). It is frequently used in combination with valerian and other sedative plants (Bruneton, 1995). ESCOP indicates its use for tenseness, restlessness, and irritability with difficulty in falling asleep (ESCOP, 1997).

Contraindications

None known.

Side Effects

None known.

Use During Pregnancy and Lactation

No restrictions known.

Interactions with Other Drugs

None known.

Dosage and Administration

Unless otherwise prescribed: 4–8 g per day of cut herb.
Dried herb: 2 g, three to four times daily.
Infusion: 2 g in 150 ml water, three to four times daily.
Fluidextract 1:1 (g/ml): 2 ml, three to four times daily.
Tincture 1:5 (g/ml): 10 ml, three to four times daily.
Native dry extract 5:0–6:0:1 (w/w): 0.3–0.4 g, three to four times daily.

References

BAnz. See *Bundesanzeiger*.

Bergner, P. 1995. Passionflower. *Medical Herbalism* 7(1–2):13–14, 26.

Bown, D. 1995. *Encyclopedia of Herbs and Their Uses*. New York: DK Publishing, Inc. 323.

Bradley, P.R. (ed.). 1992. *British Herbal Compendium*, Vol. 1. Bournemouth: British Herbal Medicine Association.

Braun, R. et al. 1997. *Standardzulassungen für Fertigarzneimittel—Text and Kommentar*. Stuttgart: Deutscher Apotheker Verlag.

Brill, S. and E. Dean. 1994. *Identifying and Harvesting Edible and Medicinal Plants in Wild (and Not So Wild) Places*. New York: Hearst Books. 105–106.

British Herbal Pharmacopoeia (BHP). 1996. Exeter, U.K.: British Herbal Medicine Association.

Bruneton, J. 1995. *Pharmacognosy, Phytochemistry, Medicinal Plants*. Paris: Lavoisier Publishing.

Bundesanzeiger (BAnz). 1998. Monographien der Kommission E (Zulassungs- und Aufbereitungskommission am BGA für den humanmed. Bereich, phytotherapeutische Therapierichtung und Stoffgruppe). Köln: Bundesgesundheitsamt (BGA).

Der Marderosian, A. (ed.). 1999. *The Review of Natural Products*. St. Louis: Facts and Comparisons.

Deutsches Arzneibuch (DAB 1997). 1997. Stuttgart: Deutscher Apotheker Verlag.

Deutsches Homöopathisches Arzneibuch, 1st ed. (DHAB 1). 1978. Stuttgart: Deutscher Apotheker Verlag.

Ellingwood, F. 1983. *American Materia Medica, Therapeutics and Pharmacognosy*. Portland, OR: Eclectic Medical Publications [reprint of 1919 original].

ESCOP. 1997. "Passiflorae herba." *Monographs on the Medicinal Uses of Plant Drugs*. Exeter, U.K.: European Scientific Cooperative on Phytotherapy.

Hamel, P.B. and M.U. Chiltoskey. 1975. *Cherokee Plants and Their Uses—A 400 Year History*. Sylva, NC: Herald Publishing Company.

Hedrick, U.P. (ed.). 1972. *Sturtevant's Edible Plants of the World*. New York: Dover Publications.

The Homeopathic Pharmacopoeia of the United States (HPUS). 1992. Arlington, VA: Pharmacopoeia Convention of the American Institute of Homeopathy.

Leung, A.Y. and S. Foster. 1996. *Encyclopedia of Common Natural Ingredients Used in Food, Drugs, and Cosmetics*, 2nd ed. New York: John Wiley & Sons, Inc.

National Formulary (NF), 5th ed. 1926. Washington, D.C.: American Pharmaceutical Association.

Newall, C.A., L.A. Anderson, J.D. Phillipson. 1996. *Herbal Medicines: A Guide for Health-Care Professionals*. London: The Pharmaceutical Press.

Perry, M.J. 1975. *Food Use of "Wild" Plants by Cherokee Indians.* The University of Tennessee, M.S. Thesis.

Pharmacopée Française Xe Édition (Ph.Fr.X.). 1983–1990. Moulins-les-Metz: Maisonneuve S.A.

Pharmacopoeia Helvetica, 7th ed. Vol. 1–4. (Ph.Helv.VII). 1987. Bern: Office Central Fédéral des Imprimés et du Matériel.

Schilcher, H. 1997. *Phytotherapy in Paediatrics: Handbook for Physicians and Pharmacists.* Stuttgart: Medpharm Scientific Publishers. 60, 62, 128, 159.

Speck, F.G. 1941. A List of Plant Curatives Obtained from the Houma Indians of Louisiana. *Primitive Man* 14:49–75.

Tyler, V.E. 1987. *The New Honest Herbal.* Philadelphia: G.F. Stickley Co.

Uphof, J.C. 1968. *Dictionary of Economic Plants.* Würzburg: Verlag von J. Cramer.

Wichtl, M. and N.G. Bisset (eds.). 1994. *Herbal Drugs and Phytopharmaceuticals.* Stuttgart: Medpharm Scientific Publishers.

Additional Resources

British Herbal Pharmacopoeia (BHP). 1990. Bournemouth, U.K.: British Herbal Medicine Association.

———. 1983. Keighley, U.K.: British Herbal Medicine Association.

Brasseur, T. and L. Angenot. 1984. [The pharmacognosy of the passion flower] [In French]. *J Pharm Belg* 39(1):15–22.

Council of Europe. 1981. *Flavouring Substances and Natural Sources of Flavourings,* 3rd ed. Strasbourg: Maisonneuve.

Direction de la Pharmacie et du Médicament (DPM). 1992. Bulletin Officiel No. 92/11 bis. [English edition]. Paris: Direction des Journaux Officiels.

Duke, J.A. 1985. *Handbook of Medicinal Herbs.* Boca Raton: CRC Press.

Goldberg, A., P. Altaffer, M. Altaffer (eds.). 1997. *Brazilian Botanical Monographs,* 1st ed. Oakland: New World Enterprises, Inc.

Hänsel, R., K. Keller, H. Rimpler, G. Schneider (eds.). 1994. *Hagers Handbuch der Pharmazeutischen Praxis,* 5th ed. Vol. 6. Berlin-Heidelberg: Springer Verlag. 34–49.

Jaspersen-Schib, R. 1990. Sédatifs à base de plantes. *Schweiz Apoth Ztg* 128:248–251.

List, P.H. and L. Hörhammer (eds.). 1973–1979. *Hagers Handbuch der Pharmazeutischen Praxis,* Vols. 1–7. New York: Springer Verlag.

Lutomski, J., B. Malek, L. Rybacka. 1975. [Pharmacochemical investigations of the raw materials from Passiflora genus. 2. The pharmacochemical estimation of juices from the fruits of *Passiflora edulis* and *Passiflora edulis* forma flavicarpa] [In German]. *Planta Med* 27(2):112–121.

Lutomski, J. and B. Malek. 1975. [Pharmacological investigations on raw materials of the genus *Passiflora.* 4. The comparison of contents of alkaloids in some harman raw materials] [In German]. *Planta Med* 27(4):381–386.

Lutomski, J., E. Segiet, K. Szpunar, K. Grisse. 1981. Die Bedeutung der Passionsblume in der Heilkunde [The importance of the passionflower in medicine]. *Pharm Unserer Zeit* 10(2):45–49.

Meier, B. 1995. *Passiflora* herb—pharmazeutische Qualität. *Z Phytother* 16:90–99.

———. 1995. *Passiflora incarnata* L.—Passionsblume. *Z Phytother* 16:115–126.

Reynolds, J.E.F. (ed.). 1993. *Martindale: The Extra Pharmacopoeia,* 30th ed. London: The Pharmaceutical Press.

Sopranzi, N., G. De Feo, G. Mazzanti, L. Tolu. 1990. Parametri biologici ed elettroencefalografici nel ratto correlati a *Passiflora incarnata* L. [Biological and electroencephalographic parameters in rats in relation to *Passiflora incarnata* L.] *Clin Ter* 132(5):329–333.

Soulimani, R. et al. 1997. Behavioural effects of *Passiflora incarnata* L. and its indole alkaloid and flavonoid derivatives and maltol in the mouse. *J Ethnopharmacol* 57(1):11–20.

Speroni, E. and A. Minghetti. 1988. Neuropharmacological activity of extracts from *Passiflora incarnata. Planta Med* 54(6):488–491.

This material was adapted from *The Complete German Commission E Monographs—Therapeutic Guide to Herbal Medicines.* M. Blumenthal, W.R. Busse, A. Goldberg, J. Gruenwald, T. Hall, C.W. Riggins, R.S. Rister (eds.) S. Klein and R.S. Rister (trans.). 1998. Austin: American Botanical Council; Boston: Integrative Medicine Communications.

1) The Overview section is new information.

2) Description, Chemistry and Pharmacology, Uses, Contraindications, Side Effects, Interactions with Other Drugs, and Dosage sections have been drawn from the original work. Additional information has been added in some or all of these sections, as noted with references.

3) The dosage for equivalent preparations (tea infusion, fluidextract, and tincture) have been provided based on the following example:
   Unless otherwise prescribed: 2 g per day of [powdered, crushed, cut or whole] [plant part]
   Infusion: 2 g in 150 ml of water
   Fluidextract 1:1 (g/ml): 2 ml
   Tincture 1:5 (g/ml): 10 ml

4) The References and Additional Resources sections are new sections. Additional Resources are not cited in the monograph but are included for research purposes.

PEPPERMINT:

PEPPERMINT LEAF
(page 299)

PEPPERMINT OIL
(page 300)

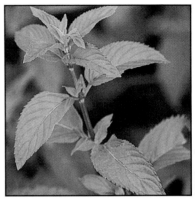

©1999 Steven Foster

Overview

Peppermint is a perennial aromatic herb that is a natural hybrid of *Mentha aquatica* L. (water mint) and *M. spicata* L. (spearmint). It is found growing wild throughout Europe and North America along stream banks and in moist wastelands where it has escaped from cultivation. A number of varieties, strains, or chemotypes are cultivated, including "Mitcham" (*rubescens* form of the *officinalis* variety), "white" (*palescens* form of the officinalis variety), "black" (var. *vulgaris*), and also the *rubescens* form of the *sylvestris* variety (Briggs, 1993; Bruneton, 1995; Grieve, 1979; Leung and Foster, 1996; Trease and Evans, 1989; Wichtl and Bisset, 1994). The material of commerce is obtained entirely from cultivation in Bulgaria, Greece, Spain, northern Europe, and the United States (BHP, 1996; Wichtl and Bisset, 1994). The U.S. is the leading producer of peppermint oil, especially in Washington, Oregon, Idaho, Wisconsin, and Indiana (Bruneton, 1995; Leung and Foster, 1996; Tyler et al., 1988).

The genus name *Mentha* is from the Greek *Mintha*, the name of a mythical nymph who metamorphosed into this plant; its species name *piperita* is from the Latin *piper*, meaning pepper, alluding to its aromatic and pungent taste (Tyler et al., 1988). Mint leaves have been used in medicine for several thousand years, according to records from the Greek, Roman, and ancient Egyptian eras (Briggs, 1993; Evans, 1991). The origin of peppermint cultivation is disputed, though there is some evidence that it was cultivated in ancient Egypt. Roman naturalist Pliny the Elder (ca. 23–79 C.E.) wrote of its uses by the Greeks and Romans. Peppermint was first recognized as a distinct species by botanist John Ray in his Synopsis Stirpium Britannicorum (second edition, 1696), and his *Historia Plantarum* (1704). It became official in the *London Pharmacopoeia* in 1721 (Briggs, 1993; Grieve, 1979; Tyler et al., 1988). Today, peppermint leaf and/or its oil are official in the national pharmacopeias of Austria, France, Germany, Great Britain, Hungary, Russia, and Switzerland, and the *European Pharmacopoeia* (BP, 1988; Bradley, 1992; DAB 10, 1991; ÖAB, 1981; Ph.Eur.3, 1997; Ph.Fr.X, 1990; Ph.Helv.VII, 1987; Ph.Hg.VII, 1986; USSR X, 1973; Wichtl and Bisset, 1994).

In Germany, peppermint leaf is one of the most economically important individual herbs, demonstrated by the fact that in 1993 nearly four thousand tons were imported, and in 1994 almost five thousand tons. It is also one of Germany's own most important medicinal plant crops (Lange and Schippmann, 1997). It is licensed as a standard medicinal tea, is official in the *German Pharmacopoeia*, and approved in the Commission E monographs (leaf and oil). It is used as a monopreparation and also as a component of many cholagogue, bile-duct, gastrointestinal, and liver remedies, and some hypnotic/sedative drugs (BAnz, 1998; Bradley, 1992; Braun et al., 1997; DAB 10, 1991; Wichtl and Bisset, 1994). In German pediatric medicine, peppermint leaf (67%) is combined with chamomile flower (33%) as an herbal tea to treat gastric upset in children. It is also used as a component of various "kidney and bladder" teas for children. Peppermint oil is used as a component of *Inhalatio composita* (45% eucalyptus oil, 45% pumilio pine oil, 10% peppermint oil) specifically indicated for coryza and nasal catarrh in children (Schilcher, 1997). In the United States, peppermint leaf is used singly and as a main component of a wide range of digestive, common cold, and decongestant dietary supplement and OTC drug products, in fluid and solid dosage forms. Peppermint leaf and peppermint oil are official in the U.S. *National Formulary.* Peppermint oil is used in the United States as a carminative in antacids, a counterirritant in topical analgesics, an antipruritic in sunburn creams, a decongestant in inhalants and lozenges, and as an antiseptic or flavoring agent in mouthwashes, gums, and toothpastes (Briggs, 1993; Leung and Foster, 1996; Tyler et al., 1988).

Most modern human studies have investigated peppermint oil rather than peppermint leaf as a treatment for stomachache (May et al., 1996), spastic colon syndrome (Somerville et al., 1984), postoperative nausea (Tate, 1997), relief of colonic muscle spasm during barium enema (Sparks et al., 1995), irritable bowel syndrome (Carling et al., 1989; Dew et al., 1984; Fernández, 1990; Koch, 1998; Lawson et al., 1988; Lech et al., 1988; Liu et al., 1997; Nash et al., 1986; Pittler and Ernst, 1998; Rees et al., 1979), prevention of abdominal distension in postoperative gynecological patients (Feng, 1997), and headaches (Gobel et al., 1994; Gobel et al., 1996). The use of peppermint oil for irritable bowel syndrome is based on preparations in enteric-coated capsules, causing a spasmolytic activity on smooth muscles of the gut. In animal tests, the probable mechanism of action has been shown to be the inhibition of smooth muscle contractions by blocking calcium influx into muscle cells (Forster et al., 1980; Giachetti et al., 1988).

In one double-blind, placebo-controlled multicenter trial, Enteroplant®, consisting of peppermint oil (90 mg) and caraway oil (50 mg) in an enteric-coated capsule, was studied in 45 patients with non-ulcerous dyspepsia. After four weeks of treatment both the intensity of pain and the global clinical impression were significantly improved for the group treated with the peppermint/caraway combination compared with the placebo group (p=0.015 and 0.008, respectively) (May et al., 1996).

In a randomized, placebo-controlled, double-blind crossover study, the effectiveness of peppermint oil against Paracetamol® (acetaminophen) and placebo was studied for use of headaches. The liquid test preparation contained 10 g of peppermint oil and ethanol (90%) (LI 170, Lichtwer Pharma, Germany); the placebo was a 90% ethanol solution to which traces of peppermint oil were added for blinding purposes. The reference preparation contained 500 mg acetaminophen. The study included analyses of 164 headache attacks of 41 male and female patients between 16 and 45 years of age suffering from tension-type headaches in accordance with the International Headache Society classification. The authors concluded that a 10% peppermint oil in ethanol solution efficiently alleviated tension-type headaches and that it was a well-tolerated and cost-effective alternative to conventional therapies (Gobel et al., 1996).

The approved modern therapeutic applications for peppermint are supportable based on its history of use in well established systems of traditional and conventional medicines, extensive phytochemical investigations, *in vitro* studies, *in vivo* pharmacological studies in animals, and human clinical studies.

Pharmacopeial grade peppermint leaf must be composed of the dried whole or cut leaf with not more than 5% stem fragments greater than 1 mm in diameter and not more than 10% leaves with brown spots caused by *Puccinia menthae*. The whole leaf must contain not less than 1.2% (ml/g) and the cut leaf must contain not less than 0.9% volatile oil. Botanical identity must be confirmed by macroscopic and microscopic examinations and organoleptic evaluation (Ph.Eur.3, 1997; Wichtl and Bisset, 1994). The ESCOP peppermint leaf monograph requires that the material comply with the *European Pharmacopoeia* (ESCOP, 1997).

European pharmacopeial grade peppermint oil is the volatile oil distilled with steam from the fresh aerial parts of the flowering plant. Its relative density must be between 0.900 and 0.916, refractive index between 1.457 and 1.467, optical rotation between −10 and −30°, among other quantitative standards. Identity must be confirmed by thin-layer chromatography (TLC), organoleptic evaluation, and quantitative analysis of internal composition by gas chromatography. It must contain 1.0–5.0% limonene, 3.5–14.0% cineole, 14.0–32.0% menthone, 1.0–9.0% menthofuran, 1.5–10.0% isomenthone, 2.8–10.0% menthylacetate, 30.0–55.0% menthol, maximum 4.0% pulegone, and maximum 1.0% carvone (Ph.Eur.3, 1997). French pharmacopeial grade peppermint oil must contain not less than 44% menthol, from 4.5–10% esters calculated as menthyl acetate, and from 15–32% carbonyl compounds calculated as menthone. TLC is used for identification, quantification of compounds, and verification of the absence of visible bands corresponding to carvone, pulegone, and isomenthone (Bruneton, 1995; Ph.Fr.X, 1990).

PEPPERMINT LEAF

Latin Name:
Mentha x *piperita*

Pharmacopeial Name:
Menthae piperitae folium

Other Names:
n/a

Description
Peppermint leaf consists of the fresh or dried leaf of *Mentha* x *piperita* L. [Fam. Lamiaceae] and its preparations in effective dosage. The herb contains at least 1.2% (v/w) essential oil. Other ingredients are tannins characteristic of Lamiaceae.

Chemistry and Pharmacology
Peppermint leaf contains luteolin, hesperidin, and rutin; caffeic, chlorogenic, and rosmarinic acids, and related tannins; choline; α- and β-carotenes; gum; minerals; resin; α and γ tocopherols; α-amyrin and squalene triterpenes; volatile oil (1.2–3%) composed mostly of monoterpenes—29–55% menthol, 10–40% menthone, 2–13% cineole, 1–11% pulegone, 1–10% menthyl acetate, 0–10% menthofuran, and 0.2–6% limonene (Bradley, 1992;

Bruneton, 1995; Budavari, 1996; ESCOP, 1997; Leung and Foster, 1996; Wichtl and Bisset, 1994).

The Commission E reported direct antispasmodic action on the smooth muscle of the digestive tract as well as choleretic and carminative activity. Note: There is a separate monograph for peppermint oil.

The *British Herbal Compendium* reported carminative, spasmolytic, and choleretic activity (Bradley, 1992). In human pharmacological studies, peppermint leaf extracts had carminative action by causing a reduction in tonus of the esophageal sphincter, thus enabling release of entrapped air (Demling and Steger, 1969).

Uses
The Commission E approved the internal use of peppermint leaf for spastic

complaints of the gastrointestinal tract, the gallbladder, and bile ducts.

The *British Herbal Compendium* indicates peppermint leaf for dyspepsia, flatulence, intestinal colic, and biliary disorders (Bradley, 1992). ESCOP indicates its use for symptomatic treatment of digestive disorders such as dyspepsia, flatulence, gastritis, and enteritis (ESCOP, 1997). The German Standard License for peppermint leaf tea indicates its use for gastrointestinal and gallbladder ailments (Braun et al., 1997).

Contraindications

In case of gallstones, first consult a physician.

Side Effects

None known.

Use During Pregnancy and Lactation

No restrictions known (McGuffin et al., 1997).

Interactions with Other Drugs

None known.

Dosage and Administration

Internal: Unless otherwise prescribed: 3–6 g per day of cut leaf for infusions and extracts.

Infusion: 2 g in 150 ml water, two to three times daily.

Fluidextract 1:1 (g/ml): 2 ml, two to three times daily.

Tincture 1:5 (g/ml): 10 ml, two to three times daily.

Tincture: 5–15 g (Erg.B.6).

Dry normalized extract 3.5–4.5:1 (w/w): 0.44–0.57 g, two to three times daily.

PEPPERMINT OIL

Latin Name:
Mentha x *piperita*

Pharmacopeial Name:
Menthae piperitae aetheroleum

Other Names:
n/a

Description

Peppermint oil consists of the essential oil of *Mentha* x *piperita* L. [Fam. Lamiaceae], obtained by steam distillation from freshly harvested, flowering sprigs, and its preparations in effective dosage. Peppermint oil contains a minimum of 4.5% and a maximum of 10% (w/w) esters, calculated as menthyl acetate, at least 44% (w/w) free alcohols, calculated as menthol, and a minimum of 15% and maximum of 32% (w/w) ketones, calculated as menthone.

Chemistry and Pharmacology

Peppermint oil contains 44–55% free alcohols (as menthol), 15–32% ketones (as menthone), 4.5–10% esters (as menthyl acetate), 3.5–14% cineole, 1.5–10% isomenthone, 1–9% menthofuran, 1–5% limonene, no more than 4% pulegone or 1% carvone, and sesquiterpenes (approximately 0.5% viridoflorol) (Bruneton, 1995; ESCOP, 1997; Leung and Foster, 1996; Ph.Eur.3, 1997, Ph.Fr.X, 1983–1990).

The Commission E reported antispasmodic, carminative, cholagogue, antibacterial, secretolytic, and cooling activity.

In human pharmacological studies peppermint oil injected into the lumen of the colon relieved colonic spasms (Leicester and Hunt, 1982). The *Indian Pharmacopoeia* reported carminative activity (IP, 1996). The volatile oil of peppermint leaf is carminative and a potent spasmolytic, acting locally to produce smooth muscle relaxation (Bradley, 1992; Leicester and Hunt, 1982).

Uses

The Commission E approved the internal use of peppermint oil for spastic discomfort of the upper gastrointestinal tract and bile ducts, irritable colon (in enteric-coated capsules), catarrhs of the respiratory tract, and inflammation of the oral mucosa; and external use for myalgia and neuralgia.

ESCOP indicates its internal use for flatulence, irritable bowel syndrome, and coughs and colds. Its external use is indicated for coughs and colds, rheumatic complaints, pruritus, urticaria, and pain in irritable skin conditions (ESCOP, 1997). Peppermint oil is used in Western and Eastern cultures to treat indigestion, nausea, sore throat, diarrhea, colds, and headaches (Leung and Foster, 1996).

Contraindications

Obstruction of bile ducts, gallbladder inflammation, severe liver damage. In case of gallstones, to be used only after consultation with a physician. Preparations containing peppermint oil should not be used on the face, particularly the nose, of infants and small children. [Ed. Note: Peppermint oil is contraindicated in infants and small children due to the potential risk of spasms of the tongue or respiratory arrest (Shultz et al., 1998).]

Side Effects

None known.

Use During Pregnancy and Lactation

No restrictions known (McGuffin et al., 1997).

Interactions with Other Drugs

None known.

Dosage and Administration

Unless otherwise prescribed: 6–12 drops per day essential oil and galenical preparations for internal and external application.
Internal: Essential oil: Average single dose 0.2 ml.
Essential oil enterically coated form: Average daily dose 0.6 ml (for IBS).
Inhalant: Add 3–4 drops of essential oil to hot water; deeply inhale the steam vapor.
External: Essential oil: Some drops rubbed in the affected skin areas (may be diluted with lukewarm water or vegetable oil).
Liniment: Oily preparation containing 5–20% essential oil in base of paraffin or vegetable oil applied locally by friction method.
Ointment or unguent: Semi-solid preparation containing 5–20% essential oil in base of petroleum jelly or lanolin spread on linen for local application.
Nasal ointment: Semi-solid preparation containing 1–5% essential oil.
Tincture: Aqueous-alcoholic preparation containing 5–10% essential oil for local application.

References

BAnz. See *Bundesanzeiger.*

Bradley, P.R. (ed.). 1992. *British Herbal Compendium,* Vol. 1. Bournemouth: British Herbal Medicine Association.

Braun, R. et al. 1997. *Standardzulassungen für Fertigarzneimittel—Text and Kommentar.* Stuttgart: Deutscher Apotheker Verlag.

Briggs, C. 1993. Peppermint: Medicinal Herb and Flavouring Agent. CPJ/RPC 89–92.

British Herbal Pharmacopoeia (BHP). 1996. Exeter, U.K.: British Herbal Medicine Association. 149.

British Pharmacopoeia (BP). 1988. (With subsequent Addenda up to 1992.) London: Her Majesty's Stationery Office.

Bruneton, J. 1995. *Pharmacognosy, Phytochemistry, Medicinal Plants*. Paris: Lavoisier Publishing.

Budavari, S. (ed.). 1996. *The Merck Index: An Encyclopedia of Chemicals, Drugs, and Biologicals*, 12th ed. Whitehouse Station, N.J.: Merck & Co, Inc.

Bundesanzeiger (BAnz). 1998. Monographien der Kommission E (Zulassungs- und Aufbereitungskommission am BGA für den humanmed. Bereich, phytotherapeutische Therapierichtung und Stoffgruppe). Köln: Bundesgesundheitsamt (BGA).

Carling, L., L.E. Svedberg, S. Hulten. 1989. Short term treatment of the irritable bowel syndrome: a placebo-controlled trial of Peppermint oil against hyoscyamine. *Opuscula Med* 34:55–57.

Demling, L. and W. Steger. 1969. Zur rechtfertigung der volksmedizin: pfefferminze und zwiebel. *Fortschr Med* 37:1305–1306.

Deutsches Arzneibuch, 10th ed. (DAB 10). 1991. (With subsequent supplements through 1996.) Stuttgart: Deutscher Apotheker Verlag.

Dew, M.J., B.K. Evans, J. Rhodes. 1984. Peppermint oil for the irritable bowel syndrome: a multicentre trial. *Br J Clin Pract* 38(11–12):394, 398.

ESCOP. 1997. "Menthae piperitae folium" and "Menthae piperitae aetheroleum." *Monographs on the Medicinal Uses of Plant Drugs*. Exeter, U.K.: European Scientific Cooperative on Phytotherapy.

Europäisches Arzneibuch, 3rd ed. (Ph.Eur.3). 1997. Stuttgart: Deutscher Apotheker Verlag. 1466–1467.

Evans, M. 1991. *Herbal Plants, History and Use*. London: Studio Editions. 105–107.

Feng, X.Z. 1997. [Effect of peppermint oil hot compresses in preventing abdominal distension in postoperative gynecological patients] [In Chinese]. *Chung Hua Hu Li Tsa Chih* 32(10):577–578.

Fernández, F. 1990. *Menta piperita* en el tratamiento de síndrome de colon irritable. *Invest Med Inter* 17:42–46.

Forster H.B., H. Niklas, S. Lutz. 1980. Antispasmodic effects of some medicinal plants. *Planta Med* 40:309–319.

Forster, H. 1983. Spasmolytische wirkung pflanzlicher carminativa [Spasmolytic effect of plant carminatives]. *Z Allg Med* 59(24):1327–1333.

Giachetti D., Taddei E., Taddei I. 1988. Pharmacological activity of essential oils on Oddi's sphincter. *Planta Med* 54(5):389–392.

Gobel H., J. Fresenius, A. Heinze, M. Dworschak, D. Soyka. 1996. Effektivität von Oleum *Menthae piperitae* und von paracetamol in der therapie des kopfschmerzes vom spannungstyp [Effectiveness of Oleum *Menthae piperitae* and paracetamol in therapy of headache of the tension type]. *Nervenarzt* 67(8):672–681.

Gobel, H., G. Schmidt, D. Soyka. 1994. Effect of peppermint and eucalyptus oil preparations on neurophysiological and experimental algesimetric headache parameters. *Cephalalgia* 14(3):182, 228–234.

Grieve, M. 1979. *A Modern Herbal*. New York: Dover Publications, Inc.

Indian Pharmacopoeia, Vol. 1. (IP 1996). 1996. Delhi: Government of India Ministry of Health and Family Welfare—Controller of Publications.

Koch, T.R. 1998. Peppermint oil and irritable bowel syndrome [in process citation]. *Am J Gastroenterol* 93(11):2304–2305.

Lange, D. and U. Schippmann. 1997. *Trade Survey of Medicinal Plants in Germany—A Contribution to International Plant Species Conservation*. Bonn: Bundesamt für Naturschutz. 32–34, 52–53, 69.

Lawson, M.J., R.E. Knight, K. Tran, G. Walker, I.C. Robers-Thompson. 1988. Failure of enteric-coated Peppermint oil in the irritable bowel syndrome: a randomized double-blind crossover study. *J Gastroent Hepatol* 3:235–238.

Lech, Y. et al. 1988. Behandling af colon irritabile med Pebermynteolie. En dobbeltblind undersogelse med placebo [Treatment of irritable bowel syndrome with peppermint oil. A double-blind study with a placebo]. *Ugeskr Laeger* 150(40):2388–2389.

Leicester, R.J. and R.H. Hunt. 1982. Peppermint oil to reduce colonic spasm during endoscopy. *Lancet* 2(8305):989.

Leung, A.Y. and S. Foster. 1996. *Encyclopedia of Common Natural Ingredients Used in Food, Drugs, and Cosmetics*, 2nd ed. New York: John Wiley & Sons, Inc.

Liu, J.H., G.H. Chen, H.Z. Yeh, C.K. Huang, S.K. Poon. 1997. Enteric-coated peppermint-oil capsules in the treatment of irritable bowel syndrome: a prospective, randomized trial. *J Gastroenterol* 32(6):765–768.

May, B., H.D. Kuntz, M. Kieser, S. Kohler. 1996. Efficacy of a fixed peppermint oil/caraway oil combination in non-ulcer dyspepsia. *Arzneimforsch* 46(12):1149–1153.

McGuffin, M., C. Hobbs, R. Upton, A. Goldberg. 1997. American Herbal Product Association's *Botanical Safety Handbook*. Boca Raton: CRC Press.

Nash, P., S.R. Gould, D.E. Bernardo. 1986. Peppermint oil does not relieve the pain of irritable bowel syndrome. *Br J Clin Pract* 40(7):292–293.

Österreichisches Arzneibuch, Vols. 1–2. (ÖAB). 1981. Wien: Verlag der Österreichischen Staatsdruckerei.

Pharmacopée Française Xe Édition (Ph.Fr.X.). 1983–1990. Moulins-les-Metz: Maisonneuve S.A.

Pharmacopoeia Helvetica, 7th ed. Vol. 1–4. (Ph.Helv.VII). 1987. Bern: Office Central Fédéral des Imprimés et du Matériel.

Pharmacopoea Hungaric, 7th ed. (Ph.Hg.VII). 1986. Budapest: Medicina Könyvkiadó.

Ph.Eur.3. See *Europäisches Arzneibuch*.

Pittler, M.H. and E. Ernst. 1998. Peppermint oil for irritable bowel syndrome: a critical review and meta-analysis. *Am J Gastroenterol* 93(7):1131–1135.

Rees, W.D., B.K. Evans, J. Rhodes. 1979. Treating irritable bowel syndrome with peppermint oil. *Br Med J* 2(6194):835–836.

Schilcher, H. 1997. *Phytotherapy in Paediatrics: Handbook for Physicians and Pharmacists.* Stuttgart: Medpharm Scientific Publishers. 46–47, 56.

Schulz, V., R. Hänsel, V.E. Tyler. 1998. *Rational Phytotherapy: A Physicians' Guide to Herbal Medicine.* New York: Springer.

Somerville, K.W., C.R. Richmond, G.D. Bell. 1984. Delayed release Peppermint oil capsules (Colpermin) for the spastic colon syndrome: a pharmacokinetic study. *Br J Clin Pharmacol* 18(4):638–640.

Sparks M.J., P. O'Sullivan, A.A. Herrington, S.K. Morcos. 1995. Does peppermint oil relieve spasm during barium enema? *Br J Radiol* 68(812):841–843.

State Pharmacopoeia of the Union of Soviet Socialist Republics, 10th ed. (USSR X). 1973. Moscow: Ministry of Health of the U.S.S.R.

Tate, S. 1997. Peppermint oil: a treatment for postoperative nausea. *J Adv Nurs* 26(3):543–549.

Trease, G.E. and W.C. Evans. 1989. *Trease and Evans' Pharmacognosy,* 13th ed. London; Philadelphia: Baillière Tindall. 421–423.

Tyler, V.E., L.R. Brady, J.E. Robbers. 1988. *Pharmacognosy,* 9th ed. Philadelphia: Lea & Febiger. 113–119.

USSR X. See *State Pharmacopoeia of the Union of Soviet Socialist Republics.*

Wichtl, M. and N.G. Bisset (eds.). 1994. *Herbal Drugs and Phytopharmaceuticals.* Stuttgart: Medpharm Scientific Publishers.

Additional Resources

Dinckler, K. 1936. Über die biologische Wirkung verschiedener Reinstoffe im äetherischen Öl von Mentha-Arten. *Pharm Zentralhalle* 77:281–290.

Direction de la Pharmacie et du Médicament (DPM). 1992. Bulletin Officiel No. 92/11 bis. [English edition]. Paris: Direction des Journaux Officiels.

Duband, F. et al. 1992. Composition aromatique et polyphenolique de l'infuse de Menthe, *Mentha x piperita* L. [Aromatic and polyphenolic composition of infused peppermint, *Mentha x piperita* L.]. *Ann Pharm Fr* 50(3):146–155.

Ergänzungsbuch zum Deutschen Arzneibuch, 6th ed. (Erg.B.6). 1953. Stuttgart: Deutscher Apotheker Verlag.

Hartke, K. and E. Mutschler (eds.). 1988. DAB 9—*Kommentar.* Vol. 3. Stuttgart: Wissen Verlagsgesellschaft. 2702–2704.

Herrmann, E.C., Jr. and L.S. Kucera. 1967. Antiviral substances in plants of the mint family (labiatae). 3. Peppermint (Mentha piperita) and other mint plants. *Proc Soc Exp Biol Med* 124(3):874–878.

Musim, M.N., I. Khadzhai, V.I. Litvinenko, A.S. Ammosov. 1976. Protyzapal'na aktyvnist' polifeol'noho preparatu, oderzhanoho z m'iaty pertsevoi [Anti-inflammatory activity of a polyphenolic preparation obtained from peppermint] *Farm Zh* (2):76–79.

Steinegger, E. and R. Hänsel. 1988. Lehrbuch der *Pharmakognosie* und Phyto*pharmazie.* Berlin-Heidelberg: Springer Verlag.

———. 1992. *Pharmakognosie,* 5th ed. Berlin: Spinger Verlag. 302–304.

The United States Pharmacopoeia, 22nd rev. (USP XXII). 1990–1992. Rockville, MD: U.S. Pharmacopoeial Convention.

Wichtl, M. 1989. In: Wichtl, M. (ed.). *Teedrogen,* 2nd ed. Stuttgart: Wissenschaftliche Verlagsgesellschaft. 372–374.

Wichtl, M. and M. Schäfer-Korting. 1993–1994. In: Hartke, K., H. Hartke, E. Mutschler, G. Rücker, M. Wichtl (eds.). DAB 10—*Kommentar.* Stuttgart: Wissenschaftliche Verlagsgesellschaft. P28–P29.

This material was adapted from *The Complete German Commission E Monographs—Therapeutic Guide to Herbal Medicines.* M. Blumenthal, W.R. Busse, A. Goldberg, J. Gruenwald, T. Hall, C.W. Riggins, R.S. Rister (eds.) S. Klein and R.S. Rister (trans.). 1998. Austin: American Botanical Council; Boston: Integrative Medicine Communications.

1) The Overview section is new information.

2) Description, Chemistry and Pharmacology, Uses, Contraindications, Side Effects, Interactions with Other Drugs, and Dosage sections have been drawn from the original work. Additional information has been added in some or all of these sections, as noted with references.

3) The dosage for equivalent preparations (tea infusion, fluidextract, and tincture) have been provided based on the following example:

   Unless otherwise prescribed: 2 g per day of [powdered, crushed, cut or whole] [plant part]
   Infusion: 2 g in 150 ml of water
   Fluidextract 1:1 (g/ml): 2 ml
   Tincture 1:5 (g/ml): 10 ml

4) The References and Additional Resources sections are new sections. Additional Resources are not cited in the monograph but are included for research purposes.

PINE NEEDLE OIL

Latin Name:
Pinus sylvestris

Pharmacopeial Name:
Pini aetheroleum

Other Names:
dwarf pine needle oil

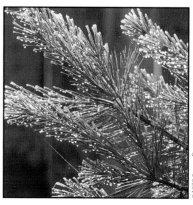

©1999 Steven Foster

Overview

Pine needle oil is steam distilled from the fresh needles, branch tips, or the combined fresh branches with needles and branch tips of *Pinus sylvestris* L. (Scots pine or Norway pine) or other essential oil-containing species of *Pinus* (DAB 1997). Scots pine is an evergreen conifer tree native to Eurasia, introduced to North America by European settlers, now cultivated extensively in the eastern United States and Canada. Its natural habitat includes the mountains of Scotland, the Scandinavian peninsulas through central Europe, south to the Mediterranean and east through eastern Siberia. More than 35 different seed sources or varieties of Scots pine are commercially recognized. Pine needle oil is produced in Austria, Russia, and Scandinavia (Leung and Foster, 1996; Koelling, 1999; PFAF, 1997). As a Christmas tree, Scots pine is probably the most cultivated species in the United States (Koelling, 1999).

Pines of all kinds have been used medicinally in many countries from the earliest times (Bown, 1995). Scots pine is the source material of Spirits of Turpentine, B.P. and Russian Turpentine. The young branches of black spruce (*P. nigra*) are the source material for "essence of spruce," and the essential oil distilled from the leaves of the dwarf pine (*P. umilio*) is the source material for "oil of pine" (Grieve, 1979). The topical antieczematic and rubefacient over-the-counter drug Pine Tar USP (syn. *pix liquida*) is obtained from the distillation of the wood of longleaf pine (*P. palustris* Mill.) or other species of pine (Bown, 1995; Budavari, 1996; Taber, 1962). The essential oil distilled from the fresh leaves of *P. pinea* and/or *P. sylvestris* is used in northern India as a component of a compound preparation (oil of pine, magnesii carbonas levis, distilled water) for inhalation to treat chronic laryngitis (Nadkarni, 1976). The steam-distilled essential oil from the balsam of *P. densiflora* Sieb. et Zucc. is official in the Chinese and Japanese pharmacopeias. *Song-jie* (its Chinese name) was first mentioned in Chinese medical literature ca. 500 C.E. as an antiarthritic and analgesic drug. Today, it is used in the traditional medicines of China, Japan, and Korea, administered as a topical paint to treat rheumatism (Bown, 1995; But et al., 1997). The Micmac of Canada prepare an aqueous infusion of the needles and twigs of white pine (*P. strobus* L.) for oral ingestion as a medicine for colds (Lacey, 1993).

In Germany, pine needle oil is official in the *German Pharmacopoeia*, the Standard Licenses for Finished Drugs Monographs, and it is also approved by Commission E. Drops of the essential oil are added to boiling water for inhalation of steam vapor as a supportive treatment for catarrhal diseases of the respiratory tract. The drops are also applied topically by carefully rubbing into the skin for rheumatic complaints (BAnz, 1998; Braun et al., 1997; DAB 1997). The Germans also prepare an aqueous infusion of pine shoots for oral ingestion for the same indications as the oil (Meyer-Buchtela, 1999). In German pediatric medicine, Pumilio pine oil is used as a component of "*Inhalatio composita*" formulation (eucalyptus oil 45%, Pumilio pine oil 45%, peppermint oil 10%), intended especially for *coryza* (acute cold and nasal inflammation) and nasal catarrh in children (Schilcher,1997). In the United States, pine needle oil, distilled from the leaves of dwarf pine (*P. mugo* Turra [syn. *P. montana* Mill.] and *P. pumilio* Haenke), is official in the *National Formulary*. It is used as a component in cough and cold medicines, vaporizer fluids, nasal decongestants, and analgesic ointments (Leung and Foster, 1996). The essential oil of Scots pine (*P. sylvestris*) is also used in aromatherapy. This plant is also used in Bach Flower Remedies (homeopathic), available in natural foods stores and herb shops (Bown, 1995; PFAF, 1997).

The approved modern therapeutic applications for pine needle oil are supportable based on its history of use in well established systems of traditional and conventional medicines, and on phytochemical investigations, and pharmacological studies.

German pharmacopeial grade pine needle oil is the steam-distilled essential oil extracted from the fresh needles, branch tips or from the combined fresh branches with needles and branch tips of P. silvestris L. or other essential oil-containing species of *Pinus*. Identification is confirmed by thin-layer chromatography (TLC) and organoleptic evaluation. Its relative density must be 0.855–0.885, refractive index 1.470–1.485, optical rotation –30.0 to ±10.0°, and acid number of maximum 1.0 (DAB 1997). Shelf life is one year when stored and packaged according to the German Standard License monograph requirements (Braun et al., 1997).

Description

The essential oil obtained from fresh needles, tips of the boughs or fresh boughs with needles and tips of *P. sylvestris* L., *P. mugo* species *pumilio* (Haenke) Franco, *P. nigra* Arnold or *P. pinaster* Soland [Fam. Pinaceae] and their preparations in effective dosage.

Chemistry and Pharmacology

Constituents include 50–97% monoterpene hydrocarbons, such as α-pinene, with lesser amounts of 3-carene, dipentene, β-pinen, D-limonene, α-terpinene, y-terpinene, cis-β-ocimene, myrcene, camphene, sabinene, and terpinolene (Schulz et al, 1998). Other constituents include bornyl acetate, borneol, 1,8-cineole, citral terpineol, T-cadinol, T-muurolol, α-cadinol, cayophyllene, chamazulen, butyric acid, valeric acid, caproic acid, and isocaproic acid (Leung and Foster, 1996).

The Commission E reported secretolytic, hyperemic, and slight antiseptic activity.

The active principles of some essential oils responsible for the antiviral and antibacterial activities are thought to be limonene, dipentene, and bornyl acetate (Leung and Foster, 1996). Pine needle oil and other essential oils can cause a decongestant effect by stimulating reflex vasoconstriction (Schulz et al., 1998).

Uses

The Commission E approved pine needle oil for catarrhal diseases of the respiratory tract, and externally only for rheumatic and neuralgic ailments. It has been used as a fragrance and flavor component in cough and cold medicines, vaporizer fluids, nasal decongestants, and analgesic ointments (Leung and Foster, 1996).

Contraindications

Bronchial asthma, whooping cough.

Side Effects

Intensified irritation may occur on skin and mucous membranes. Bronchospasms may be intensified.

Use During Pregnancy and Lactation

No restrictions known.

Interactions with Other Drugs
None known.

Dosage and Administration
Internal: Unless otherwise prescribed:
For inhalation: Add several drops to hot water, inhale vapors.
External: Apply several drops of liquid and semi-solid preparations, concentrations of 10–50%; rub into affected area.
Ointments: In the form of alcoholic solutions, gels, emulsions, or oils.

References

BAnz. See *Bundesanzeiger.*

Bown, D. 1995. *Encyclopedia of Herbs and Their Uses.* New York: DK Publishing, Inc. 329.

Braun, R. et al. 1997. *Standardzulassungen für Fertigarzneimittel—Text and Kommentar.* Stuttgart: Deutscher Apotheker Verlag.

Budavari, S. (ed.). 1996. *The Merck Index: An Encyclopedia of Chemicals, Drugs, and Biologicals,* 12th ed. Whitehouse Station, N.J.: Merck & Co, Inc.

Bundesanzeiger (BAnz). 1998. Monographien der Kommission E (Zulassungs- und Aufbereitungskommission am BGA für den humanmed. Bereich, phytotherapeutische Therapierichtung und Stoffgruppe). Köln: Bundesgesundheitsamt (BGA).

But, P.P.H. et al. (eds.). 1997. *International Collation of Traditional and Folk Medicine.* Singapore: World Scientific. 15–16.

Deutsches Arzneibuch (DAB 1997). 1997. Stuttgart: Deutscher Apotheker Verlag.

Grieve, M. 1979. *A Modern Herbal.* New York: Dover Publications, Inc.

Koelling, M.R. 1999. *History and Characteristics—Scotch Pine—Pinus sylvestris L.* Okemos, MI: National Christmas Tree Association Internet Committee. Available at: www.christree.org/treetype/scotch.html

Lacey, L. 1993. *Micmac Medicines—Remedies and Recollections.* Halifax, NS: Nimbus Publishing Ltd. 29, 36, 99, 115.

Leung, A.Y. and S. Foster. 1996. *Encyclopedia of Common Natural Ingredients Used in Food, Drugs, and Cosmetics,* 2nd ed. New York: John Wiley & Sons, Inc.

Meyer-Buchtela, E. 1999. *Tee-Rezepturen—Ein Handbuch für Apotheker und Ärzte.* Stuttgart: Deutscher Apotheker Verlag.

Nadkarni, K.M. 1976. *Indian Materia Medica.* Bombay: Popular Prakashan. 959.

Plants For A Future Database (PFAF). 1997. Cornwall, England: Plants For A Future. Available at: www.scs.leeds.ac.uk/pfaf-cgi

Schilcher, H. 1997. *Phytotherapy in Paediatrics—Handbook for Physicians and Pharmacists.* Stuttgart: Medpharm Scientific Publishers. 30–32.

Schulz, V., R. Hänsel, V.E. Tyler. 1998. *Rational Phytotherapy: A Physicians' Guide to Herbal Medicine.* New York: Springer.

Taber, C.W. 1962. *Taber's Cyclopedic Medical Dictionary,* 9th ed. Philadelphia: F.A. Davis Company. 61.

Additional Resources

Bruneton, J. 1995. *Pharmacognosy, Phytochemistry, Medicinal Plants.* Paris: Lavoisier Publishing.

Budavari, S., M.J. O'Neil, A. Smith, P.E. Heckelman (eds.). 1989. *The Merck Index: An Encyclopedia of Chemicals, Drugs, and Biologicals,* 11th ed. Rahway, N.J.: Merck & Co., Inc.

Guenther, E. 1948. *The Essential Oils,* Vols. 1–6. New York: Van Nostrand.

Kartnig, T., F. Still, F. Reinthaler. 1991. Antimicrobial activity of the essential oil of young pine shoots (Picea abies L.). *J Ethnopharmacol* 35(2):155–157.

Riechelmann, H., C. Brommer, M. Hinni, C. Martin. 1997. Response of human ciliated respiratory cells to a mixture of menthol, eucalyptus oil and pine needle oil. *Arzneimforsch* 47(9):1035–1039.

This material was adapted from *The Complete German Commission E Monographs—Therapeutic Guide to Herbal Medicines.* M. Blumenthal, W.R. Busse, A. Goldberg, J. Gruenwald, T. Hall, C.W. Riggins, R.S. Rister (eds.) S. Klein and R.S. Rister (trans.). 1998. Austin: American Botanical Council; Boston: Integrative Medicine Communications.

1) The Overview section is new information.

2) Description, Chemistry and Pharmacology, Uses, Contraindications, Side Effects, Interactions with Other Drugs, and Dosage sections have been drawn from the original work. Additional information has been added in some or all of these sections, as noted with references.

3) The dosage for equivalent preparations (tea infusion, fluidextract, and tincture) have been provided based on the following example:
Unless otherwise prescribed: 2 g per day of [powdered, crushed, cut or whole] [plant part]
Infusion: 2 g in 150 ml of water
Fluidextract 1:1 (g/ml): 2 ml
Tincture 1:5 (g/ml): 10 ml

4) The References and Additional Resources sections are new sections. Additional Resources are not cited in the monograph but are included for research purposes.

PLANTAIN

Latin Name:
Plantago lanceolata and *P. major*

Pharmacopeial Name:
Plantaginis lanceolatae herba

Other Names:
P. lanceolata: English plantain, lanceleaf plantain, narrowleaf plantain, ribwort plantain; *P. major:* common plantain, greater plantain, broadleaf plantain

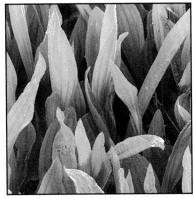

© 1999 Steven Foster

Overview

Plantain is a perennial herb widely distributed throughout Europe and Asia (Wichtl and Bisset, 1994). In India, it is found growing in the Western Himalayas from Kashmir to Simla (Nadkarni, 1976). Of the 250 known species of *Plantago* worldwide, *P. lanceolata* and *P. major* are among those with the widest geographic ranges (Der Marderosian, 1999). The material of commerce is obtained mainly from cultivation in Bulgaria, Germany, Hungary, the Netherlands, Poland, the former Yugoslavia, and the former U.S.S.R. (Wichtl and Bisset, 1994). In Germany, ribwort plantain is one of the most important medicinal plants obtained from cultivation. It is cultivated on "set-aside areas" in accordance with EEC Regulation 1765/92 in the state of Bayern (Lange and Schippmann, 1997).

Plantain herb has been used in European medicine since ancient Roman and Greek times (Grieve, 1979; Nadkarni, 1976) documented through the centuries by various herbalists including Roman naturalist Pliny the Elder (ca. 23–79 C.E.), fourteenth century English poet Geoffrey Chaucer, and seventeenth century English physician Nicholas Culpepper (Grieve, 1979).

In Germany, plantain is official in the *German Pharmacopeia*, approved in the Commission E monographs, and the tea form is official in the German Standard License monograph for oral ingestion, rinses, and gargles as well as external use as a cataplasm (BAnz, 1998; Braun et al., 1997; DAB 10, 1991–1996; Wichtl and Bisset, 1994). It is used to suppress coughs associated with bronchitis, colds, and upper respiratory inflammation, and to reduce skin inflammation (Tyler, 1994). Plantain is employed as a component in numerous antitussive and expectorant medicines, such as the instant antitussive tea Bronchostad® (Wichtl and Bisset, 1994).

A few studies have been found in the literature. Human trials have investigated its use as a treatment for chronic bronchitis (Koichev et al., 1983; Koichev, 1983; Matev et al., 1982) and also its diuretic effects (Doan et al., 1992).

German pharmacopeial grade plantain herb consists of the whole or cut, dried aerial parts of *P. lanceolata* L. It may contain no more than 5% dark-brown to blackish-brown fragments and no more than 2% other foreign matter. The pulverized dried herb must have a swelling index of not less than 6. Botanical identity must be confirmed by thin-layer chromatography (TLC), macroscopic and microscopic examinations, and organoleptic evaluation (DAB 10, 1991–1996). The Swiss pharmacopeia requires that it contain not less than 30% water-soluble extractive and not more than 10% discolored and brown leaves (Ph.Helv.VII, 1987; Wichtl and Bisset, 1994). Rare adulteration with *Digitalis lanata* is reported in the Swiss pharmacopeia though this is easily detected microscopically. Raw material adulterated with digitalis entered the supply channels in the United States undetected in the late 1990s, which resulted in significant adverse reactions.

Description

Plantain herb consists of the fresh or dried aboveground parts of *Plantago lanceolata* L. or *P. major* L. [Fam. Plantaginaceae], harvested at flowering season, and their preparations in effective dosage. Plantain contains mucilage, iridoid glycosides such as aucubin and catalpol, and tannin.

Chemistry and Pharmacology

Plantain herb contains 2–6.5% mucilage composed of polysaccharides; 6.5% tannins; iridoid glycosides, including 0.3–2.5% aucubin and 0.3–1.1% catalpol; over 1% silicic acid; phenolic carboxylic acids (protocatechuic acid); flavonoids (apigenin, luteolin); and minerals, including significant zinc and potassium (Hänsel et al., 1992–1994; Meyer-Buchtela, 1999; Wichtl and Bisset, 1994).

The Commission E reported astringent and antibacterial activity.

In vitro bacteriostatic and bactericidal activity have been shown for the cold aqueous extract and attributed to the aglycone, aucubigenin (Wichtl and Bisset, 1994). The bacteriostatic and bactericidal actions are, however, destroyed by heat, so the cold macerate form is used as a rinse, gargle, and/or cataplasm for antibacterial action (Meyer-Buchtela, 1999; Wichtl and Bisset, 1994). Experimental research using isolates of *P. lanceolata* has shown an inhibitory effect on mouse ear edema (Murai et al., 1995).

In laboratory tests, plantain reduced plasma lipid, cholesterol, β-lipoprotein, and triglyceride concentrations in rabbits with atherosclerosis; it also increased isolated guinea pig and rabbit uterine smooth muscle tone (Maksyutina et al., 1978). The iridoid glycoside aucubin has stimulated laxative actions in mice, and has also demonstrated protective effects on liver cells (Inouye et al., 1974). The effectiveness of plantain's actions is due to its mucilage and iridoid glycoside content. Plantain contains mucilage, which produces demulcent and emollient actions. The iridoid glycosides, aucubin and catalpol, show antibacterial activity when isolated from fresh plants (Tyler, 1994; Newall et al., 1996).

Uses

The Commission E approved the internal use of plantain for catarrhs of the respiratory tract and inflammatory alterations of the oral and pharyngeal mucosa. It's external application is approved for inflammatory reactions of the skin.

The German Standard License indications for use are identical to those in the Commission E monograph (Braun et al., 1997). Plantain tea is indicated for phlegm congestion (Schulz et al., 1998). Human studies have found positive results in the treatment of chronic bronchitis of a spastic or non-spastic nature with plantain (Koichev, 1983; Matev et al., 1982).

Contraindications

None known.

Side Effects

None known.

Use During Pregnancy and Lactation

No restrictions known.

Interactions with Other Drugs

None known.

Dosage and Administration

Unless otherwise prescribed: 3–6 g per day of cut herb and other galenical

preparations for internal and external use.
[Note: According to the *Pharmacopeia of Austria*, the average single dose is 1.5 g dried herb per cup of tea infusion (Meyer-Buchtela, 1999; ÖAB, 1991).]
Internal: Infusion: Steep 1.4 g of herb in 150 ml boiled water for 10 to 15 minutes, three to four times daily (Braun et al., 1997; Meyer-Buchtela, 1999).
Fluidextract 1:1 (g/ml): 1.4 ml, three to four times daily; 2–4 ml, three times daily (BHP, 1983).
Tincture 1:5 (g/ml): 7 ml, three to four times daily.
External: Cold macerate: For use as a rinse, gargle or cataplasm: Soak 1.4 g cut herb in 150 ml cold water for 1 to 2 hours, stirring often (Braun et al., 1997; Meyer-Buchtela, 1999).
Cataplasm: Prepare using the cold macerate and apply to affected area (Braun et al. 1997).
Rinse or gargle: Soak 1.4 g cut herb in 150 ml cold water for 1 to 2 hours, stirring often, three to four times daily (Braun et al., 1997; Meyer-Buchtela, 1999).

References

BAnz. See *Bundesanzeiger*.
Braun, R. et al. 1997. *Standardzulassungen für Fertigarzneimittel—Text and Kommentar*. Stuttgart: Deutscher Apotheker Verlag.
British Herbal Pharmacopoeia (BHP). 1983. Keighley, U.K.: British Herbal Medicine Association.
Bundesanzeiger (BAnz). 1998. Monographien der Kommission E (Zulassungs- und Aufbereitungskommission am BGA für den humanmed. Bereich, phytotherapeutische Therapierichtung und Stoffgruppe). Köln: Bundesgesundheitsamt (BGA).
Der Marderosian, A. (ed.). 1999. *The Review of Natural Products*. St. Louis: Facts and Comparisons.
Deutsches Arzneibuch, 10th ed. (DAB 10). 1991. (With subsequent supplements through 1996.) Stuttgart: Deutscher Apotheker Verlag.
Doan, D.D. et al. 1992. Studies on the individual and combined diuretic effects of four Vietnamese traditional herbal remedies *(Zea mays, Imperata cylindrica, Plantago major and Orthosiphon stamineus)*. *J Ethnopharmacol* 36(3):225–231.
Grieve, M. 1979. *A Modern Herbal*. New York: Dover Publications, Inc.
Hänsel, R., K. Keller, H. Rimpler, G. Schneider (eds.). 1992–1994. *Hagers Handbuch der Pharmazeutischen Praxis*, 5th ed. Vol. 4–6. Berlin-Heidelberg: Springer Verlag.
Inouye, H. et al. 1974. Purgative activities of iridoid glycosides. *Planta Med* 25:285–288.
Koichev, A. 1982. Study on the therapeutic effect of different doses from the preparation *Plantago major* in cold. *Probl Vatr Med* 10:117–124.
Koichev, A. et al. 1983. Pharmacologic-clinical study of a preparation from *Plantago major*. *Probl Pneumos Ftiziatr* 11:68–74.
Koichev, A. 1983. Complex evaluation of the therapeutic effect of a preparation from *Plantago major* in chronic bronchitis. *Probl Vatr Med* 11:61–69.
Lange, D. and U. Schippmann. 1997. *Trade Survey of Medicinal Plants in Germany—A Contribution to International Plant Species Conservation*. Bonn: Bundesamt für Naturschutz. 29–35.
Maksyutina, N.P. et al. 1978. Chemical composition and hypocholesterolemia action of some drugs from *Plantago major* leaves. Part I. Polyphenolic compounds. *Farm Zh (Kiev)* 4.
Matev, M., I. Angelova, A. Koichev, M. Leseva, G. Stefanov. 1982. [Clinical trial of *Plantago major* preparation in the treatment of chronic bronchitis] [In Bulgarian]. *Vutr Boles* 21(2):133–137.
Meyer-Buchtela, E. 1999. *Tee-Rezepturen—Ein Handbuch für Apotheker und Ärzte*. Stuttgart: Deutscher Apotheker Verlag.
Murai, M., Y. Tamayama, S. Nishibe. 1995. Phenylethanoids in the herb of *Plantago lanceolata* and inhibitory effect of arachidonic acid-induced mouse ear edema. *Planta Med* 61(5):479–480.
Nadkarni, K.M. 1976. *Indian Materia Medica*. Bombay: Popular Prakashan. 986–987.
Newall, C.A., L.A. Anderson, J.D. Phillipson. 1996. *Herbal Medicines: A Guide for Health-Care Professionals*. London: The Pharmaceutical Press.
Österreichisches Arzneibuch, 1st and 2nd suppl. (ÖAB). 1991. Wien: Verlag der Österreichischen Staatsdruckerei.
Pharmacopoeia Helvetica, 7th ed. Vol. 1–4. (Ph.Helv.VII). 1987. Bern: Office Central Fédéral des Imprimés et du Matériel.
Schulz, V., R. Hänsel, V.E. Tyler. 1998. *Rational Phytotherapy: A Physicians' Guide to Herbal Medicine*. New York: Springer.
Tyler, V.E. 1994. *Herbs of Choice: The Therapeutic Use of Phytomedicinals*. New York: Pharmaceutical Products Press.
Wichtl, M. and N.G. Bisset (eds.). 1994. *Herbal Drugs and Phytopharmaceuticals*. Stuttgart: Medpharm Scientific Publishers.

Additional Resources

Baldo, B.A., Q.J. Chensee, M.E. Howden, P.J. Sharp. 1982. Allergens from plantain (*Plantago lanceolata*). Studies with pollen and plant extracts. *Int Arch Allergy Appl Immunol* 68(4):295–304.

Bruneton, J. 1995. *Pharmacognosy, Phytochemistry, Medicinal Plants.* Paris: Lavoisier Publishing.

Chakarski, I. et al. 1982. Clinical study of a herb combination consisting of *Agrimonia eupatoria, Hypericum perforatum, Plantago major, Mentha piperita, Matricaria chamomilla* for the treatment of patients with gastroduodenitis. *Probl Vatr Med* 10:78–84.

Deutsches Arzneibuch, 10th ed. Vol. 1–6. (DAB 10). 1991. Kommentar. Stuttgart: Wissenschaftliche Verlagsgesellschaft.

Granel, C. et al. 1993. Plantain allergy (*Plantago lanceolata*): assessment of diagnostic tests. Allergol Immunopathol (Madr) 21(4):158–160.

Razina, T.G. and E.P. Zueva. 1992. [The effect of a plantain preparation on the efficacy of the irradiation of experimental animals with tumors] [In Russian]. *Radiobiologiia* 32(2):266–270.

Wren, R.C. 1988. *Potter's New Cyclopaedia of Botanical Drugs and Preparations.* Essex: The C.W. Daniel Company Ltd.

This material was adapted from *The Complete German Commission E Monographs—Therapeutic Guide to Herbal Medicines.* M. Blumenthal, W.R. Busse, A. Goldberg, J. Gruenwald, T. Hall, C.W. Riggins, R.S. Rister (eds.) S. Klein and R.S. Rister (trans.). 1998. Austin: American Botanical Council; Boston: Integrative Medicine Communications.

1) The Overview section is new information.

2) Description, Chemistry and Pharmacology, Uses, Contraindications, Side Effects, Interactions with Other Drugs, and Dosage sections have been drawn from the original work. Additional information has been added in some or all of these sections, as noted with references.

3) The dosage for equivalent preparations (tea infusion, fluidextract, and tincture) have been provided based on the following example:
    Unless otherwise prescribed: 2 g per day of [powdered, crushed, cut or whole] [plant part]
    Infusion: 2 g in 150 ml of water
    Fluidextract 1:1 (g/ml): 2 ml
    Tincture 1:5 (g/ml): 10 ml

4) The References and Additional Resources sections are new sections. Additional Resources are not cited in the monograph but are included for research purposes.

POPLAR BUD

Latin Name:
Populus species

Pharmacopeial Name:
Populi gemma

Other Names:
balm of Gilead, balm of Mecca,
tacamahac

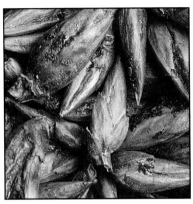

©1999 Steven Foster

Overview

About 35 species of poplar grow throughout North America, and many are used interchangeably to produce crude drugs and extracts (Hutchens, 1991). Although poplar bark is frequently harvested for medicinal preparation, the buds, which are also called balm of Gilead buds, contain a therapeutically active exudate that is approved by Commission E for the topical treatment of skin injury, hemorrhoids, frostbite, and sunburn. Buds from *Populus nigra, P. canadensis,* and *P. tacamahaca* are used therapeutically (Bradley, 1992).

Despite the lack of clinical studies on the efficacy of bud preparations, poplar buds have shown antibacterial and analgesic action and are used in treating upper respiratory infections. Poplar buds are also used as a gargle for laryngitis (Bradley, 1992; Leung and Foster, 1996). The volatile oil has demonstrated expectorant properties (Bradley, 1992).

Native American medicine includes the use of both the buds and the salicylate-rich bark to treat headaches, wounds, and as an astringent for skin conditions (Hutchens, 1991; Moerman, 1998).

Description

Poplar buds consist of the dried, unopened leaf buds of *Populus* species [Fam. Salicaceae] and their preparations in effective dosage. The herb contains essential oil, flavonoids, and phenol glycosides.

Chemistry and Pharmacology

Constituents include the volatile oils *d*-cadinene, cineole, AR-curcumene, bis-abolene, farnesene, D-α-bisabolol, β-phenethyl alcohol, acetophenone, and humulene; flavonoids (flavones: chrysin, tectochrysin, apigenin, and genkwanin; flavonols: galangin, izalpinin, quercetin, kaempferol, and several methylated derivatives; flavonones: pinocembrin and pinos-trobin, 2',6'-dihydroxy-4'-meth-oxychal-cone); and phenolic esters of two types:

esters of caffeic acid and esters of isoferulic acid (Bradley, 1992; Leung and Foster, 1996). Other constituents include the glycosides salicin, salicortin, salireposide, and benzoate derivatives, including populin, temuloidin, and tremulacin; resins, *n*-alkanes, phenolic acids, chalcones, fatty acids, and aliphatic alcohols (Bradley, 1992; Leung and Foster, 1996).

The Commission E reported antibacterial activity and stimulation of wound healing. The antibacterial acitivity is thought to be due mainly to the caffeates, and the expectorant action is attributed to the volatile oils. It has also demonstrated expectorant, antiseptic, and anti-inflammatory properties (Bradley, 1992).

Preliminary investigations into the chemical differences between species and between the buds and the bark indicate that specific constituents and levels of concentration vary enough to effect therapeutic activity. Exploration of the pharmacological actions of *P. nigra* buds indicate antibacterial, anti-fungal, anti-inflammatory, and capillary activity of the constituents (Bradley, 1992). Caffeic acids in particular are notably antibacterial (Bankova, 1990). Salycilate glycosides have been isolated from *P. tacamahaca* buds. The acetyl derivative of salicylic acid is synthesized into aspirin; these particular glycosides are analgesic and anti-inflammatory. They also occur in all preparations of poplar bark (Schulz et al., 1998; Harborne and Baxter, 1993).

Uses

The Commission E approved poplar bud for superficial skin injuries, external hemorrhoids, frostbite, and sunburn. External preparations also soothe and heal other skin conditions and injuries (sores, bruises, cuts, and pimples), and gargling with preparations from poplar bud has been shown to relieve laryngitis (Bradley, 1992; Leung and Foster, 1996).

Contraindications

Sensitivity to poplar buds, propolis, Peruvian balsam, or salicylate.

Side Effects

Occasional allergic skin reactions.

Use During Pregnancy and Lactation

No restrictions known.

Interactions with Other Drugs

None known.

Dosage and Administration

Unless otherwise prescribed: Topical application of semi-solid preparations containing 20–30% of bud exudate. Ointment: Semi-solid preparation containing 20–30% of bud exudate for external application to the skin.

References

Bankova, V.S. 1990. Synthesis of natural esters of substituted cinnamic acids. *J Nat Prod* 53: 821–824.

Bradley, P.R. (ed.). 1992. *British Herbal Compendium*, Vol. 1. Bournemouth: British Herbal Medicine Association.

Harborne, J. and H. Baxter. 1993. *Phytochemical Dictionary: A Handbook of Bioactive Compounds from Plants*. Washington: Taylor & Francis.

Hutchens, A. 1991. *Indian Herbology of North America*. Boston: Shambala.

Leung, A.Y. and S. Foster. 1996. *Encyclopedia of Common Natural Ingredients Used in Food, Drugs, and Cosmetics*, 2nd ed. New York: John Wiley & Sons, Inc.

Moerman, D.E. 1998. *Native American Ethnobotany*. Portland, OR: Timber Press.

Schulz, V., R. Hänsel, V.E. Tyler. 1998. *Rational Phytotherapy: A Physicians' Guide to Herbal Medicine*. New York: Springer.

This material was adapted from *The Complete German Commission E Monographs—Therapeutic Guide to Herbal Medicines*. M. Blumenthal, W.R. Busse, A. Goldberg, J. Gruenwald, T. Hall, C.W. Riggins, R.S. Rister (eds.) S. Klein and R.S. Rister (trans.). 1998. Austin: American Botanical Council; Boston: Integrative Medicine Communications.

1) The Overview section is new information.

2) Description, Chemistry and Pharmacology, Uses, Contraindications, Side Effects, Interactions with Other Drugs, and Dosage sections have been drawn from the original work. Additional information has been added in some or all of these sections, as noted with references.

3) The dosage for equivalent preparations (tea infusion, fluidextract, and tincture) have been provided based on the following example:
Unless otherwise prescribed: 2 g per day of [powdered, crushed, cut or whole] [plant part]
Infusion: 2 g in 150 ml of water
Fluidextract 1:1 (g/ml): 2 ml
Tincture 1:5 (g/ml): 10 ml

4) The References and Additional Resources sections are new sections. Additional Resources are not cited in the monograph but are included for research purposes.

Additional Resources

British Herbal Pharmacopoeia (BHP). 1983. Keighley, U.K.: British Herbal Medicine Association.
———. 1990. Bournemouth, U.K.: British Herbal Medicine Association.
Goodman, L.S. and A. Gilman (eds.). 1985. *The Pharmacological Basis of Therapeutics*, 7th ed. New York: MacMillan.
List, P.H. and L. Hörhammer (eds.). 1973–1979. *Hagers Handbuch der Pharmazeutischen Praxis*, Vols. 1–7. New York: Springer Verlag.
Mills, S.Y. 1985. *The Dictionary of Modern Herbalism*. Wellingborough: Thorsons.

Papay, V. et al. 1986. Isolated compounds from Hungarian propolis and *Populi gemma. Studies in Organic Chemistry* (23):233–240.
Reynolds, J.E.F. (ed.). 1989. *Martindale: The Extra Pharmacopoeia,* 29th ed. London: The Pharmaceutical Press.
Wren, R.C. 1988. *Potter's New Cyclopaedia of Botanical Drugs and Preparations*. Essex: The C.W. Daniel Company Ltd.

PSYLLIUM SEED:

PSYLLIUM SEED, BLACK
(page 316)

PSYLLIUM SEED, BLONDE
(page 317)

PSYLLIUM SEED HUSK, BLONDE
(page 318)

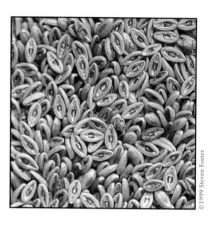

©1999 Steven Foster

Overview

Blonde psyllium (*Plantago ovata*) is a low herbaceous annual plant native to Iran and India, extensively cultivated there and in other countries, including Pakistan (Kapoor, 1990; Karnick, 1994; Nadkarni, 1976; Wichtl and Bisset, 1994). Black psyllium of the *P. afra* species is native to the western Mediterranean region, northern Africa, and western Asia, now cultivated in southern France and Spain. Black psyllium of the *P. indica* species is native to southeastern Europe and Asia Minor (Braun et al., 1997; Budavari, 1996; Leung and Foster, 1996). In commerce, blonde psyllium is obtained mainly from India, Pakistan, and Iran. Black psyllium is obtained mainly from southern France (BHP, 1996; Wichtl and Bisset, 1994).

Psyllium has a long history of medical use in both conventional and traditional systems of medicine throughout Asia, Europe, and North America. Blonde psyllium is official in the national pharmacopeias of France, Germany, Great Britain, and the United States (BP, 1988; Bradley, 1992; DAC, 1986; DAB, 1997; Newall et al., 1996; Ph.Fr.X, 1990; USP XXII, 1990–1992; Wichtl and Bisset, 1994). Psyllium monographs also appear in the *Ayurvedic Pharmacopoeia, British Herbal Pharmacopoeia, British Herbal Compendium*, ESCOP Monographs, Commission E Monographs, and the German Standard License Monographs (BAnz, 1998; BHP, 1996; Bradley, 1992; Braun et al., 1997; ESCOP, 1997; Karnick, 1994). The World Health Organization (WHO) has published a monograph on psyllium seed covering *P. afra, P. indica, P. ovata,* and *P. asiatica* (WHO, 1999). Asian psyllium seed (*P. asiatica* Linné or *P. depressa* Willd.) is official in the national pharmacopeias of China and Japan (JP XII, 1993; Tu, 1992; Yen, 1992).

In Germany, psyllium is official in the *German Pharmacopoeia* and approved in both the German Standard License and Commission E Monographs (BAnz, 1998; Braun et al., 1997; DAB 10, 1993; DAB, 1997; Wichtl and Bisset, 1994). It is used in laxatives by itself (e.g., Agiocur®-Granulat, Abführ Herbagran® Granulat-Psyllium) and in combination with senna fruit extract (e.g., Agiolax®-Granulat, Kneipplax®N) (Kneipp®, 1996; Schilcher, 1997; Wichtl and Bisset, 1994). In the United States, psyllium is used as a bulk laxative OTC drug (e.g., Metamucil®) to treat chronic constipation. The ground seeds or husks are used in dietary supplements for increased fiber, cholesterol reduction, and laxative activity (Leung and Foster, 1996; Wichtl and Bisset, 1994). In 1998, the FDA amended its soluble fiber health claim regulation to include blonde psyllium husk as a source. Psyllium products of which a single dose or serving contains at least 1.7 grams of soluble fiber can be labeled, "Consumption of the product in association with a diet low in saturated fats and cholesterol may [or might] reduce the risk of coronary heart disease" (Levy, 1998; Tips, 1998).

Modern human studies have investigated psyllium for treating irritable bowel syndrome and chronic constipation (Hotz and Plein, 1994; Tomas-Ridocci et al., 1992), maintaining remission in ulcerative colitis (Fernandez-Banares et al., 1997, 1999), its effects on serum levels of bile acids in patients with juvenile ulcerative colitis (Ejderhamm and Strandvik, 1991), hypercholesterolemia (Kwiterovich, 1995; Schectman et al., 1993; Sprecher et al., 1993; Williams et al., 1995), and its effects in the prevention of gallstones in obese patients on a reducing diet (Moran et al., 1997).

In a randomized double-blind placebo study, the effect of *P. ovata* (PO) on 20 patients with chronic constipation (CC), 10 of whom had associated irritable bowel syndrome (IBS), was investigated. Weight of feces and intestinal transit time were measured with radiopaque markers (relative impenetrability of X-rays) at the start and after 30 days of treatment. All patients treated with PO reported good results. Frequency of stools increased from 2.5 ± 1 to 8 ± 2.2 stools per week. A decrease in consistency of stools was also observed in the treated group. Fecal weight and colonic transit time were not significantly modified in the placebo group, while weight increase as well as decreased transit time were observed in the treated group. No adverse effects were observed; in particular, no flatulence, as is often seen in patients ingesting bran (Tomas-Ridocci et al., 1992).

In an open study, the effectiveness of psyllium seed husks in comparison with wheat bran on stool frequency and manifestations of irritable bowel syndrome (IBS) with constipation was investigated in 30 patients suffering from IBS group II to III. Patients received either 3.25 g psyllium seeds or 7 g wheat bran three times daily. The study comprised two treatment phases of two weeks each, separated by two weeks without any treatment, the study lasting six weeks in all. Parameters for evaluation included stool frequency and consistency as well as symptoms of pain and abdominal distention, measured by a score (1 to 4). In both treatment groups stool frequency and consistency improved by comparison to the starting point. The improvement of stool frequency was statistically significant for both substances. However, the beneficial effects of psyllium seed exceeded those of wheat bran in weeks one, two, three, five, and six. The authors concluded that psyllium seed and wheat bran are both effective for stool frequency and consistency of patients with IBS. Psyllium seeds proved to be superior to wheat bran with respect to stool frequency and abdominal distention and therefore should be preferred in treatment of IBS and constipation (Hotz and Plein, 1994).

The approved modern therapeutic applications for psyllium are supportable based on its history of use in well established systems of traditional and conventional medicines, pharmacological studies in animals, phytochemical investigations, and human clinical studies.

German pharmacopeial grade blonde psyllium seed consists of the dried ripe seed of *P. ovata* Forssk. (syn. *P. ispaghula* Roxb.) The unmilled seed must have a swelling index of at least 9. Botanical identity must be confirmed by macroscopic and microscopic examinations as well as organoleptic evaluation (DAB, 1997; Wichtl and Bisset, 1994). The *British Herbal Pharmacopoeia* requires an additional identification test by thin-layer chromatography (TLC), although the monograph states that macroscopic examination must be used to differentiate between blonde psyllium and black psyllium seed (BHP, 1996). The ESCOP psyllium monograph requires that the material comply with the German and French pharmacopeias (ESCOP, 1997).

German pharmacopeial grade black psyllium seed consists of the dried ripe whole seed of *P. afra* L. ("*P. psyllium*") or *P. indica* L. (syn. *P. arenaria* Waldstein et Kitaibel). The whole seed must have a swelling index of at least 10, contain not more than 1% foreign matter, including any green unripe seeds and/or seeds from other species of *Plantago* (e.g., *P. lanceolata* L., *P. major* L., *P. ovata* Forssk., and *P.*

sempervirens Crantz). Botanical identity must be confirmed by macroscopic examination and organoleptic evaluation (DAB 10, 1993).

PSYLLIUM SEED, BLACK

Latin Name:
Plantago psyllium

Pharmacopeial Name:
Psyllii semen

Other Names:
French psyllium

Description
Black psyllium seed consists of the dried, ripe seed of *Plantago psyllium* (syn. *P. afra* L.) and of *P. indica* L. (syn. *P. arenaria* Waldstein et Kitaibel) [Fam. Plantaginaceae] with a swelling index of at least 10, and its formulations in effective dosage. The preparation contains mucilage.

Chemistry and Pharmacology
Constituents of the seeds include 5–10% lipids with unsaturated fatty acids, sterols, and mucilaginous polysaccharide (10–15%) consisting of xylose, galacturonic acid, arabinose, and rhamnose residues (Bruneton, 1995; ESCOP, 1997). The seeds contain 15–20% protein, 5–13% fixed oil, trisaccharide planteose, and small amounts of phytosterols, triterpenes, the iridoid glucoside aucubin, and the alkaloids plantagonine, indicaine, and indicamine (ESCOP, 1997).

The Commission E reported that black psyllium seed regulates intestinal peristalsis. Psyllium seed also lowers blood cholesterol levels and LDL cholesterol in hypercholesterolemic subjects without significant changes in triglycerides and HDL cholesterol. It is also believed that the seed reduces peak levels of blood glucose by delaying intestinal absorption of sugar (ESCOP, 1997).

Uses
The Commission E approved black psyllium seed for chronic constipation and irritable bowel syndrome. It is recommended where soft stool is desired, for example, in cases of anal fissures, hemorrhoids, and post-rectal surgery.

WHO found these uses (noted above) supported by clinical data. WHO added restoration and maintenance of regularity, temporary constipation due to illness or pregnancy, and constipation due to duodenal ulcer or diverticulitis (WHO, 1999).

Contraindications
Stenosis of the esophagus or the gastrointestinal tract.

Side Effects
In rare cases allergic reactions, especially with powdered or liquid preparations.

Use During Pregnancy and Lactation
No restrictions known.

Interactions with Other Drugs
None known.

Dosage and Administration

Unless otherwise prescribed: 10–30 g per day of whole or ground seeds, other galenical preparations for oral application.

Seed: 5–10 g of seed, two to three times daily. Presoak seeds in 100–150 ml of warm water for several hours. Follow each dose by drinking at least another 200 ml of water. WHO recommends an average dose of 7.5 g dissolved in 240 ml water or juice, one to three times daily. Children 6–12 years should take one-half the adult dose (Braun et al., 1997; ESCOP, 1997; Karnick, 1994; WHO, 1999).

PSYLLIUM SEED, BLONDE

Latin Name:
Plantago ovata

Pharmacopeial Name:
Plantaginis ovatae semen

Other Names:
Indian plantago, Ispagol, pale psyllium, Spogel, Ispaghul

Description

Psyllium, consisting of the ripe seeds of *Plantago ovata* Forsskaol (syn. *P. isphagula* Roxburgh) [Fam. Plantaginaceae] and its pharmaceutical preparations. The preparation contains bulking agents.

Chemistry and Pharmacology

Constituents include mucilage, proteins, and lipids (Bruneton, 1995). The mucilage level can reach up to 30%, and is chiefly a soluble polysaccharide fraction dominated by D-xylose (Bruneton, 1995). Other constituents include aucubin, an iridoid glucoside; fructose, glucose, and sucrose; planteose, a trisaccharide; campesterol, β-sitosterol, and stigmasterol; α- and β-amyrin triterpenes; linoleic, oleic, palmitic, steric, and other fatty acids; and tannins (Bradley, 1992; Newall et al., 1996).

The Commission E reported an increase in the passage time of the bowel content in cases of diarrhea. In cases of constipation, blonde psyllium seed decreases passage time of the bowel content through increase in the volume of the stool. Commission E also noted that blonde psyllium seed lowers serum-cholesterol levels. It has been shown to slow sugar absorption, thereby reducing blood glucose (ESCOP, 1997).

Uses

The Commission E approved the use of blonde psyllium seed for chronic constipation and disorders in which easy bowel movements with a loose stool are desirable, e.g., for patients with anal fissures, hemorrhoids, following anal/rectal surgery, or during pregnancy. It was also approved as a secondary medication in the treatment of varying kinds of diarrhea and in the treatment of irritable bowel syndrome.

WHO added to these uses the following: restoration and maintenance of regularity, and constipation due to duodenal ulcer or diverticulitis (WHO, 1999).

Contraindications

Stenosis of the gastrointestinal tract. Obstruction or threatening obstruction of the bowel. Difficulties in regulating diabetes mellitus.

Side Effects

In rare cases, allergic reactions may occur.

Use During Pregnancy and Lactation

No restrictions known.

Interactions with Other Drugs

The intestinal absorption of other medication taken simultaneously may be delayed.

Warning: Diabetics who are insulin-dependent may need to reduce their insulin dosage while using psyllium seeds.

Dosage and Administration

Unless otherwise prescribed: 12–40 g per day of whole seeds or equivalent preparations, to be taken orally.

Seed: 5–10 g, three to four times daily. Presoak seeds in 100–150 ml of warm water for several hours. Follow each dose by drinking at least another 200 ml of water.

Note: Sufficient fluids must be taken with the preparation, e.g., 150 ml water to 5 g preparation. The dose should be taken a half hour to one hour after taking other medication.

Warning: Commission E (and other authorities) require the following warning: If diarrhea lasts for more than three to four days, consult a physician (Braun et al., 1997; ESCOP, 1997; Karnick, 1994; Newall et al., 1996; Wichtl and Bisset, 1994; WHO, 1999).

PSYLLIUM SEED HUSK, BLONDE

Latin Name:
Plantago ovata

Pharmacopeial Name:
Plantaginis ovatae testa

Other Names:
n/a

Description

Psyllium, consisting of the epidermis with bordering collapsed layers of *Plantago ovata* Forsskaol (syn. *P. isphagula* Roxburgh) [Fam. Plantaginaceae] and its pharmaceutical preparations. The preparation contains bulking agents.

Chemistry and Pharmacology

Constituents include a mucilaginous polysaccharide, consisting of a highly branched, acidic arabinoxylan with a xylan backbone and branches of arabinose, xylose, and 2-O-(galacturonic acid)-rhamnose residues, about 2.5% fixed oil, linoleic, leic, and palmitic acids. Other constituents include aliphatic hydrocarbons and starch (Bradley, 1992).

The Commission E reported an increase in passage time of the bowel content in cases of diarrhea. In cases of constipation, psyllium seed husk causes a decrease in passage time of the bowel content through increase in the volume of the stool. Commission E also reported that psyllium lowered the serum cholesterol level and reduced the postprandial (after eating) blood sugar increase.

Uses

The Commission E approved blonde psyllium seed husk for chronic constipation; disorders whereby easy bowel movements with a loose stool are desirable, e.g., in patients with anal fissures, hemorrhoids, following anal/rectal surgery, during pregnancy, as a secondary medication for varying kinds of diarrhea, and in the treatment of irritable bowel syndrome. WHO added to these uses the following: restoration and maintenance of regularity, and constipation due to duodenal ulcer or diverticulitis (WHO, 1999). In a clinical study 26 patients with mild to moderate hypercholesterolemia were given 102 g per day for eight weeks. Psyllium reduced the total cholesterol by 15% and decreased LDL cholesterol by 20% (Anderson et al., 1988). Another study found psyllium lowered total cholesterol by an additional 5% and LDL cholesterol by an additional 8% in 75 patients receiving a low-fat diet (Bell et al., 1989).

Contraindications

Stenosis of the gastrointestinal tract. Obstruction or threatening obstruction of the bowel. Poorly controlled diabetes mellitus.

Side Effects

In rare cases, allergic reactions may occur.

Use During Pregnancy and Lactation

No restrictions known.

Interactions with Other Drugs

The intestinal absorption of other medication taken simultaneously may be delayed.

Warning: Insulin dosage may need to be reduced for diabetics who are insulin-dependent.

Dosage and Administration

Unless otherwise prescribed: 4–20 g per day of whole seed husk as well as other galenical preparations to be taken orally. Husk: 4–5 g, one to four times daily. Presoak the husk in 150 ml of warm water for several hours.

Powdered Husk: 4–5 g, one to four times daily. Stir into 150 ml water and drink immediately, followed by additional water.

Note: Sufficient fluids must be taken with the preparation, e.g., 150 ml water to 5 g preparation. The dose should be taken a half hour to one hour after taking other medication.

Warning: Commission E (and other authorities) require the following warning: If diarrhea lasts for more than three to four days, consult a physician (ESCOP, 1996; Newall et al., 1996; Reynolds, 1993).

References

Anderson, J.W. et al. 1988. Cholesterol-lowering effects of psyllium hydrophilic mucilloid for hypercholesterolemic men. *Arch Intern Med* 148(2):292–296.

BAnz. See *Bundesanzeiger.*

Bell, L.P., K. Hectorne, H. Reynolds, T.K. Balm, D.B. Hunninghake. 1989. Cholesterol-lowering effects of psyllium hydrophilic mucilloid. Adjunct therapy to a prudent diet for patients with mild to moderate hypercholesterolemia. *JAMA* 261(23):3419–3423.

Bradley, P.R. (ed.). 1992. *British Herbal Compendium*, Vol. 1. Bournemouth: British Herbal Medicine Association.

Braun, R. et al. 1997. *Standardzulassungen für Fertigarzneimittel—Text and Kommentar.* Stuttgart: Deutscher Apotheker Verlag.

British Herbal Pharmacopoeia (BHP). 1996. Exeter, U.K.: British Herbal Medicine Association. 114–115.

British Pharmacopoeia (BP). 1988. (With subsequent Addenda up to 1992.) London: Her Majesty's Stationery Office.

Bruneton, J. 1995. *Pharmacognosy, Phytochemistry, Medicinal Plants.* Paris: Lavoisier Publishing.

Budavari, S. (ed.). 1996. *The Merck Index: An Encyclopedia of Chemicals, Drugs, and Biologicals*, 12th ed. Whitehouse Station, N.J.: Merck & Co, Inc.

Bundesanzeiger (BAnz). 1998. Monographien der Kommission E (Zulassungs- und Aufbereitungskommission am BGA für den humanmed. Bereich, phytotherapeutische Therapierichtung und Stoffgruppe). Köln: Bundesgesundheitsamt (BGA).

Dennison, B.A. and D.M. Levine. 1993. Randomized, double-blind, placebo-controlled, two-period crossover clinical trial of psyllium fiber in children with hypercholesterolemia. *J Pediatr* 123(1):24–29.

Deutsches Arzneibuch, 10th ed., 2nd suppl. (DAB 10). 1993. Stuttgart: Deutscher Apotheker Verlag.

Deutsches Arzneibuch (DAB 1997). 1997. Stuttgart: Deutscher Apotheker Verlag.

Deutscher Arzneimittel-Codex (DAC). 1986. Stuttgart: Deutscher Apotheker Verlag.

Ejderhamm, J. and B. Strandvik. 1991. Serum bile acids in relation to disease activity and intake of dietary fibers in juvenile ulcerative colitis. *Digestion* 50(3–4):162–169.

ESCOP. 1997. "Psyllii semen," "Plantaginis ovatae semen," and "Plantaginis ovatae testa." *Monographs on the Medicinal Uses of Plant Drugs.* Exeter, U.K.: European Scientific Cooperative on Phytotherapy.

Fernandez-Banares, F. et al. 1997. Randomized clinical trial of *Plantago ovata* efficacy as compared to mesalazine in maintaining remission in ulcerative colitis. *Gastroenterology* 112:A971.

Fernandez-Banares, F. et al. 1999. Randomized clinical trial of *Plantago ovata* seeds (dietary fiber) as compared with mesalamine in maintaining remission in ulcerative colitis—Spanish Group for the Study of Crohn's Disease and Ulcerative Colitis (GETECCU). *Am J Gastroenterol* 94(2):427–433.

Hotz, J. and K. Plein. 1994. Wirkung von plantago-samenschalen in vergleich zu weizenkleie auf stuhlfrequenz und beschwerden beim colon-irritabile-syndrom mit obstipation [Effectiveness of plantago seed husks in comparison with wheat brain on stool frequency and manifestations of irritable colon syndrome with constipation]. *Med Klin* 89(12):645–651.

Japanese Pharmacopoeia, 12th ed. (JP XII). 1993. Tokyo: Government of Japan Ministry of Health and Welfare—Yakuji Nippo, Ltd. 214.

Kapoor, L.D. 1990. *Handbook of Ayurvedic Medicinal Plants.* Boca Raton: CRC Press. 267.

Karnick, C.R. 1994. *Pharmacopoeial Standards of Herbal Plants,* Vol. 1. Delhi: Sri Satguru Publications. 273–276.

Kneipp®. 1996. *Wegweiser zu den Kneipp® Mitteln* [*Guide to Kneipp® Remedies*]. Würzburg: Sebastian Kneipp Gesundheitsmittel Verlag. 70–75.

Kwiterovich, P.O. Jr. 1995. The role of fiber in the treatment of hypercholesterolemia in children and adolescents. *Pediatrics* 96(5 Pt 2):1005–1009.

Leung, A.Y. and S. Foster. 1996. *Encyclopedia of Common Natural Ingredients Used in Food, Drugs, and Cosmetics*, 2nd ed. New York: John Wiley & Sons, Inc.

Levy, B. 1998. New FDA Regulations on Antioxidants and Psyllium Seed. *HerbClip 060388.* Austin, TX: American Botanical Council.

Moran, S. et al. 1997. Efecto de la administracion de fibra en la prevencion de litiasis vesicular en obesos sometidos a dieta de reduccion. Ensayo [Effects of fiber administration in the prevention of gallstones in obese patients on a reducing diet. A clinical trial]. *Rev Gastroenterol Mex* 62(4):266–272.

Nadkarni, K.M. 1976. *Indian Materia Medica.* Bombay: Popular Prakashan. 960–967.

Newall, C.A., L.A. Anderson, J.D. Phillipson. 1996. *Herbal Medicines: A Guide for Health-Care Professionals.* London: The Pharmaceutical Press.

Pharmacopée Française Xe Édition (Ph.Fr.X). 1983–1990. Moulins-les-Metz: Maisonneuve S.A.

Reynolds, J.E.F. (ed.). 1993. *Martindale: The Extra Pharmacopoeia,* 30th ed. London: The Pharmaceutical Press.

Schectman, G., J. Hiatt, A. Hartz. 1993. Evaluation of the effectiveness of lipid-lowering therapy (bile acid sequestrants, niacin, psyllium and lovastatin) for treating hypercholesterolemia in veterans. *Am J Cardiol* 71(10):759–765.

Schilcher, H. 1997. *Phytotherapy in Paediatrics: Handbook for Physicians and Pharmacists.* Stuttgart: Medpharm Scientific Publishers. 52–53.

Sprecher, D.L. et al. 1993. Efficacy of psyllium in reducing serum cholesterol levels in hypercholesterolemic patients on high- or low-fat diets. *Ann Intern Med* 119(7 pt. 1):545–554. Comment on: 627–628.

Tips, S. 1998. How Changes in FDA Regulations Affect Antioxidant, Psyllium Claims. *Whole Foods Mag* May:32–33.

Tomas-Ridocci, M. et al. 1992. Eficacia del *Plantago ovata* como regulador del transito intestinal. Estudio doble ciego comparativo frente a placebo [The efficacy of *Plantago ovata* as a regulator of intestinal transit. A double-blind study compared to placebo]. *Rev Esp Enferm Dig* 82(1):17–22.

Tu, G. (ed.). 1992. *Pharmacopoeia of the People's Republic of China* (English Edition 1992). Beijing: Guangdong Science and Technology Press. 231.

The United States Pharmacopoeia, 22nd rev. (USP XXII). 1990–1992. Rockville, MD: U.S. Pharmacopoeial Convention.

WHO. See World Health Organization.

Wichtl, M. and N.G. Bisset (eds.). 1994. *Herbal Drugs and Phytopharmaceuticals.* Stuttgart: Medpharm Scientific Publishers.

Williams, C.L., A. Bollella, A. Spark, D. Puder. 1995. Soluble fiber enhances the hypocholesterolemic effect of the step I diet in childhood. *J Am Coll Nutr* 14(3):251–257.

World Health Organization (WHO). 1999. "Semen Plantaginis." *WHO Monographs on Selected Medicinal Plants*, Vol. 1. Geneva: World Health Organization.

Yen, K.Y. 1992. *The Illustrated Chinese Materia Medica—Crude and Prepared.* Taipei: SMC Publishing, Inc. 180.

Additional Resources

Bruneton, L.L. 1996. In: Hardman, J.G. et al. (eds.). Goodman and Gilman's *The Pharmacological Basis of Therapeutics*, 9th ed. New York: McGraw-Hill.

Burton, R. and V. Manninen. 1982. Influence of a psyllium-based fibre preparation on faecal and serum parameters. *Acta Med Scand Suppl* 668:91–94.

Deutsches Arzneibuch, 10th ed. Vol. 1–6. (DAB 10). 1991. Kommentar. Stuttgart: Wissenschaftliche Verlagsgesellschaft.

Forman, D.T., J.E. Garvin, J.E. Forestner, C.B. Taylor. 1968. Increased excretion of fecal bile acids by an oral hydrophilic colloid. *Proc Soc Exp Biol Med* 127(4):1060–1063.

Frati-Munari, A.C., M.A. Flores-Garduno, R. Ariza-Andraca, S. Islas-Andrade, A. Chavez Negrete. 1989. Efecto de diferentes dosis de mucilago de *Plantago psyllium* en la prueba de tolerancia a la glucosa [Effect of different doses of *Plantago psyllium* mucilage on the glucose tolerance test]. *Arch Invest Med (Mex)* 20(2):147–152.

Hamouz, W. 1984. Therapy of acute and chronic diarrhoea with Agiocur. *Med Klin* (79):32–33.

Hänsel, R., K. Keller, H. Rimpler, G. Schneider (eds.). 1994. *Hagers Handbuch der Pharmazeutischen Praxis*, 5th ed. Vol. 6. Berlin-Heidelberg: Springer Verlag.

Heckers, H. and D. Zielinsky. 1984. Fecal composition and colonic function due to dietary variables. Results of a long-term study in healthy young men consuming 10 different diets. *Motility (Lisbon)* 24–29.

Karawya, M.S., S.I. Balbaa, M.S. Afifi. 1971. Investigation of the carbohydrate contents of certain mucilaginous plants. *Planta Med* 20(1):14–23.

Kay, R.M. and S.M. Strasberg. 1978. Origin, chemistry, physiological effects and clinical importance of dietary fibre. *Clin Invest Med* 1(1):9–24.

Kies, C. 1983. In: Furda, I. (ed.). Unconventional sources of dietary fiber. Physiological and *in vitro* functional properties. ACS Symposium Series 214. Washington DC: American Chemical Society.

Kovar, F. 1983. Was tun bei akuter, nicht bacteriell bedinger diarrhö? Symptomatische behandlung mit einem quellmittel verringert rasch die stuhlfrequenz, ohne die toxin-elimination zu stören [In German]. *Artzl Praxis* (35):1498.

Leng-Peschlow, E. 1991. *Plantago ovata* seeds as dietary fibre supplement: physiological and metabolic effects in rats. *Br J Nutr* 66(2):331–349.

Marlett, J.A., B.U. Li, C.J. Patrow, P. Bass. 1987. Comparative laxation of psyllium with and without senna in an ambulatory constipated population. *Am J Gastroenterol* 82(4):333–337.

Pharmacopoeia Helvetica, 7th ed. Vol. 1–4. (Ph.Helv.VII). 1987. Bern: Office Central Fédéral des Imprimés et du Matériel.

Qvitzau, S., P. Matzen, P. Madsen. 1988. Treatment of chronic diarrhoea: loperamide versus ispaghula husk and calcium. *Scan J Gastroenterol* 23(10):1237–1240.

Sölter, H. and D. Lorenz. 1983. Summary of clinical results with prodiem plain, a bowel-regulating agent. *Today's Therapeutic Trends* (1):45–59.

Stevens, J., P.J. VanSoest, J.B. Robertson, D.A. Levitsky. 1988. Comparison of the effects of psyllium and wheat bran on gastrointestinal transit time and stool characteristics. *J Am Diet Assoc* 88(3):323–326.

USP Drug Information, 14th ed., Vol. 2. (*USP 1994*). 1994. Rockville, MD: U.S. Pharmacopoeial Convention.

This material was adapted from *The Complete German Commission E Monographs—Therapeutic Guide to Herbal Medicines*. M. Blumenthal, W.R. Busse, A. Goldberg, J. Gruenwald, T. Hall, C.W. Riggins, R.S. Rister (eds.) S. Klein and R.S. Rister (trans.). 1998. Austin: American Botanical Council; Boston: Integrative Medicine Communications.
1) The Overview section is new information.
2) Description, Chemistry and Pharmacology, Uses, Contraindications, Side Effects, Interactions with Other Drugs, and Dosage sections have been drawn from the original work. Additional information has been added in some or all of these sections, as noted with references.
3) The dosage for equivalent preparations (tea infusion, fluidextract, and tincture) have been provided based on the following example:
Unless otherwise prescribed: 2 g per day of [powdered, crushed, cut or whole] [plant part]
Infusion: 2 g in 150 ml of water
Fluidextract 1:1 (g/ml): 2 ml
Tincture 1:5 (g/ml): 10 ml
4) The References and Additional Resources sections are new sections. Additional Resources are not cited in the monograph but are included for research purposes.

PUMPKIN SEED

Latin Name:
Cucurbita pepo

Pharmacopeial Name:
Cucurbitae peponis semen

Other Names:
n/a

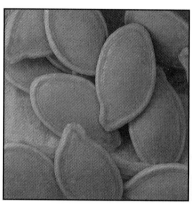

©1999 Steven Foster

Overview

Pumpkin is an herbaceous, monoecious, annual vine native to America, now cultivated worldwide in warm and temperate regions (Bombardelli and Morazzoni,
1997; Wichtl and Bisset, 1994). The material of commerce comes mainly from
medicinal cultivars (*Cucurbitae semen c.v. peponis medicinalis*) grown in southeastern Europe, mainly Austria, Hungary, and the former Yugoslavia (BHP, 1996; Wichtl
and Bisset, 1994), China, Mexico, and the former U.S.S.R. (Wichtl and Bisset,
1994). Pumpkin has been cultivated in Mexico and North America since at least
14,000 B.C.E. based on archaeological evidence (Bombardelli and Morazzoni, 1997).

Pumpkin seed has been used in traditional medicine as an anthelmintic (an agent
used to expel intestinal worms), taeniacide (an agent which kills tapeworms) and as
a diuretic (Bombardelli and Morazzoni, 1997). Its modern clinical uses are comparable to its traditional uses in North American aboriginal medicine. For example,
the Cherokee people used pumpkin seed as an anthelmintic and also as a pediatric
urinary aid to treat bed-wetting. The Iroquois people prepared an infusion of the
seeds as a diuretic given to children with reduced urination. The Menominee people of Wisconsin used the seed to facilitate the passage of urine (Moerman, 1998).
The seeds have been reported to eliminate both tapeworms and roundworms
(Budavari, 1996; Tyler, 1993). An amino acid, curcubitacin, is thought to be
responsible for the seed's anthelmintic actions (Tyler, 1993). To use pumpkin seed
as an anthelmintic agent, one method of preparation is to pound or grind 200–400
g of unpeeled seeds into a pulp, then mix the pulp with milk and honey until
reaching a porridge-like consistency. Ingestion on an empty stomach in the morning, in two doses, is recommended, followed by castor oil 2–3 hours later. Another
method is to combine 150 g of unpeeled, crushed pumpkin seeds with senna electuary. An electuary is a preparation made by mixing the drug (e.g., senna) with
honey or syrup to form a pasty mass (Weiss, 1988).

Pumpkin seeds are considered an alternative treatment for stage 1 and 2 benign
prostatic hyperplasia (BPH). In stage 1 BPH, urination is frequent, and causes
numerous interruptions of sleep during the night. There may be a delay in beginning urination, and also post-void dribbling. Stage 2 symptoms indicate bladder
function debility, and include urgency and incomplete emptying of the bladder. In
addition, Commission E also approves the use of pumpkin seed for the treatment
of irritable bladder; the seeds may help to reduce childhood incidence of bladder
stones in areas where the condition is endemic. A study in Thailand demonstrated
that pumpkin seeds reduced oxalcrystalluria (formation of bladder stones due to
the accumulation of oxalate crystals) in boys between the ages of 2 and 7, while
increasing pyrophosphate, glycosaminoglycans, and potassium values (Suphakarn
et al., 1987).

Countries where men have traditionally consumed pumpkin seeds to reduce prostate enlargement include Bulgaria, Turkey, and the Ukraine (Tyler, 1993; Weiss, 1988), but as with many promising herbal remedies, while efficacy is established empirically, it has not been proven scientifically. Similarly, how pumpkins seeds may or may not work in BPH is not currently known. One theory suggests that the fatty oil content of the seeds, at a 50% concentration, may precipitate diuresis (Tyler, 1993) and may be of benefit not only in prostate hyperplasia but also in irritable bladder. Others postulate that delta-7 sterols in the fatty oils block dihydrotestosterone from androgen receptors, which may prevent the hyperproliferation of prostate cells (Schulz et al., 1998). This theory is somewhat supported by a small, open study in which six patients who were scheduled for radical prostatectomies agreed to take pumpkin seed sterols for three to four days before the operation. When the prostatectomies were performed, tissue removed from the patients taking the sterols contained much less dihydrotestosterone, compared to dihydrotestosterone levels in the tissues taken from the control group (Schilcher, 1992).

Clinical studies on the effects of pumpkin seed preparations in BPH patients are generally lacking. However, in one study, 53 BPH patients participated in a three-month double-blind study. Results showed that urinary flow, frequency, time spent urinating, post-void dribbling and backwash, and subjective feelings about their symptoms significantly improved in the participants given the pumpkin seed preparation (Carbin et al., 1990). The success of this study indicates that follow-up studies are warranted.

In Germany, pumpkin seed is official in the *German Pharmacopeia*, tenth edition, approved in the Commission E monographs, and also official in the German Standard License monographs (Braun et al., 1997; DAB 10, 1991–1996; Wichtl and Bisset, 1994). It is used as a component of a few urological and prostate drug preparations (e.g., Prosta Fink N®, by Fink and Prostamed®, by Klein) (Weiss, 1988; Wichtl and Bisset, 1994). In German pediatric medicine, pumpkin seed preparations (e.g., Granufink® Kürbis-Granulat, by Fink) are used to treat irritable bladder and also enuresis nocturna (bedwetting). Granufink® is a granulated and sugar-coated pumpkin seed from a medicinal cultivar of pumpkin (e.g., *Cucurbita pepo* L. convar. *citrullinina* Greb. var. *styriaca* Greb.) (Schilcher, 1997). In the United States, pumpkin seed was listed in the *United States Pharmacopeia* fifth through tenth editions (Bombardelli and Morazzoni, 1997).

German pharmacopeial grade pumpkin seed consists of the whole, dried, ripe seed of *C. pepo* and/or different cultivars of this species. Botanical identification must be confirmed by macroscopic and microscopic examinations plus organoleptic evaluation. It must not smell or taste rancid (DAB 10, 1991–1996). The *British Herbal Pharmacopoeia* requirements are comparable to the DAB though it requires an additional identification test by a thin-layer chromatography (TLC) method (BHP, 1996). The German Standard License quantitative standards include not less than 35% diethyl ether-soluble extractive and not less than 0.1% total sterols (Wichtl and Bisset, 1994).

Description
Pumpkin seed consists of the ripe, dried seed of *C. pepo* L. and cultivated varieties of *C. pepo* L. [Fam. Cucurbitaceae] and its preparations in effective dosage. The seed contains cucurbitin, phytosterol in free and bound forms, β- and γ-tocopherol, and minerals, including selenium.

Chemistry and Pharmacology
Pumpkin seed contains amino acids (e.g., cucurbitin); approximately 1% phytosterols in free and bound forms;

squalene; chlorophyll pigments (chlorophyll b and pheophytin a); 4–5% minerals including selenium, zinc, calcium, copper, iron, manganese, phosphorous, and potassium; approximately 30% pectins; approximately 25–51% proteins (Bombardelli and Morazzoni, 1997; Wichtl and Bisset, 1994); approximately 30–50% oil, composed mainly of fatty acids including palmitic, stearic, oleic, and linoleic acids; tocopherols (β- and γ-tocopherol); carotenoids (lutein and β-carotene). Due to a broad genetic diversity, the oil content of pumpkin seed is highly variable depending on the taxon (Bombardelli and Morazzoni, 1997; Murkovic et al., 1996a; Murkovic et al., 1996b).

The Commission E reported that due to the lack of suitable models, there are not enough pharmacological studies to substantiate the empirically found clinical activity.

The *British Herbal Pharmacopoeia* reported prostatic action (BHP, 1996). *The Merck Index* reports its therapeutic category as anthelmintic (Budavari, 1996). The constituents tocopherol and selenium may have a protective function towards the oxidative degradation of lipids, vitamins, hormones, and enzymes. Protein fractions of pumpkin seed are thought to function as trypsin inhibitors (Krishnamoorthi et al., 1990; Wichtl and Bisset, 1994). A recent review of studies on the therapeutic activity concluded that pumpkin seed inhibits 5α-reductase *in vitro*. *In vivo*, it has demonstrated anti-androgenic and anti-inflammatory activity (Bombardelli and Morazzoni, 1997).

Uses

The Commission E approved pumpkin seed for irritable bladder and micturition problems of benign prostatic hyperplasia stages 1 and 2.

The German Standard License indicates its use for supportive treatment in functional disorders of the bladder and for difficult urination (Braun et al., 1997). Childhood enuresis nocturna and irritable bladder have been treated

successfully with pumpkin seed (Schilcher, 1997). It has also been used to eradicate tapeworm (Weiss, 1998).

Contraindications
None known.

Side Effects
None known.

Use During Pregnancy and Lactation
No restrictions known.

Interactions with Other Drugs
None known.

Dosage and Administration
Unless otherwise prescribed: 10 g per day of whole and coarsely ground seed and other galenical preparations for internal uses.

Seed: 10 g coarsely ground or well chewed seed taken with fluid (Commission E).

The German Standard License lists a higher dosage: 1–2 heaping tablespoons (15–30 g) coarsely ground or well chewed seed, taken with fluids, in the morning and evening. It is recommended to remove the testa (outer covering) from hard seeds beforehand (Braun et al., 1997).

Note: This medication relieves only the symptoms associated with an enlarged prostate without reducing the enlargement. Please consult a physician at regular intervals (Commission E).

References

British Herbal Pharmacopoeia (BHP). 1996. Exeter, U.K.: British Herbal Medicine Association.

Bombardelli, E. and P. Morazzoni. 1997. *Curcubita pepo* L. *Fitoterapia* 68(4).

Braun, R. et al. 1997. *Standardzulassungen für Fertigarzneimittel—Text and Kommentar.* Stuttgart: Deutscher Apotheker Verlag.

Budavari, S. (ed.). 1996. *The Merck Index: An Encyclopedia of Chemicals, Drugs, and Biologicals,* 12th ed. Whitehouse Station, N.J.: Merck & Co, Inc.

Carbin, B.E., B. Larsson, O. Lindahl. 1990. Treatment of benign prostatic hyperplasia with phytosterols. *Br J Urol* 66(6):639–641.

Deutsches Arzneibuch, 10th ed. (DAB 10). 1991–1996. (With subsequent supplements through 1996.) Stuttgart: Deutscher Apotheker Verlag.

Krishnamoorthi, R., Y.X. Gong, M. Richardson. 1990. A new protein inhibitor of trypsin and activated Hageman factor from pumpkin (*Cucurbita maxima*) seeds. *FEBS Lett* 273(1–2):163–167.

Moerman, D.E. 1998. *Native American Ethnobotany*. Portland, OR: Timber Press, Inc.

Murkovic, M., A. Hillebrand, J. Winkler, W. Pfannhauser. 1996a. Variability of vitamin E content in pumpkin seeds (Cucurbita pepo L.). *Z Lebensm Unters Forsch* 202(4):275–278.

Murkovic, M., A. Hillebrand, J. Winkler, E. Leitner, W. Pfannhauser. 1996b. Variability of fatty acid content in pumpkin seeds (*Cucurbita pepo* L.). *Z Lebensm Unters Forsch* 203(3):216–219.

Schilcher, H. 1997. *Phytotherapy in Paediatrics: Handbook for Physicians and Pharmacists.* Stuttgart: Medpharm Scientific Publishers.

———. 1992. Phytotherapie in der Uroligie. Stuttgart: Hippokrates Verlag.

Schulz, V., R. Hänsel, V.E. Tyler. 1998. *Rational Phytotherapy: A Physicians' Guide to Herbal Medicine.* New York: Springer.

Suphakarn, V.S., C. Yarnnon, P. Ngunboonsri. 1987. The effect of pumpkin seeds on oxalcrystalluria and urinary compositions of children in hyperendemic area. *Am J Clin Nutr* 45(1):115–121.

Tyler, V. 1993. *The Honest Herbal: A Sensible Guide to the Use of Herbs and Related Remedies*, 3rd ed. New York: Pharmaceutical Products Press.

Weiss, R.F. 1988. *Herbal Medicine*. Beaconsfield, England: Beaconsfield Publishers.

Wichtl, M. and N.G. Bisset (eds.). 1994. *Herbal Drugs and Phytopharmaceuticals*. Stuttgart: Medpharm Scientific Publishers.

Additional Resources

Braun, R. et al. 1997. *Standardzulassungen für Fertigarzneimittel—Text and Kommentar.* Stuttgart: Deutscher Apotheker Verlag.

Deutsches Arzneibuch, 10th ed. Vol. 1–6. (DAB 10). 1991. Kommentar. Stuttgart: Wissenschaftliche Verlagsgesellschaft.

Polanowski A, et al. 1987. Protein inhibitors of trypsin from the seeds of Cucurbitaceae plants. *Acta Biochim Pol* 34(4):395–406.

Weidhase, R.A. and B. Parthier. 1983. Peptide hydrolase activities in seedlings and hormone-treated cotyledons of pumpkin (*Cucurbita pepo*). *Biomed Biochim Acta* 42(7–8):897–906.

This material was adapted from *The Complete German Commission E Monographs—Therapeutic Guide to Herbal Medicines*. M. Blumenthal, W.R. Busse, A. Goldberg, J. Gruenwald, T. Hall, C.W. Riggins, R.S. Rister (eds.) S. Klein and R.S. Rister (trans.). 1998. Austin: American Botanical Council; Boston: Integrative Medicine Communications.

1) The Overview section is new information.

2) Description, Chemistry and Pharmacology, Uses, Contraindications, Side Effects, Interactions with Other Drugs, and Dosage sections have been drawn from the original work. Additional information has been added in some or all of these sections, as noted with references.

3) The dosage for equivalent preparations (tea infusion, fluidextract, and tincture) have been provided based on the following example:
   Unless otherwise prescribed: 2 g per day of [powdered, crushed, cut or whole] [plant part]
   Infusion: 2 g in 150 ml of water
   Fluidextract 1:1 (g/ml): 2 ml
   Tincture 1:5 (g/ml): 10 ml

4) The References and Additional Resources sections are new sections. Additional Resources are not cited in the monograph but are included for research purposes.

ROSEMARY LEAF

Latin Name:
Rosmarinus officinalis

Pharmacopeial Name:
Rosmarini folium

Other Names:
garden rosemary

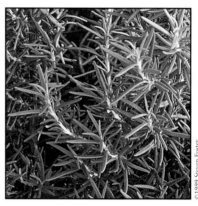

©1999 Steven Foster

Overview

Rosemary is a bushy evergreen shrub, native to the Mediterranean basin and Portugal, now cultivated in France, Spain, Portugal, Morocco, South Africa, India, China, Australia, the United Kingdom, the United States, and along the Crimean peninsula in Transcaucasia (Leung and Foster, 1996). The material of commerce comes from Spain, France, Morocco, and Tunisia (BHP, 1996; Wichtl and Bisset, 1994).

The modern approved indications for its use in Chinese, European and Indian medicines, as well as general unofficial use in dietary supplements in the United States, derive from traditional Greek medicine. Rosemary has been used in Europe since ancient times as a tonic, stimulant, and carminative to treat dyspepsia, headaches, and nervous tension (Leung and Foster, 1996). The ancient Greeks also used it to strengthen memory function; scholars wore garlands of rosemary during examinations in order to improve memory and concentration (Bown, 1995; Grieve, 1979). In China, rosemary preparations have been used for centuries for the same purposes as in traditional Greek medicine, especially to treat headaches (Leung and Foster, 1996). In India, rosemary leaf is used as a component in Ayurvedic and Unani medicines for flatulent dyspepsia associated with psychogenic tension and migraine headaches (Karnick, 1994; Nadkarni, 1976).

In Germany, rosemary leaf is licensed as a standard medicinal tea for internal and external use. Rosemary is taken internally as a carminative or stomachic component of gastrointestinal medicines in aqueous infusions, alcoholic fluidextracts, tinctures, and medicinal wine. The aqueous infusion and essential oil are also used in external preparations (e.g., bath additive, embrocation, liniment, ointment), for rheumatic diseases, and circulatory problems (Leung and Foster, 1996; Wichtl and Bisset, 1994). In the United States, rosemary is a component of dietary supplement products, in aqueous infusion, alcoholic fluidextract, and tincture dosage forms. In both the United States and Germany, the leaf is used in balneotherapy and the essential oil is used in aromatherapy. Rosemary leaf was formerly official in the *United States Pharmacopeia* from 1820 until 1950 (Boyle, 1991).

The approved modern therapeutic applications for rosemary leaf are supportable based on its long history of use in well established systems of traditional medicine, *in vivo* and *in vitro* pharmacological studies in animals, and on well documented phytochemical investigations.

Pharmacopeial grade rosemary leaf must contain not less than 1.2% volatile oil, not more than 10% brown woody stems, and not less than 15% water-soluble extractive, among other quantitative standards. Botanical identification requirements are carried out by thin-layer chromatography (TLC) as well as by examination of macroscopic and microscopic characteristics (BHP, 1996; DAC, 1986; Wichtl and Bisset, 1994). The Commission E monograph also requires not less than 1.2% (v/w) volatile oil. The *French Pharmacopoeia* requires not less than 1.5% (v/m) volatile oil (Bruneton, 1995; Ph.Fr.X., 1990). The ESCOP monograph requires that the material must conform with the *French Pharmacopoeia* standards (ESCOP, 1997). The *German Pharmacopoeia* also includes a TLC identity test for the volatile oil fraction (DAB 10, 1991; Wichtl and Bisset, 1994).

Description

Rosemary leaf consists of the fresh or dried leaf, gathered while flowering, of *Rosmarinus officinalis* L. [Fam. Lamiaceae] and its preparations in effective dosage. The preparation contains at least 1.2% (v/w) essential oil in the dried leaves.

Chemistry and Pharmacology

Rosemary leaf contains phenolic acids (2–3% rosmarinic, chlorogenic, caffeic acids); phenolic diterpenoid bitter substances (up to 4.6% carnosol, rosmaridiphenol, rosmanol); triterpenoid acids (oleanolic acid, ursolic acid); flavonoids (apigenin, luteolin, nepetin, nepitrin); 1.2–2.5% volatile oil, of which 15–50% is 1,8-cineole, 15–25% α-pinene, 12–24% α-terpineol, 10–25% camphor, 5–10% camphene, 1–6% borneol, 1–5% bornyl acetate; and tannins (Bruneton, 1995; Budavari, 1996; ESCOP, 1997; Leung and Foster, 1996; Newall et al., 1996; Wichtl and Bisset, 1994).

The Commission E reported that in humans rosemary irritates the skin. It stimulates increased blood supply when applied externally. Experimentally, it has shown antispasmodic action on gall passages and small intestines, positive inotropic activity, and increased flow through the coronary artery.

The *British Herbal Pharmacopoeia* reported carminative and spasmolytic activity (BHP, 1996). A hydroalcoholic extract of rosemary showed cholagogic/choleretic properties *in vivo* in cannulated guinea pigs by producing a rapid increase of bile secretion (ESCOP, 1997; Wichtl and Bisset, 1994). Antibacterial and spasmolytic actions have been documented (Newall et al., 1996). *The Merck Index* reported emmenagogic properties (Budavari, 1996).

Uses

The Commission E approved the internal use of rosemary leaf for dyspeptic complaints and external use as supportive therapy for rheumatic diseases and circulatory problems.

ESCOP lists its internal use for improvement of hepatic and biliary function and in dyspeptic complaints and its external use as adjuvant therapy in rheumatic conditions, peripheral circulatory disorders, promotion of wound healing, and as a mild antiseptic (ESCOP, 1997). The German Standard License for rosemary leaf tea indicates its use internally for flatulence, feeling of distension, and mild cramp-like gastrointestinal and biliary upsets. Externally it is used in supportive treatment for rheumatism of the muscles and joints (Braun et al., 1997; Wichtl and Bisset, 1994). In traditional European medicine, rosemary has been used internally as a tonic, stimulant, and carminative to treat flatulent dyspepsia, stomach pains, headaches, and nervous tension (BHP, 1983; Leung and Foster, 1996; Newall et al., 1996).

Contraindications

None known.

Side Effects

None known.

Use During Pregnancy and Lactation

Not recommended during pregnancy. No restrictions known during lactation (McGuffin et al., 1997).

Interactions with Other Drugs

None known.

Dosage and Administration

Unless otherwise prescribed: 4–6 g of cut leaf for infusions, powder, dry extracts, and other galenical preparations for internal and external use; 10–20 drops of essential oil. [Ed. note: The essential oil dosage appears excessive and possibly unsafe. A more reasonable dosage for internal use would be 2 drops (1 ml).]

Internal: Infusion: 2 g in 150 ml water, three times daily.

Fluidextract 1:1 (g/ml): 2 ml, three times daily.

Tincture 1:5 (g/ml): 10 ml, three times daily.

Dry normalized extract 4.5–5.5:1 (w/w): 0.36–0.44 g, three times daily.

Rosemary wine: Macerate 20 g cut leaf in 1 liter wine for 1 to 5 days, stirring occasionally.

External: Bath additive: Decoct 50 g of leaf in 1 liter water, let stand covered for 15 to 30 minutes, strain, and add to one full bath.

Embrocation or fomentation: Saturate a cloth with hot semi-solid preparation containing 6–10% essential oil; fold and apply firmly for a moist-heat direct application to skin.

Ointment: Semi-solid preparation containing 6–10% essential oil in base of petroleum jelly or lanolin spread on linen for local application, applied as a liniment.

References

Bown, D. 1995. *Encyclopedia of Herbs and Their Uses*. New York: DK Publishing, Inc. 343.

Boyle, W. 1991. *Official Herbs: Botanical Substances in the United States Pharmacopoeias 1820–1990*. East Palestine, OH: Buckeye Naturopathic Press.

British Herbal Pharmacopoeia (BHP). 1996. Exeter, U.K.: British Herbal Medicine Association. 162–163.

———. 1983. Keighley, U.K.: British Herbal Medicine Association.

Braun, R. et al. 1997. *Standardzulassungen für Fertigarzneimittel—Text und Kommentar*. Stuttgart: Deutscher Apotheker Verlag.

Bruneton, J. 1995. *Pharmacognosy, Phytochemistry, Medicinal Plants*. Paris: Lavoisier Publishing.

Budavari, S. (ed.). 1996. *The Merck Index: An Encyclopedia of Chemicals, Drugs, and Biologicals*, 12th ed. Whitehouse Station, N.J.: Merck & Co, Inc.

Deutsches Arzneibuch, 10th ed. (DAB 10). 1991–1996. (With subsequent supplements through 1996.) Stuttgart: Deutscher Apotheker Verlag.

Deutscher Arzneimittel-Codex (DAC). 1986. Stuttgart: Deutscher Apotheker Verlag.

ESCOP. 1997. "Rosmarini folium." *Monographs on the Medicinal Uses of Plant Drugs*. Exeter, U.K.: European Scientific Cooperative on Phytotherapy.

Grieve, M. 1979. *A Modern Herbal*. New York: Dover Publications, Inc.

Karnick, C.R. 1994. *Pharmacopoeial Standards of Herbal Plants*, Vol. 2. Delhi: Sri Satguru Publications. 112.

Leung, A.Y. and S. Foster. 1996. *Encyclopedia of Common Natural Ingredients Used in Food, Drugs, and Cosmetics*, 2nd ed. New York: John Wiley & Sons, Inc.

McGuffin, M., C. Hobbs, R. Upton, A. Goldberg. 1997. *American Herbal Product Association's Botanical Safety Handbook*. Boca Raton: CRC Press.

Nadkarni, K.M. 1976. *Indian Materia Medica*. Bombay: Popular Prakashan. 1074

Newall, C.A., L.A. Anderson, J.D. Phillipson. 1996. *Herbal Medicines: A Guide for Health-Care Professionals*. London: The Pharmaceutical Press.

Pharmacopée Française Xe Édition (Ph.Fr.X.). 1983–1990. Moulins-les-Metz: Maisonneuve S.A.

Wichtl, M. and N.G. Bisset (eds.). 1994. *Herbal Drugs and Phytopharmaceuticals*. Stuttgart: Medpharm Scientific Publishers.

Additional Resources

Braun, H. and D. Frohne. 1987. *Heilpflanzenlexikon für Ärzte und Apotheker*. Stuttgart: Gustav Fischer Verlag.

British Pharmaceutical Codex (BPC). 1973. London: The Pharmaceutical Press.

Chadha, Y.R. et al. (eds.). 1952–1988. *The Wealth of India (Raw Materials)*, Vols. 1–11. New Delhi: Publications and Information Directorate, CSIR.

Felter, H.W. and J.U. Lloyd. 1985. *King's American Dispensatory*, Vols. 1–2. Portland, OR: Eclectic Medical Publications [reprint of 1898 original].

Food Chemicals Codex, 2nd ed. (FCC II). 1972. Washington, D.C.: National Academy of Sciences.

Formacék, V. and K.H. Kubeczka. 1982. *Essential oils analysis by capillary gas chromatography and carbon-13 NMR spectroscopy*. New York: John Wiley & Sons, Inc. 7–11.

Hänsel, R. 1991. *Phytopharmaka*, 2nd ed. Berlin-Heidelberg: Springer Verlag. 134, 214.

Hänsel, R., K. Keller, H. Rimpler, G. Schneider (eds.). 1992–1994. *Hagers Handbuch der Pharmazeutischen Praxis*, 5th ed. Vol. 4–6. Berlin-Heidelberg: Springer Verlag. 367–384; 490–503.

Hartke, K., H. Hartke, E. Mutschler, G. Rücker, M. Wichtl (eds.). *DAB 10—Kommentar*. Stuttgart: Wissenschaftliche Verlagsgesellschaft.

Mongold, J.J. et al. 1991. Activité cholagogue/cholérétique d'un extrait lyophilisé de *Rosmarinus officinalis* L. Plantes Méd Phytothér 25:6–11.

Paris, R.R. and H. Moyse. 1971. Matière Medicale, Vol. 3. Paris: Masson et Cie. 277–279.

Pharmacopée Française Xe Édition (Ph.Fr.X.). 1983–1990. Moulins-les-Metz: Maisonneuve S.A.

Pharmacopoeia Helvetica, 7th ed. Vol. 1–4. (Ph.Helv.VII). 1987. Bern: Office Central Fédéral des Imprimés et du Matériel.

Reynolds, J.E.F. (ed.). 1993. *Martindale: The Extra Pharmacopoeia,* 30th ed. London: The Pharmaceutical Press.

Rulffs, W. 1984. Rosmarinöl-Badezusatz. Wirksamkeitsnachweis [Rosemary oil bath additive. Proof of effectiveness]. *Münch Med Wschr* 126(8):207–208.

Steinegger, E. and R. Hänsel. 1992. *Pharmakognosie,* 5th ed. Berlin-Heidelberg: Springer Verlag.

Taddei, I., D. Giachetti, E. Taddei, P. Mantovani, E. Bianchi. 1988. Spasmolytic activity of peppermint, sage and rosemary essences and their major constituents. *Fitoterapia* 59:463–468.

Van Hellemont, J. 1986. *Compendium de Phytotherapie*. Bruxells, Belgique: Association Pharmaceutique Belge.

Weiss, R.F. 1991. *Lehrbuch der Phytotherapie*. Stuttgart: Hippokrates Verlag. 246–247.

Wichtl, M. (ed.). 1997. *Teedrogen,* 4th ed. Stuttgart: Wissenschaftliche Verlagsgesellschaft.

This material was adapted from *The Complete German Commission E Monographs—Therapeutic Guide to Herbal Medicines*. M. Blumenthal, W.R. Busse, A. Goldberg, J. Gruenwald, T. Hall, C.W. Riggins, R.S. Rister (eds.) S. Klein and R.S. Rister (trans.). 1998. Austin: American Botanical Council; Boston: Integrative Medicine Communications.

1) The Overview section is new information.

2) Description, Chemistry and Pharmacology, Uses, Contraindications, Side Effects, Interactions with Other Drugs, and Dosage sections have been drawn from the original work. Additional information has been added in some or all of these sections, as noted with references.

3) The dosage for equivalent preparations (tea infusion, fluidextract, and tincture) have been provided based on the following example:
   Unless otherwise prescribed: 2 g per day of [powdered, crushed, cut or whole] [plant part]
   Infusion: 2 g in 150 ml of water
   Fluidextract 1:1 (g/ml): 2 ml
   Tincture 1:5 (g/ml): 10 ml

4) The References and Additional Resources sections are new sections. Additional Resources are not cited in the monograph but are included for research purposes.

SAGE LEAF

Latin Name:
Salvia officinalis

Pharmacopeial Name:
Salviae folium

Other Names:
broad-leafed sage, common sage,
Dalmatian sage, garden sage,
true sage

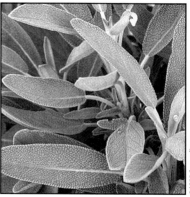

© 1999 Steven Foster

Overview

Sage is an evergreen perennial subshrub, native to the Mediterranean rim, especially around the Adriatic Sea, now cultivated in Albania, Turkey, Greece, Italy, France, the United Kingdom, and the United States (Bruneton, 1995; Budavari, 1996; Leung and Foster, 1996; Wichtl and Bisset, 1994). The material of commerce comes mainly from southeastern European countries, such as Albania and the former Yugoslavia (BHP, 1996; Wichtl and Bisset, 1994). Its cultivation in northern Europe dates back to medieval times, and it was introduced to North America during the seventeenth century (Bown, 1995). The genus name *Salvia* is derived from the Latin *salvere* (to be saved), in reference to its curative properties. This name was corrupted to *sauge* in French and *sawge* in Old English, and eventually to "sage" (Grieve, 1979).

This species was used in ancient Egyptian, Greek, and Roman medicines. Ancient Egyptians used it as a fertility drug (Bown, 1995). In the first century C.E. Greek physician Dioscorides reported that the aqueous decoction of sage stopped bleeding of wounds and cleaned ulcers and sores. He also recommended sage juice in warm water for hoarseness and cough. Pliny the Elder (ca. 23–79 C.E.) reported that sage enhanced memory functions. He prescribed decoctions, boiled in water or wine, of sage, rosemary, honeysuckle, plantain, and honey for gargles to treat sore mouths and throats (Grieve, 1979). Its uses in traditional Greek medicine spread to India, where the dried leaf (*Salbia-sefakuss* in Hindi) and fluid extract are used in traditional Indian Ayurvedic, Siddha, and Unani medicines. Eight other related Indian species of *Salvia* (e.g., *S. plebeia*) are also listed in the *Ayurvedic Pharmacopoeia* and used interchangeably with the Mediterranean species. In India, its use is indicated for flatulent dyspepsia, pharyngitis, uvulitis, stomatitis, gingivitis, and glossitis (Karnick, 1994; Nadkarni, 1976).

In Germany, sage is licensed as a standard medicinal tea to treat gastrointestinal catarrh and night sweats. The tea is also applied topically as a rinse or gargle for inflammations. Sage fluidextract, tincture, and essential oil are all used in prepared medicines for mouth and throat and as gastrointestinal remedies in fluid (e.g., juice) and solid dosage forms (e.g., capsules, drageés) (Leung and Foster, 1996; Wichtl and Bisset, 1994). In the United States, sage is used as a component of dietary supplement products for similar conditions, usually in aqueous infusion or alcoholic tincture dosage forms. Sometimes the dry herb or dry extract is used in capsules and tablets. Sage was formerly official in the *United States Pharmacopoeia* from 1840 to 1900 as a gargle in inflamed sore throat (Boyle, 1991).

Very few clinical studies have been conducted. A few German studies have investigated its perspiration-inhibiting activity (ESCOP, 1997). One open study at an outpatient clinic investigated the equivalence of efficacy and compared tolerance between an aqueous dry extract product "Sweatosan" and sage tea. Eighty patients suffering from idiopathic hyperhidrosis were treated for four weeks. Forty patients were treated with 440 mg aqueous dry extract, corresponding to 2.6 g of dry leaf, and the other 40 with an aqueous infusion, 4.5 g leaf daily. The reduction of sweat secretion reported (less than 50%) was comparable for both treatment groups, though somewhat stronger in the aqueous dry extract group (ESCOP, 1997; Rösing, 1989).

In 1997, the National Institute of Medical Herbalists in the United Kingdom sent out a questionnaire to its member practitioners on the clinical use and experience of sage. Of 49 respondents, 47 used sage in their practice and 45 used it particularly in prescriptions for menopause. Almost all references were to sage's application for hot flashes, night sweats, and its estrogenic effect. The age range of the menopause patients was 40 to 64, with an average of 49.76. Three-quarters were aged 47 to 52. Forty-three practitioners also noted its use in infections, mainly of the upper respiratory tract, 29 reported its use in sore throat, and 15 reported its use in mouth and gum disease, taken in the form of gargles and mouthwashes. Another main area emphasized by the respondents was its use as a general tonic, for fatigue, nervous exhaustion, immune system depletion, and poor memory and concentration, at any age. Dosage form preference was also reported. Sage was prescribed as tea (aqueous infusion) by 37 practitioners, alcoholic tincture by 30, fresh tincture by 14, alcoholic fluidextract by 2, fresh juice by 2, and fresh leaf by 1 (Beatty and Denham, 1998).

The approved modern therapeutic applications for sage leaf are supportable based on its history of use in well established systems of traditional medicine, on clinical data collection from medical herbalists in current practice, on phytochemical investigations, on *in vitro* and *in vivo* pharmacological studies in animals, and on some clinical studies.

Pharmacopeial grade sage leaf must contain not less than 1.5% (v/m) thujone-rich volatile oil calculated with reference to the anhydrous drug as determined by DAB (German Pharacopoeia) method V.4.5.8 (DAB, 1997; ESCOP, 1997; ÖAB, 1981; Ph.Helv.VII, 1987; Wichtl and Bisset, 1994). It must contain not less than 16% water-soluble extractive, among other quantitative standards. Botanical identity requirements are carried out by thin-layer chromatography (TLC) as well as by examination of macroscopic and microscopic characteristics (BHP, 1996). Adulteration is determined with a TLC method that can be used to examine the volatile oil composition and flavonoids profile (DAB 1997; Wichtl and Bisset, 1994). The *French Pharmacopoeia* requires between 2–3% volatile oil (Bruneton, 1995; Ph.Fr.X., 1990).

Pharmacopeial grade sage tincture (*Salviae Tinctura*) must contain not less than 0.1% thujone-rich volatile oil. Its drug-to-extract ratio is 1:10 in ethanol 70% (v/v), manufactured by percolation according to the *German Pharmacopoeia* Tincture monograph. Botanical identity of the finished tincture is determined by DAB TLC method V.6.20.2 (DAB, 1997).

Description

Sage leaf consists of the fresh or dried leaf of *Salvia officinalis* L. [Fam. Lamiaceae], and its preparations in effective dosage. The leaves contain at least 1.5% (v/w) thujone-rich essential oil, based on the dried herb. Principal components of the essential oil, in addition to thujone, are cineol and camphor. In addition, the leaves contain tannins, diterpene bitter principles, triterpenes, steroids, flavones, and flavonoid glycosides.

Chemistry and Pharmacology

Sage leaf contains 3–8% condensed catechin-type tannins (salviatannin); phenolic acids (rosmarinic, caffeic, chlorogenic, ferulic, and gallic acids);

1–3% flavonoids (apigenin and luteolin derivatives); 1.5–2.8% volatile oil, mostly monoterpenoids of which 18–60% is α-thujone, 3–10% β-thujone, 4.5–24.5% camphor, 5.5–13% cineole, 0–12% humulene, 1–6.5% α-pinene, 1.5–7% camphene, 0.5–3% limonene, max. 1% linalool, and max. 2.5% bornyl acetate; diterpenoid bitter principles carnosol, carnosic acid, and rosmanol; triterpenoids oleanolic acid and ursolic acid; and resin (Bruneton, 1995; Budavari, 1996; ESCOP, 1997; Leung and Foster, 1996; Newall et al., 1996; Wichtl and Bisset, 1994).

The Commission E reported antibacterial, fungistatic, virustatic, astringent, secretion-promoting, and perspiration-inhibiting properties.

In an open study with 80 patients both an aqueous infusion and a dried aqueous extract comparably reduced sweat secretion (ESCOP, 1997). *The Merck Index* reported its therapeutic category as antisecretory agent (Budavari, 1996). Its volatile oil has antimicrobial activity attributed to its thujone content. Its traditional uses may be explained by its volatile oil and tannin content (Jalsenjak et al., 1987; Newall et al., 1996).

Uses

The Commission E approved the internal use of sage leaf for dyspeptic symptoms and excessive perspiration, and external use for inflammations of the mucous membranes of nose and throat.

ESCOP indicates its use for inflammations such as stomatitis, gingivitis and pharyngitis, and hyperhidrosis (ESCOP, 1997). The German Standard License for sage infusion indicates its use for inflammation of the gums and the mucous membranes of the mouth and throat; pressure spots caused by prostheses and in supportive treatment of gastrointestinal catarrh (Wichtl and Bisset, 1984).

Contraindications

The pure essential oil and alcoholic extracts should not be used internally during pregnancy.

Side Effects

After prolonged ingestion of alcohol extracts or of the pure essential oil, epileptiform convulsions can occur.

Use During Pregnancy and Lactation

Not recommended (McGuffin et al., 1997).

Interactions with Other Drugs

None known.

Dosage and Administration

Unless otherwise prescribed: 4–6 g per day of cut leaf for infusions, alcoholic extracts, and distillates for gargles, rinses and other topical applications, and for internal use. Also pressed juice of fresh plants.

Internal: Dried leaf: 1–3 g, three times daily.

Infusion: 1–3 g in 150 ml water, three times daily.

Dry aqueous extract 5.5:1 (w/w): 0.18–0.36 g, three times daily.

Fluidextract 1:1 (g/ml): 1–3 ml, three times daily.

Fluidextract: 1.5–3 g (Erg.B.6).

Tincture 1:10 (g/ml): 2.5–7.5 g (Erg.B.6).

Essential oil: 0.1–0.3 ml.

Succus: Pressed juice of fresh plant in 25% alcoholic preservation.

External: Gargle or rinse: Use warm infusion: 2.5 g cut leaf in 100 ml water; or 2 to 3 drops of essential oil in 100 ml water; or use 5 ml of fluidextract diluted in 1 glass water, several times daily.

Paint: Apply the undiluted alcoholic fluidextract to the affected area with a brush or swab.

References

Beatty, C. and A. Denham. 1998. Review of Practice: Preliminary data collection for clinical audit. *Eur J Herbal Med* 4(2):32–34.

Bown, D. 1995. *Encyclopedia of Herbs and Their Uses*. New York: DK Publishing, Inc. 346.

Boyle, W. 1991. *Official Herbs: Botanical Substances in the United States Pharmacopoeias 1820–1990*. East Palestine, OH: Buckeye Naturopathic Press.

British Herbal Pharmacopoeia (BHP). 1996. Exeter, U.K.: British Herbal Medicine Association. 164.

Bruneton, J. 1995. *Pharmacognosy, Phytochemistry, Medicinal Plants*. Paris: Lavoisier Publishing.

Budavari, S. (ed.). 1996. *The Merck Index: An Encyclopedia of Chemicals, Drugs, and Biologicals*, 12th ed. Whitehouse Station, N.J.: Merck & Co, Inc.

Deutsches Arzneibuch (DAB 1997). 1997. Stuttgart: Deutscher Apotheker Verlag.

Ergänzungsbuch zum Deutschen Arzneibuch, 6th ed. (Erg.B.6). 1953. Stuttgart: Deutscher Apotheker Verlag.

ESCOP. 1997. "Salviae folium." *Monographs on the Medicinal Uses of Plant Drugs*. Exeter, U.K.: European Scientific Cooperative on Phytotherapy.

Grieve, M. 1979. *A Modern Herbal*. New York: Dover Publications, Inc.

Jalsenjak, V., S. Peljnjak, D. Kustrak. 1987. Microcapsules of sage oil: Essential oils content and antimicrobial activity. *Pharmazie* 42(6):419–420.

Karnick, C.R. 1994. *Pharmacopoeial Standards of Herbal Plants*, Vols. 1–2. Delhi: Sri Satguru Publications. Vol. 1:324–325; Vol. 2:114.

Leung, A.Y. and S. Foster. 1996. *Encyclopedia of Common Natural Ingredients Used in Food, Drugs, and Cosmetics*, 2nd ed. New York: John Wiley & Sons, Inc.

McGuffin, M., C. Hobbs, R. Upton, A. Goldberg. 1997. *American Herbal Product Association's Botanical Safety Handbook*. Boca Raton: CRC Press.

Nadkarni, K.M. 1976. *Indian Materia Medica*. Bombay: Popular Prakashan. 1094–1095.

Newall, C.A., L.A. Anderson, J.D. Phillipson. 1996. *Herbal Medicines: A Guide for Health-Care Professionals*. London: The Pharmaceutical Press.

Österreichisches Arzneibuch, 1st suppl. (ÖAB). 1981–1983. Wien: Verlag der Österreichischen Staatsdruckerei.

Pharmacopée Française Xe Édition (Ph.Fr.X.). 1983–1990. Moulins-les-Metz: Maisonneuve S.A.

Pharmacopoeia Helvetica, 7th ed. Vol. 1–4. (Ph.Helv.VII). 1987. Bern: Office Central Fédéral des Imprimés et du Matériel.

Rösing, S. 1989. Sweatosan-Studie: Untersuchungsbericht. Äquivalenz der Wirksamkeit und Vergleich der Verträglichkeit von Sweatosan und Salbeitee bei Patienten mit idiopathischer Hyperhidrosis in der dermatologischen Poliklinik. *Zyma* (unpublished).

Wichtl, M. and N.G. Bisset (eds.). 1994. *Herbal Drugs and Phytopharmaceuticals*. Stuttgart: Medpharm Scientific Publishers.

Additional Resources

Braun, R. et al. 1997. *Standardzulassungen für Fertigarzneimittel—Text and Kommentar*. Stuttgart: Deutscher Apotheker Verlag.

Brieskorn, C.H. 1991. Salbei—seine Inhaltsstoffe und sein therapeutischer Wert. *Z Phytotherapie* 12:61–69.

British Pharmaceutical Codex (BPC). 1934. London: The Pharmaceutical Press.

Council of Europe. 1989. *Plant Preparations Used as Ingredients of Cosmetic Products*, 1st ed. Strasbourg: Council of Europe.

Derbentseva, N,A, S.A. Matveenko, TIa. Omelchuk. 1965. Antymikrobna aktyvnist' preparativ z deiakykh vydiv shavlii [Antimicrobic activity of preparations from some sage species]. *Mikrobiol Zh* 27(3):76–80.

This material was adapted from *The Complete German Commission E Monographs—Therapeutic Guide to Herbal Medicines*. M. Blumenthal, W.R. Busse, A. Goldberg, J. Gruenwald, T. Hall, C.W. Riggins, R.S. Rister (eds.) S. Klein and R.S. Rister (trans.). 1998. Austin: American Botanical Council; Boston: Integrative Medicine Communications.
1) The Overview section is new information.
2) Description, Chemistry and Pharmacology, Uses, Contraindications, Side Effects, Interactions with Other Drugs, and Dosage sections have been drawn from the original work. Additional information has been added in some or all of these sections, as noted with references.
3) The dosage for equivalent preparations (tea infusion, fluidextract, and tincture) have been provided based on the following example:
   Unless otherwise prescribed: 2 g per day of [powdered, crushed, cut or whole] [plant part]
   Infusion: 2 g in 150 ml of water
   Fluidextract 1:1 (g/ml): 2 ml
   Tincture 1:5 (g/ml): 10 ml
4) The References and Additional Resources sections are new sections. Additional Resources are not cited in the monograph but are included for research purposes.

Food Chemicals Codex, 2nd ed. (FCC II). 1972. Washington, D.C.: National Academy of Sciences.

Hartke, K., H. Hartke, E. Mutschler, G. Rücker, M. Wichtl (eds.). *DAB 10—Kommentar.* Stuttgart: Wissenschaftliche Verlagsgesellschaft.

Marchenko, A.I., V.N. Pinchuk, I.V. Shvets. 1978. Primenenie mazi iz shalfeia pri lechenii treshchin guby [Use of a sage ointment in treating cracked lips]. *Stomatologiia (Mosk)* 57(1):86–87.

Reynolds, J.E.F. (ed.). 1993. *Martindale: The Extra Pharmacopoeia,* 30th ed. London: The Pharmaceutical Press.

Steinegger, E. and R. Hänsel. 1992. *Pharmakognosie,* 5th ed. Heidelberg: Springer Verlag. 343–345.

Taddei, I., D. Giachetti, E. Taddei, P. Mantovani, E. Bianchi. 1988. Spasmolytic activity of peppermint, sage and rosemary essences and their major constituents. *Fitoterapia* 59:463–468.

Takacsova, M., A. Pribela, M. Faktorova. 1995. Study of the antioxidative effects of thyme, sage, juniper and oregano. *Nahrung* 39(3):241–243.

Todorov, S. et al. 1984. Experimental pharmacological study of three species from genus *Salvia. Acta Physiol Pharmacol Bulg* 10(2):13–20.

Tucakov, J. and M. Mihajlov. 1977. Prilog uporednom farmakognozijskom proucavanju pelima (*Salvia officinalis* L.) U Pastrovicima [Comparative pharmacognostic studies on sage officinalis (*Salvia officinalis* L.) of Pastrovici]. *Glas Srp Akad Nauka [Med]* (27):47–60.

Tucker, A.O. et al. 1980. Botanical aspects of commercial sage. *Economic Bot* 34:16–19.

Van Hellemont, J. 1988. *Fytotherapeutisch Compendium,* 2nd ed. Utrecht: Bohn, Scheltema & Holkema. 539–541.

Vion Dury, J., M.D. Steinmetz, G. Jadot, Y. Millet. 1986. Effets de l'essence de sauge sur le seuil epileptogene et l'embrasement amygdalien chez le rat. Rapport preliminaire [Effects of sage essence on the epileptogenic threshold and amygdaloid body in the rat. Preliminary report] *J Toxicol Clin Exp* 6(1):29–31.

Weiss, R.F. 1991. *Lehrbuch der Phytotherapie,* 7th ed. Stuttgart: Hippokrates Verlag. 296–297.

Wichtl, M. (ed.). 1997. *Teedrogen,* 4th ed. Stuttgart: Wissenschaftliche Verlagsgesellschaft. 416–419.

Saw Palmetto Berry

Latin Name:
Serenoa repens
[syn. *Sabal serrulata*]

Pharmacopeial Name:
Sabal fructus

Other Names:
sabal

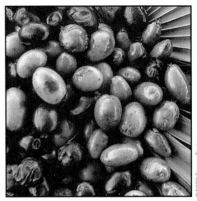

©1999 Steven Foster

Overview

Saw palmetto (SP) is a small, low-growing palm tree, native to southeastern North America, particularly Florida. The fruits (berries) were a staple food and medicine of the indigenous Floridians before European contact (Bennett and Hicklin, 1999; Duke, 1985; Hutchens, 1973; Vogel, 1970). The Seminole people of Florida use the fruit for food and the leaf stems to make medicine baskets (Moerman, 1998). They prepared an aqueous infusion of the berries for treatment of stomachache and dysentery (Duke, 1985) at a dosage of 1 teaspoon dried berries to 1 cup boiling water (Hutchens, 1973). Other sources indicate that native Americans used the fruit as a diuretic and sexual tonic (Duke, 1985; Finzelberg, 1999; Hänsel et al., 1994).

Saw palmetto berry was commonly recommended for various prostatic conditions by healthcare professionals in the early part of the twentieth century. It was an official drug, listed in two editions of the *United States Pharmacopoeia* from 1906 to 1916 and in the *National Formulary* from 1926 to 1950 (Boyle, 1991), when its use as a therapeutic option for urinary tract disorders by the medical community declined in the United States (Tyler, 1993). The berries were prescribed dispensed in an alcoholic fluidextract by physicians of the American Eclectic system of medicine (Bergner, 1997; Bone, 1998; Felter and Lloyd, 1985). *King's American Dispensatory* indicated SP's specific uses as follows: "Relaxation of parts, with copious catarrhal discharges; lack of development, or wasting away of testicles, ovaries, or mammae; prostatic irritation, with painful micturition, and dribbling of urine, particularly in the aged; tenderness of the glands, and other parts concerned in reproduction" (Felter and Lloyd, 1985). The dosage range was wide, from 1 to 60 drops, apparently based on individual diagnosis. The Eclectics described SP as the "old man's friend," as a "remedy for prostatic irritation and relaxation of tissue (rather) than for a hypertrophied prostate" (Bone, 1998; Felter and Lloyd, 1985). In the twentieth century, the *United States Dispensatory*, 23rd edition, indicated its use for the enlarged prostate of old men (Wood and Osol, 1943).

In Europe, phytotherapeutic agents have a long history of use in the treatment of benign prostatic hyperplasia (BPH). French researchers in the 1960s began to examine the chemical composition of the SP berry. A breakthrough was the development of the proprietary lipophilic (fat-soluble portion) extract of SP berries (Permixon®, Pierre Fabre, France). Rich in fatty acids and sterols, lipophilic (also called liposterolic) extracts of SP berries are currently approved by both the French and German governments for treatment of BPH (Brown, 1996; Tyler, 1993).

There are numerous controlled clinical studies that confirm the safe and effective use of SP preparations in treating the symptoms associated with BPH. There is also preliminary evidence suggesting that the herb may reduce prostate enlargement; however, evidence that SP may help prevent the onset of prostate cancer is lacking.

Many of the early clinical studies of SP for BPH were short-term (three months or less), but they did indicate a fairly rapid response to SP. One 28-day study of 110 BPH patients found 320 mg daily was effective in reducing painful urination (dysuria), nighttime urination (nocturia), and retained urine in the bladder. There was also significant improvement in urine flow rate. Forty-seven of the patients were followed for 15 to 30 months and had continued improvement (Champault et al., 1984). Another early double-blind study was conducted on 27 BPH patients between 49 and 81 years old. The authors reported a 43% increase in urine flow rate after only 60 days of treatment with 320 mg of saw palmetto extract daily, compared to 15% in the placebo group. Only one patient complained of gastric disturbances that led to discontinuation of the treatment (Tasca et al., 1985).

In a more recent three-month, multicenter open trial, 505 patients with mild to moderate symptoms of BPH were treated with Prostaserene®, an oral preparation of SP berry, at a daily dosage of 160 mg twice daily (Braeckman, 1994). At the end of the three-month period, 305 patients were available for evaluation. The quality of life score (using the International Prostate Symptom Score (IPSS), urinary flow rates, residual urinary volume, and prostate size showed significant improvement in patients taking SP after only 45 days of treatment. Serum prostate-specific antigen (PSA) concentration was not modified by taking SP, reducing the risk of masking potential prostate cancer. Only 5% of the patients completing the study reported adverse side effects. After 90 days, 88% of the patients and 88% of the physicians considered the therapy successful. This study indicates that the daily dose of 320 mg is not only effective in the reduction of BPH symptoms, but is also relatively low in adverse side effects.

In an open trial, 60 patients suffering from BPH stage I and II were treated with a twice daily dosage of 160 mg SP extract (Prostagutt® mono, Schwabe, Germany) (Redecker, 1998). Maximum urinary flow rate was defined as the main outcome measure. After three months of treatment, a significant improvement of micturition parameters was observed: an increase of 24% urinary flow rate and a reduction of both residual urine and micturition frequency. Patients reported and demonstrated subjective progress as well.

Similarly, an open multicenter trial involving 109 BPH patients treated twice daily for twelve weeks with 160 mg SP extract (Prostagutt® mono), demonstrated statistically significant and also clinically relevant improvements in micturition symptoms (Ziegler and Holscher, 1998).

In a randomized placebo-controlled clinical study conducted on 25 men with BPH given the standard dose of 320 mg per day of a proprietary SP extract (Permixon®), those with SP experienced statistically significant reductions in levels of prostatic dihydrotestosterone (DHT) and epidermal growth factor (EGF) and increased levels of testosterone (Di Silverio et al., 1998). Additionally, these levels were distinct to the periurethral regions: those with the herb had lower DHT and EGF levels in the periurethral zone. This appears to be evidence of the 5-alpha-reductase-lowering effects of SP and its more specific regionalized effects compared to the conventional drug finasteride (Proscar®) (Strauch et al., 1994).

Controversy regarding the relative efficacy of treatments for the relief of the symptoms of BPH was addressed in a 1996 French trial (Carraro et al., 1996). This six-month, double-blind, randomized equivalence study compared the effects of an SP extract (320 mg Permixon®) with those of a 5-alpha-reductase inhibitor (5 mg finasteride) in 1,098 men with moderate BPH. The IPSS was used as the primary endpoint. The study found that both Permixon® and finasteride decreased the IPSS, improved quality of life, and increased peak urinary flow rate. Finasteride markedly decreased prostate volume and serum PSA levels. The SP extract improved symptoms with little effect on volume and no change in PSA levels, and fared better than finasteride in a sexual function questionnaire and gave rise to less complaints of decreased libido and impotence.

A critical review of phytotherapeutic agents in the treatment of BPH was less positive about the efficacy of SP (Lowe and Ku, 1996), stating that no well-defined mechanism of action had been proposed, evidence for an anti-androgenic or anti-estrogenic effect was conflicting, and there were no clinical data suggesting an effect on 5-alpha-reductase activity. Clinical trials were criticized for being uncontrolled, limiting their value, and the double-blind, controlled studies had limitations in that most were of short duration (none longer than three months). Problems were attributed to the different compositions of the saw palmetto products tested. The study concluded that standardization of the preparations is needed to compare and accurately assess the effect of the different extracts.

A review of various phytomedicines used in prostate therapy in Europe was published by Buck (1996). The author reviewed clinical research on several proprietary extracts of SP (e.g., Permixon®). The article acknowledged the 5-alpha-reductase-inhibiting activity of the saw palmetto preparations, as well as other mechanisms affecting production of DHT, implicated in BPH.

A recent comparative review looked at the effectiveness and safety of phytomedicines and synthetic drugs in the treatment of BPH, with a focus on SP (Bach et al., 1997). In a three-year trial involving 309 men, saw palmetto was associated with a significant increase in urinary flow rate, and a 50% decrease in residual urine volume. In comparison, the drug finasteride showed a 30% decrease in symptom scores over three years, but urine flow improved only slightly, and residual urine volume was almost unchanged (Bach et al., 1997). Further, 10.7% of finasteride patients discontinued treatment because of side effects, compared to only 1.8% taking SP. The authors concluded that in terms of increasing urinary flow rate, the data showed a clear superiority of the SP extract in comparison to the synthetic drugs.

Saw palmetto's therapeutic efficacy and safety has been documented recently in a systematic review and meta-analysis of clinical studies (Wilt et al., 1998). This article carefully reviewed 18 studies conducted in Germany, France, and Italy. The authors searched for all studies available through the Medline database from 1966–1997, through EMBASE, Phytodok, the Cochrane Library, bibiographies in studies and review articles, and contacts with "relevant authors and drug companies." In all, 18 clinical studies involving 2,939 men were reviewed, in which patients had symptomatic BPH, the medicinal preparation was made of SP alone or with other botanicals, the trials were placebo-controlled, and the trials lasted for at least 30 days. According to the authors, some of the studies did not report results that allowed them to be included in the meta-analysis. They rated the treatment allocation concealment (for the purposes of blinding the studies) adequate in nine studies. Sixteen studies were double-blinded. Study duration ranged from 4 to 48 weeks (mean 9 weeks). Compared to placebo, SP produced lowered urinary tract scores, lower frequency of nocturia, and improvement in peak urine flow. When compared to finasteride, SP users experienced similar benefits but about a 90% lower incidence of adverse effects. Adverse effects were "mild and infrequent" and erectile dysfunction was lower when compared to finasteride, SP being 1.1% compared to finasteride at 4.9%. The authors noted that more research is needed to determine the long-term effectiveness and the ability to prevent complications associated with BPH.

During the period when the Commission E reviewed the scientific literature (1989–1991), there was no clinical evidence to support claims that SP reduces the size of an enlarged prostate. However, a recent study has detected shrinkage of the epithelial tissue in the transition zone of the gland (Marks and Tyler, 1999). Two review articles (Koch and Biber, 1994; Niederprum et al., 1994) explored the 5-alpha-reductase-inhibiting properties of the free fatty acids in SP berry. This action is critical to the herb's activity with respect to BPH and may explain a mechanism that might be associated with inhibition of prostate cancer.

Description

Saw palmetto berry consists of the ripe, dried fruit of *Serenoa repens* (Bartram) Small (syn. *Sabal serrulata* (Michaux) Nuttall ex Schultes) [Fam. Arecaceae] as well as its preparations in effective dosage. The berries contain fatty oil with fatty acids, esters, phytosterols, and polysaccharides.

Chemistry and Pharmacology

The main constituents include carbohydrates (invert sugar, mannitol, high-molecular-weight polysaccharides with galactose, arabinose, and uronic acid), fixed oils (free fatty acids and their glycerides), steroids, flavonoids, resin, pigment, tannin, and volatile oil (Newall et al., 1996). The fruits and seeds are rich in triacylglycerol-containing oil (50% of the fatty acids contain 14 or less carbons) (Bruneton, 1995).

Saw palmetto has been reported to contain diuretic, urinary antiseptic, endocrinological, and anabolic properties (Newall et al., 1996).

The fruit of SP has been shown *in vitro* to inhibit the 5-alpha-reductase and aromatoase, significant in the development of BPH (Koch and Biber, 1994). A recent animal study has shown anti-exudative and anti-inflammatory effects as well (Ziegler and Holscher, 1998). Additional research to confirm the purported hormonal and anti-inflammatory effects of SP is required.

The Commission E reported antiandrogenic and anti-exudative activity.

Uses

The Commission E approved the internal use of saw palmetto berry for urination problems in benign prostatic hyperplasia stages I and II. Traditional uses include chronic or subacute cystitis, catarrh of the genito-urinary tract, testicular atrophy, sex hormone disorders, and, specifically, prostatic enlargement in modern phytotherapy (Newall et al., 1996).

Note: The Commission E monograph states, "This medication relieves only the symptoms associated with an enlarged prostate without reducing the enlargement. Please consult a physician at regular intervals." This statement may be subject to change in light of the new research noted above (Marks and Tyler, 1999); however, additional studies are required to confirm the potential tissue-shrinking activity.

[Ed. note: Stage I of BPH is characterized by increase in frequency of urination, pollakiuria (abnormally frequent urination), nocturia, delayed onset of urination, and weak urinary stream. Stage II is characterized by the beginning of the decompensation of the bladder function accompanied by formation of residual urine and urge to urinate.]

Contraindications

None known.

Side Effects

In rare cases, stomach problems.

Use During Pregnancy and Lactation

No restrictions known.

Interactions with Other Drugs

None known.

Dosage and Administration

Internal: Unless otherwise prescribed: 1–2 g cut fruit and other equivalent galenical preparations for oral use, or 320 mg lipophilic ingredients extracted with lipophilic solvents (hexane or ethanol 90% v/v).

Fluidextract 1:1 (g/ml): 1–2 ml, twice daily.

Fluidextract 1:2 (g/ml): 2–4 ml, twice daily.

Soft native extract 10:1–14:1 (w/w) (contains approximately 85–95% fatty acids): 160 mg, twice daily.

Dry normalized extract 4:1 (w/w) (contains approximately 25% fatty acids): 400 mg, twice daily.

References

Bach, D, M. Schmitt, L. Ebeling. 1997. Phytopharmaceutical and synthetic agents in the treatment of benign prostatic hyperplasia (BPH). *Phytomedicine* 3(4):309–313.

Bennett, B.C. and J.R. Hicklin. 1998. Uses of Saw Palmetto (Serenoa repens, Arecacea) in Florida. *Econ Bot* 52(4):381–393.

Bergner, P. 1997. Electic Materia Medica: Saw Palmetto. *Medical Herbalism* 9(3):1, 16–17.

Bone, K.1998. Saw Palmetto—A Critical Review, Part 2. *MediHerb Professional Review* 61:1–4.

Boyle, W. 1991. *Official Herbs: Botanical Substances in the United States Pharmacopoeias 1820–1990.* East Palestine, OH: Buckeye Naturopathic Press.

Braeckman, J. 1994. The extract of *Serenoa repens* in the treatment of benign prostatic hyperplasia: A multicenter open study. *Curr Therapeut Res* 55:776–785.

Brown, D.J. 1996. *Herbal Prescriptions for Better Health.* Rocklin, CA: Prima Publishing. 167–172.

Bruneton, J. 1995. *Pharmacognosy, Phytochemistry, Medicinal Plants.* Paris: Lavoisier Publishing.

Buck, A.C. 1996. Phytotherapy for the prostate. *Br J Urol* 78:325–336.

Carraro, J.C. et al. 1996. Comparison of phytotherapy (Permixon) with finasteride in the treatment of benign prostate hyperplasia: a randomized international study of 1,098 patients. *Prostate* 29(4):231–240.

Champault, G., A.M. Bonnard, J. Cauquil, J.C. Patel. 1984. [The medical treatment of prostatic adenoma. A controlled study: PA-109 versus placebo in 110 patients] [In French]. *Ann Urol (Paris)* 18(6):407–410.

Di Silverio, F. et al. 1998. Effects of long-term treatment with *Serenoa repens* (Permixon®) on the concentration and regional distribution of androgens and epidermal growth factor in benign prostatic hyperplasia. *Prostate* 37(2):77–83.

Duke, J.A. 1985. *Handbook of Medicinal Herbs.* Boca Raton: CRC Press.

Felter, H.W. and J.U. Lloyd. 1985. *King's American Dispensatory*, Vols. 1–2. Portland, OR: Eclectic Medical Publications [reprint of 1898 original]. 1750–1752.

Finzelberg's Nachfolger. 1999. Product Information: ProstaFin™ SP Saw Palmetto-Extracts. Andernach: H. Finzelberg's Nachfolger & Co. KG.

Hänsel, R., K. Keller, H. Rimpler, G. Schneider (eds.). 1994. *Hagers Handbuch der Pharmazeutischen Praxis,* 5th ed. Vol. 6. Berlin-Heidelberg: Springer Verlag. 680–687.

Hutchens, A.R. 1973. *Indian Herbology of North America.* Ontario: Merco. 243–244.

Koch, E. and A. Biber. 1994. Pharmacological effects of Sabal and Urtica extracts as a basis for a rational medication of benign prostatic hyperplasia. *Urologe* 34:3–8.

Lowe, F.C. and J.C. Ku. 1996. Phytotherapy in treatment of benign prostate hyperplasia: a critical review. *Urology* 48(1):12–20.

Marks, L.S. and V.E. Tyler. 1999. *Saw palmetto* extract: newest (and oldest) treatment alternative for men with symptomatic benign prostatic hyperplasia. *Urology* 53(3):457–461.

Moerman, D.E. 1998. *Native American Ethnobotany.* Portland, OR: Timber Press, Inc. 527–528.

Newall, C.A., L.A. Anderson, J.D. Phillipson. 1996. *Herbal Medicines: A Guide for Health-Care Professionals.* London: The Pharmaceutical Press.

Niederprum, H.J., H.U. Schweikert, K.S. Zänker. 1994. Testosterone 5-α-reductase inhibition by free fatty acids from *Sabal serrulata* fruits. *Phytomedicine* 1:127–133.

Redecker, K.D. 1998. Sabal extract WS 1473 in benign prostatic hyperplasia. *Extracta Urologica.* 21(3):23–25.

Strauch, G. et al. 1994. Comparison of finasteride (Proscar®) and *Serenoa repens* (Permixon®) in the inhibition of 5-alpha reductase in healthy male volunteers. *Eur Urol* 26(3):247–252.

Tasca, A. et al. 1985. [Treatment of obstructive symptomatology caused by prostatic adenoma with an extract of Serenoa repens: Double-blind clinical study vs. placebo] [In Italian]. *Minerva Urol Nefrol* 37(1):87–91.

Tyler, V.E. 1993. *The Honest Herbal,* 3rd ed. New York: Pharmaceutical Products Press. 285–287.

Vogel, V.J. 1970 American Indian Medicine. Norman, OK: University of Oklahoma Press. 365–366.

Wilt, T.J. et al. 1998. Saw palmetto extracts for treatment of benign prostatic hyperplasia: a systematic review. *JAMA.* 280(18):1604–1609.

Wood, H.C. and A. Osol. 1943. *United States Dispensatory*, 23rd ed. Philadelphia, PA: J.B. Lippincott. 971–972.

Ziegler, H. and U. Holscher. 1998. Efficacy of saw palmetto fruit special extract WS 1473 in patients with Alken stage I–II benign prostatic hyperplasia—open mulitcentre study. *Jatros Uro* 14(3):34–43.

Additional Resources

Boccafoschi, C. and S. Annoscia. 1983. Comparison of *Serenoa repens* extract with placebo by controlled clinical trial in patients with prostatic adenomatosis. *Urologia* 50:1257–1268.

Bombardelli, E. and P. Morazzoni. 1997. *Serenoa repens* (Bartram) J.K. Small. *Fitoterapia* 68(2):99–113.

Braeckman, J., J. Bruhwyler, K. Vandekerckhove, J. Geczy. 1997. Efficacy and safety of the extract of *Serenoa repens* in the treatment of benign prostatic hyperplasia: Therapeutic equivalence between twice and once daily dosage forms. *Phytother Res* 11:558–563.

Carbin, B.E., B. Larsson, O. Lindahl. 1990. Treatment of benign prostatic hyperplasia with phytosterols. *Br J Uro* 66(6):639–641.

Carilla, E., M. Briley, F. Fauran, C. Sultan, C. Duvilliers. 1984. Binding of Permixon, a new treatment for prostatic benign hyperplasia, to the cytosolic androgen receptor in the rat prostate. *J Steroid Biochem* 20(1):521–523.

Cukier, P. et al. 1985. Permixon versus placebo: Results of a multicenter study. *C R Ther Pharmacol Clin* 4:15–21.

Di Silverio, F. et al. 1992. Evidence that *Serenoa repens* extract displays an antiestrogenic activity in prostatic tissue of benign prostatic hypertrophy patients. *Eur Urol* 21(4):309–314.

Di Silverio, F. et al. 1993. Plant extracts in BPH. *Minerva Urol Nefrol* 45(4):143–149.

Emili, E. et al. 1983. Clinical results with a new drug therapy against benign prostatic hypertrophy (Permixon). *Urologia* 50:1042–1048.

Gerber, G.S., G.P. Zagaja, G.T. Bales, G.W. Chodak, B.A. Contreras. 1998. Saw Palmetto (Serenoa repens) in men with lower urinary tract symptoms: Effects on urodynamic parameters and voiding symptoms. *Urology* 51(6):1003–1007.

Gerber, G.S. et al. 1997. *Serenoa repens* (saw palmetto) in men with benign prostatic hyperplasia (BPH): Effects on voiding symptoms, urodynamic parameters and serum prostate specific antigen (PSA). (92nd Annual Meeting of the American Urological Association) *J Urol* 157(4):331.

Liang, T. and S. Liao. 1992. Inhibition of steroid 5μ-reductase by specific aliphatic unsaturated fatty acids. *Biochem J* 285(Pt. 2):557–562.

Mandressi, A. et al. 1987. Treatment of uncomplicated benign prostatic hypertrophy (BPH) by an extract of *Serenoa repens*. Clinical results. *J Endocrinol Invest* 10(suppl. 2):49.

McGuffin, M., C. Hobbs, R. Upton, A. Goldberg. 1997. American Herbal Product Association's *Botanical Safety Handbook*. Boca Raton: CRC Press.

Metzker, H., M. Kieser, U. Hölscher. 1996. Efficacy of a combined *Sabal-Urtica* preparation in the treatment of benign prostatic hyperplasia. *Urologie* [B] 36:292–300.

Pannunzio, E. et al. 1987. *Serenoa repens* in the treatment of human benign prostatic hypertrophy (BPH). J Urol 137(4) Part 2:226A.

Rhodes, L. et al. 1993. Comparison of finasteride (Proscar"), a 5a reductase inhibitor, and various commercial plant extracts in *in vitro* and *in vivo* 5a reductase inhibition. *Prostate* 22(1):43–45.

Roveda, S. and P. Colombo. 1994. Clinical controlled trial on therapeutic bioequivalence and tolerability of *Serenoa repens* oral capsules 160 mg or rectal capsules 640 mg. *Arch Medicina Interna* 46(2):61–75.

Semino, M. et al. 1992. [Symptomatic treatment of benign prostatic hyperplasia (BHP): A comparative study of Prazosin and *Serenoa repens*] [In Spanish] Arch Esp Urol 45(3):211–213.

Sökeland J. and J. Albrecht. 1997. [A combination of *Sabal* and *Urtica* extracts vs. finasteride in benign prostatic hyperplasia (stage I to II acc. to Alken): A comparison of therapeutic efficacy in a one year double-blind study] [In German]. *Urologe A* 36(4):327–333.

Sultan, C. et al. 1984. Inhibition of androgen metabolism and binding by a liposterolic extract of *Serenoa repens* B in human foreskin fibroblasts. *J Steroid Biochem* 20(1):515–519.

This material was adapted from *The Complete German Commission E Monographs—Therapeutic Guide to Herbal Medicines*. M. Blumenthal, W.R. Busse, A. Goldberg, J. Gruenwald, T. Hall, C.W. Riggins, R.S. Rister (eds.) S. Klein and R.S. Rister (trans.). 1998. Austin: American Botanical Council; Boston: Integrative Medicine Communications.

1) The Overview section is new information.

2) Description, Chemistry and Pharmacology, Uses, Contraindications, Side Effects, Interactions with Other Drugs, and Dosage sections have been drawn from the original work. Additional information has been added in some or all of these sections, as noted with references.

3) The dosage for equivalent preparations (tea infusion, fluidextract, and tincture) have been provided based on the following example:
   Unless otherwise prescribed: 2 g per day of [powdered, crushed, cut or whole] [plant part]
   Infusion: 2 g in 150 ml of water
   Fluidextract 1:1 (g/ml): 2 ml
   Tincture 1:5 (g/ml): 10 ml

4) The References and Additional Resources sections are new sections. Additional Resources are not cited in the monograph but are included for research purposes.

SENNA:

SENNA LEAF
(page 343)

SENNA POD (FRUIT)
(page 345)

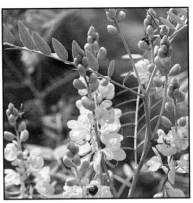

©1999 Steven Foster

Overview

Sennas are herbaceous subshrubs and both varieties used, Alexandrian and Tinnevelly, have desert origins (Bruneton, 1995). Alexandrian senna is native to northern and northeastern Africa, growing wild in semidesert and sudanosahelian zones of Africa, including Egypt, Morocco, Mauritania, Mali, and Sudan. It is cultivated in the valley of the Nile in Sudan, southern China, and India. Tinnevelly senna is native to southern India and northeastern Africa, grows wild in southern Arabia, on the coast of East Africa from Mozambique to Somaliland, and Asia. It is now cultivated on a large scale in southern and northwestern India and in Pakistan (Bruneton, 1995; Iwu, 1990; Leung and Foster, 1996; Remington et al., 1918; Wichtl and Bisset, 1994). The Tinnevelly senna of commerce is obtained mainly from India, and Alexandrian is obtained mainly from Egypt and Sudan (BHP, 1996; Wichtl and Bisset, 1994).

Senna is the most widely used anthranoid drug today and has been used for centuries in Western and Eastern systems of medicine as a laxative, usually taken as a tea or swallowed in powdered form (Bradley, 1992; Leung and Foster, 1996; Der Marderosian, 1999). Besides its wide use in conventional Western medicine, senna leaf remains an important drug used in traditional Chinese medicine and traditional Indian Ayurvedic and Unani medicine (IP, 1996; Kapoor, 1990; Karnick, 1994; Tu, 1992). Its name is derived from the Arabic *sena*. Its medical use was first described in the writings of Arabian physicians Serapion and Mesue in the ninth century C.E. (Chevallier, 1996; Grieve, 1979; Der Marderosian, 1999; Remington et al., 1918). Today, senna leaf and fruit are official in national pharmacopeias worldwide, including those of Austria, China, France, Germany, Great Britain, Hungary, India, Japan, Russia, Switzerland, the United States, the *European Pharmacopoeia*, and many others (BP, 1988; Bradley, 1992; DAB 10, 1991; IP, 1996; JP XII, 1993; ÖAB, 1981; Ph.Eur.3, 1998; Ph.Fr.X, 1994; Ph.Helv.VII, 1987; Ph.Hg.VII, 1986; Tu, 1992; USP XXII, 1990; USSR X, 1973; Wichtl and Bisset, 1994).

In Germany, senna leaf, Alexandrian senna pod, and Tinnevelly senna pod are licensed as Standard Medicinal Teas available only in the pharmacy, official in the *German Pharmacopoeia*, and approved in the Commission E monographs. They are used alone and in more than 110 prepared drugs, mostly laxatives and biliary remedies (BAnz, 1998; Bradley, 1992; Braun et al., 1997; DAB 10, 1991; Meyer-Buchtela, 1999; Wichtl and Bisset, 1994). In the United States, senna leaf, fruit, and extract are used in OTC laxatives (e.g., Correctol®, ExLax®, Senokot®, Smooth Move®).

Modern human studies have investigated the use of senna for severe constipation (Pers and Pers, 1983), for chronic constipation in long-stay elderly patients (Kinnunen et al., 1993; MacLennan and Pooler, 1974; Passmore et al., 1993), for constipation in childhood (Perkin, 1977; Sondheimer and Gervaise, 1982), for managing morphine-induced constipation (Ramesh et al., 1998), for bowel preparation prior to intravenous urography (Bailey et al., 1991), to improve colonoscopy preparation with lavage (Ziegenhagen et al., 1991; Ziegenhagen et al., 1992), for preparation prior to radiographic examination of the colon (Brouwers et al., 1980; Slanger, 1979), in management of constipation in the immediate postpartum period (Shelton, 1980), in management of postoperative constipation in anorectal surgery (Corman, 1979), to improve the visibility of abdominal organs in ultrasound examination (Heldwein et al., 1987), for disorders characterized by slow intestinal transit time or constipation (Bossi et al., 1986), and as a laxative for terminal cancer patients treated with opiates (Agra et al., 1998).

The approved modern therapeutic applications for senna are supportable based on its history of use in well established systems of traditional and conventional medicine, extensive phytochemical investigations, *in vitro* and *in vivo* pharmacological studies in animals, and human clinical studies.

Pharmacopeial grade senna leaf must consist of the dried leaflets of Alexandrian or Tinnevelly senna, or a mixture of both species. It must contain not less than 2.5% of hydroxyanthracene glycosides, calculated as sennoside B. Botanical identification must be confirmed by thin-layer chromatography (TLC), macroscopic and microscopic examinations, and organoleptic evaluation. The stomatal index (a calculation of the percentage of stomata—holes in the leaf's skin through which the plant breathes—comprising the number of epidermal cells, including the stomata, each stoma being counted as one cell) for Alexandrian senna is 10–15, usually 12.5 and for Tinnevelly senna it is 14–20, usually 17.5 (BP, 1988; IP, 1996; Ph.Eur.3, 1998; Tu, 1992). The *Japanese Pharmacopoeia* additionally requires a purity standard of not more than 5.0% rachis (the main axis of the compound leaf) and fruits contained in the senna leaf (JP XII, 1993). The *French Pharmacopoeia* additionally requires a test for absence of known adulterants, namely *Cassia auriculata* (Bruneton, 1995; Ph.Fr.X, 1994). The ESCOP monograph requires the material to comply with the *European Pharmacopoeia* (ESCOP, 1997).

Pharmacopeial grade senna leaf standardized dry extract (*Sennae folii extractum siccum normatum*) must be manufactured from *European Pharmacopoeia* (Ph.Eur.) grade Sennae folium in accordance with the Ph.Eur. Extracta monograph. It must contain minimum 5.5% and maximum 8.0% hydroxyanthracene glycosides calculated as sennoside B with reference to the dry extract, with an allowed deviation of ±10% (Ph.Eur.3, 1998).

Pharmacopeial grade senna pod must consist of the dried fruit of Alexandrian or Tinnevelly senna, or both. It must contain not less than 3.4% (Alexandrian senna pod) and not less than 2.2% (Tinnevelly senna pod) hydroxyanthracene glycosides, calculated as sennoside B. Botanical identification must be confirmed by TLC, macroscopic and microscopic examinations, and organoleptic evaluation (BP, 1988; IP, 1996; Ph.Eur.3, 1998). The *Japanese Herbal Medicines Codex*, however, requires not less than 2.2% of total anthraquinone glycosides calculated as sennoside A (JHMC, 1993). The ESCOP monographs require the material to comply with the *European Pharmacopoeia* (ESCOP, 1997).

SENNA LEAF

Latin Name:
Senna alexandrina

Pharmacopeial Name:
Sennae folium

Other Names:
Alexandrian senna, Khartoum senna, Tinnevelly senna

Description

Senna leaf consists of the dried leaflets (pinnulae) of *Cassia senna* L. (*C. acutifolia* Del.) [Fam. Fabaceae], known as Alexandrian or Khartoum senna, or of *C. angustifolia* Vahl, known as Tinnevelly senna, and their preparations in effective dosage. [Currently accepted nomenclature for all three cultivars is *Senna alexandrina* Miller.] The leaves contain anthranoids, mainly of the bianthrone type. The content of anthranoids of the emodin and aloe-emodin type is usually higher in senna pod. The preparation must conform to the currently valid pharmacopeia.

Chemistry and Pharmacology

Senna leaf contains 1.5–3% hydroxyanthracene glycosides, mainly sennosides A and B, which are rhein-dianthrones, and smaller amounts of sennosides C and D, which are rhein-aloe-emodin-heterodianthrones; naphthalene glycosides; flavonoids (derivatives of kaempferol and isorhamnetin); 10–12% mineral matter; 7–10% mucilage (galactose, arabinose, rhamnose, and galacturonic acid); about 8% polyol (pinitol); sugars (glucose, fructose, and sucrose); and resins (Bradley, 1992; Bruneton, 1995; ESCOP, 1997; Leung and Foster, 1996; Newall et al., 1996; Wichtl and Bisset, 1994).

The Commission E reported 1,8-dihydroxy-anthracene derivatives have a laxative effect. This effect is due to the sennosides, specifically their active metabolite in the colon, rheinanthrone. The effect is caused by inhibiting stationary and stimulating propulsive contractions in the colon. This results in an accelerated intestinal passage and, because of the shortened contact time, a reduction in liquid absorbed through the lumen. In addition, stimulation of active chloride secretion increases water and electrolyte content of the contents of the intestine.

Systematic studies pertaining to the kinetics of senna leaf preparations are not available. However, it must be supposed that the aglycones contained in the drug are absorbed in the upper small intestine. The β-glycosides are prodrugs that are neither absorbed nor cleaved in the upper gastrointestinal tract. They are degraded in the colon by bacterial enzymes to rheinanthrone, the laxative metabolite. The systemic availability of rheinanthrone is very low. Animal experiments reveal that less than 5% is passed in the urine in oxidized form or in conjugated form as rhein and sennodine. The major amount of rheinanthrone (more than 90%) is bound to the feces in the colon and excreted as a polymer.

Active metabolites, such as rhein, infiltrate in small amounts into the milk ducts. A laxative effect on nursing infants has not been observed. The placental permeability for rhein is very small, as was observed in animal experiments.

Drug preparations (i.e., preparations from whole senna leaf) have a higher general toxicity than the pure glycosides, presumably due to the content of aglycones. Experiments with senna leaf preparations are not available. A senna extract showed mutagenic toxicity *in vitro*. The pure substance, sennoside A,

B, showed no mutagenic toxicity *in vitro*. An *in vivo* study with a defined extract of senna pod revealed no mutagenicity. Preparations with an anthranoid content of 1.4–3.5% (calculated as the sum of specific individual compounds) were used. These were potentially equivalent to 0.9–2.9% rhein, 0.05–0.15% aloe-emodin, and 0.001–0.006% emodin. The results appear to be also applicable for specific senna leaf preparations. Some positive results have been observed for aloe-emodin, and emodin. A study for carcinogenicity was performed with an enriched sennoside fraction containing about 40.8% anthranoids, of which 35% were sennosides (calculated as the sum of the individually determined compounds), equivalent to about 25.2% of the calculated potential rhein, 2.3% potential aloe-emodin, and 0.007% potential emodin. The tested substance contained 142 ppm free aloe-emodin and 9 ppm free emodin. The study was conducted over 104 weeks. Rats received up to 25 mg/kg body weight and showed no substance-dependent increase of tumors.

Uses
The Commission E approved the internal use of senna leaf for constipation.

The World Health Organization (WHO) approves senna leaf for short-term use in occasional constipation (WHO, 1999).

The *British Herbal Compendium* indicates its use for constipation and conditions in which easy defecation with soft stools is desirable, such as anal fissure or hemorrhoids (Bradley, 1992). ESCOP indicates it for short-term use in cases of occasional constipation (ESCOP, 1997); the German Standard License for senna leaf tea indicates its use for constipation; conditions in which easy bowel evacuation with soft stools is desirable, for example in cases of anal fissures, hemorrhoids, and after recto-anal operations; for bowel clearance before X-ray examinations; and before and after abdominal surgery

(Bradley, 1992; Wichtl and Bisset, 1994).

Contraindications
Intestinal obstruction, acute intestinal inflammation, e.g., Crohn's disease, colitis ulcerosa, appendicitis, abdominal pain of unknown origin. Children under 12 years of age.

Side Effects
In single incidents, cramp-like discomforts of the gastrointestinal tract. These cases require a dosage reduction.

With chronic use or abuse: Disturbance of electrolyte balance, especially potassium deficiency, albuminuria and hematuria. Pigment implantation into the intestinal mucosa (*pseudomelanosis coli*) is harmless and usually reverses on discontinuation of the drug. Potassium deficiency can lead to disorders of heart function and muscular weakness, especially with concurrent use of cardiac glycosides, diuretics, or corticosteroids.

Use During Pregnancy and Lactation
Due to insufficient toxicological investigation, this herb should not be used during pregnancy or lactation.

Interactions with Other Drugs
In cases of chronic use or abuse, loss of potassium may potentiate cardiac glycosides and have an effect on anti-arrhythmic medications.

Potassium deficiency may be exacerbated by simultaneous administration of thiazide diuretics, corticoadrenal steroids, or licorice root.

Dosage and Administration
Unless otherwise prescribed: 0.6–2.0 g (corresponding to 20–30 mg hydroxyanthracene derivatives calculated as sennoside B) per day of cut or powdered herb or dried extracts for teas, decoctions, cold macerates, or elixirs.

Liquid or solid forms of medication exclusively for oral use.

The correct dosage is the smallest dose necessary to maintain a soft stool.

Note: The form of administration should be smaller than the daily dose.

Dried leaf: 0.6–2.0 g.

Infusion or decoction: 0.6–2.0 g in 150 ml hot water for 10 to 30 minutes.

Cold macerate: 0.6–2.0 g in 150 ml cold water for 10 to 12 hours, strain, then heat before drinking.

Fluidextract 1:1 (g/ml): 0.6–2.0 ml.

Elixir: 0.6–2.0 ml sweetened fluidextract.

Dry hydroalcoholic extract (5.5–8.0% hydroxyanthracene glycosides): 0.25–0.55 g.

Special caution for use: Stimulating laxatives must not be used for more than one to two weeks without medical advice.

Overdosage: Electrolyte and fluid imbalance.

Special warnings: Use of a stimulating laxative for longer than the recommended period can cause intestinal sluggishness.

This preparation should be used only if no effects can be obtained through changes in diet or the use of bulk-forming products.

SENNA POD (FRUIT)

Latin Name:
Senna alexandrina

Pharmacopeial Names:
Sennae fructus acutifoliae, Sennae fructus angustifoliae

Other Names:
Alexandrian senna pod, Tinnevelly senna pod

Description
Alexandrian senna pod consists of the dried fruits of *Cassia senna* L. (*C. acutifolia* Del. [syn. *S. alexandrina*]) [Fam. Fabaceae] and their preparations in effective dosage. Tinnevelly senna pod consists of dried fruits of *C. angustifolia* Vahl and their preparations in effective dosage. [Currently accepted nomenclature for both cultivars is *Senna alexandrina* Miller.] Sufficient pharmacological-toxicologic studies are available for preparations containing 1.4–3.5% anthranoids (calculated as sum of individually determined compounds), equivalent to 0.9–2.3% potential rhein, 0.05–0.15% potential aloe-emodin, and 0.001–0.006% potential emodin. The preparation must conform to the currently valid pharmacopeia.

Chemistry and Pharmacology
Senna pod contains 2.2–3.5% hydroxyanthracene glycosides, mainly sennosides A and B, which are rhein-dianthrones, and smaller amounts of sennosides C and D, which are rhein-aloe-emodin-heterodianthrones; naphthalene glycosides; flavonoids (derivatives of kaempferol and isorhamnetin); mineral matter; mucilage (galactose, arabinose, rhamnose, galacturonic acid); polyol (pinitol); sugars (glucose, fructose, sucrose) (Bradley, 1992; Bruneton, 1995; ESCOP, 1997; Leung and Foster, 1996; Newall et al., 1996).

The Commission E reported 1,8-dihydroxy-anthracene derivatives have a laxative effect. This effect is due to the sennosides, specifically their active metabolite in the colon, rheinanthrone. The effect is caused by inhibiting stationary and stimulating propulsive contractions in the colon. This results in an accelerated intestinal passage and, because of the shortened contact time, a reduction in liquid absorbed through the lumen. In addition, stimulation of the active chloride secretion increases the water and electrolyte content of the stool.

Systematic studies pertaining to the kinetics of senna pod preparations are not available. However, it must be supposed that the aglycones contained in the drug are already absorbed in the upper small intestine. The β-glycosides are prodrugs that are neither absorbed nor cleaved in the upper gastrointestinal tract. They are degraded in the colon by bacterial enzymes to rheinanthrone, the laxative metabolite. The systemic availability of rheinanthrone is very low. Animal experiments revealed that less than 5% is passed in the urine in oxidized form or conjugated form as rhein and sennodine. The major amount of rheinanthrone (more than 90%) is bound to the feces in the colon and excreted as polymers.

Active metabolites, such as rhein, infiltrate in small amounts into the milk ducts. A laxative effect on nursing infants has not been observed. The placental permeability for rhein is very small, as was observed in animals.

Drug preparations (i.e., preparations from whole senna pod) have a higher general toxicity than the pure glycosides, presumably due to the content of aglycones. Experiments with senna leaf preparations are not available. A senna extract showed mutagenic toxicity *in vitro*; the pure substance, sennoside A, B, was negative. An *in vivo* study with a defined extract of senna pod revealed no mutagenicity. Preparations with an anthranoid content of 1.4–3.5% were used (calculated as the sum of specific individual compounds) that were potentially equivalent to 0.9–2.9% rhein, 0.05–0.15% aloe-emodin, and 0.001–0.006% emodin. The results appear to be also applicable for specific senna leaf preparations. Some positive results have been observed for aloe-emodin and emodin. A study for carcinogenicity was performed with an enriched sennoside fraction containing about 40.8% anthranoids, of which 35% were sennosides (calculated as sum of the individually determined compounds), equivalent to about 25.2% of the calculated potential rhein, 2.3% potential aloe-emodin, and 0.007% potential emodin. The tested substance contained 142 ppm free aloe-emodin and 9 ppm free emodin. The study was conducted over 104 weeks. Rats received up to 25 mg/kg body weight and showed no substance-dependent increase of tumors.

Uses

The Commission E approved the internal use of senna pod for constipation.

The World Health Organization (WHO) approves senna pod for short-term use in occasional constipation (WHO, 1999).

The *British Herbal Compendium* indicates its use for constipation and conditions in which easy defecation with soft stools is desirable, such as anal fissure or hemorrhoids (Bradley, 1992). ESCOP indicates it for short-term use in cases of occasional constipation (ESCOP, 1997). The German Standard License for senna pod tea indicates its use for constipation; conditions in which easy bowel evacuation with soft stools is desirable, for example, in cases of anal fissures, hemorrhoids, and after recto-anal operations; for bowel clearance before X-ray examinations; and before and after abdominal surgery (Bradley, 1992).

Contraindications

Intestinal obstruction, acute intestinal inflammation, e.g., Crohn's disease, colitis ulcerosa, appendicitis, abdominal pain of unknown origin. Children under 12 years of age.

Side Effects

In single incidents, cramp-like discomforts of the gastrointestinal tract. These cases require a dosage reduction.

With chronic use or abuse: Disturbance of electrolyte balance, especially potassium deficiency, albuminuria and hematuria. Pigment implantation into the intestinal mucosa (*pseudomelanosis coli*) is harmless and usually reverses on discontinuation of the drug. Potassium deficiency can lead to disorders of heart function and muscular weakness, especially with concurrent use of cardiac glycosides, diuretics, or corticosteroids.

Use During Pregnancy and Lactation

During the first trimester of pregnancy, senna pod preparations should be used only if a therapeutic effect cannot be obtained with a change in diet or through the use of swelling laxatives. Active metabolites, such as rhein, infiltrate into the milk ducts. A laxative effect on nursing infants has not been observed.

Interactions with Other Drugs

In cases of chronic use or abuse, loss of potassium may potentiate cardiac glycosides and have an effect on antiarrhythmic medications. Potassium deficiency may be exacerbated by simultaneous administration of thiazide diuretics, corticosteroids, or licorice root.

Dosage and Administration

Unless otherwise prescribed: 0.6–2.0 g (corresponding to 20–30 mg hydroxyanthracene derivatives calculated as sennoside B) per day of cut or powdered fruit or dried extracts for teas, decoctions, cold macerates, or elixirs. Liquid or solid forms of medication exclusively for oral use. The correct dosage is the smallest dose necessary to maintain a soft stool.

Note: The form of administration should be smaller than the daily dose. Dried pods (powdered or whole): 0.6–2.0 g.

Infusion or decoction: 0.6–2.0 g in 150 ml warm or hot water for 10 to 30 minutes.

Cold macerate: 0.6–2.0 g in 150 ml cold water for two to three hours, strain, then heat before drinking.

Fluidextract 1:1 (g/ml): 0.6–2.0 ml.
Elixir: 0.6–2.0ml sweetened fluidextract.
Dry hydroalcoholic extract (5.5–8.0% hydroxyanthracene glycosides): 0.25–0.55 g.

Special caution for use: Stimulating laxatives must not be used for more than one to two weeks without medical advice.

Overdosage: Electrolyte and fluid imbalance.

Special warnings: Use of a stimulating laxative for longer than the recommended period can cause intestinal sluggishness.

This preparation should be used only if no effects can be obtained through changes in diet or use of bulk-forming products.

References

Agra, Y. et al. 1998. Efficacy of senna versus lactulose in terminal cancer patients treated with opioids. *J Pain Symptom Manage* 15(1):1–7.

Bailey, S.R., P.N. Tyrrell, M. Hale. 1991. A trial to assess the effectiveness of bowel preparation prior to intravenous urography. *Clin Radiol* 44(5):335–337.

BAnz. See *Bundesanzeiger*.

Bossi, S. et al. 1986. [Clinical study of a new preparation from plantago seeds and senna pods] [In Italian]. *Acta Biomed Ateneo Parmense* 57(5–6):179–186.

Bradley, P.R. (ed.). 1992. *British Herbal Compendium*, Vol. 1. Bournemouth: British Herbal Medicine Association.

Braun, R. et al. 1997. *Standardzulassungen für Fertigarzneimittel—Text and Kommentar*. Stuttgart: Deutscher Apotheker Verlag.

British Herbal Pharmacopoeia (BHP). 1996. Exeter, U.K.: British Herbal Medicine Association. 168.

British Pharmacopoeia (BP). 1988. (With subsequent Addenda up to 1992.) London: Her Majesty's Stationery Office.

Brouwers, J.R., W.P. van Ouwerkerk, S.M. de Boer, L. Thoman. 1980. A controlled trial of senna preparations and other laxatives used for bowel cleansing prior to radiological examination. *Pharmacology* 20(suppl 1):58–64.

Bruneton, J. 1995. *Pharmacognosy, Phytochemistry, Medicinal Plants*. Paris: Lavoisier Publishing.

Bundesanzeiger (BAnz). 1998. Monographien der Kommission E (Zulassungs- und Aufbereitungskommission am BGA für den humanmed. Bereich, phytotherapeutische Therapierichtung und Stoffgruppe). Köln: Bundesgesundheitsamt (BGA).

Chevallier, A. 1996. Encyclopedia of Medicinal Plants. New York: DK Publishing. 72.

Corman, M.L. 1979. Management of postoperative constipation in anorectal surgery. *Dis Colon Rectum* 22(3):149–151.

Der Marderosian, A. (ed.). 1999. *The Review of Natural Products*. St. Louis: Facts and Comparisons.

Deutsches Arzneibuch, 10th ed. (DAB 10). 1991. (With subsequent supplements through 1996.) Stuttgart: Deutscher Apotheker Verlag.

ESCOP. 1997. "Sennae folium," "Sennae fructus acutifoliae," and "Sennae fructus angustifoliae." *Monographs on the Medicinal Uses of Plant Drugs*. Exeter, U.K.: European Scientific Cooperative on Phytotherapy.

Europäisches Arzneibuch, 3rd ed., 1st suppl. (Ph.Eur.3). 1998. Stuttgart: Deutscher Apotheker Verlag. 612–617.

Grieve, M. 1979. *A Modern Herbal*. New York: Dover Publications, Inc.

Heldwein, W. et al. 1987. Evaluation of the usefulness of dimethicone and/or senna extract in improving the visualization of abdominal organs. *JCU J Clin Ultrasound* 15(7):455–458.

Indian Pharmacopoeia, Vol. 1. (IP 1996). 1996. Delhi: Government of India Ministry of Health and Family Welfare—Controller of Publications. 675–678.

Iwu, M.M. 1990. *Handbook of African Medicinal Plants*. Boca Raton: CRC Press. 143–144.

Japanese Herbal Medicines Codex (JHMC). 1993. Tokyo: Government of Japan Ministry of Health and Welfare—Yakuji Nippo, Ltd. 252–254.

Japanese Pharmacopoeia, 12th ed. (JP XII). 1993. Tokyo: Government of Japan Ministry of Health and Welfare—Yakuji Nippo, Ltd. 255–257.

Kapoor, L.D. 1990. *Handbook of Ayurvedic Medicinal Plants*. Boca Raton: CRC Press. 104.

Karnick, C.R. 1994. *Pharmacopoeial Standards of Herbal Plants*. Delhi: Sri Satguru Publications.

Kinnunen, O., I. Winblad, P. Koistinen, J. Salokannel. 1993. Safety and efficacy of a bulk laxative containing senna versus lactulose in the treatment of chronic constipation in geriatric patients. *Pharmacology* 47(suppl 1):253–255.

Leung, A.Y. and S. Foster. 1996. *Encyclopedia of Common Natural Ingredients Used in Food, Drugs, and Cosmetics*, 2nd ed. New York: John Wiley & Sons, Inc.

MacLennan, W.J. and A.F. Pooler. 1974–1975. A comparison of sodium picosulphate ("Laxoberal") with standardized senna ("Senokot") in geriatric patients. Curr Med Res Opin 2(10):641–647.

Meyer-Buchtela, E. 1999. *Tee-Rezepturen—Ein Handbuch für Apotheker und Ärzte*. Stuttgart: Deutscher Apotheker Verlag.

Newall, C.A., L.A. Anderson, J.D. Phillipson. 1996. *Herbal Medicines: A Guide for Health-Care Professionals*. London: The Pharmaceutical Press.

Österreichisches Arzneibuch, Vols. 1–2. (ÖAB). 1981. Wien: Verlag der Österreichischen Staatsdruckerei.

Passmore, A.P., K.W. Davies, C. Stoker, M.E. Scott. 1993. Chronic constipation in long stay elderly patients: a comparison of lactulose and a senna-fibre combination. *BMJ* 307(6907):769–771.

Passmore, A.P., K.W. Davies, P.G. Flanagan, C. Stoker, M.G. Scott. 1993. A comparison of Agiolax and lactulose in elderly patients with chronic constipation. *Pharmacology* 47(suppl 1):249–252.

Perkin, J.M. 1977. Constipation in childhood: a controlled comparison between lactulose and standardized senna. *Curr Med Res Opin* 4(8):540–543.

Pers, M. and B. Pers. 1983. A crossover comparative study with two bulk laxatives. *J Int Med Res* 11(1):51–53.

Pharmacopée Française Xe Édition (Ph.Fr.X). 1994. Moulins-les-Metz: Maisonneuve S.A.

Pharmacopoeia Helvetica, 7th ed. Vol. 1–4. (Ph.Helv.VII). 1987. Bern: Office Central Fédéral des Imprimés et du Matériel.

Pharmacopoea Hungaric, 7th ed. (Ph.Hg.VII). 1986. Budapest: Medicina Könyvkiadó.

Ph.Eur.3. See *Europäisches Arzneibuch*.

Ramesh, P.R., K.S. Kumar, M.R. Rajagopal, P. Balachandran, P.K. Warrier. 1998. Managing morphine-induced constipation: a controlled comparison of an Ayurvedic formulation and senna. *J Pain Symptom Manage* 16(4):240–244.

Remington, J.P. et al. 1918. *The Dispensatory of the United States of America*, 20th ed. Philadelphia; London: J.B. Lippincott Co. 990–996.

Shelton, M.G. 1980. Standardized senna in the management of constipation in the puerperium: a clinical trial. *S Afr Med J* 57(3):78–80.

Slanger, A. 1979. Comparative study of a standardized senna liquid and castor oil in preparing patients for radiographic examination of the colon. *Dis Colon Rectum* 22(5):356–359.

Sondheimer, J.M. and E.P. Gervaise. 1982. Lubricant versus laxative in the treatment of chronic functional constipation of children: a comparative study. *J Pediatr Gastroenterol Nutr* 1(2):223–226.

State Pharmacopoeia of the Union of Soviet Socialist Republics, 10th ed. (USSR X). 1973. Moscow: Ministry of Health of the U.S.S.R.

Tu, G. (ed.). 1992. *Pharmacopoeia of the People's Republic of China* (English Edition 1992). Beijing: Guangdong Science and Technology Press. 57–58.

The United States Pharmacopeia, 22nd rev. (USP XXII). 1990. Rockville, MD: U.S. Pharmacopoeial Convention.

USSR X. See *State Pharmacopoeia of the Union of Soviet Socialist Republics*.

WHO. See World Health Organization.

Wichtl, M. and N.G. Bisset (eds.). 1994. *Herbal Drugs and Phytopharmaceuticals*. Stuttgart: Medpharm Scientific Publishers.

World Health Organization (WHO). 1999. "Sennae folium" and "Sennae fructus." *WHO Monographs on Selected Medicinal Plants*, Vol. 1. Geneva: World Health Organization.

Ziegenhagen, D.J., E. Zehnter, W. Tacke, T. Gheorghiu, W. Kruis. 1992. Senna vs. bisacodyl in addition to Golytely lavage for colonoscopy preparation—a prospective randomized trial. *Z Gastroenterol* 30(1):17–19.

Ziegenhagen, D.J., E. Zehnter, W. Tacke, W. Kruis. 1991. Addition of senna improves colonoscopy preparation with lavage: a prospective randomized trial. *Gastrointest Endosc* 37(5):547–549.

Additional Resources

British Pharmaceutical Codex (BPC). 1973. London: The Pharmaceutical Press.

Deutsches Arzneibuch, 9th ed. Vol. 3. (DAB 9). 1988. Kommentar. Stuttgart: Wissenschaftliche Verlagsgesellschaft. 3110–3114.

Deutsches Arzneibuch, 10th ed. Vol. 1–6. (DAB 10). 1991. Kommentar. Stuttgart: Wissenschaftliche Verlagsgesellschaft.

Hänsel, R., K. Keller, H. Rimpler, G. Schneider (eds.). 1992. *Hagers Handbuch der Pharmazeutischen Praxis*, 5th ed. Vol. 4. Berlin-Heidelberg: Springer Verlag. 701–725.

Kobashi, K., T. Nishimura, M. Kusaka, M. Hattori, T. Namba. 1980. Metabolism of sennosides by human intestinal bacteria. *Planta Med* 40(3):225–236.

Morton, J.F. 1977. *Major Medicinal Plants*: Botany, Culture, and Uses. Springfield, IL: Chas. C. Thomas. 147–149.

National Formulary (NF), 5th ed. 1926. Washington, D.C.: American Pharmaceutical Association. 13, 229.

Norme Française (NF). 1989. NF T 75-348. Paris: Direction des Journaux Officiels.

Reynolds, J.E.F. (ed.). 1996. *Martindale: The Extra Pharmacopoeia*, 31st ed. London: Royal Pharmaceutical Society. 1240–1241.

Steinegger, E. and R. Hänsel. 1992. *Pharmakognosie*, 5th ed. Berlin-Heidelberg: Springer Verlag. 425–428.

Trease, G.E. and W.C. Evans. 1989. *Trease and Evans' Pharmacognosy*, 13th ed. London; Philadelphia: Baillière Tindall.

The United States Pharmacopeia, 21st rev. (USP XXI). 1985. Rockville, MD: U.S. Pharmacopoeial Convention.

U.S.A. Dept. of Health and Human Services: Food and Drug Administration. 1985. *Code of Federal Regulations 21* (CFR 21). Part 334. Laxative Drug Products for Over-the-Counter Human Use, Tentative Final Monograph. *Federal Register* 50(10):2124, 2151–2158.

USP Committee of Revision. 1893. *The Pharmacopoeia of the United States of America*, 7th decennial rev. (1890). Philadelphia: USP Committee of Revision. 218.

Wagner, H., S. Bladt, E.M. Zgainski. 1984. *Plant Drug Analysis*. Berlin-Heidelberg: Springer Verlag. 111.

These monographs, published by the Commission E in 1993, were modified based on new scientific research. They contain more extensive pharmacological and therapeutic information taken directly from the Commission E.

This material was adapted from *The Complete German Commission E Monographs—Therapeutic Guide to Herbal Medicines*. M. Blumenthal, W.R. Busse, A. Goldberg, J. Gruenwald, T. Hall, C.W. Riggins, R.S. Rister (eds.) S. Klein and R.S. Rister (trans.). 1998. Austin: American Botanical Council; Boston: Integrative Medicine Communications.

1) The Overview section is new information.

2) Description, Chemistry and Pharmacology, Uses, Contraindications, Side Effects, Interactions with Other Drugs, and Dosage sections have been drawn from the original work. Additional information has been added in some or all of these sections, as noted with references.

3) The dosage for equivalent preparations (tea infusion, fluidextract, and tincture) have been provided based on the following example:
   Unless otherwise prescribed: 2 g per day of [powdered, crushed, cut or whole] [plant part]
   Infusion: 2 g in 150 ml of water
   Fluidextract 1:1 (g/ml): 2 ml
   Tincture 1:5 (g/ml): 10 ml

4) The References and Additional Resources sections are new sections. Additional Resources are not cited in the monograph but are included for research purposes.

SHEPHERD'S PURSE

Latin Name:
Capsella bursa pastoris

Pharmacopeial Name:
Bursae pastoris herba

Other Names:
pick-pocket, witches' pouches

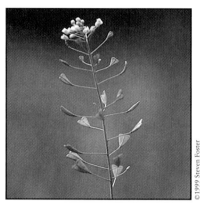
©1999 Steven Foster

Overview

Shepherd's purse is a small annual or biennial herb native to Europe (Karnick, 1994), found growing as a weed in farmland, fallow land, and along roadsides worldwide (Wichtl, 1996). It is also cultivated in India (Karnick, 1994) and other temperate and warm regions around the world (Bown, 1995). The material of commerce is collected mainly from wild plants in southeastern Europe (BHP, 1996), particularly from Bulgaria, Hungary, former Yugoslavia, and the former U.S.S.R. (Wichtl and Bisset, 1994).

The use of shepherd's purse as a food dates back at least eight thousand years. Archaeobotanical remains containing shepherd's purse seeds were recovered during excavation of the Catal Huyuk site in Turkey (ca. 5950 B.C.E.). Seeds were also recovered from the stomach of the Tollund man (ca. 500 B.C.E.–400 C.E.) (Bown, 1995). Its common name is derived from the purse shape of the plant's seed pods. Traditionally, shepherd's purse has been used as an antihemorrhagic agent and to treat diarrhea and acute cystitis (Newall et al., 1996). Nineteenth century American Eclectic physicians used shepherd's purse to treat hematuria (blood in the urine) and menorrhagia and as an external treatment for bruises, strains, and arthritis (Ellingwood, 1983). The plant was used during World War I to stop hemorrhaging when other medicines were not available. Through the end of the nineteenth century and well into the twentieth, traditional herbalists used shepherd's purse for inflammation of the genitourinary tract, for cystitis accompanied by white discharge (Grieve, 1979), to stop hemorrhage following childbirth, and internal bleeding in the lungs and colon (Hutchens, 1991).

Clinical studies that correlate with pharmacological studies to humans have not been conducted. Use during heavy menstrual bleeding, however, seems justified through empirical evidence. Efforts to determine a bioactive hemostatic principle in shepherd's purse point to an unspecified peptide (Schulz et al., 1998). Most recently, shepherd's purse has been investigated for its possible use as a biomonitor of heavy metals contamination in the environment. The authors of this study reported that it may become a particularly useful plant for monitoring short-term changes in pollution levels in urban areas (Aksoy et al., 1999).

In Germany, shepherd's purse is approved in the Commission E monographs (BAnz, 1998) and the tea form is official in the Standard License monographs (Braun et al., 1997) for treatment of menorrhagia, metrorrhagia, and nosebleeds. In extract form, it is found in a few anti-dysmenorrhea drugs (Wichtl and Bisset, 1994). An ethanolic infusion of the dried aerial parts is also official in the *German Homeopathic Pharmacopoeia* (GHP, 1993). Its modern uses in Indian Ayurvedic medicine (Karnick, 1994) and in traditional Chinese medicine (Huang, 1999) are closely comparable to its approved uses in Germany. In China, a decoction of the dried whole plant is used as an antihypertensive drug and also as a hemostatic agent for treatment of chyluria (fat globules in the urine) and hematuria (Huang, 1999).

Pharmacopeial grade shepherd's purse consists of the dried, aerial parts of *Capsella bursa-pastoris* (L.) Medikus, harvested near the end of the flowering period when the seed pods are present. Botanical identification must be confirmed by thin-layer chromatography (TLC), macroscopic and microscopic examinations, and organoleptic evaluations. It must contain not less than 12% water-soluble extractive (BHP, 1996). The German Standard License requires that it consist of the quickly dried aerial parts, collected from dry locations during high summer, containing not less than 18% water-soluble extractive. Botanical identification must be confirmed by TLC, macroscopic and microscopic examinations, and organoleptic evaluations (Braun et al., 1997).

Description

Shepherd's purse herb consists of the fresh or dried, aboveground parts of *C. bursa pastoris* (L.) Medikus [Fam. Cruciferae] and its preparations in effective dosage.

Chemistry and Pharmacology

Shepherd's purse contains flavonoids, including luteolin and quercetin 7-rutinosides and luteolin 7-galactoside; glucosinolates (e.g., sinigrin) (Iurisson, 1973; Wichtl and Bisset, 1994); minerals, including relatively high amounts of potassium salts; amino acids (e.g., proline); a peptide with hemostyptic action (Park, 1967; Wichtl and Bisset, 1994); bursic acid, citric acid; vitamins A and K (Huang, 1999); approximately 0.02% volatile oil (e.g., camphor) (Miyazawa et al., 1979). The previously reported occurrence of biogenetic amines and saponins is disputed (Wichtl, 1996).

In pharmacological studies, shepherd's purse has been found to have anti-inflammatory and diuretic actions. Intraperitoneal administration of shepherd's purse extract to rats blocked the formation of stress-induced ulcers and reduced recovery time (Kuroda and Takagi, 1969). Antineoplastic, central nervous system-depressant, and hypotensive effects have also been observed, and *in vitro* tests have shown smooth-muscle stimulant effects. Cardiac activity includes increased coronary blood flow, negative chronotropic effects, positive inotropic effects, and coronary vasodilation in laboratory animals (Kuroda and Takagi, 1969; Iurisson, 1971).

The Commission E reported muscarine-like effects with dose-dependent lowering and elevation of blood pressure, positive inotropic and chronotropic cardiac effects, and increased uterine contraction; parenteral application only.

The *British Herbal Pharmacopoeia* reported anti-hemorrhagic action (BHP, 1996). *In vitro* studies conclude that shepherd's purse acts as a smooth muscle stimulant (Kuroda and Takagi, 1969; Iurisson, 1971).

Uses

The Commission E approved the internal use of shepherd's purse for symptomatic treatment of mild menorrhagia and metrorrhagia. Topical application is approved for nosebleeds and its external use is also approved for superficial skin wounds and bruising.

The German Standard License for shepherd's purse tea indicates its use as supportive treatment for nosebleeds and excessive menstrual bleeding (Braun et al., 1997). In India, it is applied topically to injured varicose veins as an antihemorrhagic agent (Karnick, 1994).

Contraindications

Individuals with a history of kidney stones should use cautiously (McGuffin et al., 1997).

Side Effects

None known.

Use During Pregnancy and Lactation

Not recommended during pregnancy (McGuffin et al., 1997). No restrictions known during lactation.

Interactions with Other Drugs

None known.

Dosage and Administration

Unless otherwise prescribed: 10–15 g per day of cut herb for tea and other equivalent galenical preparations for internal use and 5–8 g per day for topical use.

Internal: Infusion: Steep 2–4 g in 150 ml boiled water for 15 minutes, two to four times daily between meals (Braun et al., 1997; Meyer-Buchtela, 1999). Fluidextract 1:1 (g/ml), in 25% alcohol: 1–4 ml, three times daily (BHP, 1983; Karnick, 1994; Newall et al., 1996). Note: Excessive doses of the extract may cause heart palpitations (McGuffin et al., 1997).

Topical use: Infusion: Steep 3–5 g in 180 ml (^{3}/$_4$ cup) boiled water for 10 to 15 minutes (Commission E), applied to injured area (Karnick, 1994). Fluidextract: daily dosage: 5–8 g (Erg.B.6), applied to injured area (Karnick, 1994).

References

Aksoy, A., W.H. Hale, J.M. Dixon. 1999. *Capsella bursa-pastoris* (L.) Medic. as a biomonitor of heavy metals. *Sci Total Environ* 226(2–3):177–186.

BAnz. See *Bundesanzeiger*.

Bown, D. 1995. *Encyclopedia of Herbs and Their Uses*. New York: DK Publishing, Inc. 99, 254.

Braun, R. et al. 1997. *Standardzulassungen für Fertigarzneimittel—Text and Kommentar*. Stuttgart: Deutscher Apotheker Verlag.

British Herbal Pharmacopoeia (BHP). 1983. Keighley, U.K.: British Herbal Medicine Association.

British Herbal Pharmacopoeia (BHP). 1996. Exeter, U.K.: British Herbal Medicine Association. 169–170.

Bundesanzeiger (BAnz). 1998. Monographien der Kommission E (Zulassungs- und Aufbereitungskommission am BGA für den humanmed. Bereich, phytotherapeutische Therapierichtung und Stoffgruppe). Köln: Bundesgesundheitsamt (BGA).

Ellingwood, F. 1983. *American Materia Medica, Therapeutics and Pharmacognosy*. Portland, OR: Eclectic Medical Publications [reprint of 1919 original].

Ergänzungsbuch zum Deutschen Arzneibuch, 6th ed. (Erg.B.6). 1953. Stuttgart: Deutscher Apotheker Verlag.

German Homeopathic Pharmacopoeia (GHP). 1993. Translation of the German *Homöopathisches Arzneibuch* (HAB 1), 5th suppl. 1991 to the 1st ed. 1978. Stuttgart. Deutscher Apotheker Verlag. 273–274.

Grieve, M. 1979. *A Modern Herbal*. New York: Dover Publications, Inc.

Huang, K.C. 1999. *The Pharmacology of Chinese Herbs*, 2nd ed. Boca Raton: CRC Press. 354.

Hutchens, A. 1991. *Indian Herbology of North America*. Boston: Shambala.

Iurisson, S. 1971. [Determination of active substances of *Capsella bursa pastoris*] [In Russian]. *Tartu Riiliku Ulikooli Toim* (270):71–79.

_____. 1973. [Flavonoid substances of *Capsella bursa pastoris* (L.) Medic] [In Russian]. *Farmatsiia (Moscow)* 22(5):34–35.

Karnick, C.R. 1994. *Pharmacopoeial Standards of Herbal Plants*, Vols. 1–2. Delhi: Sri Satguru Publications. Vol. 1:86–87; Vol. 2:119.

Kuroda, K. and K. Takagi. 1969. Studies on *Capsella bursa pastoris*. II. Diuretic, anti-inflammatory and anti-ulcer action of ethanol extracts of the herb. *Arch Int Pharmacodyn Ther* 178(2):392–399.

McGuffin, M., C. Hobbs, R. Upton, A. Goldberg. 1997. American Herbal Product Association's *Botanical Safety Handbook*. Boca Raton: CRC Press. 23.

Meyer-Buchtela, E. 1999. *Tee-Rezepturen—Ein Handbuch für Apotheker und Ärzte*. Stuttgart: Deutscher Apotheker Verlag.

Miyazawa, M., A. Uetake, H. Kameoka. 1979. [The constituents of the essential oils from *Capsella bursa-pastoris* Medik] [In Japanese]. *Yakugaku Zasshi* 99(10):1041–1043.

Newall, C.A., L.A. Anderson, J.D. Phillipson. 1996. *Herbal Medicines: A Guide for Health-Care Professionals*. London: The Pharmaceutical Press. 245–246.

Park, R.J. 1967. The occurrence of mustard oil glucosides in *Lepidium hyssopifolium, L. bonariense*, and *Capsella bursa-pastoris*. *Aust J Chem* 20:2799–2801.

Schulz, V., R. Hänsel, V.E. Tyler. 1998. *Rational Phytotherapy: A Physicians' Guide to Herbal Medicine*. New York: Springer.

Wichtl, M. and N.G. Bisset (eds.). 1994. *Herbal Drugs and Phytopharmaceuticals*. Stuttgart: Medpharm Scientific Publishers. 112–114.

Wichtl, M. 1996. Monographien-Kommentar. In: Braun, R. et al. 1997. *Standardzulassungen für Fertigarzneimittel—Text and Kommentar.* Stuttgart: Deutscher Apotheker Verlag.

Additional Resources

Farnsworth, N.R., A.S. Bingel, G.A. Cordell, F.A. Crane, H.H. Fong. 1975. Potential value of plants as sources of new antifertility agents I. *J Pharm Sci* 64(4):535–598.

Kuroda, K. and K. Takagi. 1969. Studies on *Capsella bursa pastoris.* I. General pharmacology of ethanol extract of the herb. *Arch Int Pharmacodyn Ther* 178(2):382–391.

Kuroda, K. and K. Takagi. 1968. Physiologically active substance in *Capsella bursa-pastoris*. *Nature* 220(168):707–708.

Moerman, D.E. 1998. *Native American Ethnobotany*. Portland, OR: Timber Press. 136.

Wichtl, M. (ed.). 1989. *Teedrogen,* 2nd ed. Stuttgart: Wissenschaftliche Verlagsgesellschaft.

Wren, R.C. 1988. *Potter's New Cyclopaedia of Botanical Drugs and Preparations.* Essex: The C.W. Daniel Company Ltd.

This material was adapted from *The Complete German Commission E Monographs—Therapeutic Guide to Herbal Medicines.* M. Blumenthal, W.R. Busse, A. Goldberg, J. Gruenwald, T. Hall, C.W. Riggins, R.S. Rister (eds.) S. Klein and R.S. Rister (trans.). 1998. Austin: American Botanical Council; Boston: Integrative Medicine Communications.

1) The Overview section is new information.

2) Description, Chemistry and Pharmacology, Uses, Contraindications, Side Effects, Interactions with Other Drugs, and Dosage sections have been drawn from the original work. Additional information has been added in some or all of these sections, as noted with references.

3) The dosage for equivalent preparations (tea infusion, fluidextract, and tincture) have been provided based on the following example:
   Unless otherwise prescribed: 2 g per day of [powdered, crushed, cut or whole] [plant part]
   Infusion: 2 g in 150 ml of water
   Fluidextract 1:1 (g/ml): 2 ml
   Tincture 1:5 (g/ml): 10 ml

4) The References and Additional Resources sections are new sections. Additional Resources are not cited in the monograph but are included for research purposes.

SOY:

SOY LECITHIN

(page 355)

SOY PHOSPHOLIPID

(page 356)

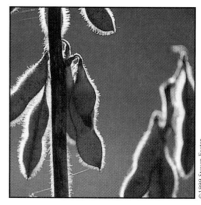

©1999 Steven Foster

Overview

The Commission E has published two positive monographs (in 1988 and in 1994) on soy lecithin, which consists of soybean phospholipids, and soy phospholipid containing 73–79% (3-sn-phosphatidyl)choline. The monographs differ in that the former refers to phospholipids extracted from soybeans, while the latter pertains to preparations consisting of a specific concentration of those phospholipids: 73–79%. Generally, lecithin removed from soybeans contains about 76% phosphatidylcholine (Schulz et al., 1998).

Phospholipids contain mostly linoleic acid (LA), a fatty acid essential to cell membrane formation. Linoleic acid is obtained primarily from food; a small amount is synthesized in the liver. When liver function is compromised, linoleic acid is deficient. Dietary supplementation with soy phospholipids may help patients with liver disease, alcoholism, or chronic parenteral nutrition reduce their risk of LA deficiency. Soy phospholipid 73–79% (3-sn-phosphatydyl)choline products, in addition, are reported to reduce symptoms of liver disease, chronic hepatitis, or liver dysfunction due to malnutrition, such as loss of appetite and abdominal pain (Schulz et al., 1998).

Soy may also lower blood lipids. Soy is recommended for hypercholesteremia in patients whose cholesterol levels do not respond to exercise or weight loss regimens. A recent meta-analysis of 38 studies noted that when dietary meat protein was supplanted with vegetable protein, risks for coronary artery disease were reduced (Anderson et al., 1995). The soy-based diets reduced serum levels of total cholesterol, LDL cholesterol, and triglyceride, without affecting HDL cholesterol (Manson et al., 1992; Anderson et al., 1995).

The full extent of soy phospholipid effects has not been determined. Published studies suggest that phospholipids may be useful in the treatment of menopause and post-menopausal conditions, cancer, hypertension, aging, and benign prostatic hyperplasia (Holt, 1996).

Soy cultivation is believed to have begun in China; the emperor Shen-nong, who compiled the *Medical Bible of the Yellow Emperor (Huang-di nei jing)* sometime between 2967 and 2597 B.C.E., counted soybean among the five sacred crops. Since then, both ancient Chinese and contemporary Chinese medical literature have claimed health benefits from soy. During the Ming Dynasty (1368–1644 B.C.E.), in his 52-volume *Chinese Materia Medica*, Li-Shi Zhen recommended soybeans for the treatment of kidney disease, edema, and poisoning. Today soy may be recommended for skin diseases, gastrointestinal disorders, leg ulcer, vitamin deficiency, and pregnancy toxemia (Holt, 1996).

Soy Lecithin

Latin Name:
Glycine max

Pharmacopeial Name:
Lecithinum ex soya

Other Names:
n/a

Description
Soy lecithin consists of the phospholipids extracted from the seeds of *Glycine max* (L.) Merrill [Fam. Fabaceae] and its preparations in effective dosage. Soy lecithin contains (3-sn-phosphatidyl)choline, phosphatidylethanolamine, and phosphatidylinositol.

Chemistry and Pharmacology
The main constituents are a natural mixture of phosphatides, mainly phosphatidylcholine (20–31.6%), phosphatidylethanolamine and phosphatidylinositol, in combination with fatty acids, carbohydrates, and other substances (DAB, 1998; Der Marderosian, 1999; Der Marderosian et al., 1988; FCC III, 1981; CFR 21, 1998). Soybean lecithin contains 11.7% palmitic, 4% stearic, 8.6% palmitoleic, 9.8% oleic, 55.0% linoleic, 4.0% linolenic, and 5.5% C20 to C22 acids (Budavari, 1996; Der Marderosian, 1999). Pharmacopeial grade soy lecithin must contain a minimum 20% and maximum 31.6% phosphatidyl choline, calculated on the dried substance. Its iodine number value must be between 76 and 85, its acid value maximum 35, and peroxide value maximum 10 (DAB, 1998).

The Commission E reported lipid-lowering activity.

The Merck Index reported its therapeutic category as lipotropic (Budavari, 1996). Soy lecithin is reported to act as an emulsifier aiding in the absorption of fats (Ringer, 1998). It appears to act by improving the metabolism of cholesterol in the digestive system (Der Marderosian, 1999).

Uses
The Commission E approved soy lecithin for moderate disturbances of fat metabolism, especially hypercholesterolemia if dietary measures are not sufficient.

Lecithin has been used as a treatment in cases of poor nutrition, rickets, anemia, diabetes, and tuberculosis (Taber, 1962). Lecithin is used to treat hypercholesterolemia, neurologic disorders, and liver disorders, including diabetic fatty liver and toxic liver damage (Der Marderosian, 1999). The FDA permits the use of lecithin in food with no limitations other than its production by current good manufacturing practice (CFR 21, 1998).

Contraindications
None known.

Side Effects
None known.

Use During Pregnancy and Lactation
No restrictions known.

Interactions with Other Drugs
None known.

Dosage and Administration
Unless otherwise prescribed: Preparations from soy beans for oral intake

containing total phospholipids in their natural mixture composition correspon-ding to 3.5 g (3-sn-phosphatidyl)-choline per day.

SOY PHOSPHOLIPID WITH 73–79% (3-SN-PHOSPHATIDYL)CHOLINE

Latin Name:
Glycine max

Pharmacopeial Name:
Sojae Lecithinum

Other Names:
lecithin enriched extract from soybean

Description

Lecithinum ex soja, lecithin from soybean, extracted from *Glycine max* (L.) Merrill [Fam. Fabaceae], enriched extract with 73–79% (3-sn-phosphatidyl)choline. The extract also includes phosphatidylethanolamine (maximum 7%), phosphatidylinositic acid (less than 0.5%), oil (2–6%), and vitamin E (0.2–0.5%). The range includes both production and analytical variances.

Chemistry and Pharmacology

Lecithin extract from soybeans consists of 76% (average) phosphatidylcholine and phosphoglycerides, of which the fatty acid linoleic acid predominates. The quota of phospholipids, the chief constituents of cell membrane, is in major part obtained by eating (0.5–3 g per day from food) and in lesser degree from synthesis by the liver.

A deficiency in phospholipids is the inevitable result of chronic parenteric nutrition. Under pharmacodynamic characteristics are "hepatoprotective" effects in numerous experimental models, e.g., protection against ethanol, alkyl alcohols, tetrachlorides, paracetamol, and galactosamine. Furthermore, in chronic models (ethanol, thioacetamide, organic solvents), there

appears to be a defense against steatosis and fibrosis of the liver. The compound works by speeding regeneration and stabilization of membranes, stopping lipid peroxidation presumably by collagen synthesis.

The pharmacokinetics of orally administered lecithin have been examined in animal studies in which the phosphatidylcholine was radioactively marked, the marking on a fatty acid in position 1 or position 2, choline, or a phosphorus. The respective marker substitutions show the pharmacokinetics. Phospholipids are degraded to lyso-phosphatidylcholine in the intestine and absorbed primarily in this form. In the gut wall phospholipids are in part resynthesized, then circulated through the lymphatic system. In part, the resynthesized phosphatidylcholine is processed in the liver to form fatty acids, choline, and glycerine-3-phosphate. In plasma, phosphatidylcholine and other phosphoglycerides are tightly bound to lipoproteins or albumin, or to both.

Phosphatidylcholine and other phosphoglycerides are degraded chiefly through a series of so-called phospholipases to fatty acids, choline and "glycerin" metabolites to be in turn resynthesized in the liver and other organs. The administered metabolites integrate within a few hours into body phospholipids. Their removal corresponds to the excretion of phospholipids and their corresponding metabolites.

Commission E noted the following results from toxicological studies: doses of phosphatidylcholine of up to 10 g/kg body weight in mice and rats and 4.5 g/kg body weight in rabbits given intravenously, intraperitoneally, and orally in a single dose are not toxic. The "no-effect" dosage over 48 weeks administration to rats lies upward of 3,750 mg/kg body weight per day. Repeated intravenous application over 12 weeks places the lowest systemic toxic dosage between 0.1 and 1 g/kg body weight and lowest local toxic dosage at over 1 g/kg body weight in rats, and application over four weeks to dogs places the lowest toxic dosage at more than 0.1 g/kg body weight in dogs. Doses of up to 3,750 mg/kg body weight in pregnant animals, animal embryos, and animal neonates showed no pathology of toxicity to reproduction. The lowest teratogenic or embryo-toxic dosage in rats in oral and intravenous administration was more than 1 g/kg body weight. In rabbits teratogenic dosages were greater than 1 g/kg body weight for oral administration and greater than 0.5 g/kg body weight in intravenous administration. Various *in vitro* tests cannot demonstrate any mutagenic potential. Carcinogenicity has not been tested.

Uses

The Commission E approved the internal use of soy phospholipid for less severe forms of hypercholesterolemia in which diet and other non-medical interventions (e.g., exercise, weight control) have not shown results; improvement of subjective complaints, such as loss of appetite and feeling of pressure in the region of liver in toxic nutritional liver disease and chronic hepatitis; prerequisite to the therapy of chronic liver disease is the recognition and avoidance of noxious agents—in the case of alcoholic liver disease, alcohol abstinence. In chronic hepatitis adjuvant therapy with phospholipids of soybeans is only indicated when improvement of symptoms is discernible from other therapy.

Contraindications
None known.

Side Effects
Occasional gastrointestinal effects, i.e., stomach pain, loose stool, and diarrhea.

Use During Pregnancy and Lactation
No restrictions known.

Interactions with Other Drugs
None known.

Dosage and Administration
Unless otherwise prescribed:
Daily dosage:
1.5–2.7 g phospholipids from soybean with 73–79% (3-sn-phosphatidyl) choline in a single dose.
Duration of treatment: Medication containing arbutin should not be taken for longer than a week or more than five times a year without consulting a physician.

References
Anderson, J.W., B.M. Johnstone, M.E. Cook-Newell. 1995. Meta-analysis of the effects of soy protein intake on serum lipids. *N Engl J Med* 333(5):276–282.

Budavari, S. (ed.). 1996. *The Merck Index: An Encyclopedia of Chemicals, Drugs, and Biologicals,* 12th ed. Whitehouse Station, N.J.: Merck & Co, Inc.

CFR 21. See U.S.A. Dept. of Health and Human Services: Food and Drug Administration.

Der Marderosian, A. (ed.). 1999. *The Review of Natural Products.* St. Louis: Facts and Comparisons.

Der Marderosian, A. et al. 1988. *Natural Product Medicine.* Philadelphia: George F. Stickley Co. 121–122, 140, 313–315.

Deutsches Arzneibuch (DAB 1998). 1998. Stuttgart: Deutscher Apotheker Verlag.

Food Chemicals Codex, 3rd ed. (FCC III). 1981. Washington, D.C.: National Academy of Sciences. 166–167.

Holt, S. 1996. *Soya for Health: The Definitive Medical Guide*. New York: Mary Ann Liebert, Inc.

Manson, J.E. et al. 1992. The primary prevention of myocardial infarction. *N Engl J Med* 326(21):1406–1416.

Ringer, D.L. 1998. *Physicians' Guide to Nutriceuticals™*. Omaha, NE: Nutritional Data Resources, L.P. 193.

Schulz, V., R. Hänsel, V.E. Tyler. 1998. *Rational Phytotherapy: A Physicians' Guide to Herbal Medicine*. New York: Springer.

Taber, C.W. 1962. *Taber's Cyclopedic Medical Dictionary*, 9th ed. Philadelphia: F.A. Davis Company. L-15.

U.S.A. Dept. of Health and Human Services: Food and Drug Administration. 1998. *Code of Federal Regulations 21* (CFR 21). Part 184.1400. Washington, D.C.: Office of the Federal Register National Archives and Records Administration. 488.

Additional Resources

Emmert, J.L., T.A. Garrow, D.H. Baker. 1996. Development of an experimental diet for determining bioavailable choline concentration and its application in studies with soybean lecithin. *J Anim Sci* 74(11):2738–2744.

Guarini, P. et al. 1998. Effects of dietary fish oil and soy phosphatidylcholine on neutrophil fatty acid composition, superoxide release, and adhesion. *Inflammation* 22(4):381–391.

Hänsel, R., K. Keller, H. Rimpler, G. Schneider (eds.). 1992–1994. *Hagers Handbuch der Pharmazeutischen Praxis*, 5th ed. Vol. 4–6. Berlin-Heidelberg: Springer Verlag.

Jannace, P.W., R.H. Lerman, J.I. Santos, J.J. Vitale. 1992. Effects of oral soy phosphatidylcholine on phagocytosis, arachidonate concentrations, and killing by human polymorphonuclear leukocytes. *Am J Clin Nutr* 56(3):599–603.

Oosthuizen W. et al. 1998. Lecithin has no effect on serum lipoprotein, plasma fibrinogen and macro molecular protein complex levels in hyperlipidaemic men in a double-blind controlled study. *Eur J Clin Nutr* 52(6):419–424.

Renaud, C., C. Cardiet, C. Dupont. 1996. Allergy to soy lecithin in a child. *J Pediatr Gastroenterol Nutr* 22(3):328–329.

Sirtori, C.R. et al. 1985. Cholesterol-lowering and HDL-raising properties of lecithinated soy proteins in type II hyperlipidemic patients. *Ann Nutr Metab* 29(6):348–357.

Steinegger, E. and R. Hänsel. 1992. *Pharmakognosie*, 5th ed. Heidelberg: Springer Verlag.

Teuscher, E. 1997. *Biogene Arzneimittel*, 5th ed. Stuttgart: Wissenschaftliche Verlagsgesellschaft.

Tompkins, R.K. and L.G. Parkin. 1980. Effects of long-term ingestion of soya phospholipids on serum lipids in humans. *Am J Surg* 140(3):360–364.

Wilson, T.A., C.M. Meservey, R.J. Nicolosi. 1998. Soy lecithin reduces plasma lipoprotein cholesterol and early atherogenesis in hypercholesterolemic monkeys and hamsters: beyond linoleate. *Atherosclerosis* 140(1):147–153.

The soy phospholipid monograph, published by the Commission E in 1994, was modified based on new scientific research. It contains more extensive pharmacological and therapeutic information taken directly from the Commission E.

This material was adapted from *The Complete German Commission E Monographs—Therapeutic Guide to Herbal Medicines*. M. Blumenthal, W.R. Busse, A. Goldberg, J. Gruenwald, T. Hall, C.W. Riggins, R.S. Rister (eds.) S. Klein and R.S. Rister (trans.). 1998. Austin: American Botanical Council; Boston: Integrative Medicine Communications.

1) The Overview section is new information.
2) Description, Chemistry and Pharmacology, Uses, Contraindications, Side Effects, Interactions with Other Drugs, and Dosage sections have been drawn from the original work. Additional information has been added in some or all of these sections, as noted with references.
3) The dosage for equivalent preparations (tea infusion, fluidextract, and tincture) have been provided based on the following example:
   Unless otherwise prescribed: 2 g per day of [powdered, crushed, cut or whole] [plant part]
   Infusion: 2 g in 150 ml of water
   Fluidextract 1:1 (g/ml): 2 ml
   Tincture 1:5 (g/ml): 10 ml
4) The References and Additional Resources sections are new sections. Additional Resources are not cited in the monograph but are included for research purposes.

St. John's Wort

Latin Name:
Hypericum perforatum

Pharmacopeial Name:
Hyperici herba

Other Names:
Hypericum, Klamathweed

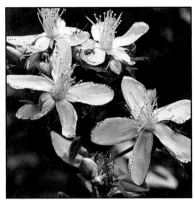

©1999 Steven Foster

Overview

St. John's wort (SJW) is a perennial herb native to Europe, North Africa, and western Asia. It has been introduced and naturalized in parts of Africa, Asia, Australia, and the Americas, and is found growing wild in neglected fields, dry pastures, rangelands, and along country roads (Bombardelli and Morazzoni, 1995; Leung and Foster, 1996; Snow, 1996; Upton, 1997; Wichtl and Bisset, 1994). In European medicine, SJW was traditionally obtained from Eastern European countries, where it is still wild collected (BHP, 1996; Braun et al., 1997; Wichtl and Bisset, 1994). It is cultivated in at least four provinces in Germany (Lange and Schippmann, 1997). The SJW used in Indian Ayurvedic medicine is distributed in the temperate western Himalayas, Kashmir, and Simla (Karnick, 1994; Nadkarni, 1976). SJW was initially brought to the northeastern United States by European colonists (Pickering, 1879; Upton, 1997). It is harvested from naturalized plants in the Pacific Northwest and eastern states (Upton, 1997). Since the mid-1990s, in order to meet new demands on supply, it has been quickly brought into large-scale cultivation in Europe, North and South America, Australia, and China.

Many of SJW's therapeutic applications (except antiviral use), including its uses as a vulnerary, diuretic, and treatment for neuralgic conditions, stem from traditional Greek medicine, originally documented by ancient Greek medical herbalists Hippocrates (ca. 460–377 B.C.E.), Theophrastus (ca. 372–287 B.C.E.), Dioscorides (first century C.E.), and Galen (ca. 130–200 C.E.) (Bombardelli and Morazzoni, 1995; Hobbs, 1990; Leung and Foster, 1996; Upton, 1997). Since the time of Swiss physician Paracelsus (ca. 1493–1541 C.E.) it has been used to treat psychiatric disorders. At that time it was described as "arnica for the nerves" (Reuter, 1998). The aerial flowering parts of SJW have been used in traditional European medicine for centuries to treat neuralgia, anxiety, neurosis, and depression (Rasmussen, 1998). The traditional way to take SJW was as herbal tea, an aqueous extract whose single dose corresponded to 2–3 g of dried crude drug (Schulz et al., 1997). In the nineteenth and twentieth centuries, American Eclectic physicians prescribed SJW to treat hysteria and nervous affections with depression. It was prescribed externally to treat wounds, bruises, sprains, and much more (Ellingwood, 1983; Felter and Lloyd, 1983; Felter, 1985; King, 1866; Snow, 1996; Upton, 1997). Today, St. John's wort is official in the national pharmacopeias of Czechoslovakia, France, Poland, Romania, and Russia (Bruneton, 1995; Hobbs, 1989; Newall et al., 1996; Ph.Fr.X, 1990; Reynolds, 1993; Upton, 1997; USSR X, 1973).

In Germany, SJW is listed in the *German Drug Codex*, approved as a medicine in the Commission E monographs, and licensed as a standard medicinal tea infusion (BAnz, 1998; Braun et al., 1997; DAC, 1991; Meyer-Buchtela, 1999; Schilcher, 1997; Wichtl and Bisset, 1994). It is used in psychiatric drugs in forms including dampoule (Hyperforat®), coated tablet (LI 160, Jarsin®, Lichtwer Pharma, Berlin), juice (Kneipp® Johanniskraut Pflanzensaft N), tea (Kneipp® Johanniskraut-Tee), and tincture (Psychotonin®M). It is used in some urological preparations affecting micturition (e.g., Inconturina®) (Kneipp®, 1996; Schilcher, 1997; Wichtl and Bisset, 1994). In German pediatric medicine, SJW aqueous infusions, alcoholic fluidextracts, and some proprietary products (such as Sedariston®, a combination of SJW and valerian (*Valeriana officinalis*) extracts), are used to treat depressive states in young people. For example, SJW is a component of a sedative tea for children, composed of 30% lemon balm leaf (*Mellissa officinalis*), 30% lavender flower (*Lavandula officinalis*), 30% passion flower herb (*Passiflora* species), and 10% SJW herb (Schilcher, 1997).

In the United States it is used in a wide range of dietary supplements in forms including alcoholic tincture, aqueous infusion (oral), oil infusion (topical), and dry standardized extract in capsules and tablets (Leung and Foster, 1996; Upton, 1997). In 1998, the *United States Pharmacopeia* Drug Information division issued a therapeutic monograph and consumer information bulletin stating that the USP Advisory Panels do not recommend or support the use of SJW because they believe that there have not been enough quality studies to prove that it is effective. However, USP noted that research indicated the safety of SJW (USP-DI, 1998). The USP also published an identification monograph that included guidelines for assessing the identity and purity of raw material in bulk or powder form (USP, 1999a).

Since 1979, there have been about 30 controlled trials with *Hypericum* extracts, involving thousands of patients with mild to moderate depressive disorders. Most studies lasted 28 to 42 days with daily dosages of 900 mg of an extract standardized to 0.3% hypericin (Jarsin®, LI 160, Lichtwer Pharma, Berlin). Up to 1997, there have been at least 15 controlled studies on a methanolic extract of SJW (LI 160) and 12 controlled studies on four additional preparations made from ethanolic extracts of SJW (Schulz et al., 1998). They have confirmed the antidepressant action of SJW extracts in humans (Bombardelli and Morazzoni, 1995; Linde et al., 1996; Reuter, 1998; Upton, 1997).

These studies on SJW do not meet the criteria for conventional antidepressant drugs according to the regulatory guidelines of the European Union, thereby keeping SJW from being accepted for treatment for major depression (De Smet and Nolen, 1996). However, some of these same deficiencies relate to studies on conventional antidepressants when they are first marketed (Cott, 1999). Studies that compare treatment with SJW to treatment with a synthetic antidepressant have not lasted longer than six weeks and have been compared using about one-half the usual dose of the antidepressant (75 mg imipramine instead of 150 mg). In addition, they have not been conducted with severely depressed patients. Yet SJW has been shown to be safe, with very few side effects, compared with synthetic antidepressants: out of 3,250 patients, only allergic reactions (0.5%), gastrointestinal upset (0.6%), and fatigue (0.4%) were observed (De Smet and Nolen, 1996). Evidence of the antidepressant activity of SJW extracts can be found in reviews by Bombardelli and Morazzoni (1995), Linde et al. (1996), and Upton (1997). No significant modern human studies investigating SJW's other therapeutic uses have been found (e.g., orally for dyspeptic complaints and topically for burns, lesions, wounds, and myalgia).

The constituents and mechanism of action responsible for the antidepressant properties of SJW have been investigated, with various authors citing different mechanisms (Bombardelli and Morazzoni, 1995; Rasmussen, 1998; Reuter, 1995, 1998). However, a recent randomized, double-blind, placebo-controlled, multicenter study on 147 male and female patients with mild to moderate depression indicated that hyperforin may be the primary active ingredient, or at least it plays a key role in the antidepressant activity. Patients received 300 mg of either a placebo, a SJW extract standardized to 0.5% hyperforin (WS 5573, W. Schwabe, Germany), or a SJW extract standardized to 5% hyperforin (WS 5572, Schwabe), three times daily for 42 days. While there was a reduction in depression scores in both the 0.5% hyperforin group and the placebo group, results were statistically significant for improvement of depressive symptoms only in the patients receiving the extract with 5% hyperforin (Laakmann et al., 1998a, 1998b). Of particular interest is the finding that patients with severe depression (n=56) experienced greater reduction of symptoms than mild to moderately depressed patients receiving the same dosage (although there is more room for improvement in severely depressed patients). The authors of this study concluded that the antidepressant activity of SJW is due to its hyperforin content. Other experimental studies have also shown the relevance of hyperforin (Chatterjee et al., 1998; Bhattacharya et al., 1998). However, additional animal and human research is being conducted to clarify the importance of hyperforin, since most of the studies on St. John's wort were conducted on preparations standardized to hypericin, not hyperforin, content. Nevertheless, a representative of the leading manufacturer of the most clinically tested hypericin-based SJW extract (i.e., LI 160 from Lichtwer Pharma) has written that this product showed hyperforin levels of 1% to 6% upon analysis; new studies by Lichtwer on LI 160 will be carried out on an extract standardized to hyperforin values of approximately 4% (Schulz, 1998).

Although additional research is warranted, the modern therapeutic application of SJW for mild to moderate depression is supported by its history of use in traditional medicine, *in vitro* studies (Cott, 1997; Wonnemann et al., 1999), *in vivo* experiments in animals (Butterweck et al., 1999; Okpanyi and Weischer, 1987), pharmacodynamic studies in humans (Kugler et al., 1990; Schulz and Jobert, 1993), pharmacokinetic studies in humans (Staffeldt et al., 1993; Weiser, 1991), human clinical studies (Hänsgen et al., 1994; Hübner et al., 1994; Cott, 1997; Fugh-Berman and Cott, 1999), meta-analyses (Linde et al., 1996) and extensive phytochemical investigations (Bombardelli and Morazzoni, 1995; Brantner et al., 1994).

A major three-year, multicenter clinical study on the antidepressant effect of SJW is being carried out in the United States under the auspices of the National Institutes of Health. This is the first clinical study to test SJW directly against a modern selective serotonin reuptake inhibitor (SSRI) (sertraline, Zoloft®) and placebo. The trial consists of 330 patients (110 in each arm—SJW, sertraline, placebo) and the duration of treatment will last six months, the longest trial on SJW to date. Patients are required to test a minimum of 20 points on the Hamilton Depression Scale, thus being classed as moderately to severely depressed.

A small study has investigated the possible use of SJW for seasonal affective disorder (SAD), a condition of depressive mood associated with winter months and lack of sunlight (Kasper, 1997). In an open study, 22 patients diagnosed with SAD were given SJW extract (300 mg three times daily) with additional bright light or the same dose of SJW in dim light conditions. As determined by a standard method for measuring depression symptoms (Hamilton Depression Scale), subjects in both groups experienced a significant reduction in depression score, there being no difference in the bright and dim light groups. Therefore, no conclusion for the effectiveness of SJW in SAD can be drawn from the results of this study.

Pharmacopeial grade SJW consists of the dried flowering tops or aerial parts of *Hypericum perforatum* L., harvested shortly before or during the flowering period. It must contain not less than 12% water soluble extractive. Botanical identity must be confirmed by thin-layer chromatography (TLC), macrocopic and microscopic examinations, and organoleptic (sensory) evaluation (BHP, 1996). The *German Drug Codex* additionally required not less than 0.4% dianthrones of the hypericin group, calculated as hypericin (DAC, 1986; Wichtl and Bisset, 1994). The German Standard License monograph requires the material to conform with the *German Drug Codex* requirements (Braun et al., 1997). However, the German Federal Institute for Drugs and Medical Devices (BfArM) declared that hypericin would no longer be used as a required marker compound for the chemical standardization of

St. John's wort (Bühler, 1995). The *United States Pharmacopeia* requires not less than 0.2% of hypericin and pseudohypericin combined and not less than 3.0% of hyperforin (USP, 1999b). The ESCOP monograph requires the material to conform with either the *French Pharmacopoeia* or the *German Drug Codex* (ESCOP, 1997).

Description

St. John's wort consists of the dried, aboveground parts of *H. perforatum* L. [Fam. Hypericaceae], gathered during flowering season, and their preparations in effective dosage.

Chemistry and Pharmacology

St. John's wort herb contains 6.5–15% catechin-type tannins and condensed-type proanthocyanidins (catechin, epicatechin, leucocyanidin); 2–5% flavonoids, mostly hyperoside (0.5–2%), rutin (0.3–1.6%), quercitrin (0.3%), isoquercitrin (0.3%), quercetin, and kaempferol; biflavonoids (approximately 0.26% biapigenin); phloroglucinol derivatives (up to 4% hyperforin); phenolic acids (caffeic, chlorogenic, ferulic); 0.05–1.0% volatile oils, mainly higher *n*-alkanes; 0.05–0.15% naphthodianthrones (hypericin and pseudohypericin); sterols (β-sitosterol); vitamins C and A; xanthones (up to 10 ppm); and choline (Bruneton, 1995; ESCOP, 1997; Leung and Foster, 1996; Newall et al., 1996; Wichtl and Bisset, 1994).

The Commission E reported that a mild antidepressant action of the herb and its preparations has been observed and reported by many physicians. Although the Commission E categorized St. John's wort as an MAO inhibitor, this was based on *in vitro* research and not conducted in animal systems. Subsequent research has indicated either no or very slight MAO activity in St. John's wort or its preparations. The Commission E recognized the anti-inflammatory action of topical oily *Hypericum* preparations.

The *British Herbal Pharmacopoeia* reported antidepressant action (BHP, 1996). In numerous controlled double-blind and open studies using hydroalcoholic SJW preparations, a significant improvement of mood, and loss of interest and activity and other depressive syndrome symptoms, such as sleep, concentration, and somatic complaints, has been reported (ESCOP, 1997).

Uses

In December 1984, the Commission E approved the internal use of St. John's wort for psychovegetative (psychoautonomic) disturbances, depressive moods, anxiety, and nervous unrest. Oily *Hypericum* preparations are approved for dyspeptic complaints. External use of oily preparations of St. John's wort is approved for treatment and post-therapy of acute and contused injuries, myalgia, and first-degree burns.

ESCOP indicates its use for mild to moderate depressive states, restlessness, anxiety, and irritability (ESCOP, 1997). The German Standard License for St. John's wort tea lists it for nervous excitement and sleep disturbances (Wichtl and Bisset, 1994). With the exception of its antiviral use, other modern applications date back two thousand years (Hobbs, 1990).

Since the 1984 monograph was based on general clinical use and only one clinical study (out of more than 27 that had been published up to 1997) had been published at that time, the Commission was relatively accurate in its evaluation of the therapeutic effects of SJW. However, given that most the recent research has focused on antidepressant activity of SJW, it is reasonable to conclude that this use should be the only primary use, when administered in proper form and dosage (Schulz et al., 1998). SJW may benefit the other uses (psychovegetative disturbances, anxiety, and nervous unrest) only within the framework of its general antidepressant activity (Schulz et al., 1998).

Contraindications

None known.

Side Effects

Commission E noted that photosensitization is possible, especially in fair-skinned individuals. However, animal and human research has indicated that photosensitization is not likely to occur at the recommended dosage levels. Based on experimental studies (animal and human), it would take approximately 30 to 50 times the recommended daily dose of 900 mg of the standardized extract to produce severe phototoxic effects in humans (Schulz et al., 1998).

Use During Pregnancy and Lactation

No restrictions known (McGuffin et al., 1997).

Interactions with Other Drugs

Commission E reported that none were known (in 1984). ESCOP also noted that none were reported (ESCOP, 1997).

Dosage and Administration

The original Commission E monograph (1984) noted the following dosage: "Unless otherwise prescribed: 2–4 g per day of chopped or powdered herb for internal use, or 0.2–1 mg of total hypericin in other forms of preparation application. Liquid and semi-solid preparations for external use. Preparations made with fatty oils for external and internal use." Although the original Commission E monograph specified minimum levels of hypericin, this is no longer required on the label of German products (Ahuis, 1998). In Germany, the current required dosage is 300 mg, three times daily of a hydroalcoholic St. John's wort extract. The registration for infusions (tea) of St. John's wort has recently been withdrawn due to a lack of evidence of efficacy (BfArM, 1998).

Based on the available research, the approved effective equivalent preparations are as follows:

Internal: Fluidextract 1:1 (g/ml): 2 ml, twice daily.

Native dry extract 5–7:1: 300 mg, three times daily.

External: Oily macerate (Oleum hyperici): macerate fresh flowering tops in olive oil or wheat-germ oil for several weeks, stirring often; strain through a cloth and press pulp; for direct application to affected areas.

References

Ahuis, F. 1998. Neues über Johanniskraut [News on St. John's Wort]. *Deutsche Apotheker Zeitung* 138:1783–1785.

BAnz. See *Bundesanzeiger*.

BfArM. 1998. Meeting of BfArM, Johanniskraut, No. 113. *BPI* [Federal Manufacturers Association]. 151.

Bhattacharya, S.K., A. Chakrabarti, S.S. Chatterjee. 1998. Activity profiles of two hyperforin-containing *Hypericum* extracts in behavioral models. *Pharmacopsychiatry* 31 (suppl. 1):22–29.

Bombardelli, E. and P. Morazzoni. 1995. *Hypericum perforatum*. Fitoterapia. 66(1):43–68.

Brantner, A., T. Kartnig, F. Quehenberger. 1994. Vergleichende phytochemische Untersuchungen an *Hypericum perforatum* L. und *Hypericum maculatum* Crantz. *Sci Pharm* 62:261–276.

Braun, R. et al. 1997. *Standardzulassungen für Fertigarzneimittel—Text and Kommentar*. Stuttgart: Deutscher Apotheker Verlag.

British Herbal Pharmacopoeia (BHP). 1996. Exeter, U.K.: British Herbal Medicine Association.

Bruneton, J. 1995. *Pharmacognosy, Phytochemistry, Medicinal Plants*. Paris: Lavoisier Publishing.

Bühler. 1995. Communication from BfArM (German Federal Institute of Drugs and Medical Devices to German Nonprescription Drug Association (BAH), Sept. 11.

Bundesanzeiger (BAnz). 1998. Monographien der Kommission E (Zulassungs- und Aufbereitungskommission am BGA für den humanmed. Bereich, phytotherapeutische Therapierichtung und Stoffgruppe). Köln: Bundesgesundheitsamt (BGA).

Butterweck, V., G. Jürgenliemk, A. Nahrstedt, H. Winterhoff. 1999. Flavonoid-Fraktionen und Hyperosid aus *Hypericum perforatum* L. zeigen anti-depressive Aktivität im Forced Swimming Test nach PORSOLT. *Zeitschrift für Phytotherapie* 20:86–87.

Chatterjee, S.S., M. Noldner, E. Koch, C. Erdelmeier. 1998. Antidepressant activity of *Hypericum perforatum* and Hyperforin: the neglected possibility. *Pharmacopsychiatry* 31 (suppl. 1):7–15.

Cott, J.M. 1999. Personal communication to M. Blumenthal, Aug. 27.

Cott, J.M. and A. Fugh-Berman. 1998. Is St. John's Wort (*Hypericum perforatum*) an effective anti-depressant? *J Nerv Ment Dis* 186(8):500–501.

Cott, J.M. 1997. *In vitro* receptor binding and enzyme inhibition by *Hypericum perforatum* extract. *Pharmacopsychiatry* 30 (suppl. 2):108–112.

De Smet, P.A. and W.A. Nolen. 1996. St. John's wort as an antidepressant. *BMJ* 313(7052):241–242.

Deutscher Arzneimittel-Codex (DAC). 1986. Stuttgart: Deutscher Apotheker Verlag. J010/1–5.

Deutscher Arzneimittel-Codex, 3rd suppl. (DAC). 1991. Stuttgart: Deutscher Apotheker Verlag.

Ellingwood, F. 1983. *American Materia Medica, Therapeutics and Pharmacognosy.* Portland, OR: Eclectic Medical Publications [reprint of 1919 original].

ESCOP. 1997. "Hyperici Herba." *Monographs on the Medicinal Uses of Plant Drugs.* Exeter, U.K.: European Scientific Cooperative on Phytotherapy.

Felter, H.W. 1985. *The Eclectic Materia Medica, Pharmacology and Therapeutics* Portland, OR: Eclectic Medical Publications [reprint of the 1922 original]. 424.

Felter, H.W. and J.U. Lloyd. 1983. *King's American Dispensatory,* 18th ed., 3rd rev. Portland, OR: Eclectic Medical Publications [reprint of 1898 original]. 1083–1039.

Fugh-Berman A. and J.M. Cott. 1999. Dietary supplements and natural products as psychotherapeutic agents. *Psychosom Med* (in press, Sept.; Oct.).

Hänsgen, K.D., J. Vesper, M. Ploch. 1994. Multicenter double-blind study examining the antidepressant effectiveness of the *Hypericum* extract LI 160. *J Geriatr Psychiatr Neurol* 7(suppl. 1):S15–S18.

Hobbs, C. 1989. St. John's wort: *Hypericum perforatum* L. A review. *HerbalGram* 18/19:24–33.

———. 1990. St. John's wort—ancient herbal protector. Pharmacy History 32(4):166.

Hübner, W.D., S. Lande, H. Podzuweit. 1994. *Hypericum* treatment of mild depressions with somatic symptoms. *J Geriatr Psychiatr Neurol* 7(suppl. 1):S12–S14.

Karnick, C.R. 1994. *Pharmacopoeial Standards of Herbal Plants,* Vols. 1–2. Delhi: Sri Satguru Publications. Vol. 1:189–192; Vol. 2:125.

Kasper, S. 1997. Treatment of seasonal affective disorder (SAD) with *Hypericum* Extract. *Pharmacopsych* 30:S89–93.

King, J. 1866. *The American Dispensatory,* 7th ed. Cincinnati: Moore, Wilstach, & Baldwin.

Kneipp®, 1996. *Wegweiser zu den Kneipp® Mitteln [Guide to Kneipp® Remedies].* Würzburg: Sebastian Kneipp Gesundheitsmittel-Verlag. 48–49, 168, 172.

Kugler, J. W. et al. 1990. Therapie depressiver Zustände. *Hypericum*-Extrakt Steigerwald als Alternative zur Benzodiazepin-Behandlung. *Z Allg Med* 66:21–29.

Laakmann, G., A. Deniel, M. Kieser. 1998a. Clinical significance of Hyperforin for the efficacy of *Hypericum* extracts on depressive disorders of different severities. *Phytomedicine* 5(6):435–442.

Laakmann, G., C. Schule, T. Baghai, M. Kieser. 1998b. St. John's wort in mild to moderate depression: the relevance of hyperforin for the clinical efficacy. *Pharmacopsychiatry* 31(suppl. 1):54–59.

Lange, D. and U. Schippmann. 1997. *Trade Survey of Medicinal Plants in Germany—A Contribution to International Plant Species Conservation.* Bonn: Bundesamt für Naturschutz. 29–35.

Leung, A.Y. and S. Foster. 1996. *Encyclopedia of Common Natural Ingredients Used in Food, Drugs and Cosmetics,* 2nd ed. New York: John Wiley & Sons, Inc.

Linde, K. et al. 1996. St. John's wort for depression—an overview and meta-analysis of randomised clinical trials. *BMJ* 313(7052):253–258.

McGuffin, M., C. Hobbs, R. Upton, A. Goldberg. 1997. American Herbal Product Association's *Botanical Safety Handbook.* Boca Raton: CRC Press.

Meyer-Buchtela, E. 1999. *Tee-Rezepturen—Ein Handbuch für Apotheker und Ärzte.* Stuttgart: Deutscher Apotheker Verlag.

Nadkarni, K.M. 1976. *Indian Materia Medica.* Bombay: Popular Prakashan. 673.

Newall, C.A., L.A. Anderson, J.D. Phillipson. 1996. *Herbal Medicines: A Guide for Health-Care Professionals.* London: The Pharmaceutical Press.

Okpanyi, S.N. and M.L. Weischer. 1987. Tierexperimentelle untersuchungen zur psychotropen wirksamkeit eines *Hypericum*-extraktes [Animal experiments on the psychotropic action of a *Hypericum* extract]. *Arzneimittelforschung* 37:10–13.

Pharmacopée Française Xe Édition (Ph.Fr.X). 1983–1990. Moulins-les-Metz: Maisonneuve S.A.

Pickering, C. 1879. *Chronological History of Plants.* Boston: Little Brown & Co.

Rasmussen, P. 1998. St. John's wort—A review of its use in depression. *Australian J Med Herbalism* 10(1):8–13.

Reuter, H.D. 1995. St. John's wort as a herbal antidepressant. *Eur J Herbal Med* Part I:1(3):19–24; Part II:1(4):15–21.

———. 1998. In: Lawson, L.D. and R. Bauer (eds.). 1998. *Phytomedicines of Europe—Chemistry and Biological Activity.* Washington, D.C.: American Chemical Society. 287–298.

Reynolds, J.E.F. (ed.). 1993. *Martindale: The Extra Pharmacopoeia,* 30th ed. London: The Pharmaceutical Press.

Schilcher, H. 1997. *Phytotherapy in Pediatrics—Handbook for Physicians and Pharmacists.* Stuttgart: Medpharm Scientific Publishers. 61–62.

Schulz, V. 1998. Hyperforin values: By no means just "traces." [letter]. *Deutsche Apotheker Zeitung* 138(6).

Schulz, V., W.D. Hübner, M. Ploch. 1997. Clinical trials with phyto-psychopharmacological agents. *Phytomed* 4(4):379–387.

Schulz, H. and M. Jobert. 1993. Der Einfluss von Johanniskraut-Extrakt auf das Schlaf-EEG bei älteren Probandinnen. *Nervenheilkunde* 12:323–327.

Schulz, V., R. Hänsel, V.E. Tyler. 1998. *Rational Phytotherapy: A Physicians' Guide to Herbal Medicine.* New York: Springer. 50–65.

Staffeldt, B. et al. 1993. Pharmakokinetik von Hypericin und Pseudohypericin nach oraler Einnahme des Johanniskraut-Extraktes LI 160 bei gesunden Probanden. *Nervenheilkunde* 12:331–338.

Snow, J.M. 1996. *Hypericum perforatum* L. (Hyperiaceae). *Protocol J Botanical Med* 2(1):16–21.

State Pharmacopoeia of the Union of Soviet Socialist Republics, 10th ed. (USSR X). 1973. Moscow: Ministry of Health of the U.S.S.R.

Upton, R. (ed.). 1997. St. John's Wort (*Hypericum perforatum*). *American Herbal Pharmacopoeia* (AHP). Santa Cruz: American Herbal Pharmacopoeia. 1–32 (published in *HerbalGram* 40).

USP-DI Update. 1998. St. John's Wort and Powdered St. John's Wort. Rockville, MD: United States Pharmacopeia Convention, May.

USP. 1999a. St. John's Wort and Powdered St. John's Wort. *United States Pharmacopeia 24-National Formulary 19.* Rockville, MD: United States Pharmacopeia Convention, Inc.

USP. 1999b. Powdered St. John's wort extract monograph. *Pharmacopeial Forum* 25(2).

USSR X. See *State Pharmacopoeia of the Union of Soviet Socialist Republics.*

Weiser, D. 1991. Pharmakokinetik von Hypericin nach oraler Einnahme des Johanniskraut-Extraktes LI 160. *Nervenheilkunde* 10:318–319.

Wichtl, M. and N.G. Bisset (eds.). 1994. *Herbal Drugs and Phytopharmaceuticals.* Stuttgart: Medpharm Scientific Publishers.

Wonnemann, M., C. Schäfer, W.E. Müller. 1999. Johanniskrautextrakt: Effekte auf GABA- und glutamaterge Rezeptorsysteme. *Zeitschrift für Phytotherapie* 20:77–82.

Additional Resources

British Herbal Pharmacopoeia (BHP). 1983. Keighley, U.K.: British Herbal Medicine Association.

Constantine, G.H. and J. Karchesy. 1999. Variations in Hypericin concentrations in *Hypericum perforatum* L. and commercial products. Pharm Biol 36(5):365–367.

Cracchiolo, C. 1998. Pharmacology of St. John's wort: botanical and chemical aspects. *Sci Rev Alt Med* 2(1):29–35.

Denke, A., W. Schneider, E.F. Elstner. 1999. Biochemical activities from *Hypericum perforatum* L.: 2nd Communication: Inhibition of metenkphaline- and tyrosine-dimerization. *Arzneimforsch/Drug Res* 49(2):109–114.

Denke, A., H. Schempp, E.Mann, W. Schneider, E.F. Elstner. 1999. Biochemical activities from *Hypericum perforatum* L.: 4th communication: Influence of different cultivation methods. *Arzneim-Forsch/Drug Res* 49(2):120–125.

Erdelmeier, C.A. 1998. Hyperforin, possibly the major non-nitrogenous secondary metabolite of *Hypericum perforatum* L. *Pharmacopsych* 31(Suppl 1):2–6.

Gaedcke, F. 1997. Johanniskraut und dessen Zubereitungen. *Deut Apoth Zeit* No. 42/97.

Grush, L.R., A. Nierenberg, B. Keefe, L.S. Cohen. 1998. St. John's wort during pregnancy [letter]. *JAMA* 280:1566.

Halama, P. 1991. Wirksamkeit des *Hypericum*—Extraktes LI 160 bei 50 Patienten einer psychiatrischen Fachpraxis. *Nervenheilkunde* 10:305–307.

Hänsel, R., K. Keller, H. Rimpler, G. Schneider (eds.). 1993. *Hagers Handbuch der Pharmazeutischen Praxis,* 5th ed. Vol. 5. Berlin-Heidelberg: Springer Verlag. 474–495.

Hippius, H. 1998. St John's wort (*Hypericum perforatum*)—A herbal antidepressant. [In Process Citation]. *Curr Med Res Opin* 14(3):171–184.

Kleber, E., T. Obry, S. Hippeli, W. Schneider, E.F. Elstner. 1999. Biochemical activities of extracts from *Hypericum perforatum* L. 1st Communication: Inhibition of dopamine-beta-hydroxylase. *Arzneim-Forsch/Drug Research* 49(2):106–109.

Lust, J. 1974. *The Herb Book.* New York: Bantam Books. 344.

Martinez, B., S. Kasper, S. Ruhrmann, H.J. Moller. 1994. *Hypericum* in the treatment of seasonal affective disorders. *J Geriatr Psychiatry Neurol* 7(Suppl 1):S29–S33.

Mediherb, Pty. Ltd. 1996. *Hypericum*—New uses for an old wort. Mediherb Professional Newsletter Part 1:44, Part 2:45, Part 3:46.

Müller, W.E. et al. 1998. Hyperforin represents the neuro-transmitter reuptake inhibiting constituent of *Hypericum* extract. *Phamacopsych* 31(Suppl 1):16–21.

Müller, W.E., M. Rolli, C. Schafer, U. Hafner. 1997. Effects of hypericum extract (LI 160) in biochemical models of antidepressant activity. *Pharmacopsychiatry* 30(Suppl):102–107.

Norme Française (NF). 1989. NF T 75-348. Paris: Direction des Journaux Officiels.

Reh, C., P. Laux, N. Schenk. 1992. *Hypericum*—Extrakt bei Depressionen—eine wirksame Alternative. *Therapiewoche* 42(25):1576–1581.

Reuter, H.D. 1993. *Hypericum* als pflanzliches Antidepressivum. *Z Phytother* 14:239–254.

Schellenberg, R., S. Sauer, W. Dimpfel. 1998. Pharmacodynamic effects of two different *Hypericum* extracts in healthy volunteers measured by quantitative EEG. *Pharmacopsych* 31 (suppl. 1):44–53.

Schemp, H., A.Denke, E.Mann, W. Schneider, E.F. Elstner. 1999. Biochemical Activities from *Hypericum perforatum* L. 3rd communication: Modulation of peroxidase activity as a simple method for standardization. *Arzneim-Forsch/Drug Res* 49(2):115–119.

Sharpley, A.L., C.L. McGavin, R. Whale, P.J. Cowen. 1998. Antidepressant-like effect of *Hypericum perforatum* (St John's wort) on the sleep polysomnogram. [In Process Citation]. *Psychopharmacology (Berl)* 139(3):286–287.

Smyshliaeva, A.V. and IuB Kudriashov. 1992. Mod-
ifikatsiia luchevogo porazheniia zhivotnykh vod-
nym ekstraktom *Hypericum perforatum* L.
Soobshchenie 1 [The modification of a radiation
lesion in animals with an aqueous extract of
Hypericum perforatum L. 1.]. *Biol Nauki*
(4):7–9.

Sommer, H. 1991. Besserung psychovegetativer
Beschwerden durch *Hypericum* im Rahmen
einer multizentrischen Doppelblindstudie. *Nervenheilkunde* 10:308–310.

Vorbach, E.U., K.H. Arnold, W.D. Hübner. 1997.
Efficacy and tolerability of St. John's wort
extract LI 160 versus imipramine in patients
with severe depressive episodes according to
ICD-10. *Pharmacopsych* 30 Suppl:81–85.

Wheatley D. 1997. LI 160, an extract of St. John's
wort, versus amitriptyline in mild to moderately
depressed outpatients—a controlled 6-week clinical trial. *Pharmacopsych* 30: Suppl:77–80.

This material was adapted from *The Complete German Commission E Monographs—Therapeutic Guide to
Herbal Medicines*. M. Blumenthal, W.R. Busse, A. Goldberg, J. Gruenwald, T. Hall, C.W. Riggins, R.S. Ris-
ter (eds.) S. Klein and R.S. Rister (trans.). 1998. Austin: American Botanical Council; Boston: Integrative
Medicine Communications.

1) The Overview section is new information.

2) Description, Chemistry and Pharmacology, Uses, Contraindications, Side Effects, Interactions with
   Other Drugs, and Dosage sections have been drawn from the original work. Additional information has
   been added in some or all of these sections, as noted with references.

3) The dosage for equivalent preparations (tea infusion, fluidextract, and tincture) have been provided
   based on the following example:
   Unless otherwise prescribed: 2 g per day of [powdered, crushed, cut or whole] [plant part]
   Infusion: 2 g in 150 ml of water
   Fluidextract 1:1 (g/ml): 2 ml
   Tincture 1:5 (g/ml): 10 ml

4) The References and Additional Resources sections are new sections. Additional Resources are not cited
   in the monograph but are included for research purposes.

Stinging Nettle:

Stinging Nettle herb and leaf
(page 370)

Stinging Nettle root
(page 372)

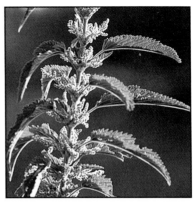

© 1999 Steven Foster

Overview

Stinging nettle is a perennial herb, found growing wild throughout the temperate zones of both hemispheres worldwide (Bombardelli and Morazzoni, 1997; Leung and Foster, 1996). The material of commerce comes mostly from wild plants collected in Albania, Bulgaria, Hungary, Germany, the former U.S.S.R., and the former Yugoslavia, though it is also cultivated somewhat (Bombardelli and Morazzoni, 1997; Wichtl and Bisset, 1994). The genus name *Urtica* comes from the Latin verb *urere*, meaning "to burn," because of its urticate (stinging) hairs. The species name *dioica* means "two houses" because the plant usually has either male or female flowers (Bombardelli and Morazzoni, 1997).

Herb and Leaf:

Stinging nettle herb has been used since ancient times. Greek physicians Dioscorides (first century C.E.) and Galen (ca. 130–200 C.E.) reported nettle leaf had diuretic and laxative action and was useful for asthma, pleurisy, and for the treatment of spleen-related illness. Roman naturalist Pliny the Elder (ca. 23–79 C.E.) reported hemostatic properties (Bombardelli and Morazzoni, 1997).

In traditional African medicine the herb is used as a snuff powder for nosebleeds, excessive menstruation, and to treat internal bleeding. It is applied on burns (List and Hörhammer, 1979). In India, the *Ayurvedic Pharmacopoeia* lists stinging nettle herb for uterine hemorrhage, cutaneous eruptions, infantile and psychogenic eczema, and nosebleed, at dosage 2–4 g herb or 3–4 ml fluidextract, always in combination with other herbs (Karnick, 1994). It is also taken in syrup or tincture form to treat urticaria (nettle rash) (Nadkarni, 1976). Stinging nettle is also widely used in North American aboriginal medicines. People of the Hesquiat, Sanpoil, Shuswap, and Tainarna nations use it as an antirheumatic drug (Moerman, 1998; Palmer, 1975; Smith, 1973; Turner and Efrat, 1982; Ray, 1933). It is also used as a gynecological aid by women of the Cowlitz, Cree, Kwakiutl, Lummi, Quinault, and Squaxin nations. It is taken as an aqueous infusion during childbirth to relax the muscles. The plant juice is taken by pregnant women who are overdue and the tips of the plant are chewed by women during labor (Gunther, 1973; Leighton, 1985; Moerman, 1998; Turner and Bell, 1973; Turner and Efrat, 1982).

In Germany, stinging nettle herb is licensed as a standard medicinal tea for diuretic action. It is also used as a component of prepared medicines intended for supportive treatment of rheumatic ailments and irrigation therapy in inflammatory conditions of the lower urinary tract (Wichtl and Bisset, 1994). Stinging nettle herb is used in German homeopathy in treatments for urticaria, herpes, eczema, hypersensitive reactions in the skin and joints, and burns (List and Hörhammer, 1979). In the United States, stinging nettle herb is used as a component in a wide range of dietary supplements. It is also used during and following birth and during lactation in traditional women's tonic formulas. It is prescribed by naturopathic physicians and licensed acupuncturists as a component in formulas used to treat hayfever and other allergies.

Modern clinical studies have investigated the use of stinging nettle herb to treat allergic rhinitis (Mittman, 1990), rheumatic complaints (Ramm and Hansen, 1995), acute arthritis (Chrubasik et al., 1997), and as a diuretic (Kirchhoff, 1983).

In a double-blind randomized study, 98 individuals with allergic rhinitis compared the effects of a freeze-dried stinging nettle herb powder (Eclectic Institute, U.S.A.) with placebo. Sixty-nine individuals completed the study. Assessment was based on daily symptom diaries and global response recorded at the follow-up visit after one week of therapy. The extract was rated higher than placebo in the global assessments. In the diary data, however, stinging nettle extract was rated only slightly better. The study reported that the extract produced positive, though limited results in the treatment of allergic rhinitis (Mittman, 1990).

In a multicenter study, 152 patients with degenerative, rheumatic diseases were given 1.54 g nettle herb dry extract (6.4–8.0:1) daily. Subjective improvement of symptoms was observed in 70% of the patients after three weeks (Ramm and Hansen, 1995). In another open randomized study, 40 patients with acute arthritis compared the effects of stewed stinging nettle herb combined with a sub-therapeutic dose of the anti-inflammatory drug Diclofenac against a standard dose of Diclofenac. Half of the patients took 50 g nettle and 50 mg Diclofenac and the other half took 200 mg Diclofenac. Thirty-seven patients completed the study. Assessment was based on the decrease in the elevated acute phase protein CRP (a protein elevated by inflammatory events and other pathological processes) and the clinical signs of acute arthritis: physical impairment, subjective pain, and pressure pain (patient assessment) and stiffness (physician assessment). All assessments were done on a verbal rating scale from 0 to 4. In both groups median scores improved by about 70% relative to the initial value. Only minor adverse effects occurred during treatment. The authors concluded that stinging nettle herb may enhance the NSAID antirheumatic effectiveness and that further investigations are needed in order to determine whether acute attacks of arthritis may respond to stewed stinging nettle herb on its own (Chrubasik et al, 1997).

In an open 14-day clinical study, 32 patients diagnosed with myocardial or chronic venous insufficiency were treated with 15 ml of nettle herb juice three times daily. A significant increase in the daily volume of urine was observed throughout the treatment, the volume in day two being 9.2% higher ($p < 0.0005$) than the baseline amount in patients with myocardial insufficiency and 23.9% higher ($p < 0.05$) in those with chronic venous insufficiency. Minor decreases in body weights (approximately 1%) and systolic blood pressure were also observed. Serum parameters were unaffected and the treatment was well tolerated apart from a tendency towards diarrhea. The treatment produced a distinct diuretic effect (Kirchhoff, 1983).

Pharmacopeial grade stinging nettle herb (leaf, flower, and stem) must be collected during the flowering period and contain not less than 18% water-soluble extractives, not more than 2% stem above 3 mm in diameter, and other quantitative standards. Botanical identity must be confirmed by thin-layer chromatography (TLC) as well as macrocopic and microscopic authentication (BHP, 1996). The *German Pharmacopoeia* and *German Pharmaceutical Codex* require similar standards though they do not have a water-soluble extractive requirement and the *Codex* requires not more than 10% stem fragments (DAB 10, 1994; DAC, 1986; Wichtl and Bisset, 1994). The ESCOP monograph requires that the material comply with the standards of the *German Pharmacopoeia* or the *Swiss Pharmacopoeia* (ESCOP, 1997).

Root:

Stinging nettle root is used in Germany as a component of approved medicines for treatment of benign prostatic hyperplasia (BPH). In the United States, it is used similarly though as a dietary supplement its indications for use are limited to non-therapeutic "structure and function" claims. Naturopathic physicians prescribe it for BPH.

Modern clinical studies have investigated the use of nettle root in the treatment of BPH (Belaiche and Lievoux, 1991; Bombardelli and Morazzoni, 1997; ESCOP, 1997; Krzeski et al., 1993; Leung and Foster, 1996; Schneider et al., 1995; Söke-land and Albrecht, 1997; Vontobel et al., 1985).

In a randomized, reference-controlled, multicenter, double-blind clinical trial 543 patients with Aiken's stage I to II BPH compared therapeutic equivalence between finasteride (Proscar®, Merck), and a combination nettle root-saw palmetto fruit extract (PRO® 160/120, Prostagutt® forte). For 48 weeks, patients were given 2 capsules of PRO® 160/120 or 1 capsule of finasteride per day. The primary variable was the change of the maximum urinary flow after 24 weeks of therapy. Urodynamic parameters such as average urinary flow, micturition volume, and micturition time were monitored as secondary variables. An increase in urinary flow rate was observed in both treatment groups (1.9 ml/s with PRO 160/120; 2.4 ml/s with finasteride). The average urinary flow increased, whereas the micturition time decreased in both groups to a similar extent. The International Prostate Symptom Score (IPSS) decreased from 11.3 to 8.2 after 24 weeks and to 6.5 at week 48 for the PRO 160/120 group, and from 11.8 to 8.0 and to 6.2 at week 48 for the finasteride group. Fewer adverse reactions were reported for the nettle-saw palmetto treatment group, such as diminished ejaculation volume, erectile dysfunction, and headache (Sökeland and Albrecht, 1997).

An open, prospective, multicenter observational study involving 419 specialist urological practices tested the efficacy and tolerability of a combination preparation made of stinging nettle root extract (WS 1031; Schwabe, Germany) and saw palmetto fruit (*Serenoa repens*) extract (WS 1473; Prostagutt®, Schwabe, Germany) with 2,080 patients suffering from BPH, stage I to II according to Aiken. A before-and-after comparison revealed an improvement in the pathological findings and in the obstructive and irritative symptoms. Efficacy and tolerability of the preparation were assessed by the physicians as generally "good" or "very good." Most patients in the study reported an improvement in their prostatic symptoms and general quality of life (Schneider et al., 1995).

In a double-blind study, 134 patients between the ages of 53 and 84 with symptoms of BPH were drawn from two medical centers in Warsaw. The patients were randomly assigned to receive 2 capsules of the standard dose of a stinging nettle root-pygeum bark (*Prunus africanum*) preparation (300 mg nettle with 25 mg pygeum) or 2 capsules containing half the standard dose, twice daily for eight weeks. After 28 days of treatment, urine flow, residual urine, and nocturia were significantly reduced in both treatment groups. After 56 days, further significant decreases were found in residual urine in the half-dose group, and in nocturia in both groups. Five patients reported adverse effects from the treatment, though treatment was not discontinued due to side effects. The authors concluded that half-doses of the nettle-pygeum combination extract are as safe and effective as the recommended full dose (Krzeski et al., 1993).

In a placebo controlled, double-blind study the effect on symptomatology and objective findings of stinging nettle root extract vs. placebo were investigated in 50 patients with prostatic hyperplasia. Twenty-five BPH I-II patients were given 300 mg stinging nettle root dry extract (5:1) twice daily for nine weeks, and 25 received placebo. Average age was 67 years. A significant (p<0.05) improvement of micturition volume (44% increase) and maximum urinary flow was observed,

and a highly significant (p=0.0005) decrease in serum levels of sex hormone binding globulin (SHBH) (Vontobel et al., 1985).

In another study, 67 men over 60 years of age with prostatic adenoma evaluated
the effects of a stinging nettle root alcoholic tincture (1:5, 40% ethanol) with a
daily dose of 5 ml. After six months of treatment, symptoms of nocturia were alleviated (nocturnal micturition frequency), especially in less severe cases (Belaiche
and Lievoux, 1991).

Pharmacopeial grade stinging nettle root must pass botanical identity tests as
determined by TLC as well as macroscopic and microscopic authentication. Quantitative standards include not less than 15% water-soluble extractive (BHP, 1996;
DAB, 1997; Wichtl and Bisset, 1994). The ESCOP monograph requires that the
material comply with the standards of the *German Pharmacopoeia* (ESCOP, 1997).

The approved modern therapeutic applications for stinging nettle herb, leaf and
root are supportable based on their history of clinical use in well established systems of traditional medicine, on well documented phytochemical investigations, on
pharmacological studies in animals, and on human clinical studies.

Stinging Nettle herb and leaf

Latin Name:
Urtica dioica

Pharmacopeial Name:
Urticae herba, stinging nettle herb; Urticae folium, stinging nettle leaf

Other Names:
common nettle or great stinging nettle (*U. dioica*); dwarf nettle or
small stinging nettle (*U. urens*)

Description

Stinging nettle herb consists of fresh or
dried aboveground parts of *Urtica
dioica* L., *U. urens* L. [Fam. Urticaceae],
and hybrids of these species, collected
during flowering season, and their
preparations in effective dosage. Stinging nettle leaf consists of fresh or dried
leaves of *U. dioica* L., *U. urens* L. and/or
hybrids of these species, gathered during flowering season, and their preparations in effective dosage. Stinging nettle
leaf and herb contain mineral salts,
mainly calcium and potassium salts, and
silicic acid. The preparation must conform to the currently valid pharmacopeia.

Chemistry and Pharmacology

Stinging nettle herb and leaf contain up
to 20% mineral salts, mainly calcium,
potassium, silicon (0.9–1.8%), and
nitrates; 1.0–2.7% chlorophylls α and
β; the amines acetylcholine, betaine,
choline, histamine, 5-hydroxytrypta-
mine (serotonin) (0.02%), lecithin;
choline acetyltransferase; caffeoylmalic
acid (up to 1.6%), caffeic and chlorogenic acids; the flavonoids quercetin,
isoquercitrin, rutin, kaempferol, and
isorhamnetin; acetic, butyric, citric,
formic, and fumaric organic acids;
carotenoids (β-carotene, lycopene);
leukotreines; sterols (β-sitosterol); tannins; volatile oil (38.5% ketones,
14.7% esters, 2% free alcohols); vitamins A, B_2, C, K1, folic acid, and pantothenic acid (Bradley, 1992; Bruneton,

1995; ESCOP, 1997; Leung and Foster, 1996; List and Hörhammer, 1979; Newall et al., 1996; Wichtl and Bisset, 1994).

The Commission E did not report pharmacological actions.

The *British Herbal Compendium* reported mild diuretic and hemostatic activities. Its flavonoids and high potassium content may contribute to the diuretic action (Bradley, 1992). In a multicenter study, 70% of 152 patients suffering from various rheumatic, mainly degenerative, diseases experienced subjective improvement after ingesting a nettle herb dry extract for three weeks at 1.54 g daily (Ramm and Hansen, 1995). In a clinical study with patients suffering from myocardial or chronic venous insufficiency, diuretic action was reported after ingesting nettle juice (Kirchhoff, 1983).

Uses

The Commission E approved the internal use of nettle herb and leaf as irrigation therapy for inflammatory diseases of the lower urinary tract and prevention and treatment of kidney gravel. Internal and external application: as supportive therapy for rheumatic ailments.

The German Standard License for nettle herb tea indicates its use to increase the amount of urine and to treat complaints associated with urination (Bradley, 1992; Wichtl and Bisset, 1994). In France, uses are permitted for oral and topical administration: traditionally used to treat moderate acne, and traditionally used for the symptomatic treatment of pain in the joints (Bruneton, 1995). Externally the juice of the fresh herb is used as a gargle and as a cataplasm on wounds, ulcers, and hemorrhoids (List and Hörhammer, 1979). ESCOP indicates its use as an adjuvant treatment of rheumatic conditions and as irrigation therapy in inflammatory conditions of the lower urinary tract (ESCOP, 1997).

Contraindications

None known.

Note: No irrigation therapy if edema exists due to impaired heart or kidney function.

Side Effects

None known.

Use During Pregnancy and Lactation

No restrictions known (McGuffin et al., 1997).

Interactions with Other Drugs

None known.

Dosage and Administration

Unless otherwise prescribed: 8–12 g per day of cut herb for teas and other galenical preparations for internal use, as stinging nettle spirit for external application.

Note: In irrigation therapy, intake of copious amounts of fluids must be taken.

Internal: Dried herb: 2–5 g, three times daily.

Infusion: Steep 2–5 g in 150 ml boiled water for 10 to 15 minutes, three times daily.

Decoction: 2–5 g in 150 ml cold water, then boil for 10 to 15 minutes, three times daily.

Juice (Succus Urticae herba): 5–10 ml, three times daily.

Fluidextract 1:1 (g/ml): 2–5 ml, three times daily.

Native dry extract 6.4–8.1:1 (w/w): 0.3–0.7 g, three times daily.

Normalized dry extract 3.5–4.5:1 (w/w): 0.5–1.25 g, three times daily.

External: Spirit or essence (Spiritus Urticae herba, 50% alcohol by volume): Alcoholic solution of distilled nettle, applied locally with a cloth.

Cataplasm: Semi-solid paste containing spirit of nettle herb for a moist-heat direct application to the skin used like a poultice.

STINGING NETTLE ROOT

Latin Name:
Urtica dioica

Pharmacopeial Name:
Urticae radix

Other Names:
common nettle or great stinging nettle (*U. dioica*); dwarf nettle or small stinging nettle (*U. urens*)

Description
Stinging nettle root consists of the underground parts of *Urtica dioica* L., *U. urens* L., and their hybrids [Fam. Urticaceae] and preparations from nettle root in effective dosage. The preparation contains β-sitosterol in free forms and as glycosides, as well as scopoletin.

Chemistry and Pharmacology
Stinging nettle root contains both acid and neutral polysaccharides (2 glucans, 2 glucogalacturonans, and 1 arabino-galactan); sterols (0.2–1% 3-β-sitosterol, 0.05–0.2% sitosterol-3-β-D-glucoside); 0.1–0.2% lectin *U. dioica* agglutinin or UDA composed of six isolectins; coumarin (approximately 0.002–0.01% scopoletin); phenolic acids, phenylpropanoid aldehydes, and alcohols; lignans (neo-olivil and derivatives); fatty acids; tannins; and monoterpenes and triterpenes (Bruneton, 1995; ESCOP, 1997; Leung and Foster, 1996; List and Hörhammer, 1979; Newall et al., 1996; Wichtl and Bisset, 1994).

The Commission E reported increased urinary volume, increased maximum urinary flow, and reduced residual urine activities. Note: This preparation relieves the symptoms of an enlarged prostate without reducing the enlargement. Please consult a physician at regular intervals.

The *British Herbal Pharmacopoeia* reported prostatic action (BHP, 1996). Preliminary clinical observations of men after long-term treatment with an alcoholic extract of nettle root reported improvement of bladder outlet obstruction symptoms and decrease in post-voiding residual urine (Bruneton, 1995). A study of BPH patients treated with a nettle root alcoholic fluidextract reported a 66% decrease in residual urine; another study reported a reduction of nocturnal micturition frequency in patients over 60 years of age after six months of treatment with a nettle root alcoholic tincture at 5 ml daily (ESCOP, 1997; Leung and Foster, 1996). The active substances responsible for these actions are unknown, which makes quality control and chemical or biological standardization of extracts difficult (Bruneton, 1995; Wichtl and Bisset, 1994).

Uses
The Commission E approved the internal use of nettle root for difficulty in urination in benign prostatic hyperplasia stages 1 and 2.

ESCOP indicates its use for symptomatic treatment of micturition disorders [nocturia (excessive nighttime urination), pollakisuria (frequent urination), dysuria (painful urination), or urine retention] in BPH stages 1 and 2 (ESCOP, 1997). The French Herbal Remedies Notice to Applicants for Marketing Authorization allows two uses of nettle root: as an adjunctive treatment for the bladder outlet obstruction symptoms of prostatic origin, and to enhance the renal elimination of water (Bruneton, 1995). It is used as a diuretic for conditions of dropsy and also for early stages of prostatitis. In African medicine it is used to treat diarrhea and as an anthelmintic to expel intestinal worms (List and Hörhammer, 1979).

Contraindications
None known.

Side Effects
Occasionally, mild gastrointestinal upsets.

Use During Pregnancy and Lactation
No restrictions known (McGuffin et al. 1997).

Interactions with Other Drugs
None known.

Dosage and Administration
Unless otherwise prescribed: 4–6 g per day of cut root for infusions as well as other galenical preparations for oral use.
Infusion: Steep 1.5 g in 150 ml boiled water for 10 to 20 minutes, three to four times daily.
Decoction: 1.5 g in cold water, heat to boil and keep boiling for about 1 minute, then steep covered for 10 minutes, three to four times daily.
Fluidextract 1:1 (g/ml): 1.5 ml, three to four times daily.
Tincture 1:5 (g/ml): 5.0–7.5 ml, three to four times daily.
Native dry extract 5.4–6.6:1 (w/w): 0.22–0.33 g, three to four times daily.

References
Belaiche, P. and O. Lievoux. 1991. Clinical studies on the palliative treatment of prostatic adenoma with extract of Urtica root. Phytother Res 5:267–269.

Bombardelli, E. and P. Morazzoni. 1997. Urtica dioica L.—Review. Fitoterapia 68(5):387–401.

Bradley, P.R. (ed.). 1992. British Herbal Compendium, Vol. 1. Bournemouth: British Herbal Medicine Association.

British Herbal Pharmacopoeia (BHP). 1996. Exeter, U.K.: British Herbal Medicine Association. 142–144.

Bruneton, J. 1995. Pharmacognosy, Phytochemistry, Medicinal Plants. Paris: Lavoisier Publishing.

Chrubasik, S., W. Enderlein, R. Bauer, W. Grabner. 1997. Evidence for antirheumatic effectiveness of Herba Urticae dioica in acute arthritis: A pilot study. Phytomed 4(2):105–108.

Deutsches Arzneibuch, 10th ed., 3rd suppl. (DAB 10). 1994. Stuttgart: Deutscher Apotheker Verlag.

Deutsches Arzneibuch (DAB 1997). 1997. Stuttgart: Deutscher Apotheker Verlag.

Deutscher Arzneimittel-Codex (DAC). 1986. Stuttgart: Deutscher Apotheker Verlag.

ESCOP. 1997. "Urticae herba," "Urticae folium," and "Urticae radix." Monographs on the Medicinal Uses of Plant Drugs. Exeter, U.K.: European Scientific Cooperative on Phytotherapy.

Gunther, E. 1973. Ethnobotany of Western Washington. Seattle: University of Washington Press. 28.

Karnick, C.R. 1994. Pharmacopoeial Standards of Herbal Plants, Vol. 2. Delhi: Sri Satguru Publications. 126.

Kirchhoff, H.W. 1983. Brennesselsaft als Diuretikum. Z Phytother 4:621–626.

Krzeski, T., M. Kazon, A. Borkowski, A. Witeska, J. Kuczera. 1993. Combined extracts of Urtica dioica and Pygeum africanum in the treatment of benign prostatic hyperplasia: double-blind comparison of two doses. Clin Ther 15(6):1011–1020.

Leighton, A.L. 1985. Wild Plant Use by the Woods Cree (Nihithawak) of East-Central Saskatchewan. Ottawa: National Museums of Canada.

Leung, A.Y. and S. Foster. 1996. Encyclopedia of Common Natural Ingredients Used in Food, Drugs, and Cosmetics, 2nd ed. New York: John Wiley & Sons, Inc.

List, P.H. and L. Hörhammer (eds.). 1979. Hagers Handbuch der Pharmazeutischen Praxis, Vol. 6. Berlin-Heidelberg: Springer Verlag.

McGuffin, M., C. Hobbs, R. Upton, A. Goldberg. 1997. American Herbal Product Association's Botanical Safety Handbook. Boca Raton: CRC Press.

Mittman, P. 1990. Randomised, double-blind study of freeze-dried Urtica dioica in the treatment of allergic rhinitis. Planta Med 56(1):44–47.

Moerman, D.E. 1998. Native American Ethnobotany. Portland, OR: Timber Press, Inc.

Nadkarni, K.M. 1976. Indian Materia Medica. Bombay: Popular Prakashan. 1258.

Newall, C.A., L.A. Anderson, J.D. Phillipson. 1996. Herbal Medicines: A Guide for Health-Care Professionals. London: The Pharmaceutical Press.

Palmer, G. 1975. Shuswap Indian Ethnobotany. Las Vegas, NV: University of Nevada Dept. of Anthropology. 70.

Ramm, S. and C. Hansen. 1995. Brennessel-Extrakt bei rheumatischen Beschwerden. Dtsch Apoth Ztg 135(suppl.):3–8.

Ray, V.F. 1933. The Sanpoil and Nespelem: Salishan Peoples of N.E. Washington. University of Washington Publications in Anthropology 5:219.

Schneider, H.J., E. Honold, T. Masuhr. 1995. Behandlung der benignen prostatahyperplasie. Ergebnisse einer anwendungsbeobachtung mit dem pflanzlichen kombinationspraparat aus Sabalextrakt WS 1473 und *Urtica* extrakt WS 1031 in urologischen fachpraxen [Treatment of benign prostatic hyperplasia. Results of a treatment study with the phytogenic combination of Sabal extract WS 1473 and Urtica extract WS 1031 in urologic specialty practices]. *Fortschr Med* 113(3):37–40.

Smith, G.W. 1973. Arctic Pharmacognosia. Arctic 26:324–333.

Sökeland, J. and J. Albrecht. 1997. Kombination aus *Sabal*- und *Urtica*extrakt vs. finasterid bei BPH (stad. I bis II nach Aiken). Vergleich der therapeutischen wirksamkeit in einer einjahrigen doppelblindstudie [Combination of *Sabal* and *Urtica* extract vs. finasteride in benign prostatic hyperplasia (Aiken stages I to II). Comparison of therapeutic effectiveness in a one year double-blind study]. *Urologe A* 36(4):327–333.

Turner, N. and B.S. Efrat. 1982. *Ethnobotany of the Hesquiat Indians of Vancouver Island.* Victoria, BC: British Columbia Provincial Museum.

Turner, N. and M.A. Bell. 1973. Ethnobotany of Southern Kwakiutl Indians of British Columbia. *Economic Botany* 27:257–310.

Vontobel, H.P., R. Herzog, G. Rutishauser, H. Kres. 1985. Ergebnisse einer doppelblindstudie über die wirksamkeit von ERU-Kapseln in der konservativen behandlung der benignen prostatahyperplasie [Results of a double-blind study on the effectiveness of ERU (extractum radicis Urticae) capsules in conservative treatment of benign prostatic hyperplasia]. *Urologe A* 24(1):49–51.

Wichtl, M. and N.G. Bisset (eds.). 1994. *Herbal Drugs and Phytopharmaceuticals.* Stuttgart: Medpharm Scientific Publishers.

Additional Resources

Awang, D.V. 1997. Saw palmetto, African prune and stinging nettle for benign prostatic hyperplasia (BPH). *Can Pharm J* Nov:37–40, 43–44, 62.

Bartsch, G., K. Dreikom, P.S. Schontoger. 1998. Kombination aus *Sabal*- und *Urtica*extrakt vs. finasterid bei BPH (stad. I bis II nach Aiken). Kommentar zur arbeit von J. Sökeland und J. Albrech [Combined *Sabal* and *Urtica* extract vs. finasteride in benign prostatic hyperplasia (Alken stages I to II). Comment on the contribution by J. Sökeland and J. Albrech]. *Urologe A* 37(1):83–85.

Bone, K. (ed.). 1997. Nettles for Arthritis? *Medi-Herb Monitor* Jun(22):1.

Braun, R. et al. 1997. *Standardzulassungen für Fertigarzneimittel—Text und Kommentar.* Stuttgart: Deutscher Apotheker Verlag.

Breedveld, F. 1994. Tenidap: A novel cytokine-modulating antirheumatic drug for the treatment of rheumatoid arthritis. *Scand J Rheumatol* 23(suppl. 100):31–44.

Broncano, F.J. et al. 1987. Estudio de efecto sobre musculatura lisa uterina de distintos preparados de las hojas de *Urtica dioica* L. *An R Acad Farm* 53:69–76.

———. 1987. Estudio de diferentes preparados de *Urtica dioica* L. sobre SNC. *An R Acad Farm* 53:284–291.

Dathe, G. and H. Schmidt. 1987. Phytotherapie der benignen prostatahyperplasie. Doppelblindstudie mit extractum radicis Urticae (ERU). *UrologeB* 27:223–226.

Dingle, J.T. 1979. Recent studies on the control of joint damage. *Ann Rheum Dis* 38(3):201–214.

Direction de la Pharmacie et du Médicament (DPM). 1992. Bulletin Officiel No. 92/11 bis. [English edition]. Paris: Direction des Journaux Officiels.

Fischer, M. and D. Wilbert. 1992. *Benigne Prostatahyperplasie III. Klinische und Experimentelle Urologie* 22. München-Bern-Wien: Zuckschwerdt. 79–84.

Fisher, C.N. 1997. Nettles—An aid to the treatment of allergic rhinitis. *Eur J Herbal Med* 3(2):34–35.

Fournier, P. 1948. *Le Livre des Plantes Médicinal et Vénéneuse de France,* Vol. 3. Paris: Lechevalier Éditeur. 138–146.

Goetz, P. 1989. Die behandlung der benignen prostatahyperplasie mit Brennesselwurzeln. *Z Phytother* 10:175–158.

Hartmann, R.W., M. Mark, F. Soldati. 1996. Inhibition of 5 α-reductase and aromatase by PHL-00801 (Prostatonin) a combination of PY 102 (*Pygeum africanum*) and UR 102 (*Urtica dioica*) extracts. *Phytomedicine* 3(2):121–128.

Hirano, T., M. Homma, K. Oka. 1994. Effects of stinging nettle root extracts and their steroidal components on the Na+,K(+)-ATPase of the benign prostatic hyperplasia. *Planta Med* 60(1):30–33.

Hryb, D.J., M.S. Khan, N.A. Romas, W. Rosner. 1995. The effect of extracts of the roots of the stinging nettle (*Urtica dioica*) on the interaction of SHBG with its receptor on human prostatic membranes. *Planta Med* 61(1):31–32.

Jaspersen-Schib, R. 1989. Die Brennessel—eine Modedroge—oder mehr? *Schweiz Apoth Ztg* 127:443–445.

Lichius, J.J. and C. Muth. 1997. The inhibiting effects of *Urtica dioica* root extracts on experimentally induced prostatic hyperplasia in the mouse. *Planta Med* 63(4):307–310.

Lutomski, J. and H. Speichert. 1983. Die Brennessel in heilkunde und ernährung [Stinging nettle in medicine and nutrition]. *Pharm Unserer Zeit* 12(6):181–186.

Madaus, G. 1979. *Lehrbuch der Biologischen Heilmittel,* 2nd ed. Vol. 3. Hildesheim-NewYork: G. Olms Verlag. 2746–2754.

Obertreis, B., K. Giller, T. Teucher, B. Behnke, H. Schmitz. 1996. Antiphlogistische effekte von extrakum-*Urticae* dioica foliorum im vergleich zu kaffeoyläpfelsäure [Anti-inflammatory effect of *Urtica dioica* folia extract in comparison to caffeic malic acid]. *Arzneimforsch* 46(1):52–56.

Obertreis, B., T. Ruttkowski, T. Teucher, B. Behnke, H. Schmitz. 1996. *Ex-vivo-in-vitro* hemmung der lipopolysaccharid-stimulierten tumor-nekrose-faktor-alpha und interleukin-1β-sekretion in humanem vollblut durch extractum Urticae dioica foliorum [Ex-vivo in-vitro inhibition of lipopolysaccharide stimulated tumor necrosis factor-alpha and interleukin-1 β secretion in human whole blood by extractum *Urticae dioicae* foliorum] *Arzneimforsch* 46(4):389–394.

Pharmacopoeia Helvetica, 7th ed. Vol. 1–4. (Ph.Helv.VII). 1987. Bern: Office Central Fédéral des Imprimés et du Matériel.

Ramm, S. and C. Hansen. 1996. Brennesselblätter-extrakt bei arthrose und rheumatoider arthritis. *Therapiewoche* 28:3–6.

Reynolds, J.E.F. (ed.). 1982. *Martindale: The Extra Pharmacopoeia,* 28th ed. London: The Pharmaceutical Press.

Ritschel, W.A., U. Kastner, A.S. Hussain, H.P. Koch. 1990. Pharmacokinetics and bioavailability of β-sitosterol in the beagle dog. *Arzneimforsch* 40(4):463–468.

Rückle, E. 1950. *Brenneselwurzeltee bei Beginnender Prostatitis.* Stuttgart: Hippokrates Verlag. 55–56.

Rutishauser, G. (ed.). 1992. *Benigne Prostatahyperplasie III. Klinische und Experimentelle Urologie* 22. München-Bern-Wien: W. Zuckschwerdt Verlag.

Schilcher, H. 1984. Pflanzliche Urologika. *Dtsch Apoth Ztg* 124:2429–2436.

———. 1988. Möglichkeiten und grenzen der phytotherapie am beispiel pflanzlicher Urologika. Teil 2: Adnexerkrankungen des mannes und der frau und urolithiasis. *Urologe B* 28:90–95.

———. 1988. Urtica-arten die brennessel. *Z Phytother* 9:160–164.

———. 1992. Phytotherapie in der Urologie. Stuttgart: Hippokrates. 20–21, 84–88.

Schilcher, H. and S. Effenberger. 1986. Scopoletin und β-sitosterol zwei geeignete leitsubstanzen für *Urticae* radix. *Dtsch Apoth Ztg* 126:79–81.

Schilcher, H., R. Boesel, S. Effenberger, S. Segebrecht. 1989. Neue untersuchungsergebnisse mit aquaretisch, antibakteriell und prostatotrop wirksamen arzneipflanzen. *Z Phytother* 10:77–82.

Schottner, M., D. Gansser, G. Spiteller. 1997. Lignans from the roots of *Urtica dioica* and their metabolites bind to human sex hormone binding globulin (SHBG). *Planta Med* 63(6):529–532.

Sommer, H. et al. 1989. Influence of an herbal mixture on respiratory diseases of horses. *Tierarztlich-Umschau* 41:846–848.

Teucher, T., B. Obertreis, T. Ruttkowski, H. Schmitz. 1996. Zytokin-sekretion im vollblut gesunder probanden nach oraler einnahme eines *Urtica dioica* L.-blattextraktes [Cytokine secretion in whole blood of healthy subjects following oral administration of *Urtica dioica* L. plant extract] *Arzneimforsch* 46(9):906–910.

Tita, B., P. Faccendini, U. Bello, L. Martinoli, P. Bolle. 1993. *Urtica dioica* L.: Pharmacological effect of ethanol extract. *Pharmacol Res* 27(suppl. 1):21–22.

Wagner, H. and F. Willer. 1992. Chemie und Pharmakologie der Polysaccharide und Lektine von *Urtica dioica*-Wurzeln. In: Rutishauser, G. (ed.). *Benigne Prostatahyperplasie III. Klinische und Experimentelle Urologie* 22. München-Bern-Wien: W. Zuckschwerdt Verlag. 125–132.

Wagner, H., F. Willer, B. Kreher. 1989. Biologisch aktive Verbindungen aus dem Wasserextrakt von *Urtica dioica* [Biologically active compounds from the aqueous extract of *Urtica dioica*]. *Planta Med* 55(5):452–454.

Wagner, H., F. Willer, R. Samtleben, G. Boos. 1994. Search for the antiprostatic principle of stinging nettle (*Urtica dioica*) roots. *Phytomed* 1:213–224.

Weiss, R.F. 1988. *Herbal Medicine.* Beaconsfield, England: Beaconsfield Publishers.

———. 1991. *Lehrbuch der Phytotherapie,* 7th ed. Stuttgart: Hippokrates. 335–336.

Wichtl, M. and M. Schäfer-Korting. 1994. *DAB 10— Kommentar,* part 3. Stuttgart: Wissenschaftliche Verlagsgesellschaft. B53.

Wylie, G. et al. 1995. A comparative study of Tenidap, a cytokine-modulating anti-rheumatic drug, and diclofenac in rheumatoid arthritis: a 24-week analysis of a 1-year clinical trial. *Br J Rheumatol* 34(6):554–563.

This material was adapted from *The Complete German Commission E Monographs—Therapeutic Guide to Herbal Medicines.* M. Blumenthal, W.R. Busse, A. Goldberg, J. Gruenwald, T. Hall, C.W. Riggins, R.S. Rister (eds.) S. Klein and R.S. Rister (trans.). 1998. Austin: American Botanical Council; Boston: Integrative Medicine Communications.

1) The Overview section is new information.

2) Description, Chemistry and Pharmacology, Uses, Contraindications, Side Effects, Interactions with Other Drugs, and Dosage sections have been drawn from the original work. Additional information has been added in some or all of these sections, as noted with references.

3) The dosage for equivalent preparations (tea infusion, fluidextract, and tincture) have been provided based on the following example:
   Unless otherwise prescribed: 2 g per day of [powdered, crushed, cut or whole] [plant part]
   Infusion: 2 g in 150 ml of water
   Fluidextract 1:1 (g/ml): 2 ml
   Tincture 1:5 (g/ml): 10 ml

4) The References and Additional Resources sections are new sections. Additional Resources are not cited in the monograph but are included for research purposes.

THYME

Latin Name:
Thymus vulgaris

Pharmacopeial Name:
Thymi herba

Other Names:
common thyme, garden thyme

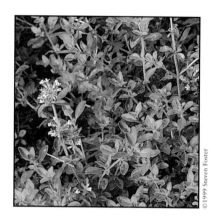

©1999 Steven Foster

Overview

Thyme is cultivated throughout the world for culinary, cosmetic, and medicinal purposes, the manufacture of perfume, and for red and white thyme oil. Common thyme (*Thymus vulgaris*) and Spanish thyme (*T. zygis*) are used interchangeably for medicinal purposes. Crude dried or fresh herb may be brewed as tea or extracted into an alcohol macerate. Common thyme contains 0.4–3.4% of the volatile oil; Spanish thyme contains 0.7–1.38%. The red or white thyme oil is manufactured commercially for use in cough drops, mouthwashes, liniment, toothpaste, detergent, and perfume. Because white thyme oil is a distilled red thyme oil product, red thyme oil is generally preferred (Leung and Foster, 1996).

Thyme in its crude herb form is carminative, antibiotic, anthelmintic, astringent, expectorant, and antitussive (Leung and Foster, 1996; Newall et al., 1996). It has been used in traditional medicine to treat heartburn, gastritis, asthma, laryngitis, pertussis, and bronchitis (Newall et al., 1996). Extracts demonstrate *in vitro* anti-inflammatory effects on guinea pig tracheal smooth muscle tissue (Leung and Foster, 1996), and the volatile oil in the herb most likely exerts spasmolytic effects on bronchial tissues in humans (Tyler, 1994). The herb is approved by Commission E in the treatment of bronchitis, whooping cough, and upper respiratory inflammation.

Like the herb's infusions and extracts, thyme oil is also carminative, expectorant, and possesses antimicrobial and anthelmintic properties, due to concentrated thymol and carvacrol content (Leung and Foster, 1996), but it is extremely toxic. As an ingredient in toothpaste, thyme oil has been blamed for cases of inflamed lips and tongue reported in the toothpaste users. Signs of toxicity escalate from nausea to respiratory arrest (Newall et al., 1996). For these reasons, the herb is preferred to the oil.

Thyme was known to classic Rome; it was added to cheeses and alcoholic beverages. In the seventeenth century, herbalist Nicholas Culpepper wrote that thyme teas and infusions were useful for whooping cough, shortness of breath, gout, and mild stomach pains. He suggested that a thyme ointment be used to eliminate abscesses and warts. Thyme oil was used as a rubefacient and counterirritant, and was part of an herbal cigarette that was smoked to relieve stomach upset, headache, and fatigue. Thyme essence was used in perfumes and embalming oils (Grieve, 1979).

Thyme's common name may be derived from a Greek word meaning to fumigate, because the Greeks used thyme as an incense. It may also have come from the Greek word *thumus*, meaning courage. In medieval times, thyme was regarded as a plant that could impart courage and vigor, and women often embroidered a sprig of thyme on gifts for their favorite knight (Grieve, 1979).

Description

Thyme consists of the stripped and dried leaves and flowers of *T. vulgaris* L., *T. zygis* L. [Fam. Lamiaceae], or both species, and their preparations in effective dosage. The herb contains at least 0.5% phenols, calculated as thymol based on the dried herb.

Chemistry and Pharmacology

Constituents include essential oil containing the phenols thymol and carvacrol; terpenoids; glycosides of phenolic monoterpenoids; eugenol and aliphatic alcohols; the flavonoids thymonin, cirsilineol, and 8-methoxycirsilineol; biphenyl compounds of monoterpenoid origin; caffeic and rosmarinic acids; and saponins (ESCOP, 1997). Other constituents include tannins, labiatic acid, ursolic acid, and oleanolic acid (Leung and Foster, 1996). Thyme also contains apigenin, luteolin, and 6-hydroxyluteolin glycosides, as well as di-, tri-, and tetramethoxylated flavones, which are all substituted in the 6-position (5,4'-dihydroxy-6,7,3'-trimethoxyflavone and its 8-methoxylated derivative, 5,6,4'-trihydroxy-7,8,3'-trimethoxyflavone, 5,4'-dihydroxy-6,7,8-trimethoxyflavone, 5,4'-dihydroxy-6,7-dimethoxyflavone) (Bruneton, 1995).

The Commission E reported bronchoantispasmodic, expectorant, and antibacterial activity.

In vitro experiments found that the flavonoids thymonin, cirsilineol, and 8-methoxy-cirsilineol may be responsible for the bronchospasmolytic effect of thyme (ESCOP, 1997). *In vivo*, rosmarinic acid demonstrated inhibitory properties in reduction of edema, inhibition of passive curtaneous anaphylaxis, and impairment of *in vivo* activation by heat-killed *Corynebacterium parvum* of mouse macrophages. This activity demonstrates that its activity may relate to complement activation (ESCOP, 1997).

Uses

The Commission E approved thyme for symptoms of bronchitis and whooping cough and catarrhs of the upper respiratory tracts. It has also been used as to improve digestion (Stecher, 1968) and to treat pertussis, stomatitis, and halitosis (ESCOP, 1997; Wichtl and Bisset, 1994).

Contraindications

None known.

Side Effects

None known.

Use During Pregnancy and Lactation

Not recommended during pregnancy. No restrictions known during lactation.

Interactions with Other Drugs

None known.

Dosage and Administration

Unless otherwise prescribed: Cut herb, powder, liquid extract or dry extract for infusions and other galenical preparations. Liquid and solid medicinal forms for internal and external application. NOTE: Combinations with other herbs that have expectorant action could be appropriate.

Internal:
Infusion: 1 to 2 g of herb for 1 cup of tea, several times daily as needed. Fluidextract 1/1 (g/ml): 1 to 2 ml, one to three times daily.

External:
Compress: 5% infusion for compresses.

References

Bruneton, J. 1995. *Pharmacognosy, Phytochemistry, Medicinal Plants*. Paris: Lavoisier Publishing.

ESCOP. 1997. "Thymi herba." *Monographs on the Medicinal Uses of Plant Drugs*. Exeter, U.K.: European Scientific Cooperative on Phytotherapy.

Grieve, M. 1979. *A Modern Herbal.* New York: Dover Publications, Inc.

Hutchens, A. 1991. *Indian Herbology of North America.* Boston: Shambala.

Leung, A.Y. and S. Foster. 1996. *Encyclopedia of Common Natural Ingredients Used in Food, Drugs, and Cosmetics,* 2nd ed. New York: John Wiley & Sons, Inc.

Newall, C.A., L.A. Anderson, J.D. Phillipson. 1996. *Herbal Medicines: A Guide for Health-Care Professionals.* London: The Pharmaceutical Press.

Stecher, P.G. (ed.). 1968. *The Merck Index: An Encyclopedia of Chemicals and Drugs,* 8th ed. Rahway, N.J.: Merck & Co., Inc.

Tyler, V.E. 1994. *Herbs of Choice: The Therapeutic Use of Phytomedicinals.* New York: Pharmaceutical Products Press.

Wichtl, M. and N.G. Bisset (eds.). 1994. *Herbal Drugs and Phytopharmaceuticals.* Stuttgart: Medpharm Scientific Publishers.

Additional Resources

Braun, R. et al. 1997. *Standardzulassungen für Fertigarzneimittel—Text and Kommentar.* Stuttgart: Deutscher Apotheker Verlag.

British Herbal Pharmacopoeia (BHP). 1983. Keighley, U.K.: British Herbal Medicine Association.

Deutsches Arzneibuch, 10th ed. Vol. 1–6. (DAB 10). 1991. Kommentar. Stuttgart: Wissenschaftliche Verlagsgesellschaft.

Englberger, W. et al. 1988. Rosmarinic acid: a new inhibitor of complement C3-convertase with anti-inflammatory activity. *Int J Immunopharm* 10(6):729–737.

McGuffin, M., C. Hobbs, R. Upton, A. Goldberg. 1997. American Herbal Product Association's *Botanical Safety Handbook.* Boca Raton: CRC Press.

Österreichisches Arzneibuch, Vols. 1–2, 1st suppl. (ÖAB). 1981–1983. Wien: Verlag der Österreichischen Staatsdruckerei.

Pharmacopoeia Helvetica, 7th ed. Vol. 1–4. (Ph.Helv.VII). 1987. Bern: Office Central Fédéral des Imprimés et du Matériel.

Van den Broucke, C.O. et al. 1983. Action spasmolytique des flavones de differentes especes de Thymus. *Plantes Med Phytother* (16):310–317.

Van den Broucke, C.O. and J.A. Lemli. 1981. Pharmacological and chemical investigation of thyme liquid extracts. *Planta Med* 41(2):129–135.

———. 1983. Spasmolytic activity of the flavonoids from *Thymus vulgaris. Pharm Weekbl* 5(1):9–14.

Wichtl, M. (ed.). 1989. *Teedrogen,* 2nd ed. Stuttgart: Wissenschaftliche Verlagsgesellschaft.

Wren, R.C. 1988. *Potter's New Cyclopaedia of Botanical Drugs and Preparations.* Essex: The C.W. Daniel Company Ltd.

This material was adapted from *The Complete German Commission E Monographs—Therapeutic Guide to Herbal Medicines.* M. Blumenthal, W.R. Busse, A. Goldberg, J. Gruenwald, T. Hall, C.W. Riggins, R.S. Rister (eds.) S. Klein and R.S. Rister (trans.). 1998. Austin: American Botanical Council; Boston: Integrative Medicine Communications.

1) The Overview section is new information.

2) Description, Chemistry and Pharmacology, Uses, Contraindications, Side Effects, Interactions with Other Drugs, and Dosage sections have been drawn from the original work. Additional information has been added in some or all of these sections, as noted with references.

3) The dosage for equivalent preparations (tea infusion, fluidextract, and tincture) have been provided based on the following example:

Unless otherwise prescribed: 2 g per day of [powdered, crushed, cut or whole] [plant part]
Infusion: 2 g in 150 ml of water
Fluidextract 1:1 (g/ml): 2 ml
Tincture 1:5 (g/ml): 10 ml

4) The References and Additional Resources sections are new sections. Additional Resources are not cited in the monograph but are included for research purposes.

TURMERIC ROOT

Latin Name:
Curcuma longa

Pharmacopeial Name:
Curcumae longae rhizoma

Other Names:
Curcuma, Indian saffron, *Haridra* (Sanskrit), *Jianghuang* (Chinese), *Kyoo* or *Ukon* (Japanese)

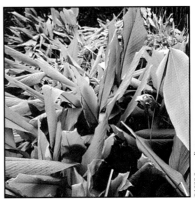

©1999 Steven Foster

Overview

Turmeric is a perennial rhizomatous shrub native to southern Asia (Leung and Foster, 1996; Wichtl and Bisset, 1994), extensively cultivated in all parts of India (API, 1989), mainly in Madras, Bengal, and Bombay (Kapoor, 1990). It is also cultivated in southern mainland China, Taiwan, Japan, Burma, Indonesia (Yen, 1992), and throughout the African continent (Iwu, 1993). The material of commerce in Europe is obtained mainly from India, Indonesia, and somewhat from China (Wichtl, 1996). India produces most of the world supply (Leung and Foster, 1996). Turmeric is an herb of major importance in the East and, until recently, one of relatively minor importance in the West (Govindarajan, 1980). It is a member of the ginger family (Zingiberaceae); the Chinese name, *jianghuang*, literally means "yellow ginger."

Traditional use of turmeric has varied somewhat regionally, though its use as a digestive aid and choleretic is almost universal (Grieve, 1979). Its modern approved applications in European medicine stem from its traditional uses in Asia. Turmeric is used extensively in the Indian systems of medicine (Ayurveda, Unani, and Siddha) and is official in the *Ayurvedic Pharmacopoeia* of India (API, 1989; Nadkarni, 1976). In Western terms, it is used as a carminative and stomachic (Kapoor, 1990; Nadkarni, 1976) for the treatment of digestive disorders such as flatulence, bloating, and appetite loss (Schulz et al., 1998). Turmeric is prepared in a variety of internal (e.g., boiled powder, fresh juice, confection) and external (e.g., paste, oil, ointment, lotion) dosage forms, as it is also applied topically for ulcers, wounds, eczema, and inflammations (Nadkarni, 1976). In both the Ayurvedic and Siddha systems of medicine, a turmeric paste is used topically to treat ulcers and scabies (Charles and Charles, 1992). In Ayurvedic medicine, turmeric also has a long history of use for its anti-inflammatory and antiarthritic effects. According to James Duke, turmeric is a safer, more natural, and less expensive cyclooxygenase (COX) inhibitor than pharmaceutical COX-inhibitor drugs (Duke, 1999). Turmeric is also used extensively in traditional Chinese medicine. It is official in the *Pharmacopoeia of the People's Republic of China* (Tu, 1992) as well as in the *Japanese Herbal Medicines Codex* (JSHM, 1993). As in India, it is used in China, Japan, and Korea for a range of indications including abdominal fullness, kidney pain, and amenorrhea (But et al., 1997; Yen, 1992). In China, the aqueous decoction dosage form is ingested orally and applied topically (But et al., 1997).

Several clinical studies have been found in the literature. Turmeric has been investigated for its cholagogous influence on the secretion of bile, pancreatic, and gastric juices (Baumann et al., 1971; Baumann, 1975). In a multicenter, randomized, double-blind study, the efficacy of turmeric rhizome for treatment of dyspepsia was investigated. The trial was conducted in six Thai hospitals and included

116 adult patients diagnosed with acid dyspepsia, flatulent dyspepsia, and/or atonic dyspepsia. Each patient received two capsules of drug or placebo, four times daily for seven days. Eighty-seven percent of the patients receiving turmeric capsules responded favorably whereas 53% of the patients receiving placebo responded to treatment. The authors concluded that the differences in efficacy between drug and placebo were statistically significant and clinically important (Thamlikitkul et al., 1989). In a subsequent controlled clinical trial, researchers at Ratchaburi Hospital in Thailand compared the effects of turmeric against a liquid antacid drug in the treatment of gastric ulcer (Kositchaiwat et al., 1993). In a small study, the antimutagenic effects of turmeric were investigated in 16 chronic cigarette smokers in comparison with six non-smokers, who served as the control group. The smokers were given 1.5 g of turmeric per day for 30 days, which resulted in a significant reduction in the urinary excretion of mutagens. The authors concluded that regular dietary intake of turmeric provides effective antimutagen action and may be useful in chemoprevention (Polasa et al., 1992).

In a pilot study, conducted by the Medical and Cancer Research and Treatment Centre of Nagercoil, India, a turmeric paste was used for the treatment of scabies in 814 patients. The researchers concluded that turmeric paste is a very inexpensive, readily available, effective and acceptable mode of treatment for scabies without noticable toxicity or adverse reactions (Charles and Charles, 1992). In another study, researchers at the Swami Prakashananda Ayurveda Research Centre, in India, investigated an alcoholic extract of turmeric as well as turmeric oil and oleoresin fractions for their effects on cytogenetic damage in patients suffering from oral submucous fibrosis. All three forms of turmeric in this study were found to decrease the number of micronucleated cells in both exfoliated oral mucosal cells and in circulating lymphocytes (Hastak et al., 1997).

In Germany, turmeric is listed in the *Drug Codex*, approved in the Commission E monographs, and the tea form is official in the Standard License monographs (Braun et al., 1997; DAC, 1986; Wichtl and Bisset, 1994). A small amount of turmeric is used as a component in numerous multi-ingredient cholagogue and biliary remedies (Wichtl and Bisset, 1994). The *German Drug Codex* monograph requires turmeric to contain not less than 3.0% curcuminoids, calculated as curcumin, and not less than 3.0% volatile oil. Macroscopic and microscopic examinations and a thin-layer chromatography test are required for botanical authentication (DAC, 1986; Wichtl and Bisset, 1994). The German Standard License monograph requires that the material conform with the qualitative and quantitative requirements of the DAC (Braun et al., 1997).

Chinese pharmacopeial grade turmeric consists of the dried rhizome of *Curcuma longa* L., collected in the winter when the aerial part of the plant has withered. It is washed clean, boiled or steamed thoroughly, then cut into thick slices to dry in the sun, then separated from the fibrous root. It must contain not less than 7.0% (ml/g) volatile oil. Botanical identity must be confirmed by macroscopic and microscopic examinations, organoleptic evaluation, and a color reaction test using filter paper, ethanol, ether, solution of boric acid, and ammonia (Tu, 1992). Indian pharmacopeial grade turmeric consists of the dried and cured rhizomes of *C. longa* L., harvested after 9 to 10 months when the lower leaves turn yellow. The curing process includes boiling and drying steps. It must contain not less than 4.0% v/w volatile oil, not less than 12% water-soluble extractive, and not less than 8% alcohol-soluble extractive. Botanical identity must be confirmed by macroscopic and microscopic examinations as well as by two different color reaction tests (API, 1989). Japanese pharmacopeial grade turmeric consists of the unpeeled or peeled (without the cork layer) rhizome of *C. longa* L., cured with boiling water, then sun dried. Botanical identity must be confirmed by macroscopic and organoleptic evaluations as well as by two different color reaction tests (JSHM, 1993).

Description

Turmeric root consists of the finger-like, often tuber-like, scalded, and dried rhizomes of *C. longa* L. (syn. *C. domestica* Valeton and *C. aromatica* Salisbury) [Fam. Zingiberaceae] and their preparations in effective dosage. The preparation contains not less than 3% dicinnamoylmethane derivatives, calculated as curcumin, and not less than 3% volatile oil, both calculated on a dry-weight basis of the preparation.

Chemistry and Pharmacology

Turmeric contains 3–7.2% volatile oil, composed mainly of sesquiterpenes such as α- and β-turmerone, αr-turmerone, α-curcumen, and zingiberene, and minor amounts of monoterpenes such as cineol (Kapoor, 1990; Leung and Foster, 1996; Wichtl, 1996); 3–5% curcuminoids (dicinnomoyl derivatives), mainly curcumin (Budavari, 1996; Iwu, 1993; Wichtl, 1996), demethoxycurcumin, bis-demethoxycurcumin, and cyclocurcumin (But et al., 1997; Kiuchi et al., 1993); 3.5% minerals (e.g., potassium); carotene; vitamin C (Kapoor, 1990; Leung and Foster, 1996); a water-soluble peptide (e.g., 0.1% 5–kDa peptide–turmerin) (Srinivas et al., 1992); 45–55% gelatinized starch, composed of polysaccharides such as the immunologically active arabinogalactans (Bruneton, 1995; Wichtl, 1996), particularly the phagocytosis–activating polysaccharides ukonan A and C (Gonda et al., 1992; Gonda et al., 1993).

Note: Under proper storage conditions the volatile oil content still diminishes by approximately 0.5% per year. Therefore, product shelf life should be determined based on this known rate of volatilization, calculating the difference between the volatile oil content on the date of packaging against the minimum amount required in the drug codex or pharmacopeial monograph (Braun et al., 1997).

The Commission E reported that the choleretic action of curcumin is experimentally well documented. Further indications exist for a cholecystokinetic and a clear anti-inflammatory action.

Turmeric has anti-inflammatory and cytotoxic effects (But et al., 1997). Curcumin, isolated from turmeric, has demonstrated anti-thrombotic action while preserving prostacyclin, an inflammatory mediator (Srivastava et al., 1985; Srivastava et al., 1986). An ethereal extract of turmeric inhibited arachidonic–induced platelet aggregation in human blood platelets (Srivastava, 1989). Turmeric has also demonstrated antioxidant, antimutagen, and anticarcinogen effects in experimental animals (Polassa et al., 1992). The isolated constituent αr-turmerone has been shown to arrest the reproduction and killer activity of human lymphocytes, which may contribute to its anti-inflammatory activity (Wichtl and Bisset, 1994). Curcuminoids, isolated from turmeric, have displayed topoisomerase I and II enzyme inhibition activity (Roth et al., 1998). *In vitro* and *in vivo* experiments have found that turmeric has antihepatotoxic and antibacterial effects (Kiso et al., 1983).

While the chemistry of turmeric is well studied, its mechanism of action is not fully understood (Tyler, 1994). The rhizome contains an anti-inflammatory and choleretic volatile oil. Anti-inflammatory actions may be due to leukotriene inhibition (Ammon et al., 1992; Leung and Foster, 1996). Its curcuminoids (e.g., curcumin) and volatile oil are both partly responsible for the anti-inflammatory activity. Curcumin is, however, more effective by parenteral injection than by oral ingestion (Ammon and Wahl, 1991). The curcuminoids, despite poor absorption when taken orally, are generally thought to be responsible for the rhizome's bile-stimulating actions (Tyler, 1994). The isolated consituent curcumin has displayed anti-inflammatory and antitumor activity, and may be protective against some cancers, such as colon cancer. In laboratory tests, curcumin's antitumor actions appear to be due to interactions with arachidonate metabolism (Rao et al., 1995). Currently, turmeric is being investigated as an antioxidant. Both the rhizome, and isolated curcumin, have shown that they are able to protect DNA breakage caused by singlet oxygen. Singlet oxygen is known to have potential genotoxic and mutagenic actions. The protective, antioxidant effects of turmeric and curcumin were greater than those of vitamins E and A (Subramanian et al., 1994). An aqueous extractive of turmeric has been shown to be more effective than isolated curcumin in protecting human lymphocyte DNA from damage induced by smoke condensate (Srinivas and Shalini, 1991). A water-soluble peptide, turmerin, isolated from turmeric, has also demonstrated effective antioxidant, DNA-protectant and antimutagen actions. Turmerin contains three residues of methionine, which may be partly responsible for the antioxidant effects (Srinivas et al., 1992). More recently, an antioxidant protein has been isolated from the aqueous extract of turmeric (Selvam et al., 1995).

Uses
The Commission E approved turmeric root for dyspeptic conditions.

The German Standard License indicates the use of turmeric tea infusion as a stomach and intestine remedy for the treatment of digestive complaints, especially functional disturbances of the gall systems (Braun et al., 1997). In both Ayurvedic and Unani medicine it is used as a stomachic and tonic (Kapoor, 1990). *The Pharmacopoeia of the People's Republic of China* indicates its use for treatment of pricking pain in the chest and hypochondrium (abdominal pain), mass formation in the abdomen, and amenorrhea (to stimulate menstrual discharge and relieve pain), among other conditions (Tu, 1992).

Contraindications
Obstruction of bile passages. In case of gallstones, first consult a physician. Note: The *Botanical Safety Handbook* states that use of turmeric root should be avoided by people with bile duct

obstruction or gallstones; it should not be administered to people who suffer from stomach ulcers or hyperacidity (McGuffin et al., 1997).

Side Effects
None known.

Use During Pregnancy and Lactation
Not recommended during pregnancy (McGuffin et al., 1997). No restrictions known during lactation.

Interactions with Other Drugs
None known.

Dosage and Administration
Unless otherwise prescribed: 1.5–3 g per day of cut root as well as other equivalent galenical preparations for internal use.
Powder: 1–3 g (API, 1989); 1–4 g (Kapoor, 1990); 0.5–1 g, several times daily (Wichtl and Bisset, 1994).
Infusion: Steep approximately 1.3 g root in 150 ml boiled water for 10 to 15 minutes, twice daily (Braun et al., 1997).
Fluidextract 1:1 (g/ml): 1.5–3 ml.
Tincture 1:5 (g/ml): 10 ml (Stansbury, 1999).

References
Ammon, H.P. and M.A. Wahl. 1991. Pharmacology of *Curcuma longa*. Planta Med 57(1):1–7.
Ammon, H.P., M.I. Anazodo, H. Safayhi, B.N. Dhawan, R.C. Srimal. 1992. Curcumin: a potent inhibitor of leukotriene B4 formation in rat peritoneal polymorphonuclear neutrophils. *Planta Med* 58(2):226
Ayurvedic Pharmacopoeia of India (API). 1989. New Delhi: Government of India—Ministry of Health and Family Welfare—Department of Health. 45–46.

Baumann, J.C., K. Heintze, H.W. Muth. 1971. Klinisch-experimentelle untersuchungen der gallen-, pankreas- und magensaftsekretion unter den phytocholagogen wirkstoffen einer *Carduus marianus–Chelidonium–Curcuma* suspension [Clinico-experimental studies on the secretion of bile, pancreatic and gastric juice under the influence of phytocholagogous agents of a suspension of *Carduus marianus*, *Chelidonium* and *Curcuma*]. *Arzneimforsch* 21(1):98–101.

Baumann, J.C. 1975. Über die wirkung von *Chelidonium*, *Curcuma*, *Absinth* und *Carduus marianus* auf die galle-und pankreassekretion bei hepatopathien [Effect of *Chelidonium*, *Curcuma*, *Absinth* and *Carduus marianus* on the bile and pancreatic secretion in liver diseases]. *Med Monatsschr* 29(4):173–180.

Braun, R. et al. 1997. *Standardzulassungen für Fertigarzneimittel—Text and Kommentar.* Stuttgart: Deutscher Apotheker Verlag.

Bruneton, J. 1995. *Pharmacognosy, Phytochemistry, Medicinal Plants.* Paris: Lavoisier Publishing.

Budavari, S. (ed.). 1996. *The Merck Index: An Encyclopedia of Chemicals, Drugs, and Biologicals,* 12th ed. Whitehouse Station, N.J.: Merck & Co., Inc. 450, 1674.

But, P.P.H. et al. (eds.). 1997. *International Collation of Traditional and Folk Medicine.* Singapore: World Scientific. 207–208.

Charles, V. and S.X. Charles. 1992. The use and efficacy of *Azadirachta indica* ADR ('Neem') and *Curcuma longa* ('Turmeric') in scabies. A pilot study. *Trop Geogr Med* 44(1–2):178–181.

Deutscher Arzneimittel-Codex (DAC). 1986. Stuttgart: Deutscher Apotheker Verlag.

Duke, J.A. 1999. Clippings from my COX box. *Journal of Medicinal Food* 1(4):293–298.

Gonda, R., M. Tomoda, K. Takada, N. Ohara, N. Shimizu. 1992. The core structure of ukonan A, a phagocytosis-activating polysaccharide from the rhizome of *Curcuma longa*, and immunological activities of degradation products. *Chem Pharm Bull* (Tokyo) 40(4):990–993.

Gonda, R., M. Tomoda, N. Ohara, K. Takada. 1993. Arabinogalactan core structure and immunological activities of ukonan C, an acidic polysaccharide from the rhizome of *Curcuma longa*. *Biol Pharm Bull* 16(3):235–238.

Govindarajan, V.S. 1980. Turmeric—chemistry, technology, and quality. *Crit Rev Food Sci Nutr* 12(3):199–301.

Grieve, M. 1979. *A Modern Herbal.* New York: Dover Publications, Inc.

Hastak, K. et al. 1997. Effect of turmeric oil and turmeric oleoresin on cytogenetic damage in patients suffering from oral submucous fibrosis. *Cancer Lett* 116(2):265–269.

Iwu, M.M. 1993. *Handbook of African Medicinal Plants.* Boca Raton: CRC Press. 164–166.

The Japanese Standards for Herbal Medicines (JSHM). 1993. Tokyo: Yakuji Nippo, Ltd. 279.

Kapoor, L.D. 1990. CRC *Handbook of Ayurvedic Medicinal Plants.* Boca Raton: CRC Press. 149–150.

Kiso, Y., Y. Suzuki, N. Watanabe, Y. Oshima, H. Hikino. 1983. Antihepatotoxic principles of *Curcuma longa* rhizomes. *Planta Med* 49(3):185–187.

Kiuchi, F. et al. 1993. Nematocidal activity of turmeric: synergistic action of curcuminoids. *Chem Pharm Bull* (Tokyo) 41(9):1640–1643.

Kositchaiwat, C., S. Kositchaiwat, J. Havanondha. 1993. *Curcuma longa* Linn. in the treatment of gastric ulcer comparison to liquid antacid: a controlled clinical trial. *J Med Assoc Thai* 76(11):601–605.

Leung, A.Y. and S. Foster. 1996. *Encyclopedia of Common Natural Ingredients Used in Food, Drugs and Cosmetics,* 2nd ed. New York: John Wiley & Sons, Inc. 499–501.

McGuffin, M., C. Hobbs, R. Upton, A. Goldberg. 1997. American Herbal Product Association's *Botanical Safety Handbook.* Boca Raton: CRC Press. 39.

Nadkarni, K.M. 1976. *Indian Materia Medica.* Bombay: Popular Prakashan. 414–418.

Polasa, K., T.C. Raghuram, T.P. Krishna, K. Krishnaswamy. 1992. Effect of turmeric on urinary mutagens in smokers. *Mutagenesis* 7(2):107–109.

Rao, C.V., A. Rivenson, B. Simi, B.S. Reddy. 1995. Chemoprevention of colon carcinogenesis by dietary curcumin, a naturally occurring plant phenolic compound. *Cancer Res* 55(2):259–266.

Roth, G.N., A. Chandra, M.G. Nair. 1998. Novel bioactivities of *Curcuma longa* constituents. *J Nat Prod* 61(4):542–545.

Schulz, V., R. Hänsel, V.E. Tyler. 1998. *Rational Phytotherapy: A Physicians' Guide to Herbal Medicine.* New York: Springer.

Selvam, R., L. Subramanian, R. Gayathri, N. Angayarkanni. 1995. The anti-oxidant activity of turmeric (*Curcuma longa*). *J Ethnopharmacol* 47(2):59–67.

Srinivas, L. and V.K. Shalini. 1991. DNA damage by smoke: protection by turmeric and other inhibitors of ROS. *Free Radic Biol Med* 11(3):277–283.

Srinivas, L., V.K. Shalini, M. Shylaja. 1992. Turmerin: a water-soluble antioxidant peptide from turmeric (*Curcuma longa*). *Arch Biochem Biophys* 292(2):617–623.

Srivastava, K.C. 1989. Extracts from two frequently consumed spices—cumin (*Cucinum cyminum*) and turmeric (*Curcuma longa*)—inhibit platelet aggregation and alter eicosanoid biosynthesis in human blood platelets. *Prostaglandins Leukot Essent Fatty Acids* 37(1):57–64.

Srivastava, R., M. Dikshit, R.C. Srimal, B.N. Dhawan. 1985. Anti-thrombotic effect of curcumin. *Thrombosis Res* 40(3):413–417.

Srivastava, R., V. Puri, R.C. Srimal, B.N. Dhawan. 1986. Effect of curcumin on platelet aggregation and vascular prostacyclin synthesis. *Arzneimforsch* 36(4):715–717.

Stansbury, J.E. 1999. Cancer prevention diet—the potential of protective phytochemicals. *Nutrition Science News* 4(8):380–386.

Subramanian, M., M. Sreejayan, N. Rao, T.P. Devasagayam, B.B. Singh. 1994. Diminution of singlet oxygen-induced DNA damage by curcumin and related antioxidants. *Mutat Res* 311(2):249–255.

Thamlikitkul, V. et al. 1989. Randomized double blind study of *Curcuma domestica* Val. for dyspepsia. *J Med Assoc Thai* 72(11):613–620.

Tu, G. (ed.). 1992. *Pharmacopoeia of the People's Republic of China* (English Edition 1992). Beijing: Guangdong Science and Technology Press. 202–203.

Tyler, V.E. 1994. *Herbs of Choice: The Therapeutic Use of Phytomedicinals.* New York: Pharmaceutical Products Press.

Wichtl, M. and N.G. Bisset (eds.). 1994. *Herbal Drugs and Phytopharmaceuticals.* Stuttgart: Medpharm Scientific Publishers. 173–175.

Wichtl, M. 1996. *Monographien—Kommentar.* In: Braun, R. et al. 1997. *Standardzulassungen für Fertigarzneimittel—Text and Kommentar.* Stuttgart: Deutscher Apotheker Verlag.

Yen, K.Y. 1992. *The Illustrated Chinese Materia Medica—Crude and Prepared.* Taipei, Taiwan: SMC Publishing, Inc. 82.

Additional Resources

Ferreira, L.A. et al. 1992. Antivenom and biological effects of ar-turmerone isolated from *Curcuma longa. Toxicon* 30(10):1211–1218.

Jentzsch, K., T. Gonda, H. Höller. 1959. Papierchromatographische Unterscheidung von *Curcuma domestica* Val. und *Curcuma xanthorrhiza* Roxb. *Pharm Acta Helv* 34(4):181–188.

Jiangsu Institute of Modern Medicine. 1977. *Zhong Yao Da Ci Dian* (Encyclopedia of Chinese Materia Medica), Vol. 3. Shanghai: Shanghai Scientific and Technical Publications.

Leung, A.Y. 1984. *Chinese Herbal Remedies.* New York: Universe Books. [Republished as: Chinese Healing Foods and Herbs. 1993. Glen Rock: AYSL Corp.]

Qureshi, S., A.H. Shah, A.M. Ageel. 1992. Toxicity studies on *Alpinia galanga* and *Curcuma longa. Planta Med* 58(2):124–127.

Randhawa, G.S. and R.K. Mahey. 1988. *Herbs, Spices, and Medicinal Plants: Recent Advances in Botany, Horticulture, and Pharmacology,* Vol. 3. Phoenix: Oryx Press.

Srimal, R.C. and B.N. Dhawan. 1973. Pharmacology of diferuloyl methane (curcumin), a nonsteroidal anti-inflammatory agent. *J Pharm Pharmacol* 25(6):447–452.

This material was adapted from *The Complete German Commission E Monographs—Therapeutic Guide to Herbal Medicines.* M. Blumenthal, W.R. Busse, A. Goldberg, J. Gruenwald, T. Hall, C.W. Riggins, R.S. Rister (eds.) S. Klein and R.S. Rister (trans.). 1998. Austin: American Botanical Council; Boston: Integrative Medicine Communications.

1) The Overview section is new information.

2) Description, Chemistry and Pharmacology, Uses, Contraindications, Side Effects, Interactions with Other Drugs, and Dosage sections have been drawn from the original work. Additional information has been added in some or all of these sections, as noted with references.

3) The dosage for equivalent preparations (tea infusion, fluidextract, and tincture) have been provided based on the following example:
Unless otherwise prescribed: 2 g per day of [powdered, crushed, cut or whole] [plant part]
Infusion: 2 g in 150 ml of water
Fluidextract 1:1 (g/ml): 2 ml
Tincture 1:5 (g/ml): 10 ml

4) The References and Additional Resources sections are new sections. Additional Resources are not cited in the monograph but are included for research purposes.

USNEA

Latin Name:
Usnea barbata, U. florida, U. hirta,
U. plicata

Pharmacopeial Name:
Usnea species

Other Names:
beard-moss, old man's beard,
tree moss, usnea lichen

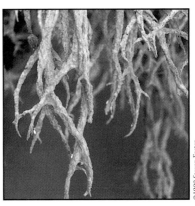

©1999 Steven Foster

Overview

Usnea is not a plant but rather a fruticose lichen—a combination of two kinds of organisms, fungus and alga, growing in a symbiotic union. Some *Usnea* species reproduce by soredia, whereby a moldlike fungus captures and entraps microscopic green algae, resulting in a new stable thallus of a specific structure with no resemblance to its fungal or algal antecedents. Usnea has vague species limits with considerable morphological variation within single populations, making species identification difficult or even impossible. It grows on the bark and wood of coniferous (e.g., Douglas fir and ponderosa pine) and deciduous hardwood (e.g., oak, and apple and other fruit trees) host trees in orchards and damp forests throughout the northern hemisphere in Asia, Europe, and North America (Hale and Cole, 1988; Hobbs, 1986; Kjeldsen, 1997). Usnea lichen prefers old-growth trees and its habitat is diminishing due to logging (Cabrera, 1996). It is almost depleted from many natural locations and has now been put under protected status in Germany, where it is listed in Annex 1 of the German Federal Ordinance on the Conservation of Species (BArtSchV) whereby a permit is necessary for both import and export of any wild collected material (Lange and Schippmann, 1997). Germany has imported most of its *Usnea barbata* supply from Indonesia up through 1991 (Lange and Schippmann, 1997), though German importers have been sourcing from the Pacific Northwest of North America since at least 1992. The government of Nepal has recently placed some lichens, including *U. barbata*, under protected status, banning its export in unprocessed forms (Bhattarai, 1999).

Usnea is used today in traditional Chinese medicine, contemporary homeopathic and naturopathic medicines, and in various systems of traditional medicine worldwide (Sharnoff and Sharnoff, 1998). The current genus name *Usnea* is not in the literature of the ancient Greeks or Romans and may have originated at the time of the Arabian school of medicine and pharmacy. The *Formulary of Al-Kindi* (ca. 850 C.E.) calls *Alectoria usneoides* "ushna" (Cabrera, 1996; Hobbs, 1986; Levey, 1966).

Usnea lichen has a recorded history of therapeutic use dating back over three thousand years in Chinese medicine (Cabrera, 1996; Tilford, 1997). Early Chinese herbalists reported the oral ingestion of *U. longissima* to have expectorant action and also indicated its topical application in powder form to treat surface infections or external ulcers. It is still in use today in tincture form to treat tuberculosis lymphedenitis (Cabrera, 1996; Hobbs, 1986). *U. diffracta* Vain. is used today in Chinese, Japanese, and Korean medicines. In China, it is prepared as an aqueous decoction for oral ingestion to treat pulmonary tuberculosis and chronic bronchitis. For topical application, in decoction or powder form, it is also used to treat infectious wounds. In Japan and Korea the decoction is used to treat scrofula and swelling, among other conditions (But et al., 1997). In the former Soviet Far East,

U. filipendula is used as a topical powder to treat wounds. This material has tested positive for antibacterial activity (Sharnoff and Sharnoff, 1998). In North American aboriginal medicines usnea is used as an expectorant drug (Kjeldsen, 1997). Additionally, the Nitinaht people use *U. longissima* externally as a wound dressing material and the Makah people use it as a dermatological aid for boils (Moerman, 1998).

In Germany, usnea is approved in the Commission E monographs and its preparations are used for mild inflammation of the oral and pharyngeal mucosa. It is usually taken in lozenge form (BAnz, 1998). In the United States, it is dispensed by licensed practitioners (e.g., acupuncturists and naturopaths) to treat urinary tract infections and upper respiratory infections, usually in an alcoholic fluidextract dosage form (Hobbs, 1986). *Usnea longissima, U. florida, U. diffracta,* and *U. barbata* are the species most commonly used by North American medical herbalists, though other local species are also used comparably. It is orally ingested as an aqueous infusion and alcoholic tincture to treat lung infections, tuberculosis, urinary tract infections, *Candida albicans,* and strep throat (Summers, 1998). Usnea is also the most common source material for antibiotic and antifungal lichen acids, particularly usnic acid (Hobbs, 1986), which is used as a component in antibiotic salves and deodorants (Sharnoff and Sharnoff, 1998). *Usnea barbata* is classified in the *Homeopathic Pharmacopoeia of the United States* (HPUS) as an OTC Class C drug prepared as a 1:10 (w/v) alcoholic tincture, in 65% v/v alcohol, and is used by homeopaths for headaches and sunstroke (Cabrera, 1996; Hobbs, 1986; HPUS, 1992). It is used by naturopaths to treat bronchitis, pleurisy, and other respiratory infections, as well as urinary tract, kidney, and bladder infections (HRPI, 1995).

Usnea lichens are also used as biological indicators of air quality, due to their measurable uptake and bioaccumulation of toxic pollutants. Lichens are like sponges that absorb much of which they are in contact. Most lichens are extremely vulnerable to air pollution. When lichens disappear, they give early warning of harmful conditions. Lichen sensitivity can vary with climate, the composition and proportion of airborne pollutants, and topographic exposure. Lichens can be used to monitor levels of sulfur dioxide and a number of toxic metals. Lichens accumulate lead in particular and acid rain appears to affect lichen propagules severely (Kjeldsen, 1997; Popblet et al., 1997; Sharnoff and Sharnoff, 1998).

Usnea lichens and/or their isolated derivatives have been the subject of several pharmacological studies due to their old medical uses in European medicine (Dobrescu et al., 1993). The approved modern therapeutic applications for *Usnea* are supportable based on its history of use in well established systems of traditional and conventional medicines, extensive phytochemical investigations, and pharmacological studies.

Description

Usnea consists of the dried thallus of *Usnea* species, primarily *U. barbata* (L.) Wiggers emend. Mot., *U. florida* (L.) Fries, *U. hirta* (L.) Hoffmann and *U. plicata* (L.) Fries [Fam. Usneaceae] and preparations of Usnea in effective dosage. The herb contains lichenic acid.

Chemistry and Pharmacology

Usnea contains lichenic acids, including usnic acid and its derivatives, diffractaic acid (Budavari, 1996; But et al., 1997); other lichenic acids including barbatic

and lobaric acids; vitamin C (Hobbs, 1986); fatty acids, including linoleic, oleic, and arachidonic acids; and sterols (But et al., 1997).

The Commission E reported antimicrobial activity.

U. barbata contains usnic acid, which has demonstrated a broad antibiotic spectrum (Dobrescu et al., 1993). Usnic acid and diffractaic acid, isolated from *U. diffracta,* have both demonstrated analgesic action in mice (Okuyama et al., 1995). Fractions containing usnic acid and isolichenin, isolated from *U. fasciata,* have demonstrated moderate activity against sarcoma 180 and Ehrlich tumor cells (Periera et al., 1994).

Uses

The Commission E approved usnea for mild inflammations of the oral and pharyngeal mucosa.

Usnea preparations are used clinically by North American herbalists for antibacterial action against gram positive bacteria in local or systemic infections and for antifungal action against *Candida albicans* (Cabrera, 1996).

Contraindications

None known.

Side Effects

None known.

Use During Pregnancy and Lactation

No restrictions known.

Interactions with Other Drugs

None known.

Dosage and Administration

Unless otherwise prescribed: Preparations of herb for lozenges and equivalent solid forms of medication.

Lozenges with preparations equivalent to 100 mg herb: 1 lozenge, three to six times daily (Commission E).

Tincture, 1:3 (g/ml), 70% alcohol: 3 ml, three times daily (Cabrera, 1996).

References

BAnz. See *Bundesanzeiger*.

Bhattarai, N.K. 1999. Medicinal plants and the Plant Research Division of Nepal. *Med Plant Conserv* 5:7–8.

Budavari, S. (ed.). 1996. *The Merck Index: An Encyclopedia of Chemicals, Drugs, and Biologicals,* 12th ed. Whitehouse Station, N.J.: Merck & Co, Inc. 1687.

Bundesanzeiger (BAnz). 1998. Monographien der Kommission E (Zulassungs- und Aufbereitungskommission am BGA für den humanmed. Bereich, phytotherapeutische Therapierichtung und Stoffgruppe). Köln: Bundesgesundheitsamt (BGA).

But, P.P.H. et al. (eds.). 1997. *International Collation of Traditional and Folk Medicine.* Singapore: World Scientific. 6–7.

Cabrera, C. 1996. Materia Medica—Usnea spp. *Eur J Herbal Med* 2(2):11–13.

Dobrescu, D. et al. 1993. Contributions to the complex study of some lichens—*Usnea genus.* Pharmacological studies on *Usnea barbata* and *Usnea hirta* species. *Rom J Physiol* 30(1–2):101–107.

Hale, M.E. and M. Cole. 1988. *Lichens of California.* Berkeley, CA: University of California Press.

Herbal Research Publications, Inc. (HRPI). 1995. *Naturopathic Handbook of Herbal Formulas: A Practical and Concise Herb User's Guide.* Ayer, MA: Herbal Research Publications, Inc. 124.

Hobbs, C. 1986. *Usnea: The Herbal Antibiotic.* Capitola, CA: Botanica Press.

The Homeopathic Pharmacopoeia of the United States (HPUS). 1992. Arlington, VA: Pharmacopoeia Convention of the American Institute of Homeopathy.

This material was adapted from *The Complete German Commission E Monographs—Therapeutic Guide to Herbal Medicines.* M. Blumenthal, W.R. Busse, A. Goldberg, J. Gruenwald, T. Hall, C.W. Riggins, R.S. Rister (eds.) S. Klein and R.S. Rister (trans.). 1998. Austin: American Botanical Council; Boston: Integrative Medicine Communications.

1) The Overview section is new information.

2) Description, Chemistry and Pharmacology, Uses, Contraindications, Side Effects, Interactions with Other Drugs, and Dosage sections have been drawn from the original work. Additional information has been added in some or all of these sections, as noted with references.

3) The dosage for equivalent preparations (tea infusion, fluidextract, and tincture) have been provided based on the following example:
Unless otherwise prescribed: 2 g per day of [powdered, crushed, cut or whole] [plant part]
Infusion: 2 g in 150 ml of water
Fluidextract 1:1 (g/ml): 2 ml
Tincture 1:5 (g/ml): 10 ml

4) The References and Additional Resources sections are new sections. Additional Resources are not cited in the monograph but are included for research purposes.

Kjeldsen, C. 1997. *Mycology—Biology 339 Sonoma State University*. Oklahoma City, OK: Custom Academic Publishing Company (CAPCO). 23–32.

Lange, D. and U. Schippmann. 1997. *Trade Survey of Medicinal Plants in Germany—A Contribution to International Plant Species Conservation*. Bonn: Bundesamt für Naturschutz. 93, 115–120.

Levey, M. 1966. *The Medical Formulary or Agrabadhin or Al-Kindi*. Madison, WI: University of Wisconsin Press.

Moerman, D.E. 1998. *Native American Ethnobotany*. Portland, OR: Timber Press. 582.

Okuyama, E., K. Umeyama, M. Yamazaki, Y. Kinoshita, Y. Yamamoto. 1995. Usnic acid and diffractaic acid as analgesic and antipyretic components of *Usnea diffracta. Planta Med* 61(2):113–115.

Periera, E.C. et al. 1994. Analysis of *Usnea fasciata* crude extracts with antineoplastic activity. Tokai *J Exp Clin Med* 19(1–2):47–52.

Poblet, A. et al. 1997. The use of epilithic Antarctic lichens (*Usnea aurantiacoatra* and *U. antartica*) to determine deposition patterns of heavy metals in the Shetland Islands, Antarctica. *Sci Total Environ* 207(2–3):187–194.

Sharnoff, S. and S. Sharnoff. 1998. *North American Lichen Project*. Available at: www.lichen.com/home.html

Summers, A. 1998. Ethnobotany of Some Common Lichens of Northern California. Rohnert Park, CA: Unpublished paper prepared for Mycology Biology 339 Course: Sonoma State University.

Tilford, G.L. 1997. *Edible and Medicinal Plants of the West*. Missoula, MT: Mountain Press Publishing Company. 148–149.

Additional Resources

Bolton, E.M. 1960. *Lichens for Vegetable Dyeing*. London: Studio Books.

Richardson, D.H.S. 1975. *The Vanishing Lichens*. Vancouver: David and Charles.

Uva Ursi leaf

Latin Name:
Arctostaphylos uva ursi

Pharmacopeial Name:
Uvae ursi folium

Other Names:
Arctostaphylos, bearberry,
beargrape

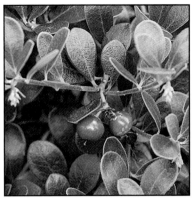

©1999 Steven Foster

Overview

Uva ursi is an evergreen perennial shrub, native to temperate regions of the northern hemisphere, growing wild in the northern latitudes of North America, Europe, and Asia (Leung and Foster, 1996; USD XI, 1858; Wichtl and Bisset, 1994). In North America its range extends from the Arctic Circle as far southward as New Jersey, Wisconsin, and Northern California. Its northerly range includes Iceland, Greenland, and Ireland (Grieve, 1979; Millspaugh, 1974; USD XI, 1858). The material of commerce comes entirely from wild plants collected throughout Europe, mainly Spain, Italy, the Balkans, and the former USSR (BHP, 1996; Leung and Foster, 1996; Wichtl and Bisset, 1994). Uva ursi leaf has been put under protected status in Germany. This species is listed in Annex 1 of the German Federal Ordinance on the Conservation of Species (BArtSchV) and a permit is necessary for both import and export of any wild collected material, excluding populations in Spain and in Scandinavian countries (Lange and Schippmann, 1997).

Uva ursi is an ancient astringent, though little used in European medicine until reported by Welsh physicians of *Myddfai* in the thirteenth century. In 1601, Clusius reported its earlier use by Galen (ca. 130–200 C.E.) as a hemostatic (Grieve, 1979; Millspaugh, 1974). In modern western medical practice, its use seems to begin with Spanish and Italian physicians (ca. 1730–1740 C.E.) for calculus complaints. Its more general adoption dates from the writings of De Haen in 1756, Gerhard of Berlin in 1763, and Murray in 1764 as a remedy in nephritic disorders (Grieve, 1979; Stille, 1874; Millspaugh, 1974). It also became official in the *London Pharmacopoeia* in 1763 (Millspaugh, 1974). In American Eclectic medicine its use was specific for relaxation of the urinary tract, with pain and mucous or bloody secretions (Felter and Lloyd, 1985). Uva ursi leaf, dry extract, and fluidextract were official in the *United States Pharmacopoeia* and *National Formulary* from 1820 to 1950. Today, uva ursi is official in the pharmacopeias of Austria, the Czech Republic, Egypt, France, Germany, Hungary, Japan, Russia, and Switzerland.

Its use in North American aboriginal medicine probably predates its acceptance into European medicine. Native Americans used uva ursi as a drug to treat inflammations of the urinary tract, especially cystitis. The dried leaf mixed with tobacco, known as *sagack-homi* in Canada and *kinnikinnick* among Western tribes, was also smoked ritually (Hutchens, 1991; Millspaugh, 1974). People of the Cherokee Nation used uva ursi to treat uterine dropsy and urinary diseases (Hamel and Chiltoskey, 1975). The Cheyenne used it as a diuretic for congested kidneys (Grinnell, 1972). The Okanagan and Thompson tribes decocted the leaves and stems for use as a urinary aid and tonic for kidneys and bladder (Moerman, 1998; Perry, 1952; Steedman, 1928).

In Germany, uva ursi leaf is licensed as a standard medicinal tea, used as a single herb and a component of many bladder and kidney teas. In dry and fluidextract form it is used for urinary tract infections (Bradley, 1992; Braun, 1997; Wichtl and Bisset, 1994). In the United States, uva ursi leaf is used as a urinary antiseptic and diuretic in a wide range of dietary supplement products.

Clinical studies on its urinary disinfectant effects have been conducted in Germany (Frohne, 1970; Newall et al., 1996). The approved modern therapeutic applications for uva ursi leaf are supportable based on its history of use in well established systems of traditional and conventional medicines, on well documented phytochemical investigations of its hydroquinone derivatives, on pharmacodynamic and pharmacokinetic studies in human urine, on pharmacological studies in animals, and on limited clinical studies.

German pharmacopeial grade uva ursi leaf must contain not less than 6% hydroquinone derivatives, calculated as anhydrous arbutin, and not more than 5% stem fragments, among other quantitative standards. Identity must be verified by thin-layer chromatography (TLC) (DAB method V.6.20.2) and macroscopic and microscopic examinations (DAB 10, 1994; Wichtl and Bisset, 1994). French pharmacopeial grade uva ursi leaf must contain not less than 7% glycosides, calculated as arbutin. Absence of known adulterants (*Buxus sempervirens, Vaccinium uliginosum, V. vitis-idaea*) must be verified by macroscopic and microscopic examination (Bruneton, 1995; Ph.Fr.X, 1990). The *Austrian Pharmacopoeia* requires not less than 5% glycoside derivatives, calculated as arbutin (ÖAB, 1981; Wichtl and Bisset, 1994), The *Japanese Pharmacopoeia* requires not less than 7.0% arbutin (JP XII, 1993), and the *Swiss Pharmacopoeia* requires not less than 8% (Ph.Helv.VII, 1987; Wichtl and Bisset, 1994).

Description

Uva ursi (bearberry) leaves, consisting of the dried leaves of *Arctostaphylos uva ursi* (L.) Sprengel [Fam. Ericaceae] and its pharmaceutical preparations.

Chemistry and Pharmacology

Uva ursi contains 6–18% (usually 7–9%) hydroquinone derivatives, mostly arbutin (hydroquinone mono-β-D-glucoside) with small amounts of the glycosides methylarbutin (up to 4%) and piceoside (P-hydroxyacetophenone glucoside), and the free aglycones hydroquinone and methylhydroquinone; 6–20% polyphenolic tannins, mainly gallotannins, ellagic tannins, catechin, and anthocyanidin derivatives; phenolic acids (approximately 0.25%) in free form, mainly gallic, P-coumaric, and syringic acids; flavonoids (approximately 1.3% hyperoside), mainly the flavonols quercetin, kaempferol, and myricetin and their glycosides, isoquercitrin, quercitrin, hyperin, and myricitrin; 0.4–0.8% triterpenes, mostly ursolic acid and uvaol; monotropein (an iridoid glucoside); resin (ursone); trace of volatile oil; and

wax (Bradley, 1992; Bruneton, 1995; Budavari, 1996; ESCOP, 1997; Leung and Foster, 1996; Newall et al., 1996; Wichtl and Bisset, 1994).

The Commission E reported that preparations made from uva ursi act antibacterially *in vitro* against *Proteus vulgaris, E. coli, Ureaplasma urealyticum, Mycoplasma hominis, Staphylococcus aureus, Pseudomonas aeruginosa*, Friedländer's pneumonia, *Enterococcus faecalis*, Streptococcus strains, and *Candida albicans*. The antimicrobial effect is associated with the aglycone hydroquinone released from arbutin (transport form) or arbutin waste products in the alkaline urine. A methanol extract of the preparation (50%) is said to have an inhibiting effect on tyrosinase activity. The forming of melanin from DOPA using tyrosinase as well as from DOPA-CHROM through auto-oxidation is also said to be inhibited by the preparation.

There are indications that after uva ursi tea (3 g/150 ml) has been taken, hydroquinone glucuronides occur predominately alongside low levels of hydroquinone.

The *British Herbal Compendium* reported its actions as urinary antiseptic and astringent (Bradley, 1992). *The Merck Index* reported its therapeutic category as urinary antiseptic. It also reports the therapeutic category of isolated arbutin as urinary anti-infective (Budavari, 1996).

Uses

The Commission E approved the use of uva ursi for inflammatory disorders of the efferent urinary tract.

The *British Herbal Compendium* lists its use for mild infections of the urinary tract (Bradley, 1992). The French marketing authorization for phytomedicines allows its use to promote the renal elimination of water and as an adjuvant to diuresis treatments in benign urinary tract infections (Bradley, 1992; DPM, 1992). The German Standard License for uva ursi medicinal tea indicates its use as support in the therapy of catarrhs of the bladder and kidney (Bradley, 1992; Braun, 1991; Wichtl and Bisset, 1994). ESCOP lists uva ursi for uncomplicated infections of the lower urinary tract, such as cystitis (ESCOP, 1997).

Contraindications

Pregnancy, lactation, children under 12.

Side Effects

Nausea and vomiting may occur in persons with sensitive stomachs.

Use During Pregnancy and Lactation

Should not be administered during pregnancy.

The occurrence of arbutin/hydroquinone in breast milk has not been researched. The preparation, therefore, should not be administered during lactation.

Interactions with Other Drugs

Uva ursi preparations should not be administered with any substances that cause acidic urine, since this reduces the antibacterial effect. An alkaline pH should be maintained by consuming a diet rich in dairy products, vegetables (especially tomatoes), fruits and fruit juices, potatoes, etc. (Tyler, 1994).

Dosage and Administration

Unless otherwise prescribed: 10–12 g per day of crushed leaf or powder corresponding to 400–840 mg hydroquinone derivatives calculated as water-free arbutin, for infusions or cold macerations; extracts and solid forms for oral administration.

Infusion: Steep 3 g in 150 ml boiling water for 15 minutes, up to four times daily, corresponding to 400–840 mg arbutin per day.

Cold macerate: Steep 3 g in 150 ml cold water for several hours, up to four times daily, corresponding to 400–840 mg arbutin per day.

Dry extract: Containing 100–210 mg hydroquinone derivatives calculated as water-free arbutin, up to four times daily.

Fluidextract 1:1 (g/ml): 3 ml, up to four times daily, corresponding to 400–840 mg arbutin per day.

(Bradley, 1992; Braun, 1991; ESCOP, 1997; Karnick, 1994; Newall et al., 1996; Wichtl and Bisset, 1994).

Duration of treatment: Medication containing arbutin should not be taken for longer than a week or more than five times a year without consulting a physician.

References

Bradley, P.R. (ed.). 1992. *British Herbal Compendium*, Vol. 1. Bournemouth: British Herbal Medicine Association.

Braun, R. et al. 1997. *Standardzulassungen für Fertigarzneimittel—Text and Kommentar*. Stuttgart: Deutscher Apotheker Verlag.

British Herbal Pharmacopoeia (BHP). 1996. Exeter, U.K.: British Herbal Medicine Association. 34.

Bruneton, J. 1995. *Pharmacognosy, Phytochemistry, Medicinal Plants*. Paris: Lavoisier Publishing.

Budavari, S. (ed.). 1996. *The Merck Index: An Encyclopedia of Chemicals, Drugs, and Biologicals*, 12th ed. Whitehouse Station, N.J.: Merck & Co, Inc.

Deutsches Arzneibuch, 10th ed., 3rd suppl. (DAB 10). 1994. Stuttgart: Deutscher Apotheker Verlag.

Direction de la Pharmacie et du Médicament (DPM). 1992. Bulletin Officiel No. 92/11 bis. [English edition]. Paris: Direction des Journaux Officiels.

Dispensatory of the United States of America, 11th ed. (USD XI). 1858. Philadelphia, PA: Lippencott. 781–782.

ESCOP. 1997. "Uvae ursi folium." *Monographs on the Medicinal Uses of Plant Drugs*. Exeter, U.K.: European Scientific Cooperative on Phytotherapy.

Felter, H.W. and J.U. Lloyd. 1985. *King's American Dispensatory*, Vols. 1–2. Portland, OR: Eclectic Medical Publications [reprint of 1898 original]. 840–841, 2038–2040.

Frohne, D. 1970. Untersuchungen zur frage der harndesinfizierenden wirkungen von Bärentraubenblatt-extrakten [The urinary disinfectant effect of extract from leaves uva ursi]. *Planta Med* 18(1):23–25.

Grieve, M. 1979. *A Modern Herbal*. New York: Dover Publications, Inc.

Grinnell, G.B. 1972. *The Cheyenne Indians—Their History and Ways of Life,* Vol. 2. Lincoln: University of Nebraska Press. 183.

Hamel, P.B. and M.U. Chiltoskey. 1975. *Cherokee Plants*. Sylva, N.C.: Herald Publishing Co. 25.

Hutchens, A.R. 1991. *Indian Herbology of North America*. Boston: Shambhala. 29–30.

Japanese Pharmacopoeia, 12th ed. (JP XII). 1993. Tokyo: Government of Japan Ministry of Health and Welfare—Yakuji Nippo, Ltd. 44–46.

Karnick, C.R. 1994. *Pharmacopoeial Standards of Herbal Plants*. Delhi: Sri Satguru Publications. 24–25.

Lange, D. and U. Schippmann. 1997. *Trade Survey of Medicinal Plants in Germany—A Contribution to International Plant Species Conservation*. Bonn: Bundesamt für Naturschutz.

Leung, A.Y. and S. Foster. 1996. *Encyclopedia of Common Natural Ingredients Used in Food, Drugs, and Cosmetics*, 2nd ed. New York: John Wiley & Sons, Inc.

Millspaugh, C.F. 1974. *American Medicinal Plants*. New York: Dover Publications, Inc. [reprint of 1892 American Plants]. 392–396.

Moerman, D.E. 1998. *Native American Ethnobotany*. Portland, OR: Timber Press, Inc. 85–89.

Newall, C.A., L.A. Anderson, J.D. Phillipson. 1996. *Herbal Medicines: A Guide for Health-Care Professionals*. London: The Pharmaceutical Press.

Österreichisches Arzneibuch, Vols. 1–2, 1st suppl. (ÖAB). 1981–1983. Wien: Verlag der Österreichischen Staatsdruckerei.

Perry, F. 1952. Ethno-Botany of the Indians in the Interior of British Columbia. *Museum of Art Notes* 2(2):36–43.

Pharmacopée Française Xe Édition (Ph.Fr.X.). 1983–1990. Moulins-les-Metz: Maisonneuve S.A.

Pharmacopoeia Helvetica, 7th ed. Vol. 1–4. (Ph.Helv.VII). 1987. Bern: Office Central Fédéral des Imprimés et du Matériel.

Stille, A. 1874. *Therapeutics and Materia Medica: A Systematic Treatise on the Action and Uses of Medicinal Agents Including Their Description and History*, 4th ed. Vol. 2. Philadelphia, PA: Lea and Blanchard. 638–639.

Steedman, E.V. 1928. The Ethnobotany of the Thompson Indians of British Columbia. *Smithsonian Institution–Bureau of American Ethnology Annual Report* 45:441–522.

USD XI. See *Dispensatory of the United States of America*.

Wichtl, M. and N.G. Bisset (eds.). 1994. *Herbal Drugs and Phytopharmaceuticals*. Stuttgart: Medpharm Scientific Publishers.

This monograph, published by the Commission E in 1994, was modified based on new scientific research. It contains more extensive pharmacological and therapeutic information taken directly from the Commission E.

This material was adapted from *The Complete German Commission E Monographs—Therapeutic Guide to Herbal Medicines*. M. Blumenthal, W.R. Busse, A. Goldberg, J. Gruenwald, T. Hall, C.W. Riggins, R.S. Rister (eds.) S. Klein and R.S. Rister (trans.). 1998. Austin: American Botanical Council; Boston: Integrative Medicine Communications.

1) The Overview section is new information.

2) Description, Chemistry and Pharmacology, Uses, Contraindications, Side Effects, Interactions with Other Drugs, and Dosage sections have been drawn from the original work. Additional information has been added in some or all of these sections, as noted with references.

3) The dosage for equivalent preparations (tea infusion, fluidextract, and tincture) have been provided based on the following example:

Unless otherwise prescribed: 2 g per day of [powdered, crushed, cut or whole] [plant part]

Infusion: 2 g in 150 ml of water

Fluidextract 1:1 (g/ml): 2 ml

Tincture 1:5 (g/ml): 10 ml

4) The References and Additional Resources sections are new sections. Additional Resources are not cited in the monograph but are included for research purposes.

Additional Resources

British Pharmaceutical Codex (BPC). 1934. London: The Pharmaceutical Press.

Deutsches Arzneibuch, 10th ed. Vol. 1–6. (DAB 10). 1991. Kommentar. Stuttgart: Wissenschaftliche Verlagsgesellschaft. B5.

Frohne, D. 1977. *Arctostaphylos uva-ursi* (L.) SPRENG. (Bärentraube). Bonn: Kooperation Phytopharmaka. Unpublished report.

———. 1986. *Arctostaphylos uva-ursi* (L.) SPRENG—Die Bärentraube. *Z Phytother* 7:45–47.

Haslam, E., T.H. Lilley, Y. Cai, R. Martin, D. Magnolato. 1989. Traditional herbal medicines—the role of polyphenols. *Planta Med* 55(1):1–8.

Kedzia, B., T. Wrocinski, K. Mrugasiewicz, P. Gorecki, H. Grzewinska. 1975. [Antibacterial action of urine containing arbutine metabolic products] [In Polish, with English summary]. *Med Dosw Mikrobiol* 27(3):305–314.

Steinegger, E. and R. Hänsel. 1988. Lehrbuch der *Pharmakognosie* und Phyto*pharmazie*, 4th ed. Heidelberg: Springer Verlag.

Weiss, R.F. 1988. *Herbal Medicine*. Beaconsfield, England: Beaconsfield Publishers.

———. 1991. *Lehrbuch der Phytotherapie*, 7th ed. Stuttgart: Hippokrates Verlag. 315–316.

Wichtl, M. (ed.). 1997. *Teedrogen*, 4th ed. Stuttgart: Wissenschaftliche Verlagsgesellschaft.

VALERIAN ROOT

Latin Name:
Valeriana officinalis

Pharmacopeial Name:
Valerianae radix

Other Names:
garden valerian, Mexican valerian, garden heliotrope, Pacific valerian, Indian valerian

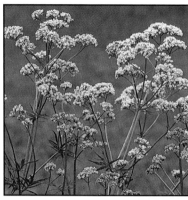

© 1999 Steven Foster

Overview

Valerian is an extremely polymorphous perennial herb represented by a complex of sub-species with natural populations dispersed over temperate and sub-polar Eurasian zones, naturalized in northeastern America, now extensively cultivated in Holland, Belgium, France, Germany, eastern Europe, Japan, and the United States (Bradley, 1992; Wichtl and Bisset, 1994). New sub-species evolve by the mechanism of polyploidy (changes in chromosome number). Twelve mainly European sub-species, such as *exaltata* (diploid), *nitida* (tetraploid), and *procurrens* (octaploid), and some transitional types have been defined (Bradley, 1992; Titz et al., 1982, 1983). Valerian is one of Germany's most important medicinal plant crops (Lange and Schippmann, 1997). The material of commerce is obtained from Belgium and France, the former U.S.S.R., and China (BHP, 1996; Leung and Foster, 1996; Wichtl and Bisset, 1994).

Its modern day therapeutic uses in Germany and the United States stem from traditional Greek medicine, originally documented by Hippocrates (ca. 460–377 B.C.E.) and later by Dioscorides (first century C.E.), author of *De Materia Medica*. Galen (ca. 130–200 C.E.) prescribed valerian for insomnia. Dioscorides and Galen referred to the drug as "phu" as an expression of aversion from its offensive odor. The current genus name, *Valeriana*, first came into use around the tenth century C.E. In the medical texts of that period, the names "Valeriana," "phu," and "fu" are used synonymously (Bown, 1995; Brown, 1995; Grieve, 1979). Although the sedative properties of valerian have been recognized for at least two thousand years, the constituents responsible for this effect and their mode of action remain unknown, despite considerable pharmacological and clinical studies confirming the empirically recognized sedative effect (ESCOP, 1997; Tyler, 1998). Today, valerian root (*Valeriana officinalis* L.s.l.) is official in the national pharmacopeias of Austria, France, Germany, Great Britain, Hungary, Russia, Switzerland, and the *European Pharmacopoeia*, among others (BP, 1988; Bradley, 1992; DAB, 1997; Newall et al., 1996; ÖAB, 1981; Ph.Eur.3, 1997; Ph.Fr.X, 1990; Ph.Helv.VII, 1987; Ph.Hg.VII, 1986; USSR X, 1973; Wichtl and Bisset, 1994). Japanese valerian root (*V. fauriei* Briquet) is official in the national pharmacopeia of Japan (JP XII, 1993). Indian valerian root (*V. jatamansi* Jones; syn. *V. wallichii* DC) is used in Indian Ayurvedic, Tibetan Buddhist, and traditional Chinese medicines (Clifford, 1984; Kapoor, 1990; Leung and Foster, 1996; Nadkarni, 1976).

In Germany, valerian is official in the *German Pharmacopoeia*, approved in the Commission E monographs, and licensed as both a standard medicinal tea infusion and as a standard medicinal tincture, 66.3 vol.% alcohol (BAnz, 1998; Bradley, 1992; Braun et al., 1997; DAB, 1997; Meyer-Buchtela, 1999; Schilcher, 1997; Wichtl and Bisset, 1994). It is used by itself in fresh pressed juice, drops, tea, and coated tablets (e.g., Baldrian-Pflanzensaft Nerventrost® and Valdispert®Dragée) but more often used in many sedative and nerve teas (e.g., Nerven- und Schlaf-Tee N and Species Sedativae ÖAB). Valerian is used in approximately sixty hypnotic/sedative drugs (Kneipp®, 1996; Schilcher, 1997; Wichtl and Bisset, 1994). For example, valerian is a main component in the licensed drug Beruhigungstee I (Sedative Tea I), composed of 40% valerian root, 20% hop strobile, 15% lemon balm leaf, 15% peppermint leaf, and 10% orange peel (Braun et al., 1997). It is also a main component in an approved Commission E "Sedative Tea," composed of 40% valerian root, 30% passion flower herb, and 30% lemon balm leaf (BAnz, 1998; Schilcher, 1997). In German pediatric medicine, valerian aqueous infusions, alcoholic tinctures diluted in milk or fruit juice, and cold macerates are used. In popular medicine, the cold macerate is considered the most efficacious (Schilcher, 1997). In the United States, valerian root is widely used in sleep aids and sedatives in alcoholic tincture, aqueous infusion, and capsules and tablets. Crude valerian root, fluidextract, alcoholic tincture, and ammoniated tincture were formerly official in the *United States Pharmacopoeia* and *National Formulary* (Grieve, 1979; Leung and Foster, 1996).

In 1992, the European-American Phytomedicines Coalition (EAPC) formally petitioned the U.S. Food and Drug Administration to review and approve valerian as an over-the-counter drug in the night-time sleep aid category (Pinco and Israelsen, 1994). At the time of publication of this book (Fall, 1999) the FDA had not yet responded to this petition. In 1998, the USP stated in a consumer information bulletin that the USP Advisory Panel did not recommend or support the use of valerian because it believed that there have not been an adequate number of clinical studies of sufficient size or duration to adequately support valerian's reported uses, although its overall safety was recognized by the USP (USP, 1998).

Modern human studies have investigated valerian's use by itself and in combination with other herbs for a variety of conditions: in combination with hops (*Humulus lupulus*) as an alternative to benzodiazepine to treat nonchronic and non-psychiatric sleep disorders (Schmitz and Jackel, 1998), its use in combination with hops as a sedative to treat disturbed sleep (Müller-Limmroth and Ehrenstein, 1977), its effects in combination with hops on vigilance (Gerhard et al., 1996), its use in combination with St. John's wort (*Hypericum perforatum*) as an alternative to diazepam to treat symptoms of anxiety (Panijel, 1985), its use in combination with camphor (*Cinnamomum camphora*), night-blooming cereus (*Echinocereus grandiflorus*), and hawthorn (*Crataegus* species) to treat functional cardiovascular disorders, hypotension, or meteorosensitivity (Busanny-Caspari et al., 1986), its effect on sleep latency and sleep quality in patients suffering from insomnia (Kamm-Kohl et al., 1984; Leathwood et al., 1982; Leathwood and Chauffard, 1982–1983, 1985), its effectiveness and tolerability in patients with insomnia (Vorbach et al., 1996), its effect on poor sleep (Lindahl and Lindwall, 1989), its effect on human sleep in healthy, young subjects (Balderer and Borbely, 1985), its effect on sleep polygraphy in poor sleepers (Schulz et al., 1994), its ability to treat nervous sleep disorders (Schmidt-Voigt, 1986), and its ability to treat control disorders of the autonomic nervous system (Boeters, 1969).

One randomized, double-blind, controlled clinical trial in parallel group design investigated the efficacy and tolerability of a hop-valerian preparation compared with a benzodiazepine preparation in patients suffering from sleep disorders according to DSM-IV criteria. (The DSM-IV is the *Diagnostic and Statistical Manual of Mental Disorders*. 1995. Washington: American Psychiatric Press). Sleep quality, fitness, and quality of life were determined by psychometric tests, psychopathologic scales, and sleep questionnaires at the beginning of the therapy, end of therapy (duration two weeks), and one week after therapy. The patient's state of health improved during therapy with both substances and a deterioration after cessation was reported for both preparations. Withdrawal symptoms were only reported in the benzodiazepine group. The authors concluded that the hop-valerian preparation in an appropriate dose is a sensible alternative to benzodiazepine for the treatment of nonchronic and non-psychiatric sleep disorders (Schmitz and Jackel, 1998).

In one double-blind, placebo-controlled, crossover study with 128 volunteers, the effects of a valerian root aqueous dry extract (approx. 3:1) on sleep latency and sleep quality were investigated. For nine nights, 400 mg of valerian extract or placebo were taken in crossover design. Compared to placebo, the extract produced significant improvements in sleep latency and in sleep quality, particularly in relatively poor sleepers (ESCOP, 1997; Leathwood and Chauffard, 1982–1983; Leathwood et al., 1983).

In a double-blind, placebo-controlled randomized study, 27 adult males and females suffering from insomnia compared a valerian extract preparation (ValerinaNatt®) with placebo on successive nights. ValerinaNatt® tablets (Pharbio Medical Sverige, Oslo, Sweden) contain 100 mg valerian extract (4:1), corresponding to 400 mg dried root, 45 mg hops extract (8.5:1), corresponding to 382 mg dried strobile, 25 mg lemon balm leaf (*Melissa officinalis*) extract (6.5:1), corresponding to 162 mg dried leaf, and 275 mg of excipient materials. The investigators stated that the valerian root extract, contained in this preparation, is composed mainly of sesquiterpenes as opposed to valepotriates. The subjects ingested either 400 mg of drug (4 tablets) or placebo each night for two nights. The results were based on a subjective evaluation method using a self-reporting scale. By comparison with placebo, the valerian preparation demonstrated a good and statistically significant effect on poor sleep (p<0.001). In the drug group, 89% reported improved sleep, 78% rated the valerian preparation better than placebo, and 44% reported perfect sleep. No adverse side effects were reported for either group (ESCOP, 1997; Lindahl and Lindwall, 1986, 1989; NetDoktor.dk, 1999; Pharbio Medical, 1999).

In a double-blind, placebo-controlled, parallel-group study, the effects of acute and repeated treatment with a valerian extract preparation (Valdispert forte®) were studied in 14 elderly female patients suffering from insomnia over a seven day period. Valdispert® forte coated tablets (Solvay Arzneimittel, Hannover, Germany) contain 45 mg valerian root dry aqueous alkaline extract (5–6:1), corresponding to 225–270 mg of dried root, and are standardized to contain 0.05 mg valerenic acid and acetoxyvalerenic acid. A daily dose of 405 mg of the valerian preparation (3 tablets, three times daily) was administered to eight subjects and the other six received placebo. Objective and subjective sleep parameters were investigated using methods including polysomnography for recording the electroencephalogram (EEG) and a self-reporting scale. Polysomnography was conducted on three nights, at one-week intervals (N0, N1, N2). N0 was one week prior to treatment, N1 was one hour before first night of treatment, and N2 was on the last night of treatment. Increased short-wave-sleep (SWS) was reported for the valerian group as well as a decrease in sleep stage 1. Rapid eye movement (REM) sleep was unaltered. Based on the EEG data, there were no significant changes in sleep latency, waking time, or sleep quality. The authors hypothesized that the valerian extract preparation increased SWS in subjects with low baseline values, which implies that sleep quality may be improved only under certain conditions (ESCOP, 1997; NetDoktor.dk, 1999; Schulz et al., 1994; Solvay Pharma, 1998; Upton, 1999).

The approved modern therapeutic applications for valerian appear to be supportable based on its history of use in well established systems of traditional and conventional medicine, extensive phytochemical investigations, many in vitro and in vivo pharmacological experiments in animals, and some human clinical studies.

Pharmacopeial grade valerian root consists of the rhizome, root, and stolons of *V. officinalis* L.s.l., dried carefully at a temperature below 40°C. The fresh undried root must contain not less than 5% (v/m) volatile oil and the dried pulverized root must contain not less than 15% water- and alcohol-soluble (40% water and 60%

ethanol) extractive. Botanical identity must be confirmed by thin-layer chromatography (TLC), macroscopic and microscopic examinations, and organoleptic evaluation (DAB 10, 1993; Ph.Eur.3, 1997; Wichtl and Bisset, 1994). The ESCOP valerian root monograph requires that the material comply with the *European Pharmacopoeia* (ESCOP, 1997).

Pharmacopeial grade valerian root dry extract is composed of the native extractive yielded from DAB-grade valerian root manufactured in accordance with the DAB Extracta monograph. The drug-to-extract ratio ranges from 3:1 to 6:1 (w/w). Identification is confirmed with TLC and organoleptic evaluation (DAB, 1997).

Description

Valerian root, consisting of fresh underground plant parts, or parts carefully dried below 40°C, of the species *V. officinalis* L. [Fam. Valerianaceae] and its preparations in effective dosage. The roots contain essential oil with monoterpenes and sesquiterpenes (valerenic acids). Preparations of valerian used therapeutically (infusion, extract, fluidextract, and tincture) no longer contain the thermolabile and chemically unstable valepotriates.

Chemistry and Pharmacology

Constituents include valtrates, didrovaltrates, and isovaltrates (Leung and Foster, 1996). Other constituents include 0.4–1.4 % monoterpenes and sesquiterpenes, caffeic, gamma-aminobutyric (GABA), and chlorogenic acids, β-sitosterol, methyl,2-pyrrolketone, choline, tannins, gum, alkaloids, and resin (Bradley, 1992; ESCOP, 1997; Newall et al., 1996).

The Commission E reported sedative and sleep-promoting activities.

Uses

The Commission E approved the internal use of valerian for restlessness and sleeping disorders based on nervous conditions.

Valerian has been reported to relieve pain, reduce spasms, and stimulate appetite (Newall et al., 1996).

The World Health Organization notes the following uses for valerian that are supported by clinical data: mild sedative and sleep-promoting agent, often used as a milder alternative or a possible substitute for stronger synthetic sedatives, e.g., benzodiazepines, in the treatment of states of nervous excitation and anxiety-induced sleep disturbances (WHO, 1999).

Contraindications

None known.

Side Effects

None known.

Use During Pregnancy and Lactation

No restrictions known.

Interactions with Other Drugs

None known.

Dosage and Administration

Unless otherwise prescribed:
Infusions: 2–3 g of fresh or dried root per cup, once to several times per day.
Tincture: $^1/_2$ –1 teaspoon (1–3 ml), once to several times per day.
Extracts: Amount equivalent to 2–3 g of preparation, once to several times per day.
External use: 100 g for one full bath; equivalent preparations.
Infusion: 2–3 g in 150 ml water.

References

Balderer, G. and A.A. Borbely. 1985. Effect of valerian on human sleep. *Psychopharmacology* (Berl) 87(4):406–409.
BAnz. See *Bundesanzeiger*.

Boeters, U. 1969. Behandlung vegetativer regula-
tionsstörungen mit valepotriaten (Valmane®)
[Treatment of control disorders of the autonomic nervous system with valepotriate]. *MMW*
111(37):1873–1876.

Bown, D. 1995. *Encyclopedia of Herbs and Their
Uses.* New York: DK Publishing, Inc. 367.

Bradley, P.R. (ed.). 1992. *British Herbal Compendium,* Vol. 1. Bournemouth: British Herbal
Medicine Association.

Braun, R. et al. 1997. *Standardzulassungen für Fertigarzneimittel—Text and Kommentar.* Stuttgart:
Deutscher Apotheker Verlag.

British Herbal Pharmacopoeia (BHP). 1996. Exeter,
U.K.: British Herbal Medicine Association.

British Pharmacopoeia (BP). 1988. (With subsequent Addenda up to 1992.) London: Her
Majesty's Stationery Office.

Brown, D.J. 1995. Valerian: Clinical Overview.
Townsend Lett Doctors May:150–151.

Bundesanzeiger (BAnz). 1998. Monographien der
Kommission E (Zulassungs- und Aufbereitungs-
kommission am BGA für den humanmed. Bere-
ich, phytotherapeutische Therapierichtung und
Stoffgruppe). Köln: Bundesgesundheitsamt
(BGA).

Busanny-Caspari, E. et al. 1986. Indikationen:
Funktionelle Herzbeschwerden, Hypotonie und
Wetterfuhligkeit. *Therapiewoche* 36:2545–2550.

Clifford, T. 1984. *Tibetan Buddhist Medicine and
Psychiatry.* York Beach, ME: Samuel Weiser, Inc.
171–186.

Deutsches Arzneibuch, 10th ed. 3rd suppl. (DAB
10). 1993. Stuttgart: Deutscher Apotheker Verlag.

Deutsches Arzneibuch (DAB 1997). 1997. Stuttgart:
Deutscher Apotheker Verlag.

ESCOP. 1997. "Valerianae radix." *Monographs on
the Medicinal Uses of Plant Drugs.* Exeter, U.K.:
European Scientific Cooperative on Phytotherapy.

Europäisches Arzneibuch, 3rd ed. (Ph.Eur.3). 1997.
Stuttgart: Deutscher Apotheker Verlag.

Gerhard, U., N. Linnenbrink, C. Georghiadou, V.
Hobi. 1996. [Vigilance-decreasing effects of two
plant-derived sedatives] [In German]. *Schweiz
Rsch Med* 85(15):473–481.

Grieve, M. 1979. *A Modern Herbal.* New York:
Dover Publications, Inc.

Japanese Pharmacopoeia, 12th ed. (JP XII). 1993.
Tokyo: Government of Japan Ministry of Health
and Welfare—Yakuji Nippo, Ltd. 151–152.

Kamm-Kohl, A.V., W. Jansen, P. Brockmann. 1984.
Moderne Baldriantherapie gegen nervöse
Störungen im Senium. *Med Welt* 35:1450–1454.

Kapoor, L.D. 1990. *Handbook of Ayurvedic Medicinal Plants.* Boca Raton: CRC Press.

Kneipp®, 1996. *Wegweiser zu den Kneipp® Mitteln
[Guide to Kneipp® Remedies].* Würzburg: Sebastian Kneipp Gesundheitsmittel-Verlag.

Lange, D. and U. Schippmann. 1997. *Trade Survey
of Medicinal Plants in Germany—A Contribution to International Plant Species Conservation.*
Bonn: Bundesamt für Naturschutz. 29–34.

Leathwood, P.D. and F. Chauffard. 1982–1983.
Quantifying the effects of mild sedatives. *J Psychiatr Res* 17(2):115–122.

———. 1985. Aqueous extract of valerian reduces
latency to fall asleep in man. *Planta Med*
51(2):144–148.

Leathwood, P.D., F. Chauffard, E. Heck, R.
Munoz-Box. 1982. Aqueous extract of valerian
root (*Valeriana officinalis* L.) improves sleep
quality in man. *Pharmacol Biochem Behav*
17(1):65–71.

Leathwood, P.D., F. Chauffard, R. Munoz-Box.
1983. Effect of *Valeriana officinalis* L. on subjective and objective sleep parameters. Sixth Eur
Congr Sleep Res, Zürich (Basel: Karger).

Leung, A.Y. and S. Foster. 1996. *Encyclopedia of
Common Natural Ingredients Used in Food,
Drugs, and Cosmetics,* 2nd ed. New York: John
Wiley & Sons, Inc.

Lindahl, O. and L. Lindwall. 1986. God sömnef-
fekt av valeriana vid jämförelse med placebo [In
Swedish]. *Läkartidningen* 83(44)3674–3675.

———. 1989. Double blind study of a valerian
preparation. *Pharmacol Biochem Behav*
32(4):1065–1066.

Meyer-Buchtela, E. 1999. *Tee-Rezepturen—Ein
Handbuch für Apotheker und Ärzte.* Stuttgart:
Deutscher Apotheker Verlag.

Müller-Limmroth, W. and W. Ehrenstein. 1977.
Untersuchungen über die Wirkung von Seda-
Kneipp auf den Schlaf schlafgestörter Menschen.
Med Klin 72:1119–1125.

Nadkarni, K.M. 1976. *Indian Materia Medica.*
Bombay: Popular Prakashan. 1260–1261.

NetDoktor.dk. 1999. Naturlaegemidler. Denmark:
NetDoktor.dk. Available at: www.netdoktor.dk/
naturlaegemidler/fakta/valerianen.htm

Newall, C.A., L.A. Anderson, J.D. Phillipson.
1996. *Herbal Medicines: A Guide for Health-
Care Professionals.* London: The Pharmaceutical
Press.

Österreichisches Arzneibuch, Vols. 1–2. (ÖAB).
1981. Wien: Verlag der Österreichischen Staatsdruckerei.

Panijel, M. 1985. Die Behandlung mittelschwerer
angstzustände. *Therapiewoche* 41:4659–4668.

Pharbio Medical. 1999. Våra produkter. Oslo,
Sweden: Pharbio Medical AS. Available at:
www.pharbio.cederroth.com

Ph.Eur.3. See *Europäisches Arzneibuch.*

Pharmacopée Française Xe Édition (Ph.Fr.X).
1983–1990. Moulins-les-Metz: Maisonneuve
S.A.

Pharmacopoeia Helvetica, 7th ed. Vol. 1–4.
(Ph.Helv.VII). 1987. Bern: Office Central
Fédéral des Imprimés et du Matériel.

Pharmacopoea Hungaric, 7th ed. (Ph.Hg.VII).
1986. Budapest: Medicina Könyvkiadó.

Pinco, R.G. and L.D. Israelson. 1994. European-
American Phytomedicines Coalition Citizen Peti-
tion to Amend FDA's Monograph on Nighttime
Sleep-aid Drug Products for Over-the-Counter
("OTC") Human Use to Include Valerian. Jun 7.

Schilcher, H. 1997. *Phytotherapy in Paediatrics: Handbook for Physicians and Pharmacists.* Stuttgart: Medpharm Scientific Publishers. 59, 62.

Schmidt-Voigt, J. 1986. Die Behandlung nervöser Schlafstörungen und innerer Unruhe mit einem rein pflanzlichen Sedativum. *Therapiewoche* 36:663–667.

Schmitz, M. and M. Jackel. 1998. [Comparative study for assessing quality of life of patients with exogenous sleep disorders (temporary sleep onset and sleep interruption disorders) treated with a hops-valerian preparation and a benzodiazepine drug] [In German]. *Wien Med Wochenschr* 148(13):291–298.

Schulz, H., C. Stolz, J. Müller. 1994. The effect of valerian extract on sleep polygraphy in poor sleepers: A pilot study. *Pharmacopsychiat* 27(4):147–151.

Solvay Pharma. 1998. Beruhigungsmittel and Antidepressiva. Hannover, Germany: Solvay Arzneimittel. Available at: www.solvay.com/de/gesundh.htm

State Pharmacopoeia of the Union of Socialist Republics, 10th ed. (USSR X) 1973. Moscow: Ministry of Health of the U.S.S.R.

Titz, W. et al. 1983. [Valepotriates and essential oil of morphologically and karyologically defined types of *Valeriana officinalis* s.l. II. Variation of some characteristic components of the essential oil] [In German]. *Sci Pharm* 51:63–86.

Titz, W., J. Jurenitsch, E. Fitzbauer-Busch, E. Wicho, W. Kubelka. 1982. [Valepotriates and essential oil of morphologically and karyologically defined types of *Valeriana officinalis* s.l. I. Comparison of Valepotriate content and composition] [In German]. *Sci Pharm* 50:309–324.

Tyler, V.E. 1998. In: Lawson, L.D. and R. Bauer (eds.). *Phytomedicines of Europe—Chemistry and Biological Activity.* Washington, D.C.: American Chemical Society. 10.

Upton, R. (ed.) 1999. *Valerian Root Analytical, Quality Control, and Therapeutic Monograph.* Santa Cruz, CA: American Herbal Pharmacopoeia.

USP Drug Information (USP). 1998. Rockville, MD: U.S. Pharmacopoeial Convention. Available at: www.usp.org/did/mgraphs/botanica/valeria2.htm

USSR X. See *State Pharmacopoeia of the Union of Soviet Socialist Republics.*

Vorbach, E.U., R. Görtelmeyer, J. Brüning. 1996. Therapie von Insomnien: Wirksamkeit und Verträglichkeit eines Baldrian-Präparates. *Psychopharmakotherapie* 3:109–115.

Wichtl, M. and N.G. Bisset (eds.). 1994. *Herbal Drugs and Phytopharmaceuticals.* Stuttgart: Medpharm Scientific Publishers.

World Health Organization (WHO). 1999. "Valerianae radix." *WHO Monographs on Selected Medicinal Plants,* Vol. 1. Geneva: World Health Organization.

Additional Resources

Boss, R. et al. 1997. *Valeriana* species. In: De Smet, P.A., K. Keller, R. Hänsel, R.F. Chandler, (eds.). *Adverse Effects of Herbal Drugs,* Vol. 3. New York: Springer Verlag.

Bravo, S.Q. et al. 1996. Polysomnographic and subjective findings in insomniacs under treatment with placebo and valerian extract (LI 156). (Proceedings of the 2nd International Congress on Phytomedicine, Munich, Germany.) *Eur J Clin Pharmacol* 50(6):552.

Diefenbach, K. et al. 1997. Valerian effects on microstructure of sleep in insomniacs. (2nd Congress of the European Assoc. for Clinical Pharmacology and Therapeutics, Berlin, Germany, Sept. 17–20.) *Eur J Clin Pharmacol* 52 (suppl.):A169.

Donath, F. and I. Roots.1996. Effects of valerian extract (Sedonium) on EEG power spectrum in male healthy volunteers after single and multiple application. (6th Annual Meeting of the German Society for Clinical Pharmacology and Therapeutics, Dresden, Germany, Sept. 5–7.) *Eur J Clin Pharmacol* 50(6):541.

DreBring, H., 1992. Insomnia: are valerian/balm combinations of equal value to Benzodiazepine? *Therapiewoche* 42:726.

This material was adapted from *The Complete German Commission E Monographs—Therapeutic Guide to Herbal Medicines.* M. Blumenthal, W.R. Busse, A. Goldberg, J. Gruenwald, T. Hall, C.W. Riggins, R.S. Rister (eds.) S. Klein and R.S. Rister (trans.). 1998. Austin: American Botanical Council; Boston: Integrative Medicine Communications.

1) The Overview section is new information.
2) Description, Chemistry and Pharmacology, Uses, Contraindications, Side Effects, Interactions with Other Drugs, and Dosage sections have been drawn from the original work. Additional information has been added in some or all of these sections, as noted with references.
3) The dosage for equivalent preparations (tea infusion, fluidextract, and tincture) have been provided based on the following example:
   Unless otherwise prescribed: 2 g per day of [powdered, crushed, cut or whole] [plant part]
   Infusion: 2 g in 150 ml of water
   Fluidextract 1:1 (g/ml): 2 ml
   Tincture 1:5 (g/ml): 10 ml
4) The References and Additional Resources sections are new sections. Additional Resources are not cited in the monograph but are included for research purposes.

Fauteck, J.D., B. Pietz, H. Winterhoff, W. Wittowski. 1996. Interaction of *Valeriana officinalis* with melatonin receptors: a possible explanation of its biological action. (Proceedings of the 2nd International Congress on Phytomedicine, Munich, Germany.)

Kohnen, R., W.D. Oswald. 1988. The effects of valerian, Propranolol and their combination on activation, performance and mood of healthy volunteers under social stress conditions. *Pharmacopsychiat* 21(6):447–448.

Lindahl, O. and L. Lindwall. 1992. Double-blind study of valopotriates by hairy root cultures of *Valeriana officinalis* var. sambucifolia. *Planta Med* 58(7):A614.

Quispe, B.S. et al. 1997. The influence of valerian on objective and subjective sleep in insomniacs. (2nd Congress of the European Assoc. for Clinical Pharmacology and Therapeutics, Berlin, Germany, Sept. 17–20.) *Eur J Clin Pharmacol* 52 (suppl.):A170.

Sanner, B., A. Strum. 1997. Treatment of sleep disorders in the elderly. *DMW (Deutsche Medizinische Wochenschrift)* 122(51–52):1599–1604.

Santos, M.S. et al. 1994. Synaptosomal GABA release as influenced by valerian root extract—involvement of the GABA carrier. *Arch Int Pharmacodyn* 327(2):220–231.

Santos, M.S. et al. 1994. The amount of GABA present in aqueous extracts of valerian is sufficient to account for [3H]GABA release in synaptosomes. *Planta Med* 60(5):475–476.

Seifert, T. 1988. Therapeutic effects of valerian in nervous disorders: A field study. *Therapeutikon* 2(94).

WALNUT LEAF

Latin Name:
Juglans regia

Pharmacopeial Name:
Juglandis folium

Other Names:
English walnut leaf, European
walnut leaf, Persian walnut leaf

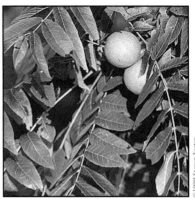

© 1999 Steven Foster

Overview

Walnut is a deciduous tree native in southeastern Europe, Asia Minor to the Indian
sub-continent, and China (HPUS, 1992; Uphof, 1968; Wichtl and Bisset, 1994),
now cultivated in temperate zones throughout Europe, North Africa, East Asia, and
North America (Wichtl, 1996). In Asia, is it found in the Himalayas and cultivated
in the Khasia hills (Karnick, 1994), Afghanistan, Kashmir, and Tibet (Nadkarni,
1976). In Europe, the material of commerce is obtained mainly from eastern and
southeastern European countries (Wichtl, 1996). Its genus name, *Juglans*, is derived
from the Latin *lupiter* (Jupiter) and *glans* (acorn) meaning "Jupiter's nuts" (Bown,
1995; Grieve, 1979).

Walnut leaf has been used medicinally for thousands of years. Roman naturalist
Pliny the Elder (ca. 23–79 C.E.) reported the cultivation of walnut in Italy by the
first century B.C.E., from trees originally transported from countries further east
(Bown, 1995; Grieve, 1979). Seventeenth century English herbalist Nicholas
Culpepper reported the use of walnut leaf in combination with onion, salt, and
honey, to draw out the venom of dogs, snakes, and spiders. Within the next few
hundred years, however, the use of walnut leaves was eventually targeted to skin
disorders. Extracts and infusions were found to be helpful in the treatment of
scrofulous diseases, herpes, eczema, and slow healing wounds (Grieve, 1979).
Nineteenth century French physician Professor Negrier reported a walnut leaf
strong infusion and/or syrup to be effective in treating scrofula in children. He also
reported using a strong decoction of the leaf as a wash, compress, or poultice for
treatment of ulcers and sore eyes (Felter and Lloyd, 1983).

In Germany, walnut leaf is listed in the *Drug Codex*, approved in the Commission E monographs, and the decoction form for external use is official in the Standard License monographs (BAnz, 1998; Braun et al., 1997; DAC, 1986; DAC,
1997; Meyer-Buchtela, 1999; Wichtl and Bisset, 1994). Walnut leaf was official in
the *German Pharmacopeia*, sixth edition (DAB 6, 1951). Today, it is used as a topical remedy for dermal inflammation and excessive perspiration of the hands and
feet. It is also a common home remedy for treatment of chronic eczema, scrofula,
and inflammation of the lids (Weiss, 1988), applied locally in bath, dressing, and/or
rinse forms (Wichtl and Bisset, 1994).

Description

Walnut leaf consists of the dried leaf of
Juglans regia L. [Fam. Juglandaceae]
and its preparations in effective dosage.
The preparation contains tannins.

Chemistry and Pharmacology

Walnut leaf contains approximately
10% tannins of the ellagitannin type;
naphthalene derivatives, especially the
monoglucosides of juglone (=5-
hydroxy-1,4-naphtholquinone) and

hydrojuglone; up to over 3% flavonoids (e.g., quercetin and kaempferol derivatives); 0.8–1.0% ascorbic acid (Bruneton, 1995; Wichtl and Bisset, 1994; Wichtl, 1996), plant acids, including gallic, caffeic, and neo-chlorogenic acids (Wichtl, 1989); and 0.001–0.03% volatile oil, mainly germacrene D (Wichtl and Bisset, 1994).

The Commision E reported astringent activity.

The primary constituents of the leaves are ellagitannins, formed from ellagic acid, itself targeted by anticancer research (Trease and Evans, 1989; Harborne and Baxter, 1993), and a naphthalene derivative, juglone. Juglone has demonstrated antiviral activities against HSV-1 virus (Harborne and Baxter, 1993), and is reportedly antifungal due to *in vitro* inhibition of *Candida albicans* and *Trichophyton rubrum* (Heisey and Gorham, 1992). However, isolated juglone may be mutagenic and carcinogenic, and further study of its therapeutic and toxic effects is recommended. Currently the advised application of walnut leaf extends only to external use (De Smet, 1993).

Its astringent activity is attributed to the tannin content. Walnut leaf has local antimycotic or bactericide action as well as insect repellent properties (Meyer-Buchtela, 1999; Roth, 1993). The steam distilled volatile oil fraction has demonstrated antifungal action (Nahrstedt et al., 1981). The isolated principle juglone has shown tumor inhibition (e.g., Ehrlich ascites tumor) effects in mice (Okada et al., 1967).

Uses

The Commission E approved the use of walnut leaf for mild, superficial inflammations of the skin and excessive perspiration of the hands and feet.

The German Standard License indicates walnut leaf aqueous decoction to be used topically as a cataplasm or partial bath for the same conditions as approved in the Commission E (Braun et al., 1997). An infusion of equal parts walnut leaf and wild pansy herb (*Viola tricolor*), for external use, is particularly

useful for skin complaints in children (Weiss, 1988). In France, walnut leaf is used topically to treat scalp itching, peeling, and dandruff, sunburn and superficial burns, and as an adjunctive emollient and itch-relieving treatment in skin disorders (Bruneton, 1995). In India, walnut leaf decoction is used externally as a wash for malignant sores and pustules (Nadkarni, 1976).

Contraindications
None known.

Side Effects
None known.

Use During Pregnancy and Lactation
No restrictions known.

Interactions with Other Drugs
None known.

Dosage and Administration
Unless otherwise prescribed: Cut leaf for decoctions and other equivalent galenical preparations for external use. Decoction: Put 2–3 g dried leaf per 100 ml cold water, bring to a boil and simmer for about 15 minutes: For use in compresses and partial baths (Braun et al., 1997; Commission E; Meyer-Buchtela, 1999).
Note: Occlusive dressings and/or topical application to large areas should be avoided (DAC, 1997; Meyer-Buchtela, 1999).

References
BAnz. See *Bundesanzeiger*.
Bown, D. 1995. *Encyclopedia of Herbs and Their Uses.* New York: DK Publishing, Inc. 145, 298.
Braun, R. et al. 1997. *Standardzulassungen für Fertigarzneimittel—Text and Kommentar.* Stuttgart: Deutscher Apotheker Verlag.
Bruneton, J. 1995. *Pharmacognosy, Phytochemistry, Medicinal Plants.* Paris: Lavoisier Publishing.

Bundesanzeiger (BAnz). 1998. Monographien der Kommission E (Zulassungs- und Aufbereitungskommission am BGA für den humanmed. Bereich, phytotherapeutische Therapierichtung und Stoffgruppe). Köln: Bundesgesundheitsamt (BGA).

De Smet, P.A. 1993. Legislatory outlook on the safety of herbal remedies. In: De Smet, P.A. (ed.). *Adverse Effects of Herbal Drugs*, Vol. 2. New York: Springer Verlag.

Deutscher Arzneimittel-Codex (DAC). 1986. Ergänzungsbuch zum Arzneibuch. Stuttgart: Deutscher Apotheker Verlag.

Deutscher Arzneimittel-Codex (DAC). 1997. Ergänzungsbuch zum Arzneibuch. Stuttgart: Deutscher Apotheker Verlag.

Deutsches Arzneibuch, 6th ed. (DAB 6). 1951. Stuttgart: Deutscher Apotheker Verlag.

Felter, H.W. and J.U. Lloyd. 1983. *King's American Dispensatory*, 18th ed., 3rd rev. Portland, OR: Eclectic Medical Publications [reprint of 1898 original]. 1090–1091.

Grieve, M. 1979. *A Modern Herbal*. New York: Dover Publications, Inc.

Harborne, J. and H. Baxter. 1993. *Phytochemical Dictionary: A Handbook of Bioactive Compounds from Plants*. Washington: Taylor & Francis.

Heisey, R.M. and B.K. Gorham. 1992. Antimicrobial effects of plant extracts on Streptococcus mutans, *Candida albicans*, *Trichophyton rubrum* and other micro-organisms. *Lett Appl Microbiol* 14:136–139.

The Homeopathic Pharmacopoeia of the United States (HPUS) *Revision Service Official Compendium*. 1992. Fairfax, VA: Pharmacopoeia Convention of the American Institute of Homeopathy.

Karnick, C.R. 1994. *Pharmacopoeial Standards of Herbal Plants*, Vol. 1. Delhi: Sri Satguru Publications. 205–206.

Meyer-Buchtela, E. 1999. Tee-Rezepturen—Ein Handbuch für Apotheker und Ärzte. Stuttgart: Deutscher Apotheker Verlag.

Nadkarni, K.M. 1976. *Indian Materia Medica*. Bombay: Popular Prakashan. 709.

Nahrstedt, A., U. Vetter, F.J. Hammerschmidt. 1981. Zur kenntnis des wasserdampfdestillates der blätter von *Juglans regia* [Composition of the steam distillation product from the leaves of *Juglans regia*]. *Planta Med* 42(4):313–332.

Okada, T.A., E. Roberts, A.F. Brodie. 1967. Mitotic abnormalities produced by juglone in Ehrlich ascites tumor cells. *Proc Soc Exp Biol Med* 126(2):583–588.

Roth, J.H. (ed.). 1993. In: Hänsel, R. *Teedrogen*, Pharmazeutisches Ring Taschenbuch Kap. 10. Stuttgart: Wissenschaftliche Verlagsgesellschaft.

Trease, G.E. and W.C. Evans. 1989. *Trease and Evans' Pharmacognosy*, 13th ed. London; Philadelphia: Baillière Tindall.

Uphof, J.C. 1968. *Dictionary of Economic Plants*, 2nd ed. New York: Verlag von J. Cramer. 289–290.

Weiss, R.F. 1988. *Herbal Medicines*. Beaconsfield, England: Beaconsfield Publishers. 332.

Wichtl, M. (ed.). 1989. *Teedrogen*, 2nd ed. Stuttgart: Wissenschaftliche Verlagsgesellschaft.

Wichtl, M. and N.G. Bisset (eds.). 1994. *Herbal Drugs and Phytopharmaceuticals*. Stuttgart: Medpharm Scientific Publishers. 281–282.

Wichtl, M. 1996. Monographien—Kommentar. In: Braun, R. et al. 1997. *Standardzulassungen für Fertigarzneimittel—Text and Kommentar*. Stuttgart: Deutscher Apotheker Verlag.

Additional Resources

Bhargava, U.C. and B.A. Westfall. 1968. Antitumor activity of *Juglans nigra* (black walnut) extractives. *J Pharm Sci* 57(10):1674–1677.

Hutchens, A. 1991. *Indian Herbology of North America*. Boston: Shambala.

Osman, N.A., S.M. Gaafar, M. Salah el-Din, G.M. Wassel, N.M. Ammar. 1987. Hazardous effect of topical cosmetic application of Deirum (*Juglans regia* L. plant) on oral tissue. *Egypt Dent J* 33(1):31–35.

This material was adapted from *The Complete German Commission E Monographs—Therapeutic Guide to Herbal Medicines*. M. Blumenthal, W.R. Busse, A. Goldberg, J. Gruenwald, T. Hall, C.W. Riggins, R.S. Rister (eds.) S. Klein and R.S. Rister (trans.). 1998. Austin: American Botanical Council; Boston: Integrative Medicine Communications.

1) The Overview section is new information.

2) Description, Chemistry and Pharmacology, Uses, Contraindications, Side Effects, Interactions with Other Drugs, and Dosage sections have been drawn from the original work. Additional information has been added in some or all of these sections, as noted with references.

3) The dosage for equivalent preparations (tea infusion, fluidextract, and tincture) have been provided based on the following example:
   Unless otherwise prescribed: 2 g per day of [powdered, crushed, cut or whole] [plant part]
   Infusion: 2 g in 150 ml of water
   Fluidextract 1:1 (g/ml): 2 ml
   Tincture 1:5 (g/ml): 10 ml

4) The References and Additional Resources sections are new sections. Additional Resources are not cited in the monograph but are included for research purposes.

WATERCRESS

Latin Name:
Nasturtium officinale

Pharmacopeial Name:
Nasturtii herba

Other Names:
green watercress, summer watercress

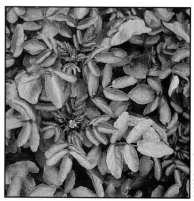

©1999 Steven Foster

Overview

Watercress is a hardy perennial herb native to Europe and temperate Asia (Uphof, 1968), cultivated and naturalized in North and South America, and the West Indies (HPUS, 1992). It is found growing wild in wetlands, particularly in calcareous regions (Grieve, 1979; HPUS, 1992). Its commercial cultivation began during the nineteenth century (Bown, 1995). The material of commerce is obtained mainly from eastern and southeastern European countries (Wichtl and Bisset, 1994). Its genus name, *Nasturtium*, is derived from the Latin *nasus tortus*, meaning convulsed or twisted nose, due to the pungent taste of its leaf (Bown, 1995; Grieve, 1979). Ancient Greek physician Hippocrates (ca. 460–377 B.C.E.) used watercress for its expectorant action (Brill and Dean, 1994). According to Grieve, it has also been used as an antiscorbutic (scurvy remedy) since ancient times (Grieve, 1979). Seventeenth century English herbalist Nicholas Culpepper reported that the bruised leaves or juice, prepared as a lotion, was used topically to treat blotches, spots, and blemishes on the skin (Grieve, 1979).

Watercress contains significant amounts of micronutrients, such as manganese, iodine, iron, and calcium (Bremness, 1994; Brill and Dean, 1994), but its main active constituents, and source of pungency, may be its glucosinolates. Glucosinolates are irritating to mucous membranes and eyes and skin, and handling plants that contain them can cause allergic dermatitis (Diamond et al., 1990). In medicinal watercress preparations, these glycosides are most likely the chemicals responsible for the plant's purported effectiveness in reducing inflammation and mucous in the upper respiratory tract. However, clinical reports that confirm these actions are lacking (Hecht et al., 1995; Hecht, 1996). Some of its beneficial effects may be due to a general stimulation of metabolism and the nervous system, including autonomous regulation (Weiss, 1988).

In Germany, watercress herb, fresh or dried, is approved in the Commission E monographs for catarrh of the respiratory tract. Watercress juice is also used as a component of several cholagogue medicines such as Cholongal Saft (Wichtl and Bisset, 1994). It is listed in the supplemental volume to the *German Pharmacopeia*, sixth edition (Erg.B.6, 1953). In German pediatric medicine, watercress is used as a disinfectant drug for antibacterial action in the treatment of lower urinary tract infections (Schilcher, 1997). The fresh aerial parts, collected during the flowering period, are also official in the *German Homeopathic Pharmacopoeia* for use in the preparation of mother tinctures and liquid dilutions thereof (GHP, 1993). In the United States, watercress herb is classified in the *Homeopathic Pharmacopoeia of the United States* as an OTC Class D drug prepared as an alcoholic tincture of the whole flowering plant, in 45% v/v alcohol (HPUS, 1992).

Description

Watercress consists of the fresh or dried aboveground parts of *Nasturtium officinale* R. Brown [Fam. Brassicaceae] and their preparations in effective dosage. The herb contains mustard glycosides and mustard oil.

Chemistry and Pharmacology

Watercress contains glucosinolates (mustard-oil glycosides) such as gluconasturtiin, a precursor of phenylethyl isothiocyanate which occurs upon hydrolysis (Chung et al., 1992), and nitriles such as 3-phenylpropionitrile, 8-methylthiooctanone nitrile (Wichtl and Bisset, 1994); minerals, including manganese, iron, phosphorus, iodine, copper, and calcium; vitamins A, C, E, and nicotinamide (Karnick, 1994; Taber, 1962).

The Commission E did not report pharmacological actions for watercress.

Watercress herb has been reported to have antibacterial (Schilcher, 1997), antiscorbutic (Nadkarni, 1976; Uphof, 1968), cholagogue (Wichtl and Bisset, 1994), and expectorant properties (Karnick, 1994).

The most recent research on watercress indicates that it may protect smokers' lungs from carcinogens present in tobacco and tobacco smoke. Diets that include watercress may help to inhibit the formation of 4- (methylnitrosamino)-1-(3-pyridyl-1-butanone), or NNK. NNK is a carcinogen present in tobacco that most likely contributes to the etiology of lung cancer, as well as of mouth and throat cancers. The constituents in watercress that cause this inhibition have not been identified, though the glucosinolate phenethyl isothiocyanate (PEITC), which is released upon chewing the leaf, is known to be a chemopreventive agent against lung cancer (Hecht et al., 1995; Hecht, 1996). Earlier animal studies demonstrated that PEITC inhibited lung tumorigenesis induced by a potent tobacco-specific carcinogenic nitrosamine. In order to determine the bioavailability of PEITC from its glucosinolate precursor, urine analysis was conducted, which has shown that PEITC is released upon ingestion of watercress leaf. This suggests that its conjugate N-acetylcysteine may be a useful biomarker compound for quantifying human exposure to PEITC in future epidemiological studies (Chung et al., 1992). Other pharmacokinetic studies have investigated the effect of watercress on the metabolism of chlorzoxazone, an *in vivo* clinical probe for CYP2E1 (Leclercq et al., 1998) and also its effects on acetaminophen metabolism in human volunteers (Chen et al., 1996).

Uses

The Commission E approved watercress for catarrh of the respiratory tract.

In Germany, it is also used to treat urinary tract infections in children (Schilcher, 1997). The powdered leaf is used in India as an expectorant to treat bronchitis and also to treat human liver fluke (*Clonorchis sinensis*) (Karnick, 1994). The fresh herb is used in naturopathy as a blood purifier (Uphof, 1968; Wichtl and Bisset, 1994) and so-called "spring cure," taken in combination with fresh dandelion and nettle herbs (Wichtl and Bisset, 1994), and is particularly useful for patients with chronic metabolic diseases and/or asthenia (Weiss, 1988).

Contraindications

Gastric and intestinal ulcers, inflammatory kidney diseases. No application for children under the age of four.

Side Effects

In rare cases, gastrointestinal complaints.

Use During Pregnancy and Lactation

Not recommended during pregnancy (McGuffin et al., 1997). No restrictions known during lactation.

Interactions with Other Drugs

None known.

Dosage and Administration

Unless otherwise prescribed: Cut herb, freshly pressed juice, and other equivalent galenical preparations.

Internal:

Dried herb: 4–6 g per day (Commission E).

Fresh herb: 20–30 g per day (Commission E).

Succus: 60–150 ml freshly pressed juice per day (Commission E).

Infusion: Steep 2 g in 150 ml boiled water for 10 minutes (Wichtl and Bisset, 1994), two to three times daily before meals.

References

Bown, D. 1995. *The Herb Society of America—Encyclopedia of Herbs & Their Uses.* New York: DK Publishing Inc. 164, 316.

Bremness, L. 1994. *Herbs.* New York: DK Publishing, Inc.

Brill, S. and E. Dean. 1994. *Identifying and Harvesting Edible and Medicinal Plants in Wild (and Not So Wild) Places.* New York: Hearst Books. 255–256.

Chen, L., S.N. Mohr, C.S. Yang. 1996. Decrease of plasma and urinary oxidative metabolites of acetaminophen after consumption of watercress by human volunteers. *Clin Pharmacol Ther* 60(6):651–660.

Chung, F.L., M.A. Morse, K.I. Eklind, J. Lewis. 1992. Quantitation of human uptake of the anticarcinogen phenethyl isothiocyanate after a watercress meal. *Cancer Epidemiol Biomarkers Prev* 1(5):383–388.

Diamond, S.P., S.G.Wiener, J.G. Marks, Jr. 1990. Allergic contact dermatitis to nasturtium. *Dermatol Clin* 8(1):77–80.

Ergänzungsbuch zum Deutschen Arzneibuch, 6th ed. (Erg.B.6). 1953. Stuttgart: Deutscher Apotheker Verlag.

German Homeopathic Pharmacopoeia (GHP), 1993. Translation of the German *Homöopathisches Arzneibuch* (HAB 1), 5th suppl. 1991 to the 1st ed. 1978. Stuttgart. Deutscher Apotheker Verlag. 291–292.

Grieve, M. 1979. *A Modern Herbal.* New York: Dover Publications, Inc.

Hecht, S.S. 1996. Chemoprevention of lung cancer by isothiocyanates. *Adv Exp Med Biol* 40(1):1–11.

Hecht, S.S., F.L. Chung, J.P. Richie, Jr. et al. 1995. Effects of watercress consumption on metabolism of a tobacco-specific lung carcinogen in smokers. *Cancer Epidemiol Biomarkers Prev* 4(8):877–884.

The Homeopathic Pharmacopoeia of the United States (HPUS). 1992. Arlington, VA: Pharmacopoeia Convention of the American Institute of Homeopathy.

Karnick, C.R. 1994. *Pharmacopoeial Standards of Herbal Plants.* Delhi: Sri Satguru Publications. Vol. 2:139.

Leclercq, I., J.P. Desager, Y. Horsmans. 1998. Inhibition of chlorzoxazone metabolism, a clinical probe for CYP2E1, by a single ingestion of watercress. *Clin Pharmacol Ther* 64(2):144–149.

McGuffin, M., C. Hobbs, R. Upton, A. Goldberg. 1997. American Herbal Product Association's *Botanical Safety Handbook.* Boca Raton: CRC Press. 78.

Nadkarni, K.M. 1976. *Indian Materia Medica.* Bombay: Popular Prakashan. 843.

Schilcher, H. 1997. *Phytotherapy in Paediatrics: Handbook for Physicians and Pharmacists.* Stuttgart: Medpharm Scientific Publishers. 55–56.

Taber, C.W. 1962. *Taber's Cyclopedic Medical Dictionary,* 9th ed. Philadelphia: F.A. Davis Company. W–2.

Uphof, J.C. 1968. *Dictionary of Economic Plants,* 2nd ed. New York: Verlag von J. Cramer. 357.

This material was adapted from *The Complete German Commission E Monographs—Therapeutic Guide to Herbal Medicines.* M. Blumenthal, W.R. Busse, A. Goldberg, J. Gruenwald, T. Hall, C.W. Riggins, R.S. Rister (eds.) S. Klein and R.S. Rister (trans.). 1998. Austin: American Botanical Council; Boston: Integrative Medicine Communications.

1) The Overview section is new information.

2) Description, Chemistry and Pharmacology, Uses, Contraindications, Side Effects, Interactions with Other Drugs, and Dosage sections have been drawn from the original work. Additional information has been added in some or all of these sections, as noted with references.

3) The dosage for equivalent preparations (tea infusion, fluidextract, and tincture) have been provided based on the following example:
   Unless otherwise prescribed: 2 g per day of [powdered, crushed, cut or whole] [plant part]
   Infusion: 2 g in 150 ml of water
   Fluidextract 1:1 (g/ml): 2 ml
   Tincture 1:5 (g/ml): 10 ml

4) The References and Additional Resources sections are new sections. Additional Resources are not cited in the monograph but are included for research purposes.

Weiss, R.F. 1988. *Herbal Medicine*. Beaconsfield, England: Beaconsfield Publishers. 274–275.

Wichtl, M. and N.G. Bisset (eds.). 1994. *Herbal Drugs and Phytopharmaceuticals*. Stuttgart: Medpharm Scientific Publishers. 353–354.

Additional Resources

Bruneton, J. 1995. *Pharmacognosy, Phytochemistry, Medicinal Plants*. Paris: Lavoisier Publishing.

Cruz, A. 1970. [Remarkable antimitotic action of watercress (*Nasturtium officinale*) on some experimental tumors] [In Portuguese]. *Hospital (Rio De J)* 77(3):943–952.

Hutchens, A. 1991. *Indian Herbology of North America*. Boston: Shambala.

WILLOW BARK

Latin Name:
Salix alba, S. purpurea L.,
S. fragilis L.

Pharmacopeial Name:
Salicis cortex

Other Names:
bay willow (*S. pentandra* L.); crack
willow (*S. fragilis* L.); purple willow
(*S. purpurea* L.); violet willow
(*S. daphnoides* Villars); white willow
(*S. alba* L.)

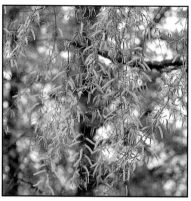

© 1999 Steven Foster

Overview

Willow is a deciduous shrub native to Britain, central and southern Europe (Karnick, 1994), Asia, and North America (Wichtl and Bisset, 1994). The material of commerce comes mainly from southeastern European countries, including Bulgaria, Hungary, Romania, the former Yugoslavia (BHP, 1996; Wichtl and Bisset, 1994), and the United Kingdom (BHP, 1996).

Some of the modern therapeutic applications for willow bark originate from its early uses in ancient Greek medicine, which were first reported by Dioscorides in his herbal *De Materia Medica* written in the first century C.E. (Bown, 1995). During the Middle Ages, willow bark was used in Europe to reduce fevers and relieve pain. Willow's anti-inflammatory and fever-reducing actions are attributed to salicylates in the bark. These glycosidic constituents were first isolated by a French chemist in 1829, and were synthesized six years later (Schulz et al., 1998). Salicylic acid, first isolated from meadowsweet leaf (*Filipendula ulmaria*; syn. *Spiraea ulmaria*), is the phytotherapeutic precursor of acetylsalicylic acid, the analgesic drug now commonly known as aspirin (Bradley, 1992; Weissman, 1991; Wichtl and Bisset, 1994).

A few human studies have been found in the literature. In one double-blind study, researchers at the Centre for Complementary Health Studies at the University of Exeter in England investigated the effect of Reumalex, an over-the-counter herbal drug containing willow bark, on 82 participants suffering with chronic arthritic pain. The subjects were randomly assigned without crossover to either Reumalex or placebo. The duration of the study was two months, resulting in a small though statistically significant improvement in pain symptoms. The researchers concluded that Reumalex exhibits a mild analgesic effect in chronic arthritis at a level appropriate for self-medication (Mills et al., 1996). In a recent pilot study, the use of Salix SST, a saliva-stimulating lozenge, was subjectively evaluated as a treatment for the relief of radiation-induced xerostomia (dryness in the mouth) in 10 patients for seven days. The researchers reported a statistically significant improvement in the dryness and general comfort of the mouth as well as improved sleep and speech (Senahayake et al., 1998). In a pharmacokinetic study in humans, three tablets containing willow bark extract (standardized to provide a total dose of 55 mg salicin) were administered to 12 male volunteers in three doses over a period of eight hours. The study calculated that the half-life of the plasma was approximately 2.5 hours (ESCOP, 1997; Pentz et al., 1989).

In Germany, willow bark is official in the *German Pharmacopeia* and approved in the Commission E monographs. It is used as a main component of some analgesic and antirheumatic drugs (Wichtl and Bisset, 1994) such as Kneipp® Rheuma-Tee N (Kneipp®, 1996). In German pediatric medicine, willow bark is used as an antipyretic component of various herbal preparations, particularly in combination with diaphoretic herbs. For example, an effective herbal tea prescribed for children with influenza is composed of 30% willow bark (*Salix* species), 40% linden flower (*Tilia* species), 10% meadowsweet flower (*F. ulmaria*), 10% German chamomile flower (*Matricaria recutita*), and 10% bitter orange peel (*Citrus aurantium*). Willow bark is also used to treat children with pain in the extremities due to cold and flu (Schilcher, 1997). Throughout the United States and Canada, willow barks of several different species are used extensively in traditional aboriginal medicines from the Seminole people in Florida to the Eskimos in Alaska. For example, the Cherokee prepare an infusion of white willow bark (*Salix alba*) as a febrifuge drug to treat fever. The Blackfoot prepare a decoction of pussy willow twigs (*S. discolor*) as an analgesic painkiller and also as a febrifuge drug. The Iroquois prepare an infusion of sandbar willow (*S. interior*) stems as an analgesic drug. The Eskimo prepare an infusion of tealeaf willow (*S. planifolia* species *pulchra*) bark also as an analgesic drug (Moerman, 1998).

German pharmacopeial grade willow bark consists of the dried, whole, cut, or powdered bark from young branches of *Salix purpurea* L., *S. daphnoides* Villars or other comparable *Salix* species, collected in the early spring. It must contain not less than 1% total salicin calculated as salicin. Botanical identity must be confirmed by thin-layer chromatography (TLC) plus macroscopic and microscopic examinations (DAB 10, 1991–1996). In addition to the two above mentioned species, the *British Herbal Pharmacopoeia* specifically allows for *S. alba* L., *S. fragilis* L., and *S. pentandra* L. and also requires that the dried bark contain not less than 10% water-soluble extractive (BHP, 1996). ESCOP requires that the material comply with the qualitative and quantitative criteria of the *German Pharmacopeia* (ESCOP, 1997).

Description

Willow bark consists of the bark of the young, two to three year-old branches harvested during early spring of *S. alba* L., *S. purpurea* L., *S. fragilis* L., and other *Salix* species [Salicaceae] and their preparations in effective dosage. The bark contains at least 1% total salicin derivatives, calculated as salicin relative to the dried herb.

Chemistry and Pharmacology

Note: As the Commission E allows for several different *Salix* species, the quantities of certain constituents may vary significantly depending on the species used (Meier et al., 1985; Meier et al., 1988; Thieme, 1965). Constituents include 1.5–11% phenolic glycosides, mainly salicylates (1.0–10.2%), including salicin and its derivatives (salicortin and tremulacin) (Bradley, 1992; Thieme, 1965; Wichtl and Bisset, 1994); 8–20% tannins, mainly catechin tannins, some gallotannins and con-

densed tannins (procyanidins); and 1–4% flavonoids, including isoquercitrin, and naringin and its glucoside (Bradley, 1992; Wichtl and Bisset, 1994). The chemistry composition of the young twigs is comparable, though in lower concentrations than the bark alone (ESCOP, 1997). The species with the highest reported salicin content are *S. purpurea*, *S. daphnoides*, and *S. fragilis* (Meier et al., 1985; Wichtl and Bisset, 1994).

The Commission E reported antipyretic, antiphlogistic, and analgesic activities.

The *British Herbal Pharmacopoeia* reported anti-inflammatory action (BHP, 1996). The *British Herbal Compendium* additionally reported analgesic, antipyretic, antirheumatic, and astringent actions (Bradley, 1992). *The Merck Index* reported analgesic action for salicin, isolated from willow bark (Budavari, 1996).

Natural salicylic acid is reported to produce fewer side effects than the synthetic acetylsalicylic acid (Meier and Liebi, 1990; Mayer and Mayer, 1949). The analgesic action of willow bark is apparently due to inhibition of prostaglandin synthesis by its salicin derivatives, which cause sensitization of peripheral pain receptors (Schilcher, 1997). Metabolites of salicin and tremulacin have demonstrated anti-inflammatory activity *in vitro* (Albrecht et al., 1990). Other *in vitro* experiments have found that salicin is stable under acidic conditions. Both saligenin and salicin have been shown to bind to human serum albumin, but saligenin has a higher affinity (ESCOP, 1997; Steinegger and Hövel, 1972).

Uses

The Commission E approved willow bark for diseases accompanied by fever, rheumatic ailments, and headaches.

The *British Herbal Compendium* indicates its use for rheumatic and arthritic conditions and feverish conditions such as the common cold or influenza (Bradley, 1992). ESCOP indicates it use for treatment of feverish conditions, symptomatic treatment of mild rheumatic complaints, and relief of headache (ESCOP, 1997). In France, it is allowed for use as an analgesic to treat headache and toothache pain as well as painful articular conditions, tendinitis, and sprains (Bradley, 1992; Bruneton, 1995).

Contraindications

See Interactions with Other Drugs. Despite concerns expressed by some health professionals, there is no evidence that willow preparations should be contraindicated in small children with flu to produce Reyes syndrome; the salicylates in willow metabolize differently than aspirin (acetylsalicylic acid).

Side Effects

See Interactions with Other Drugs.

Use During Pregnancy and Lactation

No restrictions known.

Interactions with Other Drugs

Because of willow bark's active constituents, interactions like those encountered with salicylates may arise. However, studies conducted thus far do not indicate this potential toxicity.

Dosage and Administration

Unless otherwise prescribed: Liquid and solid preparations for internal use with an average daily dosage corresponding to 60–120 mg total salicin (Commission E), which is equivalent to 6–12 g dried bark (Schilcher, 1997).

Note: Combinations with diaphoretic herbs may be very effective.

Dried bark: 1–3 g, three times daily (HPB, 1992; Karnick, 1994; Newall et al., 1996).

Decoction: Place 2–3 g finely chopped or coursely powdered bark in 150–250 ml cold water, bring to a boil and simmer for 5 minutes, three to four times daily (Meyer-Buchtela, 1999; Wichtl, 1989; Wichtl and Bisset, 1994).

Fluidextract 1:1 (g/ml), 25% ethanol: 1–2 ml, three times daily (Bradley, 1992; HPB, 1992; Karnick, 1994).

Tincture 1:5 (g/ml), 25% ethanol: 5–8 ml, three times daily (Bradley, 1992).

Dry extract: Standardized to contain 20–40 mg of total salicin, three times daily (Bradley, 1992; ESCOP, 1997).

References

Albrecht, M. et al. 1990. Anti-inflammatory activity of flavonol glycosides and salicin derivatives from the leaves of *Populus tremuloides*. *Planta Med* 56:660.

Bown, D. 1995. *Encyclopedia of Herbs and Their Uses*. New York: DK Publishing, Inc. 345.

British Herbal Pharmacopoeia (BHP). 1996. Exeter, U.K.: British Herbal Medicine Association. 188.

Bradley, P.R. (ed.). 1992. *British Herbal Compendium*, Vol. 1. Bournemouth: British Herbal Medicine Association. 224–226.

Bruneton, J. 1995. *Pharmacognosy, Phytochemistry, Medicinal Plants*. Paris: Lavoisier Publishing.

Budavari, S. (ed.). 1996. *The Merck Index: An Encyclopedia of Chemicals, Drugs, and Biologicals*, 12th ed. Whitehouse Station, N.J.: Merck & Co, Inc. 1432.

Deutsches Arzneibuch, 10th ed. (DAB 10). 1991. (With subsequent supplements through 1996.) Stuttgart: Deutscher Apotheker Verlag.

ESCOP. 1997. "Salicis cortex." *Monographs on the Medicinal Uses of Plant Drugs*. Exeter, U.K.: European Scientific Cooperative on Phytotherapy.

Health Protection Branch (HPB) *Status Manual*. 1992. Ottawa: Health Protection Branch. 212.

Karnick, C.R., 1994. *Pharmacopoeial Standards of Herbal Plants*, Vol. 1. Delhi: Sri Satguru Publications. 321–322.

Kneipp®, 1996. *Wegweiser zu den Kneipp® Mitteln [Guide to Kneipp® Remedies]*. Würzburg: Sebastian Kneipp Gesundheitsmittel-Verlag. 110–111.

Mayer, R.A. and M. Mayer. 1949. Biologische Salicyltherapie mit Cortex Salicis (Weidenrinde). *Pharmazie* 4:77–81.

Meier B., O. Sticher, A. Bettschart. 1985. Weidenrinde-Qualität. Gesamtsalicinbestimmung in Weidenrinden und Weidenpräparaten mit HPLC. *Dtsch Apoth Ztg* 125:341–347.

Meier, B. et al. 1988. Pharmaceutical aspects of the use of willows in herbal remedies. *Planta Med* 54:559–560.

Meier, B. and M. Liebi. 1990. Salicinhaltige pflanzliche Arzneimittel. Überlegungen zu Wirksamkeit und Unbedenklichkeit. *Z Phytother* 11:50–58.

Meyer-Buchtela, E. 1999. *Tee-Rezepturen—Ein Handbuch für Apotheker und Ärzte*. Stuttgart: Deutscher Apotheker Verlag.

Mills, S.Y., R.K. Jacoby, M. Chacksfield, M. Willoughby. 1996. Effect of a proprietary herbal medicine on the relief of chronic arthritic pain: a double-blind study. *Br J Rheumatol* 35(9):874–878.

Moerman, D.E. 1998. *Native American Ethnobotany*. Portland, OR: Timber Press. 500–509.

Newall, C.A., L.A. Anderson, J.D. Phillipson. 1996. *Herbal Medicines: A Guide for Health-Care Professionals*. London: The Pharmaceutical Press. 268–269.

Pentz, R. et al. 1989. Bioverfügbarkeit von Salicylsäure und Coffein aus einem phytoanalgetischen Kominationspräparat. *Dtsch Apoth Ztg* (10):92–96.

Schilcher, H. 1997. *Phytotherapy in Paediatrics: Handbook for Physicians and Pharmacists*. Stuttgart: Medpharm Scientific Publishers. 41, 63–64.

Schulz, V., R. Hänsel, V.E. Tyler. 1998. *Rational Phytotherapy: A Physicians' Guide to Herbal Medicine*. New York: Springer.

Senahayake, F., K. Piggott, J.M. Hamilton-Miller. 1998. A pilot study of *Salix* SST (saliva-stimulating lozenges) in post-irradiation xerostomia. *Curr Med Res Opin* 14(3):155–159.

Steinegger, E. and H. Hövel. 1972. Analytische und biologische untersuchungen an Salicaceen-wirkstoffen, insbesondere an salicin. II. Biologische untersuchungen [Analytic and biologic studies on Salicaceae substances, especially on salicin. II. Biological study]. *Pharm Acta Helv* 47(3):222–234.

Thieme, H. 1965. Die Phenolglykoside der Salicaceen. *Planta Med* 13:431–438.

Weissman, G. 1991. Aspirin. *Scientific Am* (Jan.):58–64.

Wichtl, M. (ed.). 1989. *Teedrogen*, 2nd ed. Stuttgart: Wissenschaftliche Verlagsgesellschaft.

Wichtl, M. and N.G. Bisset (eds.). 1994. *Herbal Drugs and Phytopharmaceuticals*. Stuttgart: Medpharm Scientific Publishers. 437–439.

Additional Resources

British Herbal Pharmacopoeia (BHP). 1983. Keighley, U.K.: British Herbal Medicine Association.

———. 1990. Exeter, U.K.: British Herbal Medicine Association.

Deutsches Arzneibuch, 10th ed. Vol. 1–6. (DAB 10). 1991. Kommentar. Stuttgart: Wissenschaftliche Verlagsgesellschaft.

Dorsch, W. et al. 1993. *Empfehlungen zu Kinderdosierngen von monographierten Arzneidrogen und ihren Zubereitungen*. Bonn: Kooperation Phytopharmaka.

This material was adapted from *The Complete German Commission E Monographs—Therapeutic Guide to Herbal Medicines*. M. Blumenthal, W.R. Busse, A. Goldberg, J. Gruenwald, T. Hall, C.W. Riggins, R.S. Rister (eds.) S. Klein and R.S. Rister (trans.). 1998. Austin: American Botanical Council; Boston: Integrative Medicine Communications.

1) The Overview section is new information.

2) Description, Chemistry and Pharmacology, Uses, Contraindications, Side Effects, Interactions with Other Drugs, and Dosage sections have been drawn from the original work. Additional information has been added in some or all of these sections, as noted with references.

3) The dosage for equivalent preparations (tea infusion, fluidextract, and tincture) have been provided based on the following example:

Unless otherwise prescribed: 2 g per day of [powdered, crushed, cut or whole] [plant part]
Infusion: 2 g in 150 ml of water
Fluidextract 1:1 (g/ml): 2 ml
Tincture 1:5 (g/ml): 10 ml

4) The References and Additional Resources sections are new sections. Additional Resources are not cited in the monograph but are included for research purposes.

Felter, H.W. and J.U. Lloyd. 1985. *King's American Dispensatory*, Vols. 1–2. Portland, OR: Eclectic Medical Publications [reprint of 1898 original].

Hänsel, R. 1991. *Phytopharmaka,* 2nd ed. New York: Springer Verlag.

Hutchens, A. 1991. *Indian Herbology of North America*. Boston: Shambala.

Meier, B. 1989. Pflanzliche versus synthetische Arzneimittel. *Schweiz Apoth Ztg* (127):472–477.

Schaffner, W. 1991. Bericht über die Pilot-Studie Zeller-Rheumadragees forte/gewisse Rheumaformen. Pharmazeutisches Institut der Universität Basel. Unpublished report for Max Zeller Söhne AG, CH-8590 Romanshorn.

Tyler, V.E. 1994. *Herbs of Choice: The Therapeutic Use of Phytomedicinals*. New York: Pharmaceutical Products Press.

Wagner, H. and M. Wiesenauer. 1995. *Phytotherapie*. New York: Gustav Fischer Verlag.

Wren, R.C. 1988. *Potter's New Cyclopaedia of Botanical Drugs and Preparations*. Essex: The C.W. Daniel Company Ltd.

Witch Hazel Leaf and Bark

Latin Name:
Hamamelis virginiana

Pharmacopeial Name:
Hamamelidis folium, witch hazel
leaf, Hamamelidis cortex,
witch hazel bark
Other Names:
Hamamelis

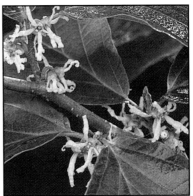

©1999 Steven Foster

Overview

Witch hazel is a deciduous shrub or small tree that flowers in the fall, native to damp woods in eastern North America from New Brunswick and Quebec to Minnesota, south to Florida, Georgia, Louisiana, and Texas (HPUS, 1992; Leung and Foster, 1996; Wichtl and Bisset, 1994). It is cultivated on a small scale in Europe (Wichtl and Bisset, 1994), though the material of commerce is obtained mainly from the eastern United States and Canada (BHP, 1996; Wichtl and Bisset, 1994).

Witch hazel preparations have a long history of traditional use in North America (Der Marderosian, 1999; Duke, 1985). The aqueous infusion of the bark was used in aboriginal medicine to treat hemorrhages, inflammations, and hemorrhoids (Millspaugh, 1974). The decoction was used in poultices for painful swellings and tumors (Grieve, 1979). These traditional uses were later adopted by nineteenth century American Eclectic physicians and the aqueous decoction form became an official preparation in the Eclectic Materia Medica. The alcoholic fluidextract form became official in the *United States Pharmacopoeia* in 1882 (Millspaugh, 1974). Today, the external use of witch hazel is well known for the astringency associated with the tannin content of its leaves and bark. In Europe, tannin-rich witch hazel extracts made from the leaf and bark are used. In the United States, the FDA has approved as an over-the-counter drug a witch hazel water, made from the steam distillate of the twigs, this preparation having virtually no tannin content. However, the product contains about 14–15% alcohol in water with a small amount of the essential oil of witch hazel. Thus, whatever astringent properties may be attributed to this type of preparation are probably due to the alcohol content, not any tannins from the herb (Tyler, 1994). However, there are reports of the distillate containing 2.5–4.2 mg/liter hamamelitannins (Zeylstra, 1998).

In a recent clinical study, a witch hazel preparation demonstrated anti-inflammatory activity on skin irritations caused by ultraviolet light. The preparation, an after-sun lotion (Eucerin®), contained a lotion base and 10% witch hazel distillate. The witch hazel lotion helped reduce inflammation by 20% after 7 hours and 27% after 48 hours compared to 11–15% for other lotions (Hughes-Formella et al., 1998). In another double-blind randomized clinical study comparing a witch hazel distillate (5.35% with 0.64 mg ketone) in a cream base to both the herb-free cream base and a 0.5% hydrocortisone cream in patients with severe ectopic eczema, the witch hazel cream was not as effective as the hydrocortisone preparation, despite what the authors confirm as the "mild, yet unmistakable anti-inflammatory effect of hamamelis cream in experimental models of inflammatory skin disease" (Korting et al., 1995). Some of these same authors had conducted an earlier randomized controlled trial comparing a witch hazel distillate (0.64 mg/2.56 mg hamamelis ketone in 100 g) with phosphatidylcholine; these were compared to a chamomile cream and a 1% hydrocortisone cream and four base preparations. The results showed an anti-inflammatory action of the hamamelis distillate on experimentally induced skin erythemas, but the hydrocortisone cream was deemed more potent, even when the herb distillate was increased by four times (Korting et al., 1993).

In Germany, witch hazel is listed in the *Drug Codex*, approved in the Commission E monographs, and the tea infusion form is official in the Standard License monographs (BAnz, 1998; Braun et al., 1997; DAC, 1986; Wichtl and Bisset, 1994). Witch hazel leaf and bark are used in some hemorrhoid teas and antiphlebitis (vein inflammation) drugs. Several witch hazel mono-preparations and combination products (e.g., with horse chestnut) are available in various dosage forms, including ointments, suppositories, coated tablets, and tinctures (Wichtl and Bisset, 1994). The mother tincture (1:10) and liquid dilutions thereof, are also official in the *German Homeopathic Pharmacopoeia* (GHP), prepared from different plant parts including the fresh leaves, the fresh bark from roots and branches, as well as a mixture of bark from the branches with tips of the shoots. The GHP also includes a monograph for an ethanolic decoction of the dried bark from stems and branches, specifying bark which contains not less than 2.5% tannins, precipitable with hide powder, calculated as pyrogallol (GHP, 1993). In the United States, witch hazel distillate, from partially dried twigs, is official in the currently valid USP (USP 24–NF 19, 1999). An alcoholic tincture (1:10 w/v, in 55% alcohol v/v) of the bark, including the root bark, is also classified in the *Homeopathic Pharmacopoeia of the United States* as an OTC Class C drug (HPUS, 1992). Witch hazel is used in several over-the-counter astringent and hemostatic preparations such as Dickinson's® witch hazel astringent cleaner towelettes with *Aloe*, Parke-Davis Tucks® hemorrhoidal pads, Preparation H® hemorrhoidal cooling gel, and Thayers® witch hazel astringent with *Aloe vera*.

European pharmacopeial grade witch hazel *leaf* consists of the dried leaves of *Hamamelis virginiana* L. containing not less than 7.0% tannins calculated with reference to the dried leaf. It may contain no more than 7% stem pieces and maximum 2% other foreign matter. Botanical identity must be confirmed by thin-layer chromatography (TLC) as well as macroscopic and microscopic examinations (Ph.Eur.3, 1997). Both the *British Herbal Pharmacopoeia* and ESCOP monographs require the leaf to conform with the requirements of the *European Pharmacopoeia* (BHP, 1996; ESCOP, 1997). The German Standard License requires that the leaf conform with the quality requirements of the *German Drug Codex* monograph (Braun et al., 1997). The *German Drug Codex* requires not less than 5.0% tannins, precipitable with hide powder (DAC, 1986, Wichtl and Bisset, 1994).

Pharmacopeial grade witch hazel *bark* consists of the dried bark from stems and branches of *H. virginiana* L. collected in the spring. The bark must contain not less than 20% ethanol (45%)-soluble extractive. Botanical identity must be confirmed by TLC as well as by macroscopic and microscopic examinations (BHP, 1996). The *German Drug Codex* requires not less than 9.0% tannins, precipitable with hide powder (DAC, 1986; Wichtl and Bisset, 1994). Witch Hazel USP is the clear, colorless distillate prepared from freshly cut and partially dried dormant twigs of *H. virginiana* L. It is prepared by macerating the twigs in water for 24 hours, then distilling it down until 800–850 mL of distillate is yielded from each 1,000 g of twigs, then adding 150 mL of alcohol to each 850 mL of distillate. It has a tannins limit of 0.03 mg tannic acid per mL, a pH between 3.0 and 5.0, and alcohol content of 14.0–15.0% (USP 24–NF 19, 1999).

Description

Witch hazel leaf consists of the dried leaf of *H. virginiana* L. [Fam. Hamamelidaceae], as well as its preparations in effective dosage. The leaf contains 3–8% tannin, mainly gallotannins. Other ingredients are flavonoids and essential oil.

Witch hazel bark consists of the dried bark of the trunk and branches of *H. virginiana* L., as well as its preparations in effective dosage. The bark contains at least 4% tannins. Characteristic ingredients of witch hazel bark are β-hamamelitannin and γ-hamamelitannin, the depside ellagitannin, catechin derivatives, and free gallic acid.

Fresh leaf and twigs of *H. virginiana* L. consist of leaves and twigs collected in spring and early summer for the production of water distillates.

Chemistry and Pharmacology

Witch hazel leaf contains 3–10% tannins (a mixture of catechins, gallotannins, plus cyanidin and delphinidin type proanthocyanidins), mainly hamamelitannin and hamamelose (Budavari, 1996; Meyer-Buchtela, 1999; Wichtl, 1989); catechins, mainly (+)-catechin, (+)-gallocatechin, (–)-epicatechin gallate, (–)-epigallocatechin gallate; phenolic acids (caffeic and gallic acids); flavonoids such as kaempferol, quercetin, quercitrin, and isoquercitrin (ESCOP, 1997; Hänsel et al., 1993); 0.01–0.5% volatile oil (Meyer-Buchtela, 1999; Wichtl, 1989), of which 40% are aliphatic alcohols, 25% are carbonyl compounds (n-hex-2-en-1-al, acetaldehyde, α- and β-ionone), 15% are aliphatic esters, and not more than 0.2% safrole (Wichtl and Bisset, 1994; Zeylstra, 1998).

Witch hazel bark contains 8–12% tannins, composed mainly of hamamelitannins (1–7%), followed by monogalloylhamamelose, free gallic acid, condensed catechin tannins, and small amounts of oligomeric proanthocyanidins; a small amount of flavonols; approximately 0.1% volatile oil with a very complex composition (Hänsel et al., 1993; Meyer-Buchtela, 1999; Wichtl, 1996).

The Commission E reported astringent, anti-inflammatory, and locally hemostatic activities.

The *British Herbal Pharmacopoeia* reported astringent action for witch hazel bark (BHP, 1996). *The Merck Index* reported its therapeutic category as astringent (Budavari, 1996). Witch hazel leaf fluidextract is vasoconstrictive in the rabbit (Bruneton, 1995). In a pharmacological study in humans a topical application of witch hazel leaf hydroglycolic extract significantly reduced skin temperature, which was interpreted as vasoconstrictive action (Diemunsch and Mathis, 1987; ESCOP, 1997). Astringent, antiseptic, and hemostatic properties of witch hazel leaf and bark infusions, ointments, and suppositories have been demonstrated in animal experiments (Wichtl and Bisset, 1994).

Uses

The Commission E approved the use of witch hazel preparations for minor skin injuries, local inflammation of skin and mucous membranes, hemorrhoids, and for varicose veins.

Witch hazel is used as an active compound in topical ointments and suppositories for the treatment of hemorrhoids (Anon., 1991; Reynolds, 1989). The German Standard License for witch hazel leaf and/or bark tea infusion, for oral ingestion or as a mouthwash, approves its use as supportive therapy for acute, non-specific diarrhea, and also to treat inflammation of the gums and mucous membranes of the mouth (Braun et al., 1997). ESCOP indicates the internal use of witch hazel leaf infusion and/or fluidextract for symptomatic treatment of conditions related to varicose veins (painful and heavy legs, and for hemorrhoids) and the external use of the decoction and/or semisolid extract for bruises, sprains, and minor injuries of the skin, local inflammations of the skin, and mucosa, hemorrhoids, and relief of neurodermatitis atopic symptoms (ESCOP, 1997). In France, witch hazel extracts and tinctures are approved for oral and topical application to treat subjective symptoms of venous insufficiency and hemorrhoids. Local application is also allowed for relief of eye irritation and for oral hygiene (Bruneton, 1995).

Contraindications
None known.

Side Effects
None known.

Use During Pregnancy and Lactation
No restrictions known (McGuffin et al., 1997).

Interactions with Other Drugs
None known.

Dosage and Administration
Unless otherwise prescribed: Cut leaves and/or bark or extracts for internal and external use, or steam distillate of fresh leaves and bark for internal and external use, as follows:

Internal (mucous membranes): Suppositories (vaginal and rectal): The amount of a preparation corresponding to 0.1–1 g drug (decoction), one to three times daily (Commission E); or, a semi-solid cylinder or cone containing 200 mg witch hazel leaf dry alcoholic extract with cocoa butter or other comparable fatty oils, one to two times daily (BPC, 1973; ESCOP, 1997; Reynolds, 1989; Zeylstra, 1998); or prepared from the concentrated infusion in a base of powdered gelatin or cocoa butter and glycerin (Cowper, 1996).

Internal (oral): Infusion: Steep 2–3 g leaf or bark in 150 ml boiled water for 10 to 15 minutes. Drink two to three times daily between meals (Braun et al., 1997; Hänsel et al., 1993; Meyer-Buchtela, 1999; Zeylstra, 1998).

Fluidextract, 1:1 (g/ml), 45% ethanol: 2–4 ml, three times daily (BHP, 1983; BPC, 1973; ESCOP, 1997).

Tincture, 1:5 (g/ml), 25% ethanol: 2–4 ml, three times daily (BPC, 1934; Karnick, 1994; Zeylstra, 1998).

External: Aqueous steam distillate (witch hazel water with preservative): For local application as needed, undiluted or diluted 1:3 with water, several times daily (Commission E).

Aromatic hydrosol (without preservative): For local application as needed, several times daily. Hydrosols may be more suitable than distillates for sensitive skin (Blackwell, 1998).

Compress: Semi-solid or fluid preparations containing 5–10% decoction or distillate are spread or soaked on linen. Fold and apply firmly to affected area. [Note: Hemorrhoidal pads are commercially available which can be folded and used as a compress on inflamed tissue].

Decoction (bark): For use as a component of compresses, place 2–3 g fine-cut or coursely powdered bark in 150 ml cold water, bring to a boil and simmer for 10 to 15 minutes (Meyer-Buchtela, 1999; Wichtl and Bisset, 1994).

Decoction (leaf): For use as a component of compresses and irrigations, boil 5–10 g in 250 ml water for 10 to 15 minutes (Commission E; ESCOP, 1997; Hänsel et al., 1993; Meyer-Buchtela, 1999).

Fluidextract 1:1 (g/ml), 45% alcohol: For use as a component of ointment, gel, or salve (Reynolds, 1989).

Gargle or mouth wash: Use the warm decoction or infusion several times daily (Braun et al., 1997).

Ointment, gel, or salve: Semi-solid preparation containing 10% decoction or fluidextract, in a base of vaseline or wool fat (anhydrous lanolin) and yellow soft paraffin, applied locally (BPC, 1973; Cowper, 1996; ESCOP, 1997; Reynolds, 1989; Zeylstra, 1998).

Poultice: Semi-solid paste containing 20–30% aqueous steam distillate or decoction, applied locally (Commission E).

Tincture 1:5 (g/ml): For use as a component of ointment, gel, or salve.

References

Anon. 1991. Drug therapy for hemorrhoids. Proven results of therapy with a hamamelis containing hemorrhoid ointment. Results of a meeting of experts. *Fortschr Med* Suppl 116:1–11.

BAnz. See *Bundesanzeiger*.

Blackwell, R. 1998. A new look at aromatic hydrosols. *Eur J Herbal Med* 4(2):13–16.

Braun, R. et al. 1997. *Standardzulassungen für Fertigarzneimittel—Text and Kommentar*. Stuttgart: Deutscher Apotheker Verlag.

British Herbal Pharmacopoeia (BHP). 1983. Keighley, U.K.: British Herbal Medicine Association. 110.

———. 1996. Exeter, U.K.: British Herbal Medicine Association. 97–98.

British Pharmaceutical Codex (BPC). 1934. London: The Pharmaceutical Press.

———. 1973. London: The Pharmaceutical Press. 218.

Bruneton, J. 1995. *Pharmacognosy, Phytochemistry, Medicinal Plants*. Paris: Lavoisier Publishing. 327.

Budavari, S. (ed.). 1996. *The Merck Index: An Encyclopedia of Chemicals, Drugs, and Biologicals*, 12th ed. Whitehouse Station, N.J.: Merck & Co, Inc. 786–787.

Bundesanzeiger (BAnz). 1998. Monographien der Kommission E (Zulassungs- und Aufbereitungskommission am BGA für den humanmed. Bereich, phytotherapeutische Therapierichtung und Stoffgruppe). Köln: Bundesgesundheitsamt (BGA).

Cowper, A.B. 1996. *Manufacturing Handbook for Herbal Medicines*. Morisset, Australia: Anne B Cowper. 31–38.

Der Marderosian, A. (ed.). 1999. *The Review of Natural Products*. St. Louis: Facts and Comparisons.

Deutscher Arzneimittel-Codex (DAC). 1986. Stuttgart: Deutscher Apotheker Verlag.

Diemunsch, A.M. and C. Mathis. 1987. Effet vasoconstricteur de l'hamamélis en application externe. *STP Pharma* 3:111–114.

Duke, J.A. 1985. *Handbook of Medicinal Herbs*. Boca Raton: CRC Press.

ESCOP. 1997. "Hamamelidis folium." *Monographs on the Medicinal Uses of Plant Drugs*. Exeter, U.K.: European Scientific Cooperative on Phytotherapy.

Europäisches Arzneibuch, 3rd ed. (Ph.Eur.3). 1997. Stuttgart: Deutscher Apotheker Verlag. 1020–1021.

German Homeopathic Pharmacopoeia (GHP). 1993. Translation of the German *Homöopathisches Arzneibuch* (HAB 1), 5th suppl. 1991 to the 1st ed. 1978. Stuttgart. Deutscher Apotheker Verlag. 489–498.

Grieve, M. 1979. *A Modern Herbal*. New York: Dover Publications, Inc.

Hänsel, R., K. Keller, H. Rimpler, G. Schneider (eds.). 1993. *Hagers Handbuch der Pharmazeutischen Praxis*, 5th ed. Vol. 5. Berlin-Heidelberg: Springer Verlag. 367–384.

The Homeopathic Pharmacopoeia of the United States (HPUS). 1992. Arlington, VA: Pharmacopoeia Convention of the American Institute of Homeopathy.

Hughes-Formella, B.J. et al. 1998. Anti-inflammatory effect of hamamelis lotion in a UVB erythema test. *Dermatology* 196(3):316–322.

Karnick, C.R. 1994. *Pharmacopoeial Standards of Herbal Plants*, Vol 2. Indian Medical Science Series, No. 37. Delhi: Sri Satguru Publications. 173–174.

Korting, H.C., M. Schafer-Korting, H. Hart, P. Laux, M. Schmid. 1993. Anti-inflammatory activity of hamamelis distillate applied topically to the skin. Influence of vehicle and dose. *Eur J Clin Pharmacol* 44(4):315–318.

Korting H.C. et al. 1995. Comparative efficacy of hamamelis distillate and hydrocortisone cream in atopic eczema. *Eur J Clin Pharmacol* 48(6):461–465.

Leung, A.Y. and S. Foster. 1996. *Encyclopedia of Common Natural Ingredients Used in Foods, Drugs, and Cosmetics*. 2nd ed. New York: John Wiley & Sons, Inc.

McGuffin M, C. Hobbs, R. Upton, A. Goldberg. 1997. American Herbal Product Association's *Botanical Safety Handbook*. Boca Raton: CRC Press.

Meyer-Buchtela, E. 1999. *Tee-Rezepturen—Ein Handbuch für Apotheker und Ärzte*. Stuttgart: Deutscher Apotheker Verlag.

Millspaugh, C.F. 1974. *American Medicinal Plants*. New York: Dover Publications, Inc [reprint of 1892 American Plants]. 227–229.

Ph.Eur.3. See *Europäisches Arzneibuch*.

Reynolds, J.E.F. (ed.). 1989. *Martindale: The Extra Pharmacopoeia*, 29th ed. London: The Pharmaceutical Press. 778–779.

Tyler, V.E. 1994. *Herbs of Choice: The Therapeutic Use of Phytomedicinals*. New York: Pharmaceutical Products Press.

United States Pharmacopeia, 24th rev. and *National Formulary*, 19th ed. (USP 24–NF19). 1999. Rockville, MD: United States Pharmacopeial Convention, Inc. 1755.

Wichtl, M. (ed.). 1989. *Teedrogen*, 2nd ed. Stuttgart: Wissenschaftliche Verlagsgesellschaft.

Wichtl, M. and N.G. Bisset (eds.). 1994. *Herbal Drugs and Phytopharmaceuticals*. Stuttgart: Medpharm Scientific Publishers. 243–247.

Wichtl, M. 1996. Monographien—Kommentar. In: Braun, R. et al. 1997. *Standardzulassungen für Fertigarzneimittel—Text and Kommentar*. Stuttgart: Deutscher Apotheker Verlag.

Zeylstra, H. 1998. *Hamamelis virginiana*. *British Journal of Phytotherapy* 5(1):23–28.

Additional Resources

Bernard, P., A. Bovis, G. Balansard. 1971. L'essai chromatographique des preparations galeniques a base de feuilles d'Hamamelis [Chromatographic assay of galenic preparations from Hamamelis leaves]. *J Pharm Belg* 26(6):661–668.

Bernard, P., P. Balansard, G. Balansard, A. Bovis. 1972. Valeur pharmacodynamique toniveineuse des preparations galeniques a base de feuilles d'hamamelis [Venitonic pharmacodynamic value of galenic preparations with a base of hamamelis leaves]. *J Pharm Belg* 27(4):505–512.

Bernard, P. 1977. Les feuilles d'hamamélis. *Plantes Méd Phytothér* 11(Spécial):184–188.

Bown, D. 1995. *Encyclopedia of Herbs and Their Uses.* New York: DK Publishing, Inc. 291.

Council of Europe. 1989. *Plant Preparations Used as Ingredients of Cosmetic Products,* 1st ed. Strasbourg: Council of Europe.

Duke, J.A. 1997. *The Green Pharmacy.* Emmaus, PA: Rodale Press.

Erdelmeier, C.A.J. et al. 1996. Antiviral and antiphlogistic activities of *Hamamelis virginiana* bark. *Planta Med* 62(3):241–245.

Hartisch, C., H. Kolodziej, F. von Bruchhausen. 1997. Dual inhibitory activities of tannins from *Hamamelis virginiana* and related polyphenols on 5-lipoxygenase and lyso-PAF: acetyl-CoA-acetyltransferase. *Planta Med* 63(2):106–110.

Hörmann, H.P. and H.C. Korting. 1994. Evidence for the efficacy and safety of topical herbal drugs in dermatology: Part 1: Anti-inflammatory agents. *Phytomed* 1:161–171.

Khory, R.N. and N.N. Katrak. 1985. *Materia Medica of India and Their Therapeutics.* Delhi: Neeraj Publishing House.

Laux, P. and R. Oschmann. 1993. Die Zaubernuss—*Hamamelis virginiana* L. *Z Phytother* 14:155–166.

Lloyd and Lloyd. 1935. History of Hamamelis extract and distillate. *J Am Pharm Assoc* 24:220.

Madaus, G. 1979. *Lehrbuch der Biologischen Heilmittel,* Vols. 1–3. Hildesheim: Georg Olms Verlag.

Malhotra, S.C. 1990. *Phytochemical Investigations of Certain Medicinal Plants Used in Ayurveda.* New Delhi: CCRA & S, Government of India.

Newall, C.A., L.A. Anderson, J.D. Phillipson. 1996. *Herbal Medicines: A Guide for Health-Care Professionals.* London: The Pharmaceutical Press.

Pharmacopée Française Xe Édition (Ph.Fr.X.). 1983–1990. Moulins-les-Metz: Maisonneuve S.A.

Pharmacopoeia Helvetica, 7th ed. (Ph.Helv.VII), Vol. 1–4. 1987. Bern: Office Central Fédéral des Imprimés et du Matériel.

Reynolds, J.E.F. (ed.). 1993. *Martindale: The Extra Pharmacopoeia,* 30th ed. London: The Pharmaceutical Press.

Sorkin, B. 1980. Hametum-Salbe, eine kortikoidfreie antiinflammatorische Salbe. *Phys Med Rehab* 21:53–57.

Steinegger, E. and R. Hänsel. 1992. *Pharmakognosie,* 5th ed. Berlin: Springer Verlag.

Van Hellemont, J. 1988. *Fytotherapeutisch Compendium,* 2nd ed. Utrecht: Bohn, Scheltema & Holkema. 284–286.

This material was adapted from *The Complete German Commission E Monographs—Therapeutic Guide to Herbal Medicines.* M. Blumenthal, W.R. Busse, A. Goldberg, J. Gruenwald, T. Hall, C.W. Riggins, R.S. Rister (eds.) S. Klein and R.S. Rister (trans.). 1998. Austin: American Botanical Council; Boston: Integrative Medicine Communications.

1) The Overview section is new information.

2) Description, Chemistry and Pharmacology, Uses, Contraindications, Side Effects, Interactions with Other Drugs, and Dosage sections have been drawn from the original work. Additional information has been added in some or all of these sections, as noted with references.

3) The dosage for equivalent preparations (tea infusion, fluidextract, and tincture) have been provided based on the following example:
Unless otherwise prescribed: 2 g per day of [powdered, crushed, cut or whole] [plant part]
Infusion: 2 g in 150 ml of water
Fluidextract 1:1 (g/ml): 2 ml
Tincture 1:5 (g/ml): 10 ml

4) The References and Additional Resources sections are new sections. Additional Resources are not cited in the monograph but are included for research purposes.

YARROW

Latin Name:
Achillea millefolium

Pharmacopeial Name:
Millefolii herba, yarrow herb
Millefolii flos, yarrow flower

Other Names:
Achillea, milfoil, millefolium

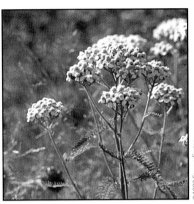

©1999 Steven Foster

Overview

Yarrow is a chemically polymorphic perennial herb from a genus of complex taxon-
omy, native to Europe, Asia, and North America, now distributed in the temperate
zone worldwide. Many species, subspecies, and microspecies have been recognized
and named (Bruneton, 1995; Budavari, 1996; Leung and Foster, 1996; Wichtl and
Bisset, 1994). Yarrow adapts itself to new surroundings and can change its mor-
phology and chemical composition significantly, depending on its environment.
New subspecies evolve by polyploidy (changes in chromosome number). The sub-
species can be differentiated by their chromosome numbers, determined by microscopic examination (Bradley, 1992; Zeylstra, 1997). The material of commerce
comes mostly from southeastern and eastern European countries and the United
Kingdom (BHP, 1996; Wichtl and Bisset, 1994). In Germany, a small amount of
yarrow is cultivated (Lange and Schippmann, 1997). The material used in
Ayurvedic medicine grows wild in the Himalayan mountains from Kashmir to
Kumaon (Nadkarni, 1976).

Yarrow has been used as medicine by many cultures for hundreds of years
(Budavari, 1996; Zeylstra, 1997). Its English common name is a corruption of the
Anglo-Saxon name *gearwe*; the Dutch, *yerw*. The genus name *Achillea* may have
been derived from the Achilles of Greek mythology, who was fabled to have had
his wounds treated by topical use of the herb. The species name *millefolium* is
derived from the many segments of its foliage. The ancient Europeans called it
Herba Militaris, the military herb—an ointment made from it was used as a vulnerary drug on battle wounds (Grieve, 1967). Yarrow flower was formerly official in
the *United States Pharmacopeia*. Today, it is official in the national pharmacopeias
of Austria, the Czech Republic, France, Germany, Hungary, Switzerland, and
Romania. Additionally, it is listed in the Indian *Ayurvedic Pharmacopoeia* for fevers
and wound healing (Karnick, 1994).

Its uses in North American aboriginal medicine are well documented. Yarrow tea
is used by healers of the Micmac nation as a diaphoretic remedy to treat fevers and
colds. The stalks are also pounded into a pulp and applied topically to bruises,
sprains, and swellings (Lacey, 1993). Yarrow has been the subject of an ongoing
study of herbal drugs used by people of the Micmac and Malecite nations of the
Canadian Maritime provinces. The study began with an examination of the observations and writings of early European settlers and missionaries. Modern phytochemical studies, using techniques including nuclear magnetic resonance
spectroscopy and combined gas chromatography-mass spectrometry, have identified a range of phytosterols and triterpenes occurring in yarrow, which may help
explain its successful therapeutic applications in Micmac and Malecite medicines
(Chandler et al., 1979; Chandler et al., 1982; Chandler and Hooper, 1982; Chandler, 1983; Hooper and Chandler, 1984). The Abnaki people use yarrow tea as a

drug to treat colds, fevers, and grippe (Rousseau, 1947). People of the Algonquin and Quebec nations use it internally to treat colds and other respiratory disorders. The powder is also used as an analgesic snuff for headaches (Black, 1980). Yarrow infusions and decoctions are used as a gastrointestinal aid by the Cherokee, Gosiute, Iroquois, and Mohegan nations (Chamberlin, 1911; Hamel and Chiltoskey, 1975; Herrick, 1977; Tantaquidgeon, 1928, 1972).

In Germany, yarrow flower is licensed as a standard medicinal tea. It is also used as a cholagogue component in numerous prepared biliary and/or gastrointestinal medicines. It is also used externally as a sitz bath to treat vegetative pelvipathia (Bradley, 1992; Braun et al., 1997; Wichtl and Bisset, 1994). In the United States, yarow is used as a diaphoretic or febrifuge component of traditional cold and flu/fever compounds marketed as dietary supplement products, often used in combination with echinacea herb, elder flower, ginger rhizome, and peppermint leaf. It is also used as a component of topical styptic preparations.

The approved modern therapeutic applications for yarrow flower are supportable based on its long history of use in well established systems of traditional medicine, on phytochemical investigations, and on pharmacological studies in animals.

German pharmacopeial grade yarrow flower must be composed of the dried aerial parts (capitulums with maximum 5% stems) harvested during the flowering period, containing not less than 0.2% (v/m) volatile oils with minimum 0.02% proazulene, calculated as chamazulene on a dry-weight basis. It must have a bitter value of maximum 5000. Botanical identity must be confirmed by thin-layer chromatograhy (TLC) as well as macroscopic and microscopic examinations (DAB, 1997; DAC, 1986; Wichtl and Bisset, 1994). The *Swiss Pharmacopoeia* also requires not less than 0.2% volatile oils, though not more than 10% peduncles of inflorescence (Ph.Helv.VII, 1987; Wichtl and Bisset, 1994). The *British Herbal Pharmacopoeia* requires not less than 15% water-soluble extractive, among other quantitative standards and identity tests (BHP, 1996).

Both the *Austrian Pharmacopoeia* and the *French Pharmacopoeia* require >0.3% volatile oil and the characterization of azulenes (Bruneton, 1995; ÖAB, 1981; Ph.Fr.X, 1990; Wichtl and Bisset, 1994). According to Bruneton, these requirements can only be fulfilled by the pink flower subspecies (*sudetica*, from mountain areas), or by other species entirely (e.g., *A. collina*), because the official species at best contains only traces of azulenes (Bruneton, 1995). The most widespread species [*Achillea millefolium* L. ssp. millefolium] is hexaploid and the volatile oil contains no chamazulene (Bradley, 1992).

Description

Yarrow herb consists of the fresh or dried aboveground parts of *A. mille-folium* L. [Fam. Asteraceae], harvested at flowering season, and its preparations in effective dosage. Yarrow flower consists of the dried inflorescence of *A. millefolium* L. *s.l.* [Fam. Asteraceae] and its preparations in effective dosage. The preparation contains essential oil and proazulene.

Chemistry and Pharmacology

Yarrow contains 3–4% condensed and hydrolysable tannins; 0.3–1.4% volatile oils, mostly linalool, borneol, camphor, β-caryophyllene, 1,8-cineole, and sesquiterpene lactones composed of guaianolides, mainly achillicin (a proazulene), achillin, leucodin, and germacranolides (dihydroparthenolide, achillifolin, millefin); flavonoids (apigenin, luteolin, isorhamnetin, rutin); amino acids (alanine, histidine, leucine, lysine); fatty acids (linoleic, palmitic, oleic); phenolic acids (caffeic, salicylic); vitamins (ascorbic acid, folic acid); alkaloids and bases (achiceine, achilleine, betaine, choline); alkanes (tricosane); polyacetylenes; saponins; sterols (β-sitosterol); sugars (dextrose, glucose, mannitol, sucrose); and coumarins (Bradley, 1992; Bruneton, 1995; Leung and Foster, 1996; Newall et al., 1996; Wichtl and Bisset, 1994).

The Commission E reported choleretic, antibacterial, astringent, and antispasmodic activities.

The *British Herbal Compendium* reported diaphoretic, antipyretic, anti-inflammatory, spasmolytic, aromatic bitter, hemostatic, hypotensive, and emmenagogic activities (Bradley, 1992). Anti-inflammatory activity was reported in laboratory mice and rats with an aqueous extract of yarrow flower heads (Leung and Foster, 1996; Newall et al., 1996). It is possible that its anti-inflammatory and antispasmodic properties are due to its flavonoids content (Bruneton, 1995). Choleretic activity has been confirmed in animal experiments. Antimicrobial activity against a range of bacteria has been reported for aqueous and ether extracts of yarrow (Wichtl and Bisset, 1994).

Uses

The Commission E approved the internal use of yarrow flower for loss of appetite and dyspeptic ailments, such as mild, spastic discomforts of the gastrointestinal tract, and externally as a sitz bath for painful, cramp-like conditions of psychosomatic origin in the lower part of the female pelvis.

The *British Herbal Compendium* lists its internal use for feverish conditions, common cold, and digestive complaints; and its topical use for slow-healing wounds and skin inflammations (Bradley, 1992). The German Standard License for yarrow tea indicates its use for mild cramp-like or spasmodic gastrointestinal-bilious complaints, for gastric catarrh, and for appetite stimulation (Bradley, 1992; Wichtl and Bisset, 1994).

Contraindications

Allergy to yarrow and other composites.

Side Effects

None known.

Use During Pregnancy and Lactation

Not recommended during pregnancy (McGuffin et al., 1997; Newall et al., 1996). No restrictions known during lactation.

Interactions with Other Drugs

None known.

Dosage and Administration

Internal: Unless otherwise prescribed: 4.5 g per day of cut herb, or 3 g of cut flower for teas and other galenical preparations; pressed juice of fresh plants.
Infusion: 1–2 g in 150 ml boiled water for 10 to 15 minutes, three times daily between meals.
Succus (pressed juice from fresh herb): 5 ml (1 teaspoon), three times daily between meals.
Fluidextract 1:1 (g/ml): 1–2 ml, three times daily between meals.
Tincture 1:5 (g/ml): 5 ml, three times daily between meals.
External: Unless otherwise prescribed: Sitz baths.
Sitz bath: 100 g yarrow per 20 liters (5 gallons) of warm or hot water, just enough to cover the hips with the knees up; wrap upper body in towels; soak 10 to 20 minutes, rinse.

References

Black, M.J. 1980. *Algonquin Ethnobotany: An Interpretation of Aboriginal Adaptation in South Western Quebec.* Ottawa: National Museums of Canada. Mercury Series No. 65.

Bradley, P.R. (ed.). 1992. *British Herbal Compendium,* Vol. 1. Bournemouth: British Herbal Medicine Association.

Braun, R. et al. 1997. *Standardzulassungen für Fertigarzneimittel—Text and Kommentar.* Stuttgart: Deutscher Apotheker Verlag.

British Herbal Pharmacopoeia (BHP). 1996. Exeter, U.K.: British Herbal Medicine Association.

Bruneton, J. 1995. *Pharmacognosy, Phytochemistry, Medicinal Plants.* Paris: Lavoisier Publishing.

Budavari, S. (ed.). 1996. *The Merck Index: An Encyclopedia of Chemicals, Drugs, and Biologicals,* 12th ed. Whitehouse Station, N.J.: Merck & Co, Inc.

Chamberlin, R.V. 1911. *The Ethnobotany of the Gosiute Indians of Utah.* Memoirs Amer Anthro Assoc 2(5):331–405.

Chandler, R.F. 1983. Vindication of Maritime Indian herbal remedies. *J Ethnopharmacol* 9(2–3):323–327.

Chandler, R.F. and S.N. Hooper. 1982. Herbal remedies of the Maritime Indians: a preliminary screening. Part III. *J Ethnopharmacol* 6(3):275–285.

Chandler, R.F. et al. 1982. Herbal remedies of the Maritime Indians: sterols and triterpenes of *Achillea millefolium* L. (Yarrow). *J Pharm Sci* 71(6):690–693.

Chandler, R.F., L. Freeman, S.N. Hooper. 1979. Herbal remedies of the Maritime Indians. *J Ethnopharmacol* 1(1):49–68.

Deutsches Arzneibuch (DAB 1997). 1997. Stuttgart: Deutscher Apotheker Verlag.

Deutscher Arzneimittel-Codex (DAC). 1986. Stuttgart: Deutscher Apotheker Verlag.

Grieve, M. 1967. *A Modern Herbal,* Vol. 2. New York; London: Hafner Publishing Co. 863–865.

Hamel, P.B. and M.U. Chiltoskey. 1975. *Cherokee Plants.* Sylva, N.C.: Herald Publishing Co. 62.

Herrick, J.W. 1977. *Iroquois Medical Botany.* Ann Arbor, MI: University Microfilms International. 470.

Hooper, S.N. and R.F. Chandler. 1984. Herbal remedies of the Maritime Indians: phytosterols and triterpenes of 67 plants. *J Ethnopharmacol* 10(2):181–194.

Karnick, C.R. 1994. *Pharmacopoeial Standards of Herbal Plants,* Vol. 2. Delhi: Sri Satguru Publications. 150.

Lacey, L. 1993. *Micmac Medicines—Remedies and Recollections.* Halifax, NS: Nimbus Publishing Ltd. 95, 116.

Lange, D. and U. Schippmann. 1997. Trade Survey of Medicinal Plants in Germany—A Contribution to International Plant Species Conservation. Bonn: Bundesamt für Naturschutz. 33.

Leung, A.Y. and S. Foster. 1996. *Encyclopedia of Common Natural Ingredients Used in Food, Drugs, and Cosmetics,* 2nd ed. New York: John Wiley & Sons, Inc.

McGuffin, M., C. Hobbs, R. Upton, A. Goldberg. 1997. American Herbal Product Association's *Botanical Safety Handbook.* Boca Raton: CRC Press.

Nadkarni, K.M. 1976. *Indian Materia Medica.* Bombay: Popular Prakashan. 20.

Newall, C.A., L.A. Anderson, J.D. Phillipson. 1996. *Herbal Medicines: A Guide for Health-Care Professionals.* London: The Pharmaceutical Press.

*Österreichisches Arzneibuch,*1st suppl. (ÖAB). 1981–1983. Wien: Verlag der Österreichischen Staatsdruckerei.

Pharmacopée Française Xe Édition (Ph.Fr.X.). 1983–1990. Moulins-les-Metz: Maisonneuve S.A.

Pharmacopoeia Helvetica, 7th ed. Vol. 1–4. (Ph.Helv.VII). 1987. Bern: Office Central Fédéral des Imprimés et du Matériel.

Rousseau, J. 1947. Ethnobotanique Abenakise. *Archives de Folklore* 11:145–182.

Tantaquidgeon, G. 1928. Mohegan Medicinal Practices. *SI-BAE Annual Report* (43):264–270.

———. 1972. Folk Medicine of the Delaware and Related Algonkian Indians. *Pennsylvania Hist and Mus Commission Anth Papers* (3):75, 128.

Wichtl, M. and N.G. Bisset (eds.). 1994. *Herbal Drugs and Phytopharmaceuticals.* Stuttgart: Medpharm Scientific Publishers.

Zeylstra, H. 1997. Just Yarrow? *Brit J Phytother* 4(4):184–189.

Additional Resources

British Herbal Pharmacopoeia (BHP). 1983. Keighley, U.K.: British Herbal Medicine Association.

Chandler, R.F., S.N. Hooper, M.J. Harvery. 1982. Ethnobotany and *Phytochemistry* of Yarrow, *Achillea millefolium,* Compositae. *Economic Botany* 36:203–223.

Coffin, A.I. 1852. *A Botanic Guide to Health and the Natural Pathology of Disease.* London: British Medico-Botanic Establishment. 88–89.

Council of Europe. 1989. *Plant Preparations Used as Ingredients of Cosmetic Products,* 1st ed. Strasbourg: Council of Europe.

Czygan, F.C. 1994. Schafgarbe: Alte Heilpflanze neu Untersucht. *PZ* 139(6):439.

Direction de la Pharmacie et du Médicament (DPM). 1992. Achillée millefeuille, *sommité fleurie.* Bulletin Officiel No. 92/11 bis. [English edition]. Paris: Direction des Journaux Officiels.

Goldberg, A.S., E.C. Mueller, E. Eigen, S.J. Desalva. 1969. Isolation of the anti-inflammatory principles from *Achillea millefolium* (Compositae). *J Pharm Sci* 58(8):938–941.

Goldberg, A.S. et al. 1970. U.S. Patent 3,552,350; through *Chem Abstr* 73:102048w.

Hänsel, R., K. Keller, H. Rimpler, G. Schneider (eds.). 1992. *Hagers Handbuch der Pharmazeutischen Praxis,* 5th ed. Vol. 4. Berlin-Heidelberg: Springer Verlag. 45–54.

Krivenko, V.V., G.P. Potebnia, V.V. Loiko. 1989. Opyt lecheniia nekotorykh zabolevanii organov pishchevareniia lekarstvennymi rasteniiami [Experience in treating digestive organ diseases with medicinal plants]. *Vrach Delo* (3):76–78.

Madaus, G. 1979. *Lehrbuch der Biologischen Heilmittel,* Vols. 1–3. Hildesheim: Georg Olms Verlag.

Mascolo, N. et al. 1987. Biological screening of Italian medicinal plants for anti-inflammatory activity. *Phytother Res* 1:28–31.

Reynolds, J.E.F. (ed.). 1993. *Martindale: The Extra Pharmacopoeia,* 30th ed. London: The Pharmaceutical Press.

Shipochliev, T. and G. Fournadjiev. 1984. Spectrum of the anti-inflammatory effect of *Arctostaphylos uva ursi* and *Achillea millefolium* L. Probl Vutr Med 12:99–107.

Spaich, W. 1977. *Moderne Phytotherapie.* Heidelberg: Haug Verlag.

Steinegger, E. and R. Hänsel. 1988. Lehrbuch der *Pharmakognosie* und Phyto*pharmazie,* 4th ed. Heidelberg: Springer Verlag. 317–319.

———. 1992. *Pharmakognosie*, 5th ed. Berlin-Heidelberg: Springer Verlag.

Tewari, J.P., M.C. Srivastava, J.L. Bajpai.1974. Phy-
topharmacologic studies of *Achillea millefolium*
Linn. *Indian J Med Sci* 28(8):331–336.

Weiss, R.F. 1988. *Herbal Medicine*. Beaconsfield,
England: Beaconsfield Publishers. 92, 315.

Wichtl, M. (ed.). 1997. *Teedrogen,* 4th ed.
Stuttgart: Wissenschaftliche Verlagsgesellschaft.

This material was adapted from *The Complete German Commission E Monographs—Therapeutic Guide to Herbal Medicines*. M. Blumenthal, W.R. Busse, A. Goldberg, J. Gruenwald, T. Hall, C.W. Riggins, R.S. Rister (eds.) S. Klein and R.S. Rister (trans.). 1998. Austin: American Botanical Council; Boston: Integrative Medicine Communications.

1) The Overview section is new information.

2) Description, Chemistry and Pharmacology, Uses, Contraindications, Side Effects, Interactions with Other Drugs, and Dosage sections have been drawn from the original work. Additional information has been added in some or all of these sections, as noted with references.

3) The dosage for equivalent preparations (tea infusion, fluidextract, and tincture) have been provided based on the following example:
Unless otherwise prescribed: 2 g per day of [powdered, crushed, cut or whole] [plant part]
Infusion: 2 g in 150 ml of water
Fluidextract 1:1 (g/ml): 2 ml
Tincture 1:5 (g/ml): 10 ml

4) The References and Additional Resources sections are new sections. Additional Resources are not cited in the monograph but are included for research purposes.

YEAST:

YEAST, BREWER'S
(page 425)

YEAST, BREWER'S/
HANSEN CBS 5926
(page 426)

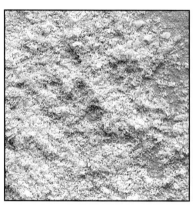

©1999 Steven Foster

Overview

Brewer's yeast is a fungus, classified under the genus *Saccharomyces*, meaning sugar (*saccharo*) fungus (*myces*). Medicinal brewer's yeast is the focus of ongoing scientific and medical study. The Hansen CBS strain binds to fibriated pathogenic bacteria. Medicinal applications relate to the treatment of acute diarrhea, the prevention of *Candida* proliferation, the treatment of acne, and the alleviation of premenstrual symptoms (PMS). Uses for disorders associated with specific diseases, such as recurrence of *Clostridium difficile* disease (CDD) and *Candida* proliferation in pediatric cystic fibrosis patients, are currently being investigated (Muller et al., 1995; McFarland et al., 1994).

Diarrhea prevention has been demonstrated through clinical studies. Tested in a multicenter, double-blind, controlled study of critically ill patients fed through tubes, Hansen CBS prevented diarrhea, even in patients for whom additional factors placed them at even higher risk than that presented by the feeding tubes alone (Bleichner et al., 1997). Beta-lactam antibiotics are also associated with causing diarrhea. In a double-blind, placebo-controlled study, high-risk patients were given either Hansen CBS or placebo within 72 hours of starting a beta-lactam antibiotic. The patients continued to take the yeast supplement for three days following the course of therapy. The resulting protection of Hansen CBS against antibiotic-induced diarrhea was 51%, with no accompanying adverse side effects (McFarland et al., 1995). Because antibiotic-induced diarrhea is common in the elderly, a placebo-controlled study was designed to determine whether or not older patients could benefit from the antidiarrheal effects of Hansen CBS as well; however, in this study the yeast supplement was not effective (Lewis et al., 1998).

A double-blind, placebo-controlled study was designed to demonstrate effects of yeast supplementation on varying types of acne in 139 subjects. According to their doctors, 74.3% of the patients were reported to have seen improvement. Over 80% of the patients felt their acne had completely healed (Weber et al., 1989).

A randomized, placebo-controlled, double-blind study of 40 patients with mild to moderate premenstral syndrome was conducted to test the effects of yeast supplementation versus placebo against PMS. At the end of the six-month study, brewer's yeast was determined more effective in reducing premenstrual symptoms than placebo (Facchinetti et al., 1997).

Yeast supplementation may also be effective in reducing preterm infant mortality in areas where nutritional deficiencies are endemic. In a recent trial, 28 preterm infants in Hungary were given a selenium-enriched yeast product. The product was found to be safe and to increase selenium levels effectively in preterm infants (Bogye et al., 1998).

Both brewer's yeast and Hansen CBS 5926 brewer's yeast are approved in Germany for the treatment of chronic acne and furunculosis (the occurrence of several boils at the same time) and loss of appetite. Hansen CBS 5926 is given in cases of acute and traveler's diarrhea and diarrhea associated with the use of a feeding tube.

Yeast, Brewer's

Latin Name:
Saccharomyces cerevisiae, Candida utilis

Pharmacopeial Name:
Faex medicinalis

Other Names:
brewer's dried yeast, debittered brewer's dried yeast, primary dried yeast

Description
Medicinal yeast consists of fresh or dried cells of *Saccharomyces cerevisiae* Meyer [Fam. Saccharomycetaceae] or of *Candida utilis* (Hennenberg) Rodden et Kreyer Van Rey [Fam. Cryptococ-caceae] and their preparations in effective dosage. Medicinal yeast contains vitamins, particularly B complex, glu-cans, and mannans.

Chemistry and Pharmacology
The main constituents include polysac-charides: long chain carbohydrates composed of glucans and mannans; not less than 40% proteins; B complex vita-mins: not less than 0.012% thiamine hydrochloride, 0.004% riboflavin, and 0.025% nicotinic acid, and not more than 0.004% folic acid (Budavari, 1996; CFR 21, 1998; Tu, 1992).

The Commission E reported antibac-terial activity and stimulation of phago-cytosis.

The *Chinese Pharmacopoeia* reports its therapeutic category as vitamin (Tu, 1992). *The Merck Index* reports its ther-apeutic category as a source of protein and vitamin B complex (Budavari, 1996). Dry yeast is one of the highest natural sources of thiamin, an essential nutrient for normal metabolism of car-bohydrates and fats (Taber, 1962).

Uses
The Commission E approved the use of brewer's yeast for loss of appetite and as a supplement for chronic forms of acne and furunculosis.

The Merck Index indicates its use as a source of vitamins (Budavari, 1996). The FDA permits the use of dried yeast as a food ingredient provided that its total folic acid content is not greater than 0.04 milligram per gram of yeast (approximately 0.008 milligram of pteroylglutamic acid per gram) (CFR 21, 1998). It has been used as a topical application to ulcers and also orally to treat putrid fevers (Nadkarni, 1976).

Contraindications
None known.

Side Effects
Migraine-like headaches may occur in sensitive individuals. The ingestion of fermentable yeast may cause flatulence.

Use During Pregnancy and Lactation
No restrictions known.

Interactions with Other Drugs
None known.

Note: Simultaneous intake of monoamine oxidase inhibitors may cause an increase in blood pressure.

Dosage and Administration

Unless otherwise prescribed: 6 g per day of medicinal yeast and galenical preparations for internal use.
Dried yeast: 2 g, three times daily.
Yeast tablets: Equivalent of 2 g dried yeast, three times daily.

YEAST, BREWER'S/HANSEN CBS 5926

Latin Name:
Saccharomyces cerevisiae Hansen CBS 5926, *S. boulardii*

Pharmacopeial Name:
Saccharomyces cerevisiae Hansen CBS 5926

Other Names:
n/a

Description

Brewer's yeast from *Saccharomyces cerevisiae* Hansen CBS 5926 (syn. *S. boulardii*) [Fam. Saccharomycetaceae] and genetically identical strains in lyophilized (freeze-dried) form. One gram of the lyophilisate contains 885 mg *S. cerevisiae* Hansen CBS 5926 corresponding to 1×10^{10} viable organisms.

Chemistry and Pharmacology

The effectiveness of brewer's yeast depends on the viability of the organism. Brewer's yeast can bind fimbriated, pathogenic bacteria. *In vitro*, growth inhibition was demonstrated by co-culturing brewer's yeast with the following organisms: *Proteus mirabilis* and *P. vulgaris*, *Salmonella typhi* and *S. typhimurium*, *Pseudomonas aeruginosa*, *Staphylococcus aureus*, *Escherichia coli*, certain *Shigella*, and *C. albicans*. Concentration dependencies for growth inhibitions were not given. Brewer's yeast can also inhibit the growth of *Clostridium difficile*, as well as the diarrhea-causing effect of enterotoxic strains of *E. coli*. On the isolated intestinal loop model, sodium and water influx into the intestinal lumen was induced by incubation with the toxin from the cholera vibrio; this reaction was reduced by 40% in the presence of brewer's yeast. Intestinal preparations were also employed to show the reversal of the increased chloride transport induced by prostaglandins E2 and I2 in the presence of brewer's yeast compared to untreated controls. An increase in the activity of the disaccharidases saccharidase, lactase, and maltase, located in the intestinal membrane, was observed in animal and human experiments. In animal experiments, the secretory immunoglobulin (sIgA) was increased in the gastrointestinal tract after oral intake of brewer's yeast. With a single oral dosage of 3 g/kg body weight of brewer's yeast, no toxic reactions were observed in mice and rats. No substance-dependent changes were observed with a dosage of 330 mg/kg body weight over six weeks (six days per week) given to dogs, and about 100 mg/kg body weight given daily over six months to rats and rabbits. The Ames test with *Salmonella typhimurium* TA 90, TA 100, TA 1335, TA 1337, and TA 1338 revealed no mutagenic effects, with or without activation of SY-mix. Experiments for embryocytic and carcinogenic effects are not available.

Uses

The Commission E approved the use of brewer's yeast Hansen CBS 5926 for symptomatic treatment of acute diarrhea, for prophylactic and symptomatic treatment of diarrhea during travel, diarrhea occurring while tube feeding, as an adjuvant for chronic forms of acne, as a dietary supplement, and as a source of B vitamins and protein (Stecher, 1968). Medically it has been used as an application to ulcers and as an internal remedy for putrid fevers. Yeast has shown therapeutic action in the cases of furunculosis, acne, and similar skin diseases (Nadkarni, 1976).

Note: In case of diarrhea, replacement of fluids and electrolytes is an important therapeutic measure, especially for children. Diarrhea of infants and small children requires consultation with a physician. Diarrheas lasting longer than two days, containing blood, or accompanied by fever, require medical attention. If during therapy with brewer's yeast microbiological tests are performed on stool samples, the intake of yeast must be reported to the laboratory, since false positive results may be reported.

Contraindications

Not to be used in case of yeast allergies.
Warning: Infants and small children are excluded from self-medication in any case.

Side Effects

Oral intake may cause flatulence. In individual cases, intolerance (incompatibilities) may occur in the form of itching, urticaria, local or general exanthemas, and Quincke's edema.

Use During Pregnancy and Lactation

No restrictions known.

Interactions with Other Drugs

The simultaneous intake of brewer's yeast and antimycotics can influence the activity of brewer's yeast.

Warning: Simultaneous intake of MAO-inhibitors may cause increased blood pressure.

Dosage and Administration

Unless otherwise prescribed:
Lyophylisate in capsules for internal use as well as addition to tubal feed mixtures.
Daily dosage (children older than 2 years/adults):
For prevention of travel diarrhea, beginning 5 days prior to journey: 250–500 mg daily.
For therapy of diarrhea: 250–500 mg daily
For diarrhea due to tube feeding: Add 500 mg brewer's yeast per liter of nutrient solution. The treatment should be continued for several days after diarrhea has ceased.
For acne: 750 mg daily.

References

Bleichner, G., H. Blehaut, H. Mentec, D. Moyse. 1997. *Saccharomyces boulardii* prevents diarrhea in critically ill tube-fed patients. A multicenter, randomized, double-blind placebo-controlled trial. *Intensive Care Med* 23(5):517–523.

Bogye, G., G. Alfthan, T. Machay. 1998. Randomized clinical trial of enteral yeast-selenium supplementation in preterm infants. *Biofactors* 8(1–2):139–142.

Budavari, S. (ed.). 1996. *The Merck Index: An Encyclopedia of Chemicals, Drugs, and Biologicals,* 12th ed. Whitehouse Station, N.J.: Merck & Co, Inc. 1726.

CFR 21. See U.S.A. Dept. of Health and Human Services: Food and Drug Administration.

Facchinetti, F. et al. 1997. Effects of a yeast-based dietary supplementation on premenstrual syndrome. A double-blind placebo-controlled study. *Gynecol Obstet Invest* 43(2):120–124.

Lewis, S.J., L.F. Potts, R.E. Barry. 1998. The lack of therapeutic effect of *Saccharomyces boulardii* in the prevention of antibiotic-related diarrhoea in elderly patients. *J Infect* 36(2):171–174.

McFarland, L.V. et al. 1995. Prevention of beta-lactam-associated diarrhea by *Saccharomyces boulardii* compared with placebo. *Am J Gastroenterol* 90(3):439–448.

McFarland, L.V. et al. 1994. A randomized placebo-controlled trial of *Saccharomyces boulardii* in combination with standard antibiotics for *Clostridium difficile* disease. *JAMA* 271(24):1913–1918.

Muller, J., N. Remus, K.H. Harms. 1995. Mycoserological study of the treatment of paediatric cystic fibrosis patients with *Saccharomyces boulardii* (*Saccharomyces cerevisiae* Hansen CBS 5926). *Mycoses* 38(3–4):119–123.

Nadkarni, K.M. 1976. *Indian Materia Medica.* Bombay: Popular Prakashan.

Stecher, P.G. (ed.). 1968. *The Merck Index: An Encyclopedia of Chemicals and Drugs*, 8th ed. Rahway, N.J.: Merck & Co., Inc.

Taber, C.W. 1962. *Taber's Cyclopedic Medical Dictionary*, 9th ed. Philadelphia: F.A. Davis Company. T22–T23.

Tu, G. (ed.). 1992. *Pharmacopoeia of the People's Republic of China* (English Edition 1992). Beijing: Guangdong Science and Technology Press. 813.

U.S.A. Dept. of Health and Human Services: Food and Drug Administration. 1998. *Code of Federal Regulations 21* (CFR 21). Parts 172.896 and 172.898. Washington, D.C.: Office of the Federal Register National Archives and Records Administration. 109–110.

Weber, G., A. Adamczyk, S. Freytag. 1989. [Treatment of acne with a yeast preparation] [In German]. *Fortschr Med* 107(26):563–566.

Additional Resources

Andre, F.E. and A. Safary. 1987. Summary of clinical findings on Engerix-B, a genetically engineered yeast derived hepatitis B vaccine. *Postgrad Med J* 63(2):169–177.

Bizeau, C., P. Galzy, M. Bastide, J.M. Bastide. 1974. [Immunofluorescent study of morphologic mutants of *Saccharomyces cerevisiae* Hansen] [In French]. *C R Acad Sci Hebd Seances Acad Sci D* 279(25):1955–1958.

Böckeler, W. and G. Thomas. 1989. In-vitro-Studien zur destabilisierenden Wirkung lyophilisierter *Saccharomyces cerevisiae* Hansen CBS 5926-Zellen auf Engerobakterien. Lässt sich diese Eigenschaft biochemisch erklären? In: Müller, J., R. Ottenjann, J. Seifert (eds.).

Ökosystem Darm. Heidelberg: Springer Verlag. 142–153.

Chavanet, P. et al. 1994. Cross-sectional study of the susceptibility of *Candida* isolates to antifungal drugs and *in vitro-in vivo* correlation in HIV-infected patients. *AIDS* 8(7):945–950.

Gedek, B. and G. Hagenhoff. 1989. Orale Verabreichung von lebensfähigen Zellen des Hefestammes *Saccharomyces cerevisiae* Hansen CBS 5926 und deren Schicksal während der Magen-Darm-Passage. *Therapiewoche* (38):33–40.

McCullough, M.J., K.V. Clemons, J.H. McCusker, D.A. Stevens. 1998. Species identification and virulence attributes of *Saccharomyces boulardii* (nom. inval.) *J Clin Microbiol* 36(9):2613–2617.

Oblack, D.L. et al. 1981. Clinical evaluation of the AutoMicrobic system Yeast Biochemical Card for rapid identification of medically important yeasts. *J Clin Microbiol* 13(2):351–355.

Petzoldt, K. and E. Muller. 1986. [Animal experiment and cell biology study of *Saccharomyces cerevisiae* Hansen CBS 5926 in the non-specific enhancement of resistance to infection] [In German]. *Arzneimforsch* 36(7):1085–1088.

Pfaller, M.A. et al. 1994. Selection of candidate quality control isolates and tentative quality control ranges for *in vitro* susceptibility testing of yeast isolates by National Committee for Clinical Laboratory Standards proposed standard methods. *J Clin Microbiol* 32(7):1650–1653.

Plein, K. and J. Hotz. 1993. Therapeutic effects of *Saccharomyces boulardii* on mild residual symptoms in a stable phase of Crohn's disease with special respect to chronic diarrhea—a pilot study. *Z Gastroenterol* 31(2):129–134.

Sinai, Y. et al. 1974. Enhancement of resistance to infectious disease by oral administration of brewer's yeast. *Infection Immunol* (9):781–787.

Surawicz, C.M. et al. 1989. Die prophylaxe antibiotika-assoziierter diarrhoen mit *Saccharomyces boulardii*. eine prospektive studie [Prevention of antibiotic-associated diarrhea by *Saccharomyces boulardii*: a prospective study]. *Gastroenterol* 96(4):981–988.

The Hansen CBS 5926 brewer's yeast monograph, published by the Commission E in 1994, was modified based on new scientific research. It contains more extensive pharmacological and therapeutic information taken directly from the Commission E.

This material was adapted from *The Complete German Commission E Monographs—Therapeutic Guide to Herbal Medicines.* M. Blumenthal, W.R. Busse, A. Goldberg, J. Gruenwald, T. Hall, C.W. Riggins, R.S. Rister (eds.) S. Klein and R.S. Rister (trans.). 1998. Austin: American Botanical Council; Boston: Integrative Medicine Communications.

1) The Overview section is new information.

2) Description, Chemistry and Pharmacology, Uses, Contraindications, Side Effects, Interactions with Other Drugs, and Dosage sections have been drawn from the original work. Additional information has been added in some or all of these sections, as noted with references.

3) The dosage for equivalent preparations (tea infusion, fluidextract, and tincture) have been provided based on the following example:
   Unless otherwise prescribed: 2 g per day of [powdered, crushed, cut or whole] [plant part]
   Infusion: 2 g in 150 ml of water
   Fluidextract 1:1 (g/ml): 2 ml
   Tincture 1:5 (g/ml): 10 ml

4) The References and Additional Resources sections are new sections. Additional Resources are not cited in the monograph but are included for research purposes.

YOHIMBE BARK

Latin Name:
Pausinystalia yohimbe

Pharmacopeial Name:
Yohimbehe cortex

Other Names:
johimbe

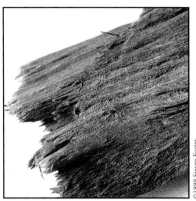

© 1999 Steven Foster

Overview

Yohimbe is a tall evergreen forest tree, reaching a height of 90 feet and width of 40 feet, native to southwestern Nigeria, Cameroon, Gabon, and the Congo. The material of commerce is collected in the wild in this same region (Bown, 1995; Keay, 1989; Leung and Foster, 1996; Reichert, 1997).

Yohimbe bark has traditionally been used in western Africa as a sexual aphrodisiac, especially in male erectile disorders, reportedly stimulating both erection and salivation. Medicinal use of yohimbe bark reached Europe in the 1890s. The majority of pharmacological data is on one of its isolated constituents, the indole alkaloid *yohimbine*, rather than on whole bark preparations (Bown, 1995; Duke, 1997; Grasing et al., 1996; Leung and Foster, 1996). Yohimbine is also found in related trees (*Pausinystalia macroceras* and *P. tillesii*) as well as in Indian snakeroot (*Rauwolfia serpentina* (L.) Benth) and quebracho (*Aspidosperma quebracho-blanco*). In Africa, *P. lane-poolei* (*pamprana, igbepo*) is also used therapeutically. A dressing of the ground bark is applied topically to yaws (an infectious tropical skin disease) and itching skin (Bown, 1995; Budavari, 1996; Duke, 1997).

In Germany, yohimbe bark is the subject of a negative (unapproved) monograph in the Commission E due to lack of data and safety concerns. In the United States, yohimbe bark is widely used in numerous aphrodisiac, athletic performance (as an alternative to anabolic steroids) and male sexual performance dietary supplements. The most commonly prescribed drug for functional impotence is yohimbine hydrochloride (e.g., Afrodex®, Aphrodyne®, Yocon®, Yohimex®, Yohydrol®), which is often combined with other drugs, including strychnine, thyroid, and methyltestosterone (Leung and Foster, 1996; Tyler, 1993). *The Merck Index* reports its therapeutic category as an α-adrenergic blocker and mydriatic (causing pupillary dilatation), its use as a pharmacological probe for the study of α_2-adrenoceptor, and its uses in veterinary medicine as an aphrodisiac and as an adrenergic blocking agent (Budavari, 1996).

No significant human studies on crude yohimbe bark or its whole extract have been conducted. Numerous studies, however, have investigated the actions of the isolated constituent yohimbine; for example, some pharmacokinetic studies have been performed in humans (Grasing et al., 1996; Owen et al., 1987) and human clinical studies have investigated its use for erectile dysfunction or male impotence (Morales et al., 1987; Reid et al., 1987; Riley, 1994). One study indicated that lower doses of yohimbine, given to patients who are fasting or eating a low-fat diet, may be more effective (Grasing et al., 1996).

There are a few studies showing that yohimbine is effective for some impotence, especially of vascular, diabetic, or psychogenic origins. It can improve the quality and staying power of erections, usually without increasing sexual excitement. The Commission E noted side effects, however, including dizziness, nervousness, and anxiety. To determine its therapeutic efficacy and evaluate the safety of yohimbine in regard to its specific use for erectile dysfunction, a systematic review and meta-analysis of randomized clinical trials was conducted (Ernst and Pittler, 1998). The authors found seven trials that fit the predefined inclusion criteria. Overall methodological quality of those studies was satisfactory. The meta-analysis demonstrated that yohimbine is superior to placebo in treating erectile dysfunction. Serious adverse reactions were infrequent and reversible. The authors concluded that the benefits seem to outweigh the risks. Therefore, yohimbine is considered to be a reasonable therapeutic option for erectile dysfunction (Ernst and Pittler, 1998). This conclusion is based not on the bark but on the isolated constituent yohimbine, which is available as a drug. A review of yohimbine and related yohimbe alkaloids details potential adverse effects and drug interactions (De Smet, 1997).

Though yohimbe bark is freely available in the United States in health and natural food stores, pharmacies, and by mail order, it should be used with caution. It is not recommended for excessive or long-term use and may potentiate pharmaceutical MAO-inhibitors. Its pharmaceutical derivative, yohimbine, can significantly increase blood pressure at oral doses of only 15–20 mg (12 mg can induce a hypertensive crisis in patients taking tricyclic antidepressants), produce unpleasant digestive and central nervous system symptoms, and may potentiate hypotensive drugs. A dose as low as 10 mg can induce mania in patients with bipolar depression (Bruneton, 1995; De Smet and Smeets, 1994; Grasing et al., 1996; McGuffin et al., 1997; Osol and Farrar, 1955; Reichert, 1997; Roth et al., 1984). An analysis of commercial yohimbe products sold in the United States revealed that few products were found with any appreciable levels of yohimbine, raising concerns about the quality control of some of these products (Betz et al., 1995).

Description

Yohimbe bark consists of the dried bark of the trunk and branches of *Pausinystalia yohimbe* (K. Schumann) Pierre ex Beille [syn. *Corynanthe yohimbi* Schumann] [Fam. Rubiaceae] and its preparations. The bark contains alkaloids. The main alkaloid is yohimbine.

Chemistry and Pharmacology

Yohimbe contains up to 6% indole alkaloids, 10–15% of which are yohimbine (quebrachine); also α-yohimbine (isoyohimbine), *allo*-yohimbine (dihydroyohimbine), yohimbinine, α-yohimbane, yohimbenine, corynantheine, and others (Betz et al., 1995; Budavari, 1996; Leung and Foster, 1996).

The Commission E did not report pharmacological actions.

Uses

The Commission E reported its unofficial use for sexual disorders, as an aphrodisiac, and for feebleness and exhaustion. The effectiveness of this herb and its preparations for the claimed applications is not sufficiently documented in the scientific literature, and thus the Commission E categorized it as an unapproved herb.

The Commission E did not find adequate documentation to support this use. The Evaluation section of the original monograph states, "The therapeutic administration of yohimbe bark and its preparations is not recommended because of insufficient proof of efficacy and the unforeseeable correlation between risk and benefit."

Contraindications

In existing liver and kidney diseases and in chronic inflammation of the sexual organs or prostate gland (McGuffin et al., 1997; Reynolds, 1989; Roth et al., 1984).

Side Effects

Therapeutic administration of yohimbine can cause nervous excitation, tremor, sleeplessness, anxiety, increased blood pressure, tachycardia, nausea, and vomiting. In case of existing liver and kidney diseases, yohimbe preparations should not be used. Interactions with psychopharmacological herbs have been reported.

Use During Pregnancy and Lactation
No data available.

Interactions with Other Drugs
May potentiate pharmaceutical MAO-inhibitors and, in high doses, potentiate hypotensive drugs (McGuffin et al., 1997).

Dosage and Administration
Evaluation: The therapeutic administration of yohimbe bark and its preparations is not recommended because of insufficient proof of efficacy and the unforeseeable correlation between risk and benefit (Commission E). Yohimbine Hydrochloride: 5.4 mg, three times daily (Rice et al., 1996); 6 mg, three times daily (Morales et al., 1987; Reid et al., 1987; Reynolds, 1989; Werbach and Murray, 1994); 15–20 mg per day, though higher doses, up to 42 mg per day, may be more effective (Werbach and Murray, 1994). Other sources state that yohimbine may be more effective at lower doses and that there are significant risks associated with doses over 10 mg (Devi, 1998; Reichert, 1997; Riley, 1994).

References
Betz, J.M., K.D. White, A. Der Marderosian. 1995. Gas chromatographic determination of yohimbine in commercial yohimbe products. *J AOAC Int* 78(5):1189–1194.
Bown, D. 1995. *Encyclopedia of Herbs and Their Uses.* New York: DK Publishing, Inc. 322.
Bruneton, J. 1995. *Pharmacognosy, Phytochemistry, Medicinal Plants.* Paris: Lavoisier Publishing.
Budavari, S. (ed.). 1996. *The Merck Index: An Encyclopedia of Chemicals, Drugs, and Biologicals,* 12th ed. Whitehouse Station, N.J.: Merck & Co, Inc.
De Smet, P.A. 1997. Yohimbe Alkaloids—General Discussion. In: De Smet, P.A., K. Keller, Hänsel R., Chandler, R.F. (eds.) 1997. *Adverse Effects of Herbal Drugs,* Vol. 3. New York: Springer Verlag. 181–205.
De Smet, P.A. and O.S. Smeets. 1994. Potential risks of health food products containing yohimbe extracts [letter]. *BMJ* 309(6959):958.
Devi, L. 1998. Yohimbine—Clinical Study Shows Effects at Different Dose Levels. *HerbClip 060481.* Austin, TX: American Botanical Council.
Duke, J.A. 1997. *The Green Pharmacy.* Emmaus, PA: Rodale Press. 176, 188, 191–192, 288.
Ernst, E. and M.H. Pittler. 1998. Yohimbine for erectile dysfunction: a systematic review and meta-analysis of randomized clinical trials. *J Urol* 159(2):433–436.
Grasing, K. et al. 1996. Effects of yohimbine on autonomic measures are determined by individual values for area under the concentration-time curve. *J Clin Pharmacol* 36(9):814–822.
Keay, R.W. 1989. *Trees of Nigeria.* Oxford: Clarendon Press.
Leung, A.Y. and S. Foster. 1996. *Encyclopedia of Common Natural Ingredients Used in Food, Drugs, and Cosmetics,* 2nd ed. New York: John Wiley & Sons, Inc.
McGuffin, M., C. Hobbs, R. Upton, A. Goldberg. 1997. American Herbal Product Association's *Botanical Safety Handbook.* Boca Raton: CRC Press.

This material was adapted from *The Complete German Commission E Monographs—Therapeutic Guide to Herbal Medicines.* M. Blumenthal, W.R. Busse, A. Goldberg, J. Gruenwald, T. Hall, C.W. Riggins, R.S. Rister (eds.) S. Klein and R.S. Rister (trans.). 1998. Austin: American Botanical Council; Boston: Integrative Medicine Communications.
1) The Overview section is new information.
2) Description, Chemistry and Pharmacology, Uses, Contraindications, Side Effects, Interactions with Other Drugs, and Dosage sections have been drawn from the original work. Additional information has been added in some or all of these sections, as noted with references.
3) The dosage for equivalent preparations (tea infusion, fluidextract, and tincture) have been provided based on the following example:
Unless otherwise prescribed: 2 g per day of [powdered, crushed, cut or whole] [plant part]
Infusion: 2 g in 150 ml of water
Fluidextract 1:1 (g/ml): 2 ml
Tincture 1:5 (g/ml): 10 ml
4) The References and Additional Resources sections are new sections. Additional Resources are not cited in the monograph but are included for research purposes.

Morales, A. et al. 1987. Is yohimbine effective in the treatment of organic impotence? Results of a controlled trial. *J Urol* 137(6):1168–1172.

Osol, A. and G.E. Farrar. 1955. *The Dispensatory of the United States of America*, 25th ed. Philadelphia, PA: J.B. Lippincott Company.

Owen, J.A. et al. 1987. The pharmacokinetics of yohimbine in man. *Eur J Clin Pharmacol* 32(6):577–582.

Reichert, R. 1997. Yohimbine Pharmacokinetics. *Quarterly Rev Nat Med* Spring:17–18.

Reid, K. et al. 1987. Double-blind trial of yohimbine in treatment of psychogenic impotence. *Lancet* 2(8556):421–423.

Reynolds, J.E.F. (ed.). 1989. *Martindale: The Extra Pharmacopoeia,* 29th ed. London: The Pharmaceutical Press.

Rice, T.F. et al. 1996. *Physicians' Desk Reference*®, 50th ed. Montvale, NJ: Medical Economics Company. 1283, 1322, 1363, 1892, 2552.

Riley, A.J. 1994. Yohimbine in the treatment of erectile disorder. *Br J Clin Pract* 48(3):133–136.

Roth, L. et al. 1984. *Giftpflanzen, Pflanzengifte.* Munich: Ecomed.

Tyler, V.E. 1993. *The Honest Herbal*, 3rd ed. Binghamton, N.Y.: Pharmaceutical Products Press. 327–329.

Werbach, M.R. and M.T. Murray. 1994. *Botanical Influences on Illness—A Sourcebook of Clinical Research.* Tarzana, CA: Third Line Press. 199–202.

Additional Resources

Clark, J.T. 1991. Suppression of copulatory behavior in the male rats following central administration of clonidine. *Neuropharmacology* (U.K.) 30(4):373–382.

Clark, J.T., E.R. Smith, J.M. Davidson. 1985. Testosterone is not required for the enhancement of sexual motivation by yohimbe. *Physiological Behav* 35(4):517–521.

———. 1985. Evidence for the modulation of sexual behavior by alpha-adrenoceptors in male rats. *Neuroendocrinology* (Switz) 41(1):36–43.

Davis, G.A. and R. Kohl. 1977. The influence of alpha receptors on lordosis in the female rat. *Pharm Biochem Behav* 6(1):47–53.

Smith, E.R. and J.M. Davidson. 1990. Yohimbine attenuates aging-induced sexual deficiencies in male rats. *Physiol Behav* 47(4):631–634.

Smith, E.R., R.L. Lee, S.L. Schnur, J.M. Davidson. 1987. Alpha 2-adrenoceptor antagonists and male sexual behavior: 1. Mating Behavior. *Physiol Behav* 41(1):7–14.

———. 1987. Alpha 2-adrenoceptor antagonists and male sexual behavior: 2. Erectile and ejaculatory reflexes. Physiol Behav 41(1):15–19.

Taber, C.W. 1962. *Taber's Cyclopedic Medical Dictionary*, 9th ed. Philadelphia, PA: F.A. Davis Company. M–59.

"QUICK-LOOK"
CROSS-REFERENCES

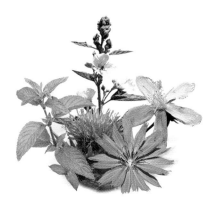

Uses

This section provides information on the appropriate use of herbs. It links medical indications cited in the text and the herbs found to be effective in their treatment. However, some of the herbs listed here may have been found effective for treatment of minor symptoms or for prevention of a condition or disease, or in some cases as adjuvant (secondary) therapy. For example, Psyllium seed husk is used as an adjuvant therapy for anal fissures—a mild laxative to soften the stool but not directly beneficial to the anal fissures.

A guide to uses by medical category is included to help identify the types of uses listed in this section. Immediately following this guide, the herbs are listed alphabetically under each use. An asterisk indicates the uses that have been added to this text and are not approved by the Commission E. This information is prepared as a guide for health professionals, researchers and consumers but should not be considered as a suggestion for self-medication. It is essential to refer to the complete monograph in order to view the role the herb may provide for each indication as well as any contraindications, side effects, and related therapeutic data.

Uses by Category

(Herbs are listed by uses as described in the monographs starting on page 438.)

Cardiovascular
Arterial Occlusive Disease
Atherosclerosis
Cardiac Insufficiency
Cardiac Symptoms
Circulatory Disorders
Geriatric Vascular Changes
High Cholesterol/Hypercholesteremia
Hyperlipidemia
Hypertension
Hypotension
Phlebitis
Post-thrombic Syndrome
Tachycardia
Tonic
Varicose Veins/Varicosis
Venous Insufficiency

Dermatological
Acne
Ano-genital Irritation
Burns
Eczema
Frostbite
Furunculosis
Gums, Inflamed
Insect Bites
Irrigation Therapy
Itching
Seborrhea
Skin Injury or Irritation
Skin, Bacterial Infections
Sunburn
Ulcers, Skin
Wounds

Endocrinology, Reproductive System, Obstetrics/ Gynecology, Prostate
Adrenocorticoid insufficiency
Amenorrhea
Breast Pain
Dysmenorrhea
Fatigue
Lactation, Poor
Menopausal Symptoms
Menorrhagia
Menstrual Disorders
Metrorrhagia
Pelvic Cramps
Premenstrual Syndrome (PMS)
Prostatitis
Sexual Disorders
Thyroid, Overactive

Information in this index is derived from the monographs on each herb listed. Readers are cautioned not to rely solely on this information when using this data for research purposes, in making clinical judgments, or when using this information as a guide for self-medication. In all such cases, the reader should always refer to the original monograph for relevant details surrounding the responsible use of the respective herb.

Urination, Diminished, Associated
with BPH Stages 1 and 2

Gastrointestinal
Anal fissures
Appetite, Loss of
Bloating, Feeling of Abdominal
    Fullness
Colon, Irritable (Irritable Bowel
    Syndrome)
Constipation
Diarrhea
Diverticulitis
Dyspepsia
Flatulence
Gargle/Mouthwash
Gastric Mucosa, Inflammation of
Gastrointestinal Disorders
Hemorrhoids
Inflammation, Gastrointestinal Tract
Nervous Stomach
Pain, Gastrointestinal
Rectum, Post-surgical Care of
Spasm, Gastrointestinal
Ulcers, Gastrointestinal

Hematology, Lymphatic, Cancer
Hematoma
Scrofula

Immunology, AIDS, Infectious Diseases
Convalescence
Debility
Fever
Free Radical Deactivation

Liver and Gallbladder
Biliary Dyskinesia
Biliary Spasm
Cirrhosis of the Liver
Gallbladder Disorders
Hepatitis
Liver Disease

Neurology, Psychiatry
Anorexia
Anxiety
Depression
Headache

Locomotor System, Degenerative
    Disorders of
Memory
Mental Concentration
Mood Disturbance
Motion Sickness
Neuralgia
Perspiration, Excessive
Restlessness
Sleep Disturbances
Stress
Tinnitus
Toothache
Vertigo

Ophthalmology
Retinal Lesion and Edema

Respiratory
Asthma
Bronchitis
Bronchospasm
Catarrh, Upper Respiratory Tract
Colds and Flu
Cough
Inflammation, Oral or Pharyngeal
Influenza
Mucous Membrane, Irritation
Nose Bleed
Respiratory Infection, Chronic
Sinusitis
Sore Throat
Whooping Cough

Rheumatological, Orthopedic, Muscles, Contusions
Arthritis
Arthrosis
Bruises, Contusions
Dislocations, Bone
Edema, Post-traumatic
Injuries
Joint Pain
Leg Cramps
Muscle Pain
Muscle Spasm
Rheumatism
Rheumatoid arthritis
Swelling, Legs
Swelling, Post-operative or
    Post-traumatic

Urinary Tract System
Bladder Irritation
Diuretic
Dysuria

Kidney Stones and Gravel
Urinary Disorders
Urinary Infection or Inflamation

Uses as Listed in Monographs

Acne
Yeast, Brewer's
Yeast, Brewer's/Hansen
   CBS 5926*

Acrocyanosis
Ginkgo Biloba leaf extract

Adrenocorticoid insufficiency
Licorice root*

Amenorrhea
Turmeric root*

Anal fissures
Cascara Sagrada bark*
Psyllium seed husk, Blonde
   (secondary)
Psyllium seed, Black
Psyllium seed, Blonde (secondary)
Senna leaf*
Senna pod*

Ano-genital Irritation
Chamomile flower, German
Oak bark

Anorexia
Blessed Thistle herb*
Gentian root*
Ginger root*

Anxiety
Hops
Kava Kava rhizome (root)
Passionflower herb
St. John's wort
Valerian root

Appetite, Loss of
Angelica root
Blessed Thistle herb
Cinnamon bark
Coriander seed
Dandelion herb
Dandelion root with herb
Devil's Claw root
Fenugreek seed
Gentian root
Hops*
Horehound herb
Iceland moss

Lavender flower*
Lemon Balm*
Onion
Orange peel, bitter
Soy Phospholipid
Valerian root*
Yarrow
Yeast, Brewer's

Arterial Occlusive Disease
Ginkgo Biloba leaf extract

Arthritis
Devil's Claw root*
Ivy leaf*
Licorice root*
Meadowsweet*
Willow bark*

Arthrosis
Devil's Claw root*

Asthma
Ephedra

Atherosclerosis
Hawthorn berry*
Hawthorn leaf with flower*
Onion

Biliary Dyskinesia
Dandelion root with herb

Biliary Spasm
Peppermint leaf
Peppermint oil

Bladder Irritation
Juniper berry*
Pumpkin seed

**Bloating, Feeling of Abdominal
Fullness**
Angelica root
Artichoke leaf*
Cinnamon bark
Cinnamon bark, Chinese
Dandelion herb
Fennel oil
Fennel seed
Gentian root
Licorice root*

*The asterisk indicates a use derived from references other than the Commission E.

Information in this index is derived from the monographs on each herb listed. Readers are cautioned not to rely solely on this information when using this data for research purposes, in making clinical judgments, or when using this information as a guide for self-medication. In all such cases, the reader should always refer to the original monograph for relevant details surrounding the responsible use of the respective herb.

Breast Pain
Chaste Tree fruit

Bronchitis
Ephedra*
Eucalyptus leaf*
Ginger root*
Horehound herb*
Ivy leaf
Thyme

Bronchospasm
Ephedra

Bruises, Contusions
Arnica flower (external)
Calendula flower* (external)
Shepherd's Purse* (external)
St. John's wort (external)
Witch Hazel leaf and bark* (external)

Burns
St. John's wort (external)
Walnut leaf*

Cardiac Insufficiency
Hawthorn berry*
Hawthorn flower
Hawthorn leaf
Hawthorn leaf with flower

Cardiac Symptoms
Hawthorn flower
Hawthorn leaf
Motherwort herb

Catarrh, Upper Respiratory Tract
Elder flower*
Eucalyptus leaf
Eucalyptus oil
Fennel oil
Fennel seed
Horehound herb*
Horseradish
Ivy leaf
Licorice root
Linden flower*
Marshmallow leaf*
Mint oil
Mullein flower
Peppermint oil
Pine needle oil
Plantain

Thyme
Watercress

Circulatory Disorders
Butcher's Broom
Ginkgo Biloba leaf extract
Hawthorn berry*
Lavender flower
Rosemary leaf

Cirrhosis of the Liver
Milk Thistle fruit

Colds and Flu
Echinacea Angustifolia herb and root/Pallida herb*
Echinacea Pallida root
Echinacea Purpurea herb
Echinacea Purpurea root*
Elder flower
Ephedra
Linden flower
Meadowsweet
Mint oil*
Myrrh*
Peppermint oil*
Willow bark*
Yarrow*

Colon, Irritable (Irritable Bowel Syndrome)
Bilberry fruit* (secondary)
Flaxseed
Peppermint oil
Psyllium seed husk, Blonde
Psyllium seed, Black
Psyllium seed, Blonde

Constipation
Buckthorn bark
Cascara Sagrada bark
Dandelion herb*
Devil's Claw root*
Flaxseed
Psyllium seed husk, Blonde
Psyllium seed, Black
Psyllium seed, Blonde
Senna leaf
Senna pod

Convalescence
Eleuthero root
Ginseng root

---

*The asterisk indicates a use derived from references other than the Commission E.

Information in this index is derived from the monographs on each herb listed. Readers are cautioned not to rely solely on this information when using this data for research purposes, in making clinical judgments, or when using this information as a guide for self-medication. In all such cases, the reader should always refer to the original monograph for relevant details surrounding the responsible use of the respective herb.

Cough
Flaxseed*
Horehound herb*
Iceland moss
Ivy leaf*
Licorice root*
Linden flower
Marshmallow leaf
Marshmallow root
Mullein flower*
Myrrh*
Peppermint oil*

Crocq's Disease
Ginkgo Biloba leaf extract

Debility
Eleuthero root
Ginseng root

Depression
Cola nut*
Ginkgo Biloba leaf extract
   (secondary)
Maté*
St. John's wort

Diarrhea
Bilberry fruit
Cinnamon bark, Chinese*
Devil's Claw root*
Mint oil*
Oak bark
Psyllium seed husk, Blonde
Psyllium seed, Blonde (secondary)
Stinging Nettle root*
Witch Hazel leaf and bark*
Yeast, Brewer's/Hansen
   CBS 5926*

Dislocations, Bone
Arnica flower (external)
Diuretic
Dandelion root with herb

Diverticulitis
Flaxseed
Psyllium seed husk, Blonde*
Psyllium seed, Black*
Psyllium seed, Blonde*

Dysmenorrhea
Black Cohosh root

Dyspepsia
Angelica root
Artichoke leaf
Blessed Thistle herb
Boldo leaf
Bromelain*
Cinnamon bark
Cinnamon bark, Chinese
Coriander seed
Dandelion herb
Dandelion root with herb
Devil's Claw root
Fennel oil
Fennel seed
Gentian root
Ginger root
Horehound herb
Juniper berry
Meadowsweet*
Milk Thistle fruit
Orange peel, bitter
Parsley herb and root*
Peppermint leaf*
Rosemary leaf
Sage leaf
St. John's wort
Turmeric root
Yarrow

Dysuria
Parsley herb and root*
Stinging Nettle root*
Watercress*

Eczema
Chamomile flower, German*
Fenugreek seed* (external)
Marshmallow root*
Walnut leaf*

Edema, Post-traumatic
Arnica flower (external)
Horsetail herb

Fatigue
Cola nut
Eleuthero root
Ginseng root
Maté
Yohimbe bark*

---

*The asterisk indicates a use derived from references other than the Commission E.

Information in this index is derived from the monographs on each herb listed. Readers are cautioned not to rely solely on this information when using this data for research purposes, in making clinical judgments, or when using this information as a guide for self-medication. In all such cases, the reader should always refer to the original monograph for relevant details surrounding the responsible use of the respective herb.

Fever
Devil's Claw root*
Elder flower*
Meadowsweet*
Willow bark
Yarrow*
Yeast, Brewer's*
Yeast, Brewer's/Hansen
CBS 5926*

Flatulence
Angelica root
Cinnamon bark
Cinnamon bark, Chinese
Coriander seed*
Dandelion herb
Dandelion root with herb*
Devil's Claw root*
Fennel oil
Fennel seed
Gentian root
Horehound herb
Licorice root*
Mint oil
Parsley herb and root*
Peppermint leaf*
Peppermint oil*
Rosemary leaf*

Free Radical Deactivation
Ginkgo Biloba leaf extract

Frostbite
Poplar bud

Furunculosis
Arnica flower (external)
Fenugreek seed* (external)
Marshmallow root* (external)
Yeast, Brewer's
Yeast, Brewer's/Hansen
CBS 5926*

Gallbladder Disorders
Boldo leaf*
Mint oil
Peppermint leaf
Sage leaf*

Gargle/Mouthwash
Chamomile flower, German
Marshmallow root* (external)
Myrrh* (external)
Poplar bud* (external)

Witch Hazel leaf and bark*
(external)

Gastric Mucosa, Inflammation of
Marshmallow root

Gastrointestinal Disorders
Dandelion root with herb*
Devil's Claw root*
Fennel seed*
Flaxseed*
Gentian root*
Lavender flower
Lemon Balm
Licorice root*
Mint oil
Orange peel, bitter*
Passionflower herb*
Peppermint oil*
Yarrow*

Geriatric Vascular Changes
Garlic
Hawthorn flower
Hawthorn leaf with flower
Onion
Walnut leaf*

Gums, Inflamed
Chamomile flower, German

Headache
Devil's Claw root*
Ephedra*
Linden flower*
Maté*
Mint oil*
Willow bark

Hematoma
Arnica flower (external)

Hemorrhoids
Bilberry fruit*
Buckthorn bark*
Butcher's Broom
Cascara Sagrada bark*
Horse Chestnut seed*
Poplar bud
Psyllium seed husk, Blonde
(secondary)
Psyllium seed, Black
Psyllium seed, Blonde (secondary)
Senna leaf

*The asterisk indicates a use derived from references other than the Commission E.

Information in this index is derived from the monographs on each herb listed. Readers are cautioned not to rely solely on this information when using this data for research purposes, in making clinical judgments, or when using this information as a guide for self-medication. In all such cases, the reader should always refer to the original monograph for relevant details surrounding the responsible use of the respective herb.

Senna pod*
Stinging Nettle herb and leaf*
(external)
Witch Hazel leaf and bark
(external)

Hepatitis
Soy Phospholipid

High Cholesterol/Hypercholesteremia
Garlic
Psyllium seed husk, Blonde*
Soy Lecithin
Soy Phospholipid

Hyperlipidemia
Garlic

Hypertension
Garlic*
Hawthorn leaf with flower*
Linden flower*

Hypotension
Hawthorn berry*
Hawthorn leaf

Inflammation, Gastrointestinal Tract
Chamomile flower, German
Dandelion herb*
Marshmallow root
Meadowsweet*
Peppermint leaf*
Sage leaf*

Inflammation, Oral or Pharyngeal
Arnica flower (external)
Bilberry fruit
Calendula flower
Chamomile flower, German
Eucalyptus leaf*
Iceland moss
Marshmallow leaf
Marshmallow root
Myrrh (external)
Oak bark
Peppermint oil
Plantain
Sage leaf (external)
Thyme*
Usnea
Witch Hazel leaf and bark*
(external)

Influenza
Echinacea Pallida root

Injuries
Arnica flower (external)
St. John's wort (external)
Witch Hazel leaf and bark*
(external)

Insect Bites
Arnica flower (external)

Irrigation Therapy
Asparagus root
Goldenrod
Horsetail herb
Stinging Nettle herb and leaf

Itching
Butcher's Broom
Oat straw

Joint Pain
Arnica flower (external)

Kidney Stones and Gravel
Asparagus root
Goldenrod
Horsetail herb
Juniper berry*
Parsley herb and root
Stinging Nettle herb and leaf

Lactation, Poor
Chaste Tree fruit*

Leg Cramps
Butcher's Broom
Horse Chestnut seed

Liver Disease
Milk Thistle fruit
Soy Phospholipid

Locomotor System, Degenerative Disorders of
Devil's Claw root

Memory
Ginkgo Biloba leaf extract

Menopausal Symptoms
Black Cohosh root

Menorrhagia
Shepherd's Purse

Menstrual Disorders
Chaste Tree fruit

*The asterisk indicates a use derived from references other than the Commission E.

Information in this index is derived from the monographs on each herb listed. Readers are cautioned not to rely solely on this information when using this data for research purposes, in making clinical judgments, or when using this information as a guide for self-medication. In all such cases, the reader should always refer to the original monograph for relevant details surrounding the responsible use of the respective herb.

Mental Concentration
Eleuthero root
Ginkgo Biloba leaf extract
Ginseng root

Metrorrhagia
Shepherd's Purse

Mood Disturbance
Hops
Lavender flower

Motion Sickness
Ginger root

Mucous Membrane, Irritation
Chamomile flower, German
Marshmallow leaf
Marshmallow root
Peppermint oil
Plantain
Witch Hazel leaf and bark

Muscle Pain
Horseradish* (external)
Peppermint oil (external)
St. John's wort (external)

Muscle Spasm
Cayenne pepper
Valerian root*

Nervous Stomach
Artichoke leaf*
Cinnamon bark, Chinese*
Ginger root*
Lavender flower
Mint oil*

Neuralgia
Devil's Claw root*
Mint oil (external)
Passionflower herb*
Peppermint oil (external)
Pine needle oil (external)

Nose Bleed
Shepherd's Purse (external)

Pain, Gastrointestinal
Coriander seed*
Flaxseed*
Licorice root*
Rosemary leaf*

Pelvic Cramps
Yarrow

Perspiration, Excessive
Sage leaf
Walnut leaf

Phlebitis
Arnica flower (external)

Post-thrombic Syndrome
Horse Chestnut seed

Premenstrual Syndrome (PMS)
Black Cohosh root
Chaste Tree fruit
Yarrow

Prostatitis
Stinging Nettle root*

Rectum, Post-surgical Care of
Buckthorn bark*
Cascara Sagrada bark*
Psyllium seed, Black
Psyllium seed, Blonde (secondary)
Senna leaf*
Senna pod*

Respiratory Infection, Chronic
Chamomile flower, German
Echinacea Purpurea herb
Horehound herb*
Licorice root*
Plantain*

Restlessness
Hops
Kava Kava rhizome (root)
Lavender flower
Linden flower
Passionflower herb
Valerian root

Retinal Lesion and Edema
Ginkgo Biloba leaf extract

Rheumatism
Arnica flower (external)
Black Cohosh root
Boldo leaf*
Dandelion herb*
Dandelion root with herb*
Devil's Claw root*
Eucalyptus oil (external)
Ginger root*
Ivy leaf*
Licorice root*
Maté*

*The asterisk indicates a use derived from references other than the Commission E.

Information in this index is derived from the monographs on each herb listed. Readers are cautioned not to rely solely on this information when using this data for research purposes, in making clinical judgments, or when using this information as a guide for self-medication. In all such cases, the reader should always refer to the original monograph for relevant details surrounding the responsible use of the respective herb.

Meadowsweet*
Parsley herb and root*
Peppermint oil*
Pine Needle oil (external)
Rosemary leaf
Stinging Nettle herb and leaf
  (internal/external)
Willow bark

Rheumatoid arthritis
Flaxseed*
Willow bark*

Scrofula
Ivy leaf*

Seborrhea
Oat straw

Sexual Disorders
Yohimbe bark*

Sinusitis
Bromelain
Ephedra*

Skin Injury or Irritation
Calendula flower*
Chamomile flower, German
Devil's Claw root* (external)
Fenugreek seed* (external)
Flaxseed* (external)
Ivy leaf* (external)
Marshmallow root* (external)
Oak bark (external)
Oat straw (external)
Peppermint oil*
Plantain (external)
Poplar bud
Shepherd's Purse
Stinging Nettle herb and leaf*
  (external)
Walnut leaf
Witch Hazel leaf and bark
Yarrow* (external)
Yeast, Brewer's/Hansen
  CBS 5926* (external)

Skin, Bacterial Infections
Chamomile flower, German
Yeast, Brewer's/Hansen
  CBS 5926*

Sleep Disturbances
Chamomile flower, German*

Hops
Lavender flower
Lemon Balm
Orange peel, bitter*
Valerian root

Sore Throat
Arnica flower
Bilberry fruit
Iceland moss
Marshmallow leaf
Mullein flower*
Oak bark

Spasm, Gastrointestinal
Angelica root
Boldo leaf
Chamomile flower, German
Cinnamon bark
Cinnamon bark, Chinese
Peppermint leaf

Stress
Kava Kava rhizome (root)

Sunburn
Poplar bud

Swelling, Legs
Butcher's Broom

Swelling, Post-operative or Post-traumatic
Bromelain
Horse Chestnut seed

Tachycardia
Hawthorn leaf with flower*
Motherwort herb
Passionflower herb*

Thyroid Overactive
Motherwort herb

Tinnitus
Ginkgo Biloba leaf extract

Tonic
Eleuthero root
Turmeric root*

Toothache
Mint oil

Ulcers, Gastrointestinal
Licorice root

*The asterisk indicates a use derived from references other than the Commission E.

Information in this index is derived from the monographs on each herb listed. Readers are cautioned not to rely solely on this information when using this data for research purposes, in making clinical judgments, or when using this information as a guide for self-medication. In all such cases, the reader should always refer to the original monograph for relevant details surrounding the responsible use of the respective herb.

Ulcers, Skin
Echinacea Purpurea herb

Urinary Disorders
Parsley herb and root

Urinary Infection or Inflammation
Asparagus root
Boldo leaf*
Echinacea Angustifolia herb and
  root/Pallida herb*
Echinacea Pallida root*
Echinacea Purpurea herb
Goldenrod*
Horseradish
Horsetail herb
Stinging Nettle herb and leaf
Uva Ursi leaf (secondary)

**Urination, Diminished, Associated
with BPH Stages 1 and 2**
Pumpkin seed
Saw Palmetto berry
Stinging Nettle root

Varicose Veins/Varicosis
Horse Chestnut seed
Witch Hazel leaf and bark

Venous Insufficiency
Bilberry fruit*
Butcher's Broom (secondary)
Horse Chestnut seed

Vertigo
Ginkgo Biloba leaf extract

Whooping Cough
Thyme

Wounds
Calendula flower
Echinacea Angustifolia herb and
  root/Pallida herb*
Echinacea Purpurea herb
Horsetail herb
Myrrh*
Shepherd's Purse (external)

*The asterisk indicates a use derived from references other than the Commission E.

Information in this index is derived from the monographs on each herb listed. Readers are cautioned not to rely solely on this information when using this data for research purposes, in making clinical judgments, or when using this information as a guide for self-medication. In all such cases, the reader should always refer to the original monograph for relevant details surrounding the responsible use of the respective herb.

CONTRAINDICATIONS

This section, condensed from the monographs, provides a list of the herbs that should be avoided with particular conditions. A guide to contraindications by medical category is included to help identify the types of contraindications listed in this chapter. Immediately following this guide, the herbs are listed alphabetically under each contraindication. It is essential to refer to the complete monograph before making any therapeutic judgements.

CONTRAINDICATIONS BY CATEGORY

(Herbs are listed by contraindications as described in the monographs starting on page 448.)

Cardiovascular
Cardiac Insufficiency
Hypertension
Hypokalemia
Pheochromocytoma

Dermatological
Collagenosis
Exanthemas, Urticarial
Irrigation Therapy with
    Concurrent Edema
Skin Injury

Endocrinology, Reproductive System, Obstetrics/ Gynecology, Prostate
Children/Infants
Diabetes Mellitus
Pheochromocytoma
Progressive Systemic Diseases
Prostate Adenoma
Thyrotoxicosis

Gastrointestinal
Abdominal Pain of Unknown Origin
Appendicitis
Colitis, Ulcerative
Crohn's Disease
Esophageal Stenosis
Gastrointestinal Inflammation
Gastrointestinal Stenosis
Ileus
Intestinal Inflammation
Intestinal Obstruction
Ulcers, Gastric and Duodenal

Hematology, Lymphatic, Cancer
Pheochromocytoma

Immunology, AIDS, Infectious Diseases
AIDS
Allergy/Hypersensitivity
Autoimmune Diseases
HIV
Infectious Diseases
Leukosis
Tuberculosis

Liver and Gallbladder
Bile Duct Inflammation
Bile Duct Obstruction
Cholestatic Liver Disorders
Cirrhosis of the Liver
    (see also Liver Disease)
Gallbladder Empyema
Gallbladder Inflammation
Gallstones
Liver Disease

Neurology, Psychiatry
Anxiety
Cerebral Circulation, Impaired
Depression
Hypertonia
Multiple Sclerosis
Restlessness

Ophthalmology
Glaucoma

Information in this index is derived from the monographs on each herb listed. Readers are cautioned not to rely solely on this information when using this data for research purposes, in making clinical judgments, or when using this information as a guide for self-medication. In all such cases, the reader should always refer to the original monograph for relevant details surrounding the responsible use of the respective herb.

Respiratory
Asthma
Whooping Cough

Urinary Tract System
Kidney Disease (Inflammation)
Kidney Insufficiency
Renal Inflammation or Disease

CONTRAINDICATIONS AS LISTED IN MONOGRAPHS

Abdominal Pain of Unknown Origin
Buckthorn bark
Cascara Sagrada bark
Senna leaf
Senna pod

AIDS
Echinacea Angustifolia herb and
root/Pallida herb
Echinacea Pallida root
Echinacea Purpurea root

Allergy/Hypersensitivity
Arnica flower
Artichoke leaf
Black Cohosh root
Blessed Thistle herb
Bromelain
Cayenne pepper
Cinnamon bark
Cinnamon bark, Chinese
Dandelion herb (rare)
Echinacea Purpurea herb
(injectible)
Echinacea Purpurea root
(injectible)
Ginkgo Biloba leaf extract
Meadowsweet
Poplar bud
Yarrow

Anxiety
Ephedra

Appendicitis
Buckthorn bark
Cascara Sagrada bark
Senna leaf
Senna pod

Asthma
Pine Needle oil

Autoimmune Diseases
Echinacea Pallida root

Bile Duct Inflammation
Eucalyptus leaf
Eucalyptus oil

Bile Duct Obstruction
Artichoke leaf
Boldo leaf

Dandelion herb
Dandelion root with herb
Eucalyptus leaf
Eucalyptus oil
Kava Kava rhizome (root)
Mint oil
Peppermint oil
Turmeric root

Cardiac Insufficiency
Oak bark

Cerebral Circulation, Impaired
Ephedra

Children/Infants
Buckthorn bark
Cascara Sagrada bark
Eucalyptus leaf
Eucalyptus oil
Fennel oil
Horseradish
Mint oil (external)
Peppermint oil (external)
Senna leaf
Senna pod
Watercress

Cholestatic Liver Disorders
Licorice root

**Cirrhosis of the Liver
(see also Liver Disease)**
Licorice root

Colitis, Ulcerative
Buckthorn bark
Cascara Sagrada bark
Senna leaf
Senna pod

Collagenosis
Echinacea Pallida root
Echinacea Purpurea herb
Echinacea Purpurea root

Crohn's Disease
Buckthorn bark

Cascara Sagrada bark
Senna leaf
Senna pod

Information in this index is derived from the monographs on each herb listed. Readers are cautioned not
to rely solely on this information when using this data for research purposes, in making clinical judgments,
or when using this information as a guide for self-medication. In all such cases, the reader should always
refer to the original monograph for relevant details surrounding the responsible use of the respective herb.

Depression
Kava Kava rhizome (root)

Diabetes Mellitus
Echinacea Purpurea herb
(injectable)
Echinacea Purpurea root
(injectable)
Psyllium seed husk, Blonde
Psyllium seed, Blonde

Esophageal Stenosis
Psyllium seed, Black
Psyllium seed, Blonde

Exanthemas, Urticarial
Chaste Tree fruit

Gallbladder Empyema
Dandelion herb
Dandelion root with herb

Gallbladder Inflammation
Mint oil
Peppermint oil

Gallstones
Artichoke leaf
Boldo leaf
Dandelion herb
Dandelion root with herb
Devil's Claw root
Ginger root
Peppermint leaf
Peppermint oil
Turmeric root
Gastrointestinal Inflammation
Eucalyptus leaf
Eucalyptus oil

Gastrointestinal Stenosis
Psyllium seed husk, Blonde
Psyllium seed, Black
Psyllium seed, Blonde

Glaucoma
Ephedra

HIV
Echinacea Pallida root
Hypertension
Eleuthero root
Ephedra

Hypertonia
Licorice root
Oak bark

Hypokalemia
Flaxseed
Licorice root

Ileus
Dandelion herb
Dandelion root with herb
Flaxseed
Psyllium seed husk, Blonde
Psyllium seed, Blonde
Senna leaf

Infectious Diseases
Oak bark

Intestinal Inflammation
Buckthorn bark
Cascara Sagrada bark
Eucalyptus leaf
Eucalyptus oil
Senna leaf
Senna pod

Intestinal Obstruction
Buckthorn bark
Cascara Sagrada bark
Senna leaf
Senna pod

Irrigation Therapy with Concurrent Edema
Goldenrod
Horsetail herb
Stinging Nettle herb and leaf

Kidney Disease (Inflammation)
Asparagus root
Juniper berry
Parsley herb and root
Watercress

Kidney Insufficiency
Licorice root

Leukosis
Echinacea Angustifolia herb and
root/Pallida herb
Echinacea Pallida root
Echinacea Purpurea herb
Echinacea Purpurea root

Liver Disease
Boldo leaf
Eucalyptus leaf
Eucalyptus oil
Mint oil
Peppermint oil

Information in this index is derived from the monographs on each herb listed. Readers are cautioned not to rely solely on this information when using this data for research purposes, in making clinical judgments, or when using this information as a guide for self-medication. In all such cases, the reader should always refer to the original monograph for relevant details surrounding the responsible use of the respective herb.

Multiple Sclerosis
Echinacea Angustifolia herb and
  root/Pallida herb
Echinacea Pallida root
Echinacea Purpurea herb
Echinacea Purpurea root

Pheochromocytoma
Ephedra

Progressive Systemic Diseases
Echinacea Angustifolia herb and
  root/Pallida herb
Echinacea Pallida root
Echinacea Purpurea herb
Echinacea Purpurea root

Prostate Adenoma
Ephedra

Renal Inflammation or Disease
Asparagus root
Horseradish
Juniper berry
Licorice root
Watercress

Restlessness
Ephedra

Skin Injury
Cayenne pepper (external)
Oak bark (external)

Thyrotoxicosis
Ephedra

Tuberculosis
Echinacea Angustifolia herb and
  root/Pallida herb
Echinacea Pallida root
Echinacea Purpurea herb
Echinacea Purpurea root

Ulcers, Gastric and Duodenal
Cola nut
Devil's Claw root
Gentian root
Horseradish
Watercress

Whooping Cough
Pine Needle oil

SIDE EFFECTS

This section, condensed from the monographs, lists potential adverse side effects of specific herbs. A guide to side effects by medical category is included to help identify the types of side effects listed in this chapter. Immediately following this guide, the herbs are listed alphabetically under each side effect. The listing of a particular herb under a corresponding side effect does not necessarily constitute a clear correlation of the herb with the effect; it means that it may be produced under certain conditions in some individuals. It is essential to refer to the complete monograph before making any therapeutic judgements. Side effects are sometimes only observed "in rare cases" and/or "in sensitive individuals." For example, nausea and vomiting are listed here as possible side effects of Uva Ursi. However, the monograph clarifies that "nausea and vomiting may occur in persons with sensitive stomachs." Thus, inclusion of a particular herb under a corresponding side effect should not be interpreted as an inevitable result of using the herb.

SIDE EFFECTS BY CATEGORY

(Herbs are listed by side effects as described in the monographs starting on page 453.)

Cardiovascular
Cardiac Arrhythmia
Edema
Heart Function, Disorders of
Hypertension
Tachycardia

Dermatological
Dermatitis
Eczema
Hives
Itching
Photosensitization
Skin Allergy
Skin Irritation

Endocrinology, Reproductive System, Obstetrics/ Gynecology, Prostate
Electrolyte Imbalance
Menstruation, Early Post-partum Return of
Mineralocorticoid Effects
Potassium Deficiency
Sodium Retention
Water Retention

Gastrointestinal
Cramps
Diarrhea
Flatulence
Gastrointestinal Disturbance
Intestinal Sluggishness
Laxative
Nausea
Vomiting

Immunology, AIDS, Infectious Diseases
Allergy, General
Fever

Neurology, Psychiatry
Convulsions
Dependency
Headache
Irritability
Restlessness
Sleep Disorder

Ophthalmology
Accommodation Disturbance, Ocular

Respiratory
Allergic Reactions, Respiratory Tract
Bronchospasm Increase
Mucous Membrane Irritation

Urinary Tract System
Albuminuria
Hematuria
Kidney Inflammation
Myoglobinuria
Urination, Difficulties in

SIDE EFFECTS AS LISTED IN MONOGRAPHS

Accommodation Disturbance, Ocular
Kava Kava rhizome (root)

Albuminuria
Buckthorn bark
Cascara Sagrada bark
Senna leaf
Senna pod

Allergic Reactions, Respiratory Tract
Fennel oil

Allergy, General
Asparagus root
Blessed Thistle herb
Bromelain
Echinacea Purpurea herb
Echinacea Purpurea root
Fennel oil
Fenugreek seed
Garlic
Ginkgo Biloba leaf extract
Kava Kava rhizome (root)
Poplar bud
Psyllium seed husk, Blonde
Psyllium seed, Black
Psyllium seed, Blonde

Bronchospasm Increase
Pine Needle oil

Cardiac Arrhythmia
Ephedra

Convulsions
Sage leaf

Cramps
Buckthorn bark
Cascara Sagrada bark
Senna leaf
Senna pod

Dependency
Ephedra

Dermatitis
Arnica flower
Ivy leaf

Diarrhea
Bromelain
Eucalyptus leaf

Eucalyptus oil
Soy Phospholipid

Eczema
Arnica flower

Edema
Licorice root

Electrolyte Imbalance
Buckthorn bark
Cascara Sagrada bark
Senna leaf
Senna pod

Fever
Echinacea Purpurea herb
(injectible)
Echinacea Purpurea root
(injectible)

Flatulence
Yeast, Brewer's

Gastrointestinal Disturbance
Black Cohosh root
Bromelain
Butcher's Broom
Cola nut
Dandelion root with herb
Eucalyptus leaf
Eucalyptus oil
Garlic
Ginkgo Biloba leaf extract
Horse chestnut seed
Horseradish
Mint oil
Saw Palmetto berry
Soy Phospholipid
Stinging Nettle root
Turmeric root
Watercress

Headache
Ephedra
Gentian root
Ginkgo Biloba leaf extract
Yeast, Brewer's

Heart Function, Disorders of
Buckthorn bark
Cascara Sagrada bark

Senna leaf

Hematuria
Buckthorn bark
Cascara Sagrada bark
Senna leaf
Senna pod

Hives
Cayenne pepper
Chaste Tree fruit

Hypertension
Ephedra
Licorice root

Intestinal Sluggishness
Buckthorn bark
Cascara sagrada bark

Irritability
Ephedra

Itching
Chaste Tree fruit

Kidney Inflammation
Juniper berry

Laxative
Milk Thistle fruit

Menstruation, Early Post-partum Return of
Chaste Tree fruit

Mineralocorticoid Effects
Licorice root

Mucous Membrane Irritation
Pine Needle oil

Myoglobinuria
Licorice root

Nausea
Butcher's Broom
Echinacea Purpurea herb
(injectible)
Echinacea Purpurea root
(injectible)
Ephedra

Eucalyptus leaf
Eucalyptus oil
Uva Ursi leaf

Photosensitization
Angelica root
Orange peel, bitter
St. John's wort

Potassium Deficiency
Buckthorn bark
Cascara Sagrada bark
Licorice root
Senna leaf
Senna pod

Restlessness
Cola nut
Ephedra

Skin Allergy
Poplar bud

Skin Irritation
Pine Needle oil

Sleep Disorder
Cola nut
Ephedra

Sodium Retention
Licorice root

Tachycardia
Ephedra

Urination, Difficulties in
Ephedra

Vomiting
Echinacea Purpurea herb
(injectible)
Echinacea Purpurea root
(injectible)
Ephedra
Eucalyptus leaf
Eucalyptus oil
Uva Ursi leaf

Water Retention
Licorice root

PHARMACOLOGICAL ACTIONS

This section, condensed from the "Chemistry and Pharmacology" section of the monographs, provides a list of pharmacological actions of specific herbs. A guide to pharmacological actions by medical category is included to help identify the types of actions listed in this chapter. Immediately following this guide, the herbs are listed alphabetically under each pharmacological action. An asterisk indicates the uses which have been added to this text and are not approved by the Commission E. In some cases, the pharmacological actions listed were demonstrated by in vitro experiments or in vivo studies (on animals) but have not been confirmed in human clinical trials. Their inclusion is intended to help health professionals understand the potential activity, risks, and/or benefits of the herb. It is essential to refer to the complete herb monograph before making any therapeutic judgements.

PHARMACOLOGICAL ACTIONS BY CATEGORY

(Herbs are listed by pharmacological actions as described in the monographs starting on page 457.)

Cardiovascular
Antihypertensive
Calcium-antagonist-like Effects
Cholesterol-lowering
Chronotropic, Positively
Circulatory Stimulant
Circulatory/Vascular Tonic
Coronary Artery Flow, Increases
Hyperemic
Inotropic, Positively
Lipid-lowering
Myocardial Circulation, Increases
Roborant
Vasodilator
Venous Tonic

Dermatological
Anti-exudative
Anti-inflammatory
Antiperspirant
Astringent
Deodorant
Granulatory
Skin Irritation, Decreases
Skin Irritation, Stimulates
Skin Metabolism, Stimulates
Wound-healing

Endocrinology, Reproductive System, Obstetrics/ Gynecology, Prostate
Adrenocorticotrophic
Antiandrogenic
Blood Sugar Regulation
Blood Supply, Increase
Endurance, Increased
Estrogen-receptor Site Binding
Glycogenolytic
Luteinizing-hormone Suppression
Prolactin Level, Decreases
Tyrosinase, Inhibiting
Uterine Contraction, Stimulates

Gastrointestinal
Antiemetic
Antiflatulent
Appetite Stimulant
Carminative
Gastric Juices, Stimulates
Gastric Ulcers, Accelerate Healing of
Intestinal Motility, Inhibiting
Intestinal Motility, Stimulating
Laxative
Lipolytic
Peristalsis, Regulation of
Salivation, Increases
Secretion of Gastric Juices
Secretolytic

Secretomotory
Smooth Muscle Contraction
Smooth Muscle Relaxant
Spasmolytic

Hematology, Lymphatic, Cancer
Antichemotactic
Cytotoxic
Diaphoretic
Fibrinolytic Activity, Increases
Hemostatic
Leucocyte Increase
Lymphocyte Increase
Platelet Aggregation, Inhibits
Prothrombin Time, Increases
Spleen Cell Increase
Thrombocyte Aggregation, Inhibits

Immunology, AIDS, Infectious Diseases
Antibacterial
Antifungal
Antimicrobial
Antimycotic
Antiparasitic
Antiseptic
Antiviral
Immunomodulation
Phagocytosis, Stimulates
Pyretic
T-Cell Production
Temperature Elevation

Liver and Gallbladder
Cholagogue
Cholecystokinetic
Choloretic
Hepatoprotective

Neurology, Psychiatry
Analgesic
Anti-anxiety

Anticonvulsant
Antidepressant
Antiphlogistic
Antipyretic
Antispasmodic
Bathmotropic, Negatively
Central Nervous System, Stimulant
Dromotropic, Positively
MAO Inhibitor
Muscarine-like
Musculotropic
Nerve Damaging
Salivation, Increases
Sedative
Soporific
Sympathomimetic

Respiratory
Analeptic, Respiratory
Anti-irritant
Antitussive
Bronchial Secretion, Increased
Bronchoantispasmodic
Demulcent
Expectorant
Mucociliary Activity, Increases
Mucous Membrane Irritant

Rheumatological, Orthopedic, Muscles, Contusions
Anti-edematous
Antirheumatic
Electrolyte-like Reaction on Capillary Wall
Muscle Relaxant

Urinary Tract System
Diuretic
Residual Urine, Reduces
Urinary Flow, Increases

PHARMACOLOGICAL ACTIONS AS LISTED IN MONOGRAPHS

Adrenocorticotrophic
Licorice root*

Analeptic, Respiratory
Cola nut
Maté

Analgesic
Arnica flower
Calendula flower*
Dandelion herb
Devil's Claw root
Ivy leaf*
Kava Kava rhizome (root)*
Maté*
Poplar bud*
Usnea*
Willow bark

Anti-anxiety
Kava Kava rhizome (root)

Anti-edematous
Bilberry fruit*
Bromelain*
Devil's Claw root*
Ginkgo Biloba leaf extract
Thyme*

Anti-exudative
Horse Chestnut seed
Saw Palmetto berry

Anti-inflammatory
Bilberry fruit*
Calendula flower
Chamomile flower, German*
Devil's Claw root*
Elder flower*
Eucalyptus leaf*
Ginger root*
Licorice root*
Meadowsweet*
Orange peel, bitter*
Poplar bud*
Pumpkin seed*
Saw Palmetto berry*
Shepherd's Purse*
St. John's wort
Turmeric root
Willow bark*

Witch Hazel leaf and bark

Anti-irritant
Marshmallow leaf
Mullein flower

Antiandrogenic
Pumpkin seed*
Saw Palmetto berry

Antibacterial
Angelica root*
Blessed Thistle herb*
Calendula flower*
Cayenne pepper*
Chamomile flower, German
Cinnamon bark
Cinnamon bark, Chinese
Ephedra
Eucalyptus oil*
Garlic
Ivy leaf*
Lemon Balm*
Mint oil
Onion
Orange peel, bitter*
Peppermint oil
Pine Needle oil*
Plantain
Poplar bud
Sage leaf
Thyme
Turmeric root*
Uva Ursi leaf
Watercress*
Yarrow
Yeast, Brewer's
Yeast, Brewer's/Hansen CBS 5926*

Antichemotactic
Echinacea Angustifolia herb and
root/Pallida herb*

Anticonvulsant
Kava Kava rhizome (root)

Antidepressant
Cola nut*
Ginseng root*
St. John's wort

---

*The asterisk indicates a pharmacological action derived from references other than the Commission E.

Information in this index is derived from the monographs on each herb listed. Readers are cautioned not to rely solely on this information when using this data for research purposes, in making clinical judgments, or when using this information as a guide for self-medication. In all such cases, the reader should always refer to the original monograph for relevant details surrounding the responsible use of the respective herb.

Antiemetic
  Artichoke leaf*
  Ginger root

Antiflatulent
  Lavender flower

Antifungal
  Angelica root*
  Calendula flower*
  Cinnamon bark
  Cinnamon bark, Chinese
  Garlic
  Ivy leaf*
  Oat straw*
  Orange peel, bitter*
  Sage leaf
  Walnut leaf*

Antihypertensive
  Onion

Antimicrobial
  Arnica flower*
  Blessed Thistle herb*
  Fennel oil
  Horseradish
  Iceland moss
  Mint oil*
  Onion*
  Sage leaf*
  Usnea
  Uva Ursi leaf*
  Yarrow*

Antimycotic
  Garlic

Antiparasitic
  Calendula flower*
  Ivy leaf*
  Yeast, Brewer's/Hansen CBS 5926*

Antiperspirant
  Sage leaf

Antiphlogistic
  Arnica flower
  Butcher's Broom
  Chamomile flower, German
  Devil's Claw root
  Goldenrod
  Willow bark

Antipyretic
  Mint oil
  Peppermint oil
  Willow bark
  Yarrow*

Antirheumatic
  Juniper berry*

Antiseptic
  Arnica flower
  Cayenne pepper*
  Eucalyptus leaf*
  Eucalyptus oil*
  Fenugreek seed
  Juniper berry*
  Myrrh*
  Pine Needle oil
  Saw Palmetto berry*
  Uva Ursi leaf*

Antispasmodic
  Angelica root
  Boldo leaf
  Chamomile flower, German
  Eucalyptus leaf
  Eucalyptus oil
  Fennel oil
  Fennel seed
  Ginger root
  Goldenrod
  Hawthorn leaf with flower*
  Ivy leaf
  Kava Kava rhizome (root)
  Licorice root
  Linden flower*
  Mint oil
  Motherwort herb*
  Passionflower herb*
  Peppermint leaf
  Peppermint oil
  Rosemary leaf
  Yarrow

Antitussive
  Ephedra

Antiviral
  Calendula flower*
  Cinnamon bark*
  Cinnamon bark, Chinese*

*The asterisk indicates a pharmacological action derived from references other than the Commission E.

Information in this index is derived from the monographs on each herb listed. Readers are cautioned not to rely solely on this information when using this data for research purposes, in making clinical judgments, or when using this information as a guide for self-medication. In all such cases, the reader should always refer to the original monograph for relevant details surrounding the responsible use of the respective herb.

Elder flower*
Garlic*
Motherwort herb*
Mullein flower*
Oak bark
Pine Needle oil*
Sage leaf
Walnut leaf*

Appetite Stimulant
Blessed Thistle herb*
Dandelion root with herb
Devil's Claw root

Astringent
Bilberry fruit
Linden flower*
Meadowsweet*
Myrrh
Oak bark
Plantain
Sage leaf
Uva Ursi leaf*
Walnut leaf
Willow bark*
Witch Hazel leaf and bark
Yarrow

Bathmotropic, Negatively
Hawthorn leaf with flower

Blood Sugar Regulation
Psyllium seed husk, Blonde

Blood Supply, Increase
Rosemary leaf (external)

Bronchial Secretion, Increased
Elder flower
Ephedra*
Gentian root

Bronchoantispasmodic
Thyme

Calcium-antagonist-like Effects
Angelica root*

Carminative
Angelica root*
Artichoke leaf*
Blessed Thistle herb*
Coriander seed*
Fennel oil*
Fennel seed*
Ginger root*

Juniper berry*
Lemon Balm
Mint oil
Myrrh*
Parsley herb and root*
Peppermint leaf
Peppermint oil
Rosemary leaf*

Central Nervous System, Stimulant
Cola nut*
Ephedra
Ginseng root*

Cholagogue
Angelica root
Dandelion herb*
Dandelion root with herb*
Ginger root
Mint oil
Peppermint oil
Watercress*

Cholecystokinetic
Turmeric root

Cholesterol-lowering
Artichoke leaf*
Fenugreek seed*
Garlic
Ginseng root*
Oak bark*
Orange peel, bitter*
Psyllium seed husk, Blonde
Psyllium seed, Blonde

Choloretic
Artichoke leaf
Boldo leaf*
Dandelion root with herb
Devil's Claw root
Horehound herb
Orange peel, bitter*
Peppermint leaf
Rosemary leaf*
Turmeric root
Yarrow

Chronotropic, Positively
Cola nut
Hawthorn leaf with flower
Maté
Shepherd's Purse

*The asterisk indicates a pharmacological action derived from references other than the Commission E.

Information in this index is derived from the monographs on each herb listed. Readers are cautioned not to rely solely on this information when using this data for research purposes, in making clinical judgments, or when using this information as a guide for self-medication. In all such cases, the reader should always refer to the original monograph for relevant details surrounding the responsible use of the respective herb.

Circulatory Stimulant
Ginkgo Biloba leaf extract*

Circulatory/Vascular Tonic
Bilberry fruit*
Horse Chestnut seed

Coronary Artery Flow, Increases
Hawthorn leaf with flower
Rosemary leaf

Cytotoxic
Motherwort herb*

Demulcent
Fenugreek seed*
Flaxseed*
Iceland moss
Licorice root*
Marshmallow leaf*
Marshmallow root
Plantain*

Deodorant
Chamomile flower, German

Diaphoretic
Angelica root*
Elder flower
Ephedra*
Goldenrod*
Linden flower

Diuretic
Angelica root*
Artichoke leaf*
Asparagus root
Butcher's Broom
Cola nut
Dandelion herb*
Dandelion root with herb
Elder flower*
Goldenrod
Horsetail herb
Juniper berry
Maté
Meadowsweet*
Parsley herb and root*
Saw Palmetto berry*
Shepherd's Purse*
Stinging Nettle herb and leaf*

Dromotropic, Positively
Hawthorn leaf with flower

Electrolyte-like Reaction on Capillary Wall
Butcher's Broom

Endurance, Increased
Eleuthero root

Estrogen-Receptor Site Binding
Black Cohosh root

Expectorant
Eucalyptus leaf
Eucalyptus oil
Horehound herb*
Ivy leaf
Licorice root
Mullein flower
Thyme
Watercress*

Fibrinolytic Activity, Increases
Garlic
Pumpkin seed*

Gastric Juices, Stimulates
Angelica root
Blessed Thistle herb
Boldo leaf
Cayenne pepper*
Cola nut
Gentian root
Ginger root

Gastric Ulcers, Accelerate Healing of
Licorice root

Glycogenolytic
Fenugreek seed*
Ginseng root*
Maté
Psyllium seed, Black*
Psyllium seed, Blonde*
Yeast, Brewer's/Hansen CBS 5926*

Granulatory
Calendula flower
Poplar bud

Hemostatic
Stinging Nettle herb and leaf*
Witch Hazel leaf and bark
Yarrow*

Hepatoprotective
Artichoke leaf*

*The asterisk indicates a pharmacological action derived from references other than the Commission E.

Information in this index is derived from the monographs on each herb listed. Readers are cautioned not to rely solely on this information when using this data for research purposes, in making clinical judgments, or when using this information as a guide for self-medication. In all such cases, the reader should always refer to the original monograph for relevant details surrounding the responsible use of the respective herb.

Dandelion root with herb*
Garlic*
Milk Thistle fruit
Soy Phospholipid
Turmeric root*

Hyperemic
Cayenne pepper
Eucalyptus oil
Fenugreek seed
Horseradish
Pine Needle oil

Immunomodulation
Arnica flower*
Echinacea Purpurea herb
Eleuthero root
Ginseng root*
Iceland moss*
Oat straw*

Inotropic, Positively
Ginger root
Hawthorn leaf with flower
Maté
Rosemary leaf
Shepherd's Purse

Intestinal Motility, Inhibiting
Passionflower herb

Intestinal Motility, Stimulating
Buckthorn bark
Cascara Sagrada bark
Cinnamon bark
Cinnamon bark, Chinese
Cola nut
Fennel oil
Fennel seed
Ginger root
Ginseng root*

Laxative
Buckthorn bark
Cascara Sagrada bark
Dandelion root with herb*
Flaxseed
Senna leaf
Senna pod

Leucocyte Increase
Echinacea Purpurea herb
Horsetail herb*

Lipid-lowering
Artichoke leaf*
Fenugreek seed*
Garlic
Onion
Soy Lecithin

Lipolytic
Cinnamon bark*
Cola nut
Coriander seed*
Maté
Pumpkin seed*

Luteinizing-Hormone Suppression
Black Cohosh root

Lymphocyte Increase
Eleuthero root

MAO Inhibitor
St. John's wort

Mucociliary Activity, Increases
Fennel seed

Mucous Membrane Irritant
Ivy leaf

Muscarine-like
Shepherd's Purse

Muscle Relaxant
Saw Palmetto berry

Musculotropic
Chamomile flower, German

Myocardial Circulation, Increases
Ginkgo Biloba leaf extract*
Hawthorn leaf with flower

Nerve Damaging
Cayenne pepper

Peristalsis, Regulation of
Psyllium seed, Black
Psyllium seed, Blonde

Phagocytosis, Stimulates
Echinacea Angustifolia herb and
   root/Pallida herb*
Echinacea Pallida root
Echinacea Purpurea herb
Echinacea Purpurea root
Marshmallow root
Yeast, Brewer's

*The asterisk indicates a pharmacological action derived from references other than the Commission E.

Information in this index is derived from the monographs on each herb listed. Readers are cautioned not to rely solely on this information when using this data for research purposes, in making clinical judgments, or when using this information as a guide for self-medication. In all such cases, the reader should always refer to the original monograph for relevant details surrounding the responsible use of the respective herb.

Platelet Aggregation, Inhibits
Eleuthero root*
Garlic
Ginkgo Biloba leaf extract*

Prolactin Level, Decreases
Chaste Tree fruit

Prothrombin Time, Increases
Bromelain*
Garlic

Pyretic
Echinacea Purpurea herb

Residual Urine, Reduces
Stinging Nettle root

Roborant
Gentian root

Salivation, Increases
Blessed Thistle herb
Gentian root
Ginger root

Secretion of Gastric Juices
Gentian root

Secretolytic
Fennel seed
Fenugreek seed
Ginger root
Licorice root
Mint oil
Peppermint oil
Pine needle oil

Secretomotory
Eucalyptus leaf
Eucalyptus oil
Sage leaf

Sedative
Hawthorn leaf with flower*
Hops*
Ivy leaf*
Kava Kava rhizome (root)
Lavender flower
Lemon Balm
Linden flower*
Motherwort herb*
Passionflower herb*
Valerian root

Skin Irritation, Decreases

Marshmallow leaf
Marshmallow root

Skin Irritation, Stimulates
Cayenne pepper
Rosemary leaf

Skin Metabolism, Stimulates
Chamomile flower, German

Smooth Muscle Contraction
Juniper berry
Shepherd's Purse*
Smooth Muscle Relaxant
Angelica root*
Boldo leaf*

Soporific
Hops
Valerian root

Spasmolytic
Artichoke leaf*
Coriander seed*
Hops*
Lemon Balm*
Parsley herb and root*
Rosemary leaf*
Thyme*

Spleen Cell Increase
Echinacea Purpurea herb

Sympathomimetic
Ephedra

T-Cell Production
Ginseng root

Temperature Elevation
Echinacea Purpurea herb

Thrombocyte Aggregation, Inhibits
Bromelain*
Onion

Tyrosinase, Inhibiting
Uva Ursi leaf

Urinary Flow, Increases
Stinging Nettle root

Uterine Contraction, Stimulates
Shepherd's Purse

---

*The asterisk indicates a pharmacological action derived from references other than the Commission E.

Information in this index is derived from the monographs on each herb listed. Readers are cautioned not to rely solely on this information when using this data for research purposes, in making clinical judgments, or when using this information as a guide for self-medication. In all such cases, the reader should always refer to the original monograph for relevant details surrounding the responsible use of the respective herb.

Vasodilator
Ginkgo Biloba leaf extract*
Ginseng root*
Hawthorn leaf with flower*
Linden flower*
Pine Needle oil
Shepherd's Purse*

Venous Tonic
Butcher's Broom
Ginkgo Biloba leaf extract*

Wound-healing
Calendula flower
Chamomile flower, German
Echinacea Purpurea herb*
Horsetail herb*
Poplar bud

*The asterisk indicates a pharmacological action derived from references other than the Commission E.

Information in this index is derived from the monographs on each herb listed. Readers are cautioned not to rely solely on this information when using this data for research purposes, in making clinical judgments, or when using this information as a guide for self-medication. In all such cases, the reader should always refer to the original monograph for relevant details surrounding the responsible use of the respective herb.

INTERACTIONS

This section, condensed from the monographs, summarizes the possible antagonistic or synergistic interactions an herb may have with conventional pharmaceutical medicines. It is essential to refer to the complete herb monograph before making any therapeutic judgments.

Alcohol
Kava Kava rhizome (root)

Alkaline drugs
Oak bark

Alkaloids
Oak bark

Antiarrythmic agents
Buckthorn bark
Cascara Sagrada bark
Senna leaf
Senna pod

Anticoagulants
Bromelain

Barbiturates
Kava Kava rhizome (root)

Caffeine-containing beverages
Cola nut

Cardiac glycosides
Buckthorn bark
Cascara Sagrada bark
Ephedra
Senna leaf
Senna pod

Corticosteroids
Buckthorn bark
Cascara Sagrada bark
Senna leaf
Senna pod

Digitalis glycosides
Licorice root

Dopamine-receptor antagonists
Chaste Tree fruit (shown in animal
experiments only)

Guanethidine
Ephedra

Halothane
Ephedra

Licorice root
Buckthorn bark
Cascara Sagrada bark
Senna leaf
Senna pod

MAO inhibitors
Ephedra
Yeast, Brewer's
Yeast, Brewer's/Hansen CBS 5926

Oxytocin
Ephedra

Psychoanaleptic drugs
Cola nut

Psychopharmacological agents
Kava Kava rhizome (root)

Secale alkaloid derivatives
Ephedra

Tetracycline
Bromelain

Thiazide diuretics
Buckthorn bark
Cascara Sagrada bark
Licorice root
Senna leaf
Senna pod

Thrombocytic aggregation inhibitors
Bromelain

Urine-acidifying agents
Uva Ursi leaf

Information in this index is derived from the monographs on each herb listed. Readers are cautioned not to rely solely on this information when using this data for research purposes, in making clinical judgments, or when using this information as a guide for self-medication. In all such cases, the reader should always refer to the original monograph for relevant details surrounding the responsible use of the respective herb.

USE DURING PREGNANCY AND LACTATION

This section, condensed from the monographs, summarizes which herbs should be avoided during pregnancy and lactation. The section is divided into a list of herbs contraindicated by the Commission E during pregnancy and a separate list of herbs not for use during lactation. In some cases, significant safety studies have not been conducted and so there are no known restrictions. It is essential to use caution when using herbs during pregnancy and lactation.

Pregnancy
Angelica root*
Black Cohosh root
Blessed Thistle herb*
Buckthorn bark
Cascara Sagrada bark
Chaste Tree fruit*
Cinnamon bark*
Cinnamon bark, Chinese*
Echinacea Purpurea herb
Echinacea Purpurea root
Ephedra*
Fennel oil
Fennel seed
Fenugreek seed*
Ginger root*
Ginseng root
Horehound herb
Horseradish
Juniper berry*
Kava Kava rhizome (root)
Licorice root*
Motherwort herb
Myrrh
Orange peel, bitter
Parsley herb and root*
Rosemary leaf*
Sage leaf*
Senna leaf
Senna pod
Shepherd's Purse
Thyme
Turmeric root
Uva Ursi leaf
Watercress
Yarrow*

Lactation
Angelica root*
Black Cohosh root
Blessed Thistle herb*
Buckthorn bark
Cascara Sagrada bark
Cinnamon bark*
Cinnamon bark, Chinese*
Ephedra*
Garlic*
Ginger root*
Horehound herb
Horseradish
Juniper berry*
Kava Kava rhizome (root)
Orange peel, bitter
Sage leaf*
Senna leaf
Senna pod
Uva Ursi leaf

* The asterisk indicates a contraindication derived from references other than the Commission E.

Information in this index is derived from the monographs on each herb listed. Readers are cautioned not to rely solely on this information when using this data for research purposes, in making clinical judgments, or when using this information as a guide for self-medication. In all such cases, the reader should always refer to the original monograph for relevant details surrounding the responsible use of the respective herb.

DURATION OF USE

This section, condensed from the monographs, summarizes how long an herb should be taken. Responsible use of some herbs, such as ephedra, requires that they be used for only a limited amount of time. In other cases, such as with hawthorn leaf with flower, efficacy depends upon taking the herb for a minimum amount of time.

Bilberry fruit	If diarrhea persists for more than 3 to 4 days, consult a physician.
Black Cohosh root	Not more than 6 months.
Bromelain	Eight to 10 days.
Buckthorn bark	Not more than 1 to 2 weeks without medical advice.
Cascara Sagrada bark	Not more than 1 to 2 weeks without medical advice.
Cayenne pepper	Externally: Not more than 2 days with 14-day interval for application in same location.
Echinacea Pallida root	Not more than 8 weeks.
Echinacea Purpurea herb	External and internal: Not more than 8 weeks. Parenteral: Not more than 3 weeks.
Eleuthero root	Generally not more than 3 months; a repeated course is feasible.
Ephedra	Short-term duration only.
Fennel oil	Not more than several weeks.
Fennel seed	Not more than several weeks without consulting a physician or pharmacist.
Ginkgo Biloba leaf extract	Depending on indication: Cognitive: Not less than 8 weeks. Intermittent claudication: Not less than 6 weeks.
Ginseng root	Generally not more than 3 months.
Hawthorn leaf with flower	Not less than 6 weeks.
Kava Kava rhizome (root)	Not more than 3 months without medical advice.
Oak bark	If diarrhea persists for more than 3 to 4 days, consult a physician; other applications: not more than 2 to 3 weeks.
Onion	If use continues for several months, the daily amount of diphenylamine should not exceed 0.035 g.
Psyllium seed and seed husk, Blonde	If diarrhea persists for more than 3 to 4 days, consult a physician.
Senna leaf and pod (fruit)	Not more than 2 weeks without medical advice.
Uva Ursi leaf	Medication containing arbutin should not be taken for more than a week or more than 5 times a year without consulting a physician.

Information in this index is derived from the monographs on each herb listed. Readers are cautioned not to rely solely on this information when using this data for research purposes, in making clinical judgments, or when using this information as a guide for self-medication. In all such cases, the reader should always refer to the original monograph for relevant details surrounding the responsible use of the respective herb.

TAXONOMY BY ENGLISH NAME

ENGLISH NAME	LATIN NAME	PHARMACOPEIAL NAME
Angelica root	*Angelica archangelica*	Angelicae radix
Arnica flower	*Arnica montana* or *A. chamissonis* subsp. *foliosa*	Arnicae flos
Artichoke leaf	*Cynara scolymus*	Cynarae folium
Asparagus root	*Asparagus officinalis*	Asparagi rhizoma
Bilberry fruit	*Vaccinium myrtillus*	Myrtilli fructus
Black Cohosh root	*Cimicifuga racemosa*	Cimicifugae racemosae rhizoma
Blessed Thistle herb	*Cnicus benedictus*	Cnici benedicti herba
Boldo leaf	*Peumus boldus*	Boldo folium
Bromelain	*Ananas comosus*	Bromelainum
Buckthorn bark	*Rhamnus frangula*	Frangulae cortex
Butcher's Broom	*Ruscus aculeatus*	Rusci aculeati rhizoma
Calendula flower	*Calendula officinalis*	Calendulae flos
Cascara Sagrada bark	*Rhamnus purshiana*	Rhamni purshianae cortex
Cayenne pepper	*Capsicum* species	Capsici fructus, Capsici fructus acer
Chamomile flower, German	*Matricaria recutita* (syn. *Chamomilla recutita*)	Matricariae flos
Chaste Tree fruit	*Vitex agnus castus*	Agni casti fructus
Cinnamon bark	*Cinnamomum verum*	Cinnamomi ceylanici cortex
Cinnamon bark, Chinese	*Cinnamomum aromaticum*	Cinnamomi cassiae cortex
Cola nut	*Cola nitida*	Colae semen
Coriander seed	*Coriandrum sativum*	Coriandri fructus
Dandelion herb	*Taraxacum officinale*	Taraxaci herba
Dandelion root with herb	*Taraxacum officinale*	Taraxaci radix cum herba
Devil's Claw root	*Harpagophytum procumbens*	Harpagophyti radix
Echinacea Angustifolia herb and root/Pallida herb	*Echinacea angustifolia/ E. pallida*	Echinaceae angustifoliae/ pallidae herba
Echinacea Pallida root	*Echinacea pallida*	Echinaceae pallidae radix
Echinacea Purpurea herb	*Echinacea purpurea*	Echinaceae purpureae herba
Echinacea Purpurea root	*Echinacea purpurea*	Echinaceae purpureae radix
Elder flower	*Sambucus nigra*	Sambuci flos
Eleuthero root	*Eleutherococcus senticosus*	Eleutherococci radix
Ephedra	*Ephedra sinica*	Ephedrae herba
Eucalyptus leaf	*Eucalyptus globulus*	Eucalypti folium
Eucalyptus oil	*Eucalyptus*	Eucalypti aetheroleum
Fennel oil	*Foeniculum vulgare*	Foeniculi aetheroleum
Fennel seed	*Foeniculum vulgare*	Foeniculi fructus
Fenugreek seed	*Trigonella foenum-graecum*	Foenugraeci semen
Flaxseed	*Linum usitatissimum*	Lini semen
Garlic	*Allium sativum*	Allii sativi bulbus
Gentian root	*Gentiana lutea*	Gentianae radix
Ginger root	*Zingiber officinale*	Zingiberis rhizoma
Ginkgo Biloba leaf extract	*Ginkgo biloba*	Ginkgo folium
Ginseng root	*Panax ginseng*	Ginseng radix
Goldenrod	*Solidago virgaurea*	Solidago, Virgaureae herba
Hawthorn berry	*Crataegus monogyna*	Crataegi fructus
Hawthorn flower	*Crataegus monogyna* or *C. laevigata*	Crataegi flos

ENGLISH NAME	LATIN NAME	PHARMACOPEIAL NAME
Hawthorn leaf	*Crataegus monogyna* or C. *laevigata*	Crataegi folium
Hawthorn leaf with flower	*Crataegus monogyna*	Crataegi folium cum flore
Hops	*Humulus lupulus*	Lupuli strobulus
Horehound herb	*Marrubium vulgare*	Marrubii herba
Horse Chestnut seed	*Aesculus hippocastanum*	Hippocastani semen
Horseradish	*Armoracia rusticana*	Armoraciae rusticanae radix
Horsetail herb	*Equisetum arvense*	Equiseti herba
Iceland moss	*Cetraria islandica*	Lichen islandicus
Ivy leaf	*Hedera helix*	Hederae helicis folium
Juniper berry	*Juniperus communis*	Juniperi fructus
Kava Kava rhizome (root)	*Piper methysticum*	Piperis methystici rhizoma
Lavender flower	*Lavandula angustifolia*	Lavandulae flos
Lemon Balm	*Melissa officinalis*	Melissae folium
Licorice root	*Glycyrrhiza glabra*	Liquiritiae radix
Linden flower	*Tilia cordata*	Tiliae flos
Marshmallow leaf	*Althaea officinalis*	Althaeae folium
Marshmallow root	*Althaea officinalis*	Althaeae radix
Maté	*Ilex paraguariensis*	Mate folium
Meadowsweet	*Filipendula ulmaria*	Spiraeae flos; meadowsweet flower, Spiraeae herba
Milk Thistle fruit	*Silybum marianum* (L.) [Fam. Asteraceae]	Cardui mariae fructus
Mint oil	*Mentha arvensis*	Menthae arvensis aetheroleum
Motherwort herb	*Leonurus cardiaca*	Leonuri cardiacae herba
Mullein flower	*Verbascum densiflorum*	Verbasci flos
Myrrh	*Commiphora molmol*	Myrrha
Oak bark	*Quercus robur* and/or *Q. petraea, Q. alba*	Quercus cortex
Oat straw	*Avena sativa*	Avenae stramentum
Onion	*Allium cepa*	Allii cepae bulbus
Orange peel, bitter	*Citrus aurantium*	Aurantii pericarpium
Parsley herb and root	*Petroselinum crispum*	Petroselini herba/radix
Passionflower herb	*Passiflora incarnata*	Passiflorae herba
Peppermint leaf	*Mentha* x *piperita*	Menthae piperitae folium
Peppermint oil	*Mentha* x *piperita*	Menthae piperitae aetheroleum
Pine Needle oil	*Pinus sylvestris*	Pini aetheroleum
Plantain	*Plantago lanceolata* and *P. major*	Plantaginis lanceolatae herba
Poplar bud	*Populus* species	Populi gemma
Psyllium seed husk, Blonde	*Plantago ovata*	Plantaginis ovatae testa
Psyllium seed, Black	*Plantago psyllium*	Psyllii semen
Psyllium seed, Blonde	*Plantago ovata*	Plantaginis ovatae semen
Pumpkin seed	*Cucurbita pepo*	Cucurbitae peponis semen
Rosemary leaf	*Rosmarinus officinalis*	Rosmarini folium
Sage leaf	*Salvia officinalis*	Salviae folium
Saw Palmetto berry	*Serenoa repens*	Sabal fructus
Senna leaf	*Senna alexandrina*	Sennae folium
Senna pod	*Senna alexandrina*	Sennae fructus acutifoliae
Shepherd's Purse	*Capsella bursa pastoris*	Bursae pastoris herba
Soy Lecithin	*Glycine max*	Lecithinum ex soya
Soy Phospholipid	*Glycine max*	Sojae Lecithinum

English Name	Latin Name	Pharmacopeial Name
St. John's wort	*Hypericum perforatum*	Hyperici herba
Stinging Nettle herb and leaf	*Urtica dioica*	Urticae herba/folium
Stinging Nettle root	*Urtica dioica*	Urticae radix
Thyme	*Thymus vulgaris*	Thymi herba
Turmeric root	*Curcuma longa*	Curcumae longae rhizoma
Usnea	*Usnea barbata, U. florida, U. hirta, U. plicata*	Usnea
Uva Ursi leaf	*Arctostaphylos uva ursi*	Uvae ursi folium
Valerian root	*Valeriana officinalis*	Valerianae radix
Walnut leaf	*Juglans regia*	Juglandis folium
Watercress	*Nasturtium officinale*	Nasturtii herba
Willow bark	*Salix alba, S. purpurea L., S. fragilis L.*	Salicis cortex
Witch Hazel leaf and bark	*Hamamelis virginiana*	Hamamelidis folium et cortex
Yarrow	*Achillea millefolium*	Millefolii herba/flos
Yeast, Brewer's	*Saccharomyces cerevisiae, Candida utilis*	Faex medicinalis
Yeast, Brewer's/Hansen CBS 5926	*Saccharomyces cerevisiae*	Saccharomyces cerevisiae Hansen CBS 5926
Yohimbe bark	*Pausinystalia yohimbe*	Yohimbehe cortex

Taxonomy by Latin Name

Latin Name	English Name	Pharmacopeial Name
Achillea millefolium	Yarrow	Millefolii herba/flos
Aesculus hippocastanum	Horse Chestnut seed	Hippocastani semen
Allium cepa	Onion	Allii cepae bulbus
Allium sativum	Garlic	Allii sativi bulbus
Althaea officinalis	Marshmallow leaf	Althaeae folium
Althaea officinalis	Marshmallow root	Althaeae radix
Ananas comosus	Bromelain	Bromelainum
Angelica archangelica	Angelica root	Angelicae radix
Arctostaphylos uva ursi	Uva Ursi leaf	Uvae ursi folium
Armoracia rusticana	Horseradish	Armoraciae rusticanae radix
Arnica montana or *A. chamissonis* subsp. *foliosa*	Arnica flower	Arnicae flos
Asparagus officinalis	Asparagus root	Asparagi rhizoma
Avena sativa	Oat straw	Avenae stramentum
Calendula officinalis	Calendula flower	Calendulae flos
Capsella bursa pastoris	Shepherd's Purse	Bursae pastoris herba
Capsicum species	Cayenne pepper	Capsici fructus, Capsici fructus acer
Cetraria islandica	Iceland moss	Lichen islandicus
Cimicifuga racemosa	Black Cohosh root	Cimicifugae racemosae rhizoma
Cinnamomum aromaticum	Cinnamon bark, Chinese	Cinnamomi cassiae cortex
Cinnamomum verum	Cinnamon bark	Cinnamomi ceylanici cortex
Citrus aurantium	Orange peel, bitter	Aurantii pericarpium
Cnicus benedictus	Blessed Thistle herb	Cnici benedicti herba
Cola nitida	Cola nut	Colae semen
Commiphora molmol	Myrrh	Myrrha
Coriandrum sativum	Coriander seed	Coriandri fructus
Crataegus monogyna	Hawthorn leaf with flower	Crataegi folium cum flore
Crataegus monogyna	Hawthorn berry	Crataegi fructus
Crataegus monogyna or *C. laevigata*	Hawthorn leaf	Crataegi folium
Crataegus monogyna or *C. laevigata*	Hawthorn flower	Crataegi flos
Cucurbita pepo	Pumpkin seed	Cucurbitae peponis semen
Curcuma longa	Turmeric root	Curcumae longae rhizoma
Cynara scolymus	Artichoke leaf	Cynarae folium
Echinacea angustifolia/ E. pallida	Echinacea Angustifolia herb and root/Pallida herb	Echinaceae angustifoliae/ pallidae herba
Echinacea pallida	Echinacea Pallida root	Echinaceae pallidae radix
Echinacea purpurea	Echinacea Purpurea root	Echinaceae purpureae radix
Echinacea purpurea	Echinacea Purpurea herb	Echinaceae purpureae herba
Eleutherococcus senticosus	Eleuthero root	Eleutherococci radix
Ephedra sinica	Ephedra	Ephedrae herba
Equisetum arvense	Horsetail herb	Equiseti herba
Eucalyptus	Eucalyptus oil	Eucalypti aetheroleum
Eucalyptus globulus	Eucalyptus leaf	Eucalypti folium
Filipendula ulmaria	Meadowsweet	Spiraeae flos, meadowsweet flower; Spiraeae herba
Foeniculum vulgare	Fennel oil	Foeniculi aetheroleum

LATIN NAME	ENGLISH NAME	PHARMACOPEIAL NAME
Foeniculum vulgare	Fennel seed	Foeniculi fructus
Gentiana lutea	Gentian root	Gentianae radix
Ginkgo biloba L.	Ginkgo Biloba leaf extract	Ginkgo folium
Glycine max	Soy Lecithin	Lecithinum ex soya
Glycine max	Soy Phospholipid	Sojae Lecithinum
Glycyrrhiza glabra	Licorice root	Liquiritiae radix
Hamamelis virginiana	Witch Hazel leaf and bark	Hamamelidis folium et cortex
Harpagophytum procumbens	Devil's Claw root	Harpagophyti radix
Hedera helix	Ivy leaf	Hederae helicis folium
Humulus lupulus	Hops	Lupuli strobulus
Hypericum perforatum	St. John's wort	Hyperici herba
Ilex paraguariensis	Maté	Mate folium
Juglans regia	Walnut leaf	Juglandis folium
Juniperus communis	Juniper berry	Juniperi fructus
Lavandula angustifolia	Lavender flower	Lavandulae flos
Leonurus cardiaca	Motherwort herb	Leonuri cardiacae herba
Linum usitatissimum	Flaxseed	Lini semen
Marrubium vulgare	Horehound herb	Marrubii herba
Matricaria recutita (syn. *Chamomilla recutita*)	Chamomile flower, German	Matricariae flos
Melissa officinalis	Lemon Balm	Melissae folium
Mentha arvensis	Mint oil	Menthae arvensis aetheroleum
Mentha x *piperita*	Peppermint oil	Menthae piperitae aetheroleum
Mentha x *piperita*	Peppermint leaf	Menthae piperitae folium
Nasturtium officinale	Watercress	Nasturtii herba
Panax ginseng	Ginseng root	Ginseng radix
Passiflora incarnata	Passionflower herb	Passiflorae herba
Pausinystalia yohimbe	Yohimbe bark	Yohimbehe cortex
Petroselinum crispum	Parsley herb and root	Petroselini herba/radix
Peumus boldus	Boldo leaf	Boldo folium
Pinus sylvestris	Pine Needle oil	Pini aetheroleum
Piper methysticum	Kava Kava rhizome (root)	Piperis methystici rhizoma
Plantago lanceolata and *P. major*	Plantain	Plantaginis lanceolatae herba
Plantago ovata	Psyllium seed, Blonde	Plantaginis ovatae semen
Plantago ovata	Psyllium seed husk, Blonde	Plantaginis ovatae testa
Plantago psyllium	Psyllium seed, Black	Psyllii semen
Populus species	Poplar bud	Populi gemma
Quercus robur and/or *Q. petraea, Q. alba*	Oak bark	Quercus cortex
Rhamnus frangula	Buckthorn bark	Frangulae cortex
Rhamnus purshiana	Cascara Sagrada bark	Rhamni purshianae cortex
Rosmarinus officinalis	Rosemary leaf	Rosmarini folium
Ruscus aculeatus	Butcher's Broom	Rusci aculeati rhizoma
Saccharomyces cerevisiae	Yeast, Brewer's/Hansen CBS 5926	Saccharomyces cerevisiae Hansen CBS 5926
Saccharomyces cerevisiae, Candida utilis	Yeast, Brewer's	Faex medicinalis
Salix alba, S. purpurea L., *S. fragilis* L.	Willow bark	Salicis cortex
Salvia officinalis	Sage leaf	Salviae folium
Sambucus nigra	Elder flower	Sambuci flos

LATIN NAME	ENGLISH NAME	PHARMACOPEIAL NAME
Senna alexandrina	Senna leaf	Sennae folium
Senna alexandrina	Senna pod	Sennae fructus acutifoliae
Serenoa repens	Saw Palmetto berry	Sabal fructus
Silybum marianum	Milk Thistle fruit	Cardui mariae fructus
Solidago virgaurea	Goldenrod	Solidago, Virgaureae herba
Taraxacum officinale	Dandelion herb	Taraxaci herba
Taraxacum officinale	Dandelion root with herb	Taraxaci radix cum herba
Thymus vulgaris	Thyme	Thymi herba
Tilia cordata	Linden flower	Tiliae flos
Trigonella foenum-graecum	Fenugreek seed	Foenugraeci semen
Urtica dioica	Stinging Nettle root	Urticae radix
Urtica dioica	Stinging Nettle herb and leaf	Urticae herba/folium
Usnea barbata, U. florida, *U. hirta, U. plicata*	Usnea	Usnea species
Vaccinium myrtillus	Bilberry fruit	Myrtilli fructus
Valeriana officinalis	Valerian root	Valerianae radix
Verbascum densiflorum	Mullein flower	Verbasci flos
Vitex agnus castus	Chaste Tree fruit	Agni casti fructus
Zingiber officinale	Ginger root	Zingiberis rhizoma

APPENDICES

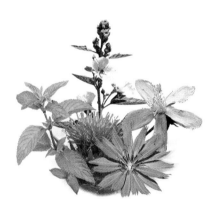

TABLE 1: TOP-SELLING HERBS IN THE UNITED STATES

This table lists the retail sales and the percent of increase in sales for the top 13 herbs in food, drug, and mass market (FDM) retail outlets. The same herbs remained best-sellers from 1997 to 1998. These herbs comprise 91% of the total retail sales for all herbs in FDM combined, and do not represent sales in health/natural food stores, multi-level marketing (MLM) companies, mail order, health professionals, or via the internet.

HERB	1998 RANKING	1997 RANKING	RETAIL SALES 1998	RETAIL SALES 1997	PERCENT CHANGE 1997 – 1998
Ginkgo	1	1	150,859,328	90,421,640	66.8
St. John's Wort*	2	5	140,358,560	48,446,328	189.7
Ginseng	3	2	95,871,544	86,216,928	11.2
Garlic	4	3	84,054,520	71,638,072	17.3
Echinacea/Goldenseal**	5	4	69,702,144	49,245,168	41.5
Saw Palmetto	6	6	32,102,622	18,446,246	74.0
Kava Kava[†]	7	13	16,584,425	2,953,650	461.5
Pycnogenol[‡]/Grape Seed	8	7	12,113,555	9,973,348	21.5
Cranberry	9	9	10,378,810	6,188,689	67.7
Valerian Root	10	10	8,650,521	6,112,876	41.5
Evening Primrose	11	8	8,552,860	7,308,980	17.0
Bilberry	12	11	6,441,501	4,560,067	41.3
Milk Thistle	13	12	4,966,170	3,038,425	63.4
Total (top 13 herbs)			$640,636,560	$404,550,417	58.4%
Total Herb Sales			$688,352,192	$442,928,512	55.4%

Source: Information Resources Inc., Grocery, Drug, Mass Data, 52 weeks ending 12/27/98.
   Herbal Supplement Category as defined by Pharmavite Corp.

*St. John's Wort jumped from 5th place to 2nd, with sales increasing by approximately 190 percent.

**Reflects sales of Echinacea and Goldenseal as individual products and in combination with each other.

[†]Kava Kava moved from 13th to 7th, with sales growing by 461 percent.

[‡]Pycnogenol® is a patented extract of French maritime pine bark.
Grapeseed is used for similar anti-oxidant and anti-inflammatory purposes, and are thus combined in this tracking survey.

TABLE 2: HERB SALES IN UNITED STATES BY RETAIL OUTLET— 12-MONTH PERIOD ENDING DECEMBER 1998 VS. 1997

This table lists the growth of herbal products by retail outlet. According to a natural products industry survey for a 12-month period ending December 1998, sales of single herbals grew 4.7% (to $412.9 million) in natural product outlets and an average of 49% (to $286.5 million) in grocery, drug, and mass merchandise stores combined. The same survey found that the sales for men's single herbal formulas advanced 73.0% (to $13.6 million) and those for women's single herbal formulas advanced 101.0% (to $4.2 million) in the same time period.

RETAIL OUTLET	PRODUCT	SALES (MILLIONS OF $)	INCREASE IN SALES (%)
Natural products outlets	Herbal singles	412.9	4.7
	Calmative herbal singles (e.g., valerian, kava, chamomile)	29.8	42.3
	Brain/circulation singles	86.6	2.7
Supermarkets	Herbal singles	65.1	56.8
	Calmative singles	4.3	249.7
Drug stores	Herbal singles	128.4	46.6
	Calmative singles	7.5	168.8
Mass merchandisers	Herbal singles	93.0	43.7
	Calmative singles	5.9	191.7
F/D/M*	Brain/circulation singles	100.5	39.4
	Men's single herbal formulas	13.6	73.0
	Women's single herbal formulas	4.2	101.0

* Food/Drug/Mass Market Combination Sales [Spence Information Services (SPINS) 1999]. [AC Nielsen ScanTrack: Spencer Information Services (SPINS) NaturalTrack, SPINS Distributor Information; 12-month ending December 1998 versus year ago.] Source: Johnston, 1999.

TABLE 3: TOP-SELLING HERBS IN GERMANY—1996

This table lists the most frequently prescribed monopreparation phytomedicines in Germany in 1996, according to the *Arzneiverordnungsreport* (Prescription Drug Report) (Schwabe, 1997). These figures include sales of phytomedicines that are prescribed by physicians.

HERB/PHYTOMEDICINE (NO. OF PRODUCTS)	THERAPEUTIC CATEGORY	RETAIL SALES (MILLIONS OF U.S. $)*	CHANGE FROM 1995 (%)
Ginkgo biloba leaf extract (5)	circulatory preparations	211.938	-8.7
St. John's wort (7)	antidepressant	71.039	+31.1
Horse chestnut seed (3)	vein preparations	51.195	+10.8
Yeast (2)	antidiarrheal, acne	33.049	+2.4
Hawthorn flower and leaf	cardiac preparations	29.057	-6.8
Myrtle (Myrtus communis) (1)	cough remedy	27.098	+0.6
Saw palmetto	urologic	24.400	+31.8
Stinging nettle root (1)	urologic	20.187	-4.4
Ivy (3)	cough remedy	19.074	+8.0
Mistletoe (1)	cancer treatment	18.060	+3.9
Milk thistle (1)	hepatoprotectant	16.867	+0.9
Bromelain— pineapple enzyme (2)	anti-inflammatory	3.219	+71.2
Echinacea (2)	immunostimulant	10.799	-20.2
Chamomile	dermatological	.278	-7.3
Chaste tree (*Vitex*) (2)	gynecological	7.987	+83.9
Greater Celandine (1)	gastrointestinal agent	6.342	-9.9
Black cohosh (1)	gynecological	.302	+1.5
Kava kava (1)	tranquilizer	.819	-38.8
Artichoke (1)	dyspepsia	5.242	+95.2
Comfrey (1)	dermatological	.880	-11.4

*Currency in U.S.$ based on 1.80 German marks (DM) (0.55 DM per $) on Jan. 26, 1998.
Sources: Schwabe, 1997. *Arzneiverordnungsreport*. Courtesy PhytoPharm Consulting GmbH, Berlin (Gruenwald, 1998).

TABLE 4: CLINICAL STUDIES CONDUCTED ON TOP-SELLING EUROPEAN PHYTOMEDICINES—1973–1997

This table lists leading phytomedicines in Germany and the number of clinical studies that have been conducted on each, as cited in *Rational Phytotherapy* (Schulz et al., 1998). Studies were conducted on a sole proprietary product (e.g., Horse Chestnut seed extract), or two proprietary standardized products (e.g., ginkgo), or specific types of preparations (e.g., aqueous or hydro-alcoholic extracts).

PHYTOMEDICINE	STUDY YEARS	NO. OF STUDIES	NO. OF PARTICIPANTS
Garlic	1986–1992	18	2920
Ginkgo	1975–1996	36*	2326
Hawthorn	1981–1996	13	791
Horse Chestnut seed	1973–1996	8	798
Kava	1989–1995	6	469
St. John's wort	1979–1997	22	1851
Valerian	1977–1996	8	560

Source: Schulz et al., 1998, with additional information added by editors.

*Clinical trials measuring cognitive effects only. Does not include other research on ginkgo (e.g., Le Bars study on effects of early stages of Alzheimer's dementia (Le Bars et al., 1997).

TABLE 5: MOST FREQUENTLY PRESCRIBED AND RESEARCHED PHYTOMEDICINE BRANDS IN GERMANY AND U.S. BRAND COUNTERPARTS

This table lists the most frequently prescribed German phytomedicines and their equivalent brand name products in the United States. ©1999 by Mark Blumenthal (based on an article published in *HerbalGram*).

HERB	EUROPEAN BRAND NAME/ MANUFACTURER	U.S. BRAND NAME/ U.S. IMPORTER	USE
Black Cohosh *Cimicifuga racemosa*	Remifemin®/Schaper & Brümmer	Remifemin®/ Enzymatic/ PhytoPharmica	menopause
Chamomile *Matricaria recutita*	Kamillosan®/Asta Medica	CamoCare®/ Abkit	dermatological
Chaste Tree *Vitex agnus-castus*	Agnolyt®/Madaus	Femaprin®/ Nature's Way	PMS
Echinacea *Echinacea purpurea*	Echinacin®/Madaus AG	Echinaguard®/ Nature's Way	colds/flu
Garlic *Allium sativum*	Kwai®/Lichtwer Pharma	Kwai®/Lichtwer Pharma	circulatory
Ginkgo *Ginkgo biloba*	Tebonin®/Schwabe	Ginkgold®/ Nature's Way	circulatory
		Ginkoba®/Pharmaton	cognitive
		Quanterra®/ Warner-Lambert	cognitive
	Kaveri®/ Lichtwer	Ginkai®/Lichtwer	cognitive
Ginseng *Panax ginseng*	Ginsana®/Pharmaton (Switzerland)	Ginsana®/ Pharmaton	tonic
Hawthorn *Cragaegus* spp.	Crataegutt®/Schwabe	HeartCare®/ Nature's Way	cardiotonic
	Faros®/Lichtwer Pharma	not imported into the U.S.	cardiotonic
Horse Chestnut *Aesculus hippocastanum*	Venostasin®/Klinge Pharma	Venastat®/Pharmaton	venous tonic
	Venoplant®/ Schwabe	not imported into the U.S.	venous tonic
Kava *Piper methysticum*	Laitan®/ Schwabe	not imported into the U.S.	anxiolytic
Milk Thistle *Silybum marianum*	Legalon®/Madaus	Thisylin®/ Nature's Way	hepatoprotectant

Herb	European Brand Name/ Manufacturer	U.S. Brand Name/ U.S. Importer	Use
Saw Palmetto *Serenoa repens*	Permixon®/Pierre Fabre (France)	Elusan® Prostate/Plantes & Médicines Inc.	BPH
	Prostagutt®/ Schwabe	ProstActive/Nature's Way	BPH
St. John's wort *Hypericum perforatum*	Jarsin®(LI 160)/ Lichtwer Pharma	Kira®/Lichtwer Pharma*	depression
	LI 160 WS/ Lichtwer-Schwabe	Quanterra® Emotional Balance/ Warner Lambert*	depression
	Kira®/Lichtwer Pharma	[not imported into the U.S.; Kira in the U.S. is Jarsin; Kira in Germany is a different SJW preparation]	depression
	Neuroplant®/Schwabe	Perika®/Nature's Way Movana®/Pharmaton	depression

COMBINATION PRODUCTS

Echinacea purpurea root Baptisia tinctoria, Thuja occidentalis	Esberitox®/Schaper & Brümmer	Esberitox®/ Enzymatic/ PhytoPharmica	immunostimulation colds/flu
Ash *(Fraxinus excelsior)* Aspen *(Populus tremula)* Goldenrod *(Solidago virgaurea)*	Phytodolor®/Steigerwald	Phytodolor®/ Enzymatic/ PhytoPharmica	rheumatoid arthritis

*Kira® is made from Lichtwer's LI 160 extract; Quanterra® is made from an extract designated LI 160 WS, a slightly different but purportedly phytoequivalent extract made by Lichtwer and Schwabe.

Product listing is in alphabetical order by the herb's common name and does not reflect market status. Tebonin® is the top-selling monopreparation phytomedicine in total sales value, ranking 3rd in all phytomedicine prescriptions written (both for monopreparations and combinations) and 29th in all prescriptions written, including prescriptions written for conventional drugs (Schulz et al., 1998). The ranking of products from Germany is based on the number of prescriptions written and does not include additional sales generated by self-medication purchases (these products are available without a prescription).

This table is for educational purposes only and does not necessarily constitute a recommendation or an endorsement of these products by the American Botanical Council. Specific brands are listed in acknowledgement of clinical studies conducted on them and/or market data indicating a high rate of prescription by German physicians.

CURRENT STATUS OF THE COMMISSION E

Since 1995 the Commission E has not issued any new monographs. The Commission's focus instead has been to serve in Germany as a Commission for Registration of phytomedicines to be sold by prescription. They are also involved in the decisions made concerning the extension of registrations of nonpresciption phytomedicines (Schulte, 1995).

The *Kooperation Phytopharmaka* (an industry-backed scientific organization) is now collecting data from studies published subsequent to the Commission E monographs. This new information is submitted for consideration in preparation of ESCOP (European Scientific Cooperative on Phytotherapy) monographs and is also considered by BfArM (German Federal Institute for Drugs and Medical Devices) in its process for the licensing and registration of phytomedicinal drug products. The licensing requirements stipulate that scientific material on phytomedicines undergoing license review must be up-to-date (Schilcher, 1998b).

The Commission E now acts primarily as a highly authoritative advisory board to the BfArM in their review of applications for marketers of phytomedicines seeking sales authorization in Germany. A phytomedicine's positive monograph is no longer the sole requirement for the registration of an herbal drug; the Commission E continues to weigh whether or not the documentation in a positive monograph reflects current information and is therefore sufficient for the herbal drug's registration. If external experts and the Commission E agree that the data in a product registration is up-to-date and accurate, then the BfArM may approve the registration. If the BfArM does not agree with the Commission E's evaluation, it must justify its position in a public report. To date, this situation has not occurred; the BfArM has always agreed with the Commission E's assessments (Schilcher, 1998a). Of the phytomedicines registered since the passing of the Second German Medicines Act in 1994, 610 are based on the approval of a positive Commission E monograph (Schilcher, 1998a). Thus, even in the view of external experts, the positive monographs are still up-to-date (Schilcher, 1997).

The focus of attention in Western Europe in the development of herbal drug monographs has shifted from the Commission E to ESCOP; however, the ESCOP monographs are scientific publications and lack official status. With no new monographs being produced or revised by the Commission E, and with the European Union's efforts to eventually harmonize drug regulations throughout Western (and perhaps Eastern) Europe, the Commission E monographs will become historical documentation and a model for future scientific documentation of herbs and phytomedicines. In addition to ESCOP, other non-governmental bodies have also published authoritative monographs. The recently published monographs by the World Health Organization (see below) have been reviewed and approved by drug regulatory agencies in dozens of countries (Farnsworth, 1999).

THE COMMISSION E MEMBERS

The Commission E is composed of leading medical and pharmaceutical experts in phytotherapy in Germany. According to the Second German Medicines Act, members of scientific committees must have experience in their respective areas of study. The Commission E is composed of 24 members, including physicians, pharmacists, non-medical practitioners, pharmacologists, toxicologists, biostatisticians, and representatives of the pharmaceutical industry, who are nominated by associations of health professionals (Keller, 1992). Fifty percent are experts from clinical/therapeutic fields (Busse, 1996). Based on the change in composition with five new commissioners in 1999, there are now 13 full university professors on the Commission (Schilcher, 1999). Commission E members are appointed for three-year terms; re-appointment is by the Minister of Health and the process is headed by a Chairman (Dr. Oelze) and a Vice President (Prof. Dr. H. Schilcher).

One of the unique features of Commission E is the interdisciplinary composition of its membership: approximately half of the members have theoretical expertise with herbs and phytomedicines and half of the members have practical experience with phytotherapy. One long-standing member wrote that the interdisciplinary nature of the Commission E is unique in the world (Schilcher, 1997).

The Commission E's scientists and physicians have authored over one thousand scientific publications, in phytotherapy, medicine, pharmacology, dentistry, health-care delivery, and medical ethics.

The distinguished physicians and scientists serving on the Commission E (this lists includes all active members and their deputies) are:

Toxicology/Pharmacology

Member: Prof. Dr. rer. nat. Hilke Winterhoff
University of Münster
Institute of Pharmacology and Toxicology

Deputy: Prof. Dr. med. Gerhard Eisenbrand
Director of the Institute of Pharmacology and Toxicology
University of Saarbrücken

Clinical Pharmacology

Member: Prof. Dr. med. Dieter Loew
Wiesbaden

Deputy: Prof. Dr. med. Ivar Roots
Director of the Institute for Clinical Pharmacology
University Clinic Charité, Berlin

Medical Statistics

Member: Prof. Dr. phil. Wilhelm Gaus
University of Ulm, Department of Biometry and Medical Documentation

Deputy: Prof. Dr. phil. nat. Berthold Schneider
University of Hanover
Institute for Biometry of Medicine

Pharmacy

Member: Prof. Dr. phil. Franz-C. Czygan
University of Würzburg
Chair of Department of Pharmaceutical Biology

Deputy: Prof. Dr. rer. nat. Gerhard Franz
University of Regensburg,
Chair of Department of Pharmaceutical Biology

Medical Practice

Members: Dr. med. Fritz Oelze
Hamburg

Dr. Manfred Bocksch
Doctor of General Medicine
Eurasburg

Priv. Doz. Dr. med. Karin Kraft
University of Bonn

Univ. Prof. Dr. rer. nat. Heinz Schilcher
Marx-Zentrum Pharmacy
Munich

Dr. med. Egon Frölich
Chief Physician of the Rheintal Clinic
Bad Krozingen

Dr. med. Heinz Leúchtgens
Chief Physician of the Kneipp-Clinic
Bad Wörishofen

Univ. Prof. Dr. med. habil. Hartwig Wilhelm Bauer
Munich

Peter A. Zizmann
Natural Practitioner
Hechingen

Deputies: Dr. med. Axel Wiebrecht
Doctor of General Medicine
Berlin

Prof. Dr. med. Heribert Frotz
Chief Physician of the Internal Section
of the Marienkrankenhaus
Bergisch-Gladbach

Prof. Dr. med. Günther Faust
Doctor of General Medicine
Mainz

Prof. Dr. rer. nat. habil. Ulrike Lindequist
Ernst-Moritz-Arndt University
Institute for Pharmaceutical Biology
Greifswald

Dr. med. Markus Wiesenauer
Weinstadt

Dr. med. Franz Eduard Brock
Chief Physician of the Hospital
Bad Wörishofen

Dr. med. Klaus Mohr
Staufenberg

Dr. rer. nat. Wolfgang Widmaier
Stuttgart

WHO MONOGRAPHS

The *WHO Monographs on Selected Medicinal Plants,* Volume 1 was published by the World Health Organization (WHO) in June 1999. In 1991 WHO published "Guidelines for the Assessment of Herbal Medicines" (Akerele, 1991), in which the international health agency called for the establishment of monographs to help set standards to document the quality of herbal products, as well as outline the therapeutic parameters for their safe and effective use.

Pharmacognosists at the College of Pharmacy of the University of Illinois at Chicago (UIC) compiled data to produce the first volume of WHO monographs. The primary editor is Gail Mahady, Ph.D., Research Assistant Professor of Pharmacognosy at UIC, along with Harry H.H.S. Fong, Ph.D., Professor of Pharmacognosy, and Norman R. Farnsworth, Ph.D., Research Professor of Pharmacognosy and Senior University Scholar. The monographs produced by the team at UIC have been peer reviewed and accepted by medicinal plant experts convened by WHO from many countries and cultures.

The first volume contains 28 monographs on 31 plant species. There are two on aloe (one for drug aloe (*Aloe ferox*), the laxative; the other for aloe gel (*A. vera*)), echinacea (one on Echinacea root, including *Echinacea angustifolia* and *E. pallida*; another on *E. purpurea* herb) and senna (*Cassia senna*), one for the fruit and one for leaf preparations. All monographs were extensively peer reviewed by an international team of scientific experts assembled by WHO. A second volume is scheduled for publication in 2000.

The WHO monographs contain most of the essential elements needed to determine baseline standards for identity and quality and to assess the relative safety and efficacy of each medicinal plant. The monographs were complete in 1996 and 1997, and thus reflect research published up to those years.

The therapeutics section includes three levels of medicinal uses: 1. Those supported by clinical data (listed in the table below), 2. Those described in pharmacopeias and traditional systems of medicine, and 3. Those described in folk medicine, not supported by experimental or clinical data.

Correlation to Commission E monographs: Of the 28 monographs published in the first volume of WHO monographs, 18 of the herbs had uses that the WHO scientists deemed supportable by clinical studies. Most of these uses closely parallel the approved uses previously deemed appropriate in positive monographs published by the Commission E. In some cases, due to the fact that new data had been published since the Commission E monographs were developed, the WHO monographs actually suggest uses not previously approved by Commission E (e.g., the use of chamomile as a sedative, as there was no scientific data to document this historical and popular use until the mid-1990s). The worldwide peer review and acceptance of the WHO monographs based on modern scientific studies becomes a form of validation and confirmation that the Commission E process is rational, scientific, and still relevant as a regulatory mechansim for assessing the therapeutic properties of herbs and phytomedicines.

TABLE 6: USES OF MEDICINAL PLANTS SUPPORTED BY CLINICAL DATA IN WHO MONOGRAPHS

COMMON NAME**	LATIN NAME	USE(S)†
Aloe*	*Aloe vera, A. ferox*	Short-term treatment of occasional constipation.
Aloe Vera gel	*Aloe vera*	None.
Astragalus root	*Astragalus membranaceus*	None.
Brucea	*Brucea javanica*	None.
Bupleurum root	*Bupleurum falcatum*	None.
Chamomile flower*	*Matricaria recutita*	Internal: Symptomatic treatment of digestive ailments such as dyspepsia, epigastric bloating, impaired digestion, and flatulence. Infusions of chamomile flowers have been used in the treatment of restlessness and in mild cases of insomnia due to nervous disorders. External: Inflammation and irritations of the skin and mucosa (skin cracks, bruises, frostbite, and insect bites), including irritations and infections of the mouth and gums, and hemorrhoids.
Cinnamon bark*	*Cinnamomum* spp.	None.
Echinacea root*	*Echinacea angustifolia E. pallida*	Administered orally in supportive therapy for colds and infections of the respiratory and urinary tract. Beneficial effects in the treatment of these infections are generally thought to be brought about by stimulation of the immune response.
Echinacea Purpurea herb*	*E. purpurea*	Administered orally in supportive therapy for colds and infections of the respiratory and urinary tract. Beneficial effects in the treatment of these infec tions are generally thought to be brought about by stimulation of the immune response. External uses include promo tion of wound healing and treatment of inflammatory skin conditions.
Ephedra/Ma huang*	*Ephedra sinica*	Treatment of nasal congestion due to hay fever, allergic rhinitis, acute coryza, common cold, and sinusitis. The drug is further used as a bronchodilator in the treatment of bronchial asthma.

Common Name**	Latin Name	Use(s)†
Garlic*	*Allium sativum*	As an adjuvant to dietetic management in treatment of hyperlipidemia, and in prevention of atherosclerotic (age-dependent) vascular changes. May be useful in treatment of mild hypertension.
Ginger*	*Zingiber officinale*	The prophylaxis of nausea and vomiting associated with motion sickness, postoperative nausea, pernicious vomiting in pregnancy, and seasickness.
Ginkgo*	*Ginkgo biloba*	Extracts (concentrated) have been used for symptomatic treatment of mild to moderate cerebrovascular insufficiency (demential syndromes in primary degenerative dementia, vascular dementia, and mixed forms of both) with the following symptoms: memory deficit, disturbance in concentration, depressive emotional condition, dizziness, tinnitus, and headache. Such extracts are also used to improve pain-free walking distance in people with peripheral arterial occlusive disease, e.g., intermittent claudication, Raynaud's disease, acrocyanosis, and post-phlebitis syndrome, and to treat inner ear disorders, e.g., tinnitus and vertigo of vascular and involutive origin.
Ginseng root*	*Panax ginseng*	Prophylactic and restorative agent for enhancement of mental and physical capacities, in cases of weakness, exhaustion, tiredness, and loss of concentration, and during convalescence.
Goldthread root	*Coptis* spp.	None.
Gotu kola herb	*Centella asiatica*	Treatment of wounds, burns, and ulcerous skin ailments, and prevention of keloid and hypertrophic scars. Extracts of the plant have been employed to treat second- and third-degree burns. Extracts have been used topically to accelerate healing, particularly in cases of chronic postsurgical and post-trauma wounds. Extracts have been administered orally to treat stress-induced stomach and duodenal ulcers.
Indian Snakeroot*	*Rauvolfia serpentina*	The principal use today is in the treatment of mild essential hypertension. Treatment is usually administered in combination with a diuretic agent to

Common Name**	Latin Name	Use(s)†
		support the drug's antihypertensive activity, and to prevent fluid retention, which may develop if Indian Snakeroot is given alone.
Licorice*	*Glycyrrhiza glabra; G. uralensis*	None.
Onion*	*Allium cepa*	Age-dependent change in blood vessels and loss of appetite.
Peony root	*Paeonia lactiflora*	None.
Platycodon	*Platycodon grandiflorum*	None.
Psyllium seed*	*Plantago* spp.	As a bulk-forming laxative used to restore and maintain regularity. Indicated in the treatment of chronic constipation, temporary constipation due to illness or pregnancy, irritable bowel syndrome, and constipation related to duodenal ulcer or diverticulitis. Also used to soften stools of those with hemorrhoids, or after anorectal surgery.
Rhubarb root*	*Rheum officinale*	Short-term treatment of occasional constipation.
Senna fruit*	*Cassia senna*	Short-term treatment of occasional constipation.
Thyme*	*Thymus vugaris*	None.
Turmeric root*	*Curcuma longa*	Treatment of acid, flatulent, or atonic dyspepsia.
Valerian*	*Valeriana officinalis*	Mild sedative and sleep-promoting agent. Often used as alternative or a possible substitute for stronger synthetic sedatives, e.g., benzodiazepines, in the treatment of states of nervous excitation and anxiety-induced sleep disturbances.

*Denotes herbs also evaluated by the Commission E.

**Original WHO monographs are listed by pharmacopeial names, e.g., Genseng Radix for ginseng root, Sannae Folium for Senna leaf, etc. English common names are substituted here, in the monograph title and occasionally in the Uses column, when WHO used the pharmacopeial name.

†References cited in original WHO text; not included here. Uses are edited slightly for space.

TABLE 7: WHO MONOGRAPHS IN FINAL STAGES OF PREPARATION— PUBLICATION IN 2000

The following 29 monographs have been compiled and reviewed by Gail Mahady and colleagues at the Univeristy of Illinois at Chicago for the World Health Organization (WHO). The monographs are nearing stages of final editing, and are scheduled to be published in 2000.

COMMON NAME	LATIN BINOMIAL
Andrographis root	*Andrographis paniculata*
Angelica root*	*Angelica polymorpha* var. *sinensis*
Basil herb, Holy	*Ocimum sanctum*
Black Cohosh*	*Cimicifuga racemosa*
Buckthorn bark*	*Rhamnus frangula*
Calendula flower*	*Calendula officinalis*
Cascara Sagrada bark*	*Rhamnus purshiana*
Devil's Claw*	*Harpagophytum procumbens*
Elder flower*	*Sambucus nigra*
Eleuthero*	*Eleutherococcus senticosus*
Eucalyptus*	*Eucalyptus globulus*
Evening Primrose	*Oenothera biennis*
Feverfew	*Tanacetum parthenium*
Hawthorn*	*Crataegus monogyna*
Horse Chestnut seed*	*Aesculus hippocastanum*
Kava*	*Piper methysticum*
Lemon Balm*	*Melissa officinalis*
Marshmallow*	*Althea officinalis*
Milk Thistle fruit*	*Silybum marianum*
Nettle herb/root*	*Urtica dioica, U. urens*
Peppermint*	*Mentha x piperita*
Pygeum bark	*Prunus (Pygeum) africana*
Saw Palmetto berry*	*Serenoa repens*
Seneca Snake root*	Polygala senega
St. John's wort*	*Hypericum perforatum*
Tea tree	*Melaleuca alternifolia*
Uva ursi leaf*	*Archtostaphylos uva-ursi*
Witch Hazel leaf*	*Hamamelis virginia*

Source: Mahady, 1999
*Denotes herbs also evaluated by the Commission E.

TABLE 8: ESCOP MONOGRAPHS

The European Scientific Cooperative on Phytotherapy (ESCOP) was formed in 1990 as an organization of scientists with expertise in various aspects of phytomedicine. In an effort to help harmonize therapeutic data on herbal drug products sold in the European Union, ESCOP has published 50 monographs on medicinal plants used in Western Europe, although, unlike those of the Commission E, ESCOP monographs are not official on a regulatory level. ESCOP monographs cover therapeutic aspects of the herbal drug; there are no data on quality control measures for determining identity or assaying purity. Such information is usually found in the respective pharmacopeias of European countries. Except for Feverfew, all herbal drugs reviewed by ESCOP also have been evaluated by Commission E. They are published in fascicules (volumes) of ten herbs.

COMMON NAME	PHARMACOPEIAL NAME	LATIN BINOMIAL
Fascicule 1		
Marshmallow root	Altheae radix	*Althaea officinalis*
Birch leaf	Betulae folium	*Betula* spp.
Boldo leaf	Boldo folium	*Peumus boldus*
Calendula flower	Calendula flos	*Calendula officinalis*
Fennel seed	Foeniculi fructus	*Foeniculum vulgare*
St. John's wort	Hyperici herba	*Hypericum perforatum*
Linseed	Lini semen	*Linum usitatissimum*
Java tea	Orthosiphonis folium	*Orthosiphon spicatus*
Thyme herb	Thymi herba	*Thymus vulgaris*
Ginger root	Zingiberis rhizoma	*Zingiber officinale*
Fascicule 2		
Devil's Claw root	Harpagophyti radix	*Harpagophytum procumbens*
Lemon Balm leaf	Melissa folium	*Melissa officinalis*
Ispaghula (Psyllium seed)	Plantaginis Ovatae semen	*Plantago psyllium*
Ispaghula (Psyllium husk)	Plantaginis Ovatae testa	*Plantago psyllium*
Sage leaf	Salviae folium	*Salvia officinalis*
Goldenrod herb	Solidaginis virgaureae herba	*Solidago virgaurea*
Feverfew leaf and herb	Tanacetii Parthenii herba/folium	*Tanacetum parthenium*
Dandelion leaf	Taraxaci folium	*Taraxacum officinale*
Dandelion root	Taraxaci radix	*Taraxacum officinale*
Nettle root	Urticae radix	*Urtica dioica*
Fascicule 3		
Garlic	Allii sativi bulbus	*Allium sativum*
Anise seed	Anisi fructu	*Pimpinella anisum*
Caraway seed	Carvi fructus	*Carum carvi*
Juniper berry	Juniperi fructus	*Juniperus communis*
Iceland moss	Lichen islandicu	*Cetraria islandica*
Peppermint oil	Menthae piperitae aetholeum	*Mentha* x *piperita*
Peppermint leaf	Menthae piperitae folium	*Mentha* x *piperita*
Senega snake root	Polygalae radix	*Polygala senega*
Cowslip root	Primulae radix	*Primula veris*
Rosemary leaf with flower	Rosmarini folium cum flore	*Rosmarinus officinalis*

COMMON NAME	PHARMACOPEIAL NAME	LATIN BINOMIAL
Fascicule 4		
Wormwood	Absinthii herba	*Artemisia absinthium*
Arnica flower	Arnicae flos	*Arnica montana*
Gentian root	Gentianae radix	*Gentiana lutea*
Hops flower	Lupuli flos	*Humulus lupulus*
Melilot	Meliloti herba	*Melilotus officinalis*
Passionflower herb	Passiflorae herba	*Passiflora* spp.
Blackcurrant leaf	Ribis nigri folium	*Ribes nigrum*
Willow bark	Salicis cortex	*Salix* spp.
Nettle leaf/herb	Urticae folium/herba	*Urtica dioica*
Valerian root	Valeriana radix	*Valeriana officinalis*
Fascicule 5		
Cape Aloes	Aloe capensis	*Aloe ferox*
Buckthorn bark (Frangula)	Frangulae cortex	*Rhamnus frangula*
Witch hazel leaf	Hamamelis folium	*Hamamelis virginiana*
Rest-harrow root	Ononidis radix	*Ononis spinosa*
Psyllium seed	Psylli semen	*Plantago psyllium*
Cascara sagrada bark	Rhamni purshiani cortex	*Rhamnus purshianus*
Senna leaf	Sennae folium	*Cassia senna*
Alexandrian senna pods	Sennae fructus acutifoliae	*Cassia senna*
Tinnevelly senna pods	Sennae fructus angustifoliae	*Cassia senna*
Uva ursi leaf	Uvae ursi folium	*Arctostaphylos uva-ursi*
Fascicule 6		
Eucalyptus oil	Eucalypti aetheroleum	*Eucalyptus globulus*
Echinacea Purpurea herb	Echinacea purpurea herba	*Echinacea purpurea*
Echinacea Purpurea root	Echinacea purpurea radix	*Echinacea purpurea*
Echinacea Pallida root	Echinacea pallidae radix	*Echinacea pallida*
Chamomile flower	Matricaria flos	*Matricaria recutita*
Centaury herb	Centaurii herba	*Centaureum erythraea*
Myrrh gum	Myrrha	*Commiphora molmol*
Horse Chestnut seed	Hippocastani semen	*Aesculus hippocastanum*
Rhubarb root	Rhei radix	*Rheum officinalis*
Hawthorn leaf with flower	Crateagi folium cum fructus	*Crataegus monogyna*

REFERENCES TO APPENDIX TABLES AND TEXT

Akerele, O. 1991. WHO Guidelines for the Assessment of Herbal Medicines. Geneva: World Health Organization. Reprinted in *HerbalGram* 28:13–20 (1993).

Busse, W. 1996. Personal communication to M. Blumenthal, Mar. 28.

ESCOP. 1997. *Monographs on the Medicinal Uses of Plant Drugs* (5 volumes). Exeter, U.K.: European Scientific Cooperative on Phytotherapy.

Farnsworth, NR. 1999. Personal communication to M. Blumenthal, Jul. 19.

Gruenwald, J. 1998. Personal communication, Jan. 25.

Johnston, B.A. 1999. Herbal Formulas Show Market Growth. *HerbalGram* 46:57.

Keller, K. 1992. Results of the revision of herbal drugs in the Federal Republic of Germany with a special focus on risk aspects. *Zeitschrift Phytother* 13:116–120.

Le Bars, P.L. et al. 1997. A placebo-controlled, double-blind, randomized trial of an extract of *Ginkgo biloba* for dementia. *JAMA* 278(16):1327–1332.

Mahady, G. Personal communication to M. Blumenthal, Aug. 6.

Schilcher, H. 1999. Personal communication to M. Blumenthal, Aug. 6.

Schilcher, H. 1997. Personal communication to M. Blumenthal, Dec. 30.

Schilcher, H. 1998a. Personal communication to M. Blumenthal, Feb. 9.

Schilcher, H. 1998b. The Phytotherapy Situation in the Republic of Germany. *Münchner Medizinische Wochenschrift.*

Schulte, G. 1995. Letter to H. Schilcher, August 25.

Schulz,V., R. Hänsel, V.E. Tyler. 1998. *Rational Phytotherapy: A Physician's Guide to Herbal Medicine.* Berlin-Heidelberg: Springer Verlag.

Schwabe, U. 1997. *Arzneiverordnungsreport* [Prescription Drug Report]. Stuttgart: Gustav Fischer Verlag.

World Health Organization (WHO). 1999. *WHO Monographs on Selected Medicinal Plants,* Vol. 1. Geneva: World Health Organization.

ABBREVIATIONS AND SYMBOLS

ASK — Bearbeitungsnummern des Bundesinstituts für Arzneimittel und Medizinprodukte,
      working numbers of the Federal Institute for Drug Agents and Medicinal Products
      for individual chemical reagents

B.Anz. — *Bundesanzeiger* (German Federal Gazette), edited by the Minister of Justice

B.C.E. — before common era. Refers to a historical date prior to 1 C.E. (A.D.)

BfArM — German Federal Institute of Drugs and Medical Devices (formerly BGA)

BGA — German Federal Health Agency (now BfArM)

C — Celsius, Centigrade

C.E. — common era. Refers to historical dates since the first year of this historical era (=A.D.)

ca — circa, approximately

cm, cm^2 — centimeter(s), square centimeter(s)

DAB 6 — *Deutsches Arzneibuch (German Pharmacopoeia)*, Sixth edition 1926

DAB 7 — *Deutsches Arzneibuch (German Pharmacopoeia)*, Seventh edition 1968

DAB 8 — *Deutsches Arzneibuch (German Pharmacopoeia)*, Eighth edition 1978;
      First Supplement 1980; Second Supplement 1983

DAB 9 — *Deutsches Arzneibuch (German Pharmacopoeia)*, Ninth edition 1986;
      First Supplement 1989; Second Supplement 1990

DAB 10 — *Deutsches Arzneibuch (German Pharmacopoeia)*, Tenth edition 1991;
      First Supplement 1992; Second Supplement 1993

DAC — *Deutscher Arzneimittel-Codex (German Drug Formulary)*

D.C. — de Candolle (botanical authority)

emend. — emendavit, as corrected (in botanical name)

Erg.B.6 — *Ergänzungsbuch zum Deutschen Arzneibuch (Supplement Volume to the
      German Pharmacopoeia)*, Sixth edition 1926. Reprinted 1953

Fam. — plant family

FIP — Federacion Internacionale Pharmaceutique (International Pharmaceutical Federation)

FIP unit — measurement of calorie content in bread units issued by the Federacion
      Internacionale Pharmaceutique

g — gram

GPU — guinea pig units, ad hoc measure used for fixed combination of pheasant's eye
      fluidextract, lily-of-the-valley powdered extract, squill powdered extract, and olean-
      der leaf powdered extract

HPLC — High performance liquid chromatography

kPa — kiloPascals

L. — Linnaeus (botanical authority)

l — liter

LD^{50} — Lethal-dosage-50, dose causing death in 50% of test animals

LD^{100} — Lethal-dosage-100, dose causing death in 100% of test animals

m/m — mass in mass measurement

m/v — mass in volume measurement

mcg — microgram

mg — milligram

mg/kg — milligrams drug per kilogram body weight

ml — milliliter

mm — millimeters

m — meters

MAO — monoamine oxidase

MMR — Molar Mass

MW — molecular weight

N — normal (solution)

nm — nanometers
Nutt. — Nuttall (botanical authority)
NYHA — New York Heart Association
ÖAB — *Österreichisches Arzneibuch (Austrian Pharmacopoeia)*, 2 volumes, 1981;
      First Supplement 1983
PA — pyrrolizidine alkaloid
Ph. Helv. VI — *Pharmacopoea Helvetica (Swiss Pharmacopeia)*, sixth edition
p.p. — pro parte, in part (in botanical name)
R — reagent
Rf — radiative frequency (in HPLC)
RN — normalized reagent
s.l. — sensu lato, in a broad sense (in botanical name)
spp. — species
syn. — synonym
var. — varietas, variety (variety of plant within species)
v/v — volume in volume measurement
v/w — volume in weight measurement
UV — ultraviolet
WHO — World Health Organization
μ — microns
μg — microgram
μl — microliter
μm — micrometer
α — alpha
β — beta
γ — gamma

WEIGHTS AND MEASURES

Metric Weight
1 kilogram (kg, kilo)   = 1000 grams
1 centigram (cg)   = 0.01 gram
1 milligram (mg)   = 0.001 gram
1 microgram (μg, mcg)   = 0.0001 gram

Avoirdupois Weight

pounds	ounces	drachma	grains
1	= 16	= 256	= 7000
	1	= 16	= 437.5
		1	= 27.34375

Apothecaries Weight

pounds	ounces	drachma	scruples	grains
1	= 12	= 96	= 288	= 5760
	1	= 8	= 24	= 480
		1	= 3	= 60
			1	= 24

1 grain   = 065 mg
1 grain   = 0.097 minims
1 minim   = 1 drop
60 drops   = 1 fluid dram

Comparison of United States, British Imperial, and Metric Systems of Liquid Measures
1 U.S. minim   = 1.04 Imperial minims
1 U.S. gallon   = 0.8237 Imperial gallon
1 U.S. pint   = 0.8237 Imperial pint
1 Imperial gallon   = 1.2009 U.S. gallons
1 Imperial pint   = 1.2009 U.S. pints
1 Imperial fluid ounce = 437.5 grains
1 U.S. gallon   = 128 fluid ounces = 61440 minims = 3.785 liters
8 pints or 6.66 Imp. pints = 8.3283 lbs. avoirdupois at 60° F
1 Imperial gallon   = 160 fluid ounces = 76800 minims = 4.5460 liters
8 Imperial pints or   = 10 lbs. avoirdupois at 60° F
  9.6072 U.S. pints

Metric to English Length
1 millimeter (mm)   = 0.04 inches (in)
1 centimeter (cm)   = 0.39 in
1 decimeter (dm)   = 3.93 in
1 meter (m)   = 39.3 in

English to Metric Length
1 inch (in) = 25.4 millimeters (mm)   = 2.54 cm
1 foot (ft) = 304.8 mm = 30.48 cm = 0.3048 m

GENERAL REFERENCES

Bradley, P.R. (ed.). 1992. *British Herbal Compendium*, Vol. 1. Bournemouth: British Herbal Medicine Association.

Braun, R. et al. 1997. *Standardzulassungen für Fertigarzneimittel—Text and Kommentar*. Stuttgart: Deutscher Apotheker Verlag.

British Herbal Pharmacopoeia (BHP). 1983. Keighley, U.K.: British Herbal Medicine Association.

British Herbal Pharmacopoeia (BHP). 1990. Bournemouth, U.K.: British Herbal Medicine Association.

British Herbal Pharmacopoeia (BHP). 1996. Exeter, U.K.: British Herbal Medicine Association.

British Pharmacopoeia (BP). 1988. (With subsequent Addenda up to 1992.) London: Her Majesty's Stationery Office.

British Pharmaceutical Codex (BPC). 1934. London: The Pharmaceutical Press.

British Pharmaceutical Codex (BPC). 1949. London: The Pharmaceutical Press.

British Pharmaceutical Codex (BPC). 1973. London: The Pharmaceutical Press.

Bruneton, J. 1995. *Pharmacognosy, Phytochemistry, Medicinal Plants.* Paris: Lavoisier Publishing.

Budavari, S. (ed.). 1996. *The Merck Index: An Encyclopedia of Chemicals, Drugs, and Biologicals,* 12th ed. Whitehouse Station, N.J.: Merck & Co, Inc.

Bundesanzeiger (BAnz). 1998. Monographien der Kommission E (Zulassungs- und Aufbereitungskommission am BGA für den humanmed. Bereich, phytotherapeutische Therapierichtung und Stoffgruppe). Köln: Bundesgesundheitsamt (BGA).

Chinese Pharmacopoeia (CHP). 1990. Beijing: Chinese Ministry of Health —People's Health Publications.

Der Marderosian, A. (ed.). 1999. *The Review of Natural Products.* St. Louis: Facts and Comparisons.

Deutsches Arzneibuch der Deutsche Demokratische Republik (DAB-DDR). 1985. Berlin: Akademie Verlag.

Deutsches Arzneibuch, 6th ed. (DAB 6). 1926. Stuttgart: Deutscher Apotheker Verlag.

Deutsches Arzneibuch, 7th ed. (DAB 7). 1968. Stuttgart: Deutscher Apotheker Verlag.

Deutsches Arzneibuch, 8th ed. (DAB 8). 1978. Stuttgart: Deutscher Apotheker Verlag.

Deutsches Arzneibuch, 9th ed. (DAB 9). 1986. Stuttgart: Deutscher Apotheker Verlag.

Deutsches Arzneibuch, 10th ed. (DAB 10). 1991. (With subsequent supplements through 1996.) Stuttgart: Deutscher Apotheker Verlag.

Deutsches Arzneibuch, 10th ed., 3rd suppl. (DAB 10). 1993. Stuttgart: Deutscher Apotheker Verlag.

Deutsches Arzneibuch, 10th ed. Vol. 1–6. (DAB 10). 1991. Kommentar. Stuttgart: Wissenschaftliche Verlagsgesellschaft.

Deutsches Arzneibuch (DAB 1997). 1997. Stuttgart: Deutscher Apotheker Verlag.

Deutsches Arzneibuch (DAB 1998). 1998. Stuttgart: Deutscher Apotheker Verlag.

Deutscher Arzneimittel-Codex (DAC). 1986. Stuttgart: Deutscher Apotheker Verlag.

Duke, J.A. 1985. *Handbook of Medicinal Herbs.* Boca Raton: CRC Press.

Ellingwood, F. 1983. *American Materia Medica, Therapeutics and Pharmacognosy.* Portland, OR: Eclectic Medical Publications [reprint of 1919 original].

ESCOP. 1997. *Monographs on the Medicinal Uses of Plant Drugs.* Exeter, U.K.: European Scientific Cooperative on Phytotherapy.

Ergänzungsbuch zum Deutschen Arzneibuch, 6th ed. (Erg.B.6). 1953. Stuttgart: Deutscher Apotheker Verlag.

Europäisches Arzneibuch, 3rd ed. (Ph.Eur.3). 1997. Stuttgart: Deutscher Apotheker Verlag.

Europäisches Arzneibuch, 3rd ed., 1st suppl. (Ph.Eur.3). 1998. Stuttgart: Deutscher Apotheker Verlag.

Europäisches Arzneibuch (Ph.Eur.). 1999. Stuttgart: Deutscher Apotheker Verlag.

Felter, H.W. and J.U. Lloyd. 1983. *King's American Dispensatory*, 18th ed., 3rd rev. Portland, OR: Eclectic Medical Publications [reprint of 1898 original].

Fleming, T. (ed.). 1998. *PDR® for Herbal Medicines*. Montvale, N.J.: Medical Economics Company, Inc.

Food Chemicals Codex, 2nd ed. (FCC II). 1972. Washington, D.C.: National Academy of Sciences.

Food Chemicals Codex, 3rd ed. (FCC III). 1981. Washington, D.C.: National Academy of Sciences.

Grieve, M. 1979. *A Modern Herbal*. New York: Dover Publications, Inc.

Hänsel, R., K. Keller, H. Rimpler, G. Schneider (eds.). 1992–1994. *Hagers Handbuch der Pharmazeutischen Praxis*, 5th ed. Vol. 4–6. Berlin-Heidelberg: Springer Verlag.

Indian Pharmacopoeia, Vol. 1. (IP 1996). 1996. Delhi: Government of India Ministry of Health and Family Welfare—Controller of Publications.

Japanese Pharmacopoeia, 12th ed. (JP XII). 1993. Tokyo: Government of Japan Ministry of Health and Welfare—Yakuji Nippo, Ltd.

Jiangsu Institute of Modern Medicine. 1977. *Zhong Yao Da Ci Dian* (Encyclopedia of Chinese Materia Medica), Vol. 3. Shanghai: Shanghai Scientific and Technical Publications.

Karnick, C.R. 1994. *Pharmacopoeial Standards of Herbal Plants*. Delhi: Sri Satguru Publications.

Lange, D. and U. Schippmann. 1997. *Trade Survey of Medicinal Plants in Germany—A Contribution to International Plant Species Conservation*. Bonn: Bundesamt für Naturschutz.

Leung, A.Y. and S. Foster. 1996. *Encyclopedia of Common Natural Ingredients Used in Food, Drugs, and Cosmetics*, 2nd ed. New York: John Wiley & Sons, Inc.

List, P.H. and L. Hörhammer (eds.). 1973–1979. *Hagers Handbuch der Pharmazeutischen Praxis*, Vols. 1–7. New York: Springer Verlag.

The Homeopathic Pharmacopoeia of the United States (HPUS). 1992. Arlington, VA: Pharmacopoeia Convention of the American Institute of Homeopathy.

McGuffin, M., C. Hobbs, R. Upton, A. Goldberg. 1997. American Herbal Product Association's *Botanical Safety Handbook*. Boca Raton: CRC Press.

Meyer-Buchtela, E. 1999. *Tee-Rezepturen—Ein Handbuch für Apotheker und Ärzte*. Stuttgart: Deutscher Apotheker Verlag.

Moerman, D.E. 1998. *Native American Ethnobotany*. Portland: Timber Press.

Nadkarni, K.M. 1976. *Indian Materia Medica*. Bombay: Popular Prakashan.

National Formulary (NF), 16th ed. 1985. Washington, D.C.: American Pharmaceutical Association.

Newall, C.A., L.A. Anderson, J.D. Phillipson. 1996. *Herbal Medicines: A Guide for Health-Care Professionals*. London: The Pharmaceutical Press.

Österreichisches Arzneibuch, Vols. 1–2. (ÖAB). 1981. Wien: Verlag der Österreichischen Staatsdruckerei.

Österreichisches Arzneibuch, Vols. 1–2, 1st suppl. (öAB). 1981–1983. Wien: Verlag der Österreichischen Staatsdruckerei.

Österreichisches Arzneibuch, 1st and 2nd suppl. (ÖAB). 1991. Wien: Verlag der Österreichischen Staatsdruckerei.

Pharmacopée FranÁaise Xe Édition (Ph.Fr.X). 1983–1990. Moulins-les-Metz: Maisonneuve S.A.

Pharmacopoeia Helvetica, 7th ed. Vol. 1–4. (Ph.Helv.VII). 1987. Bern: Office Central Fédéral des Imprimés et du Matériel.

Reynolds, J.E.F. (ed.). 1989. *Martindale: The Extra Pharmacopoeia,* 29th ed. London: The Pharmaceutical Press.

Reynolds, J.E.F. (ed.). 1993. *Martindale: The Extra Pharmacopoeia,* 30th ed. London: The Pharmaceutical Press.

Reynolds, J.E.F. (ed.). 1996. *Martindale: The Extra Pharmacopoeia,* 31st ed. London: Royal Pharmaceutical Society.

Schulz, V., R. Hänsel, V.E. Tyler. 1998. *Rational Phytotherapy: A Physicians' Guide to Herbal Medicine.* New York: Springer.

Stecher, P.G. (ed.). 1968. *The Merck Index: An Encyclopedia of Chemicals and Drugs,* 8th ed. Rahway, N.J.: Merck & Co., Inc.

Steinegger, E. and R. Hänsel. 1992. *Pharmakognosie,* 5th ed. Berlin-Heidelberg: Springer Verlag.

The United States Pharmacopeia, 20th rev. (USP). 1980. Rockville, MD: U.S. Pharmacopoeial Convention.

United States Pharmacopeia, 24th rev. and *National Formulary,* 19th ed. (USP 24–NF19). 1999. Rockville, MD: United States Pharmacopeial Convention, Inc.

Trease, G.E. and W.C. Evans. 1989. *Trease and Evans' Pharmacognosy,* 13th ed. London; Philadelphia: Bailliére Tindall.

———. 1966. *A Textbook of Pharmacognosy,* 9th ed. London: Bailliére, Tindall, and Cassell.

Tu, G. (ed.). 1992. *Pharmacopoeia of the People's Republic of China* (English Edition 1992). Beijing: Guangdong Science and Technology Press.

Tyler, V.E. 1994. *Herbs of Choice: The Therapeutic Use of Phytomedicinals.* New York: Pharmaceutical Products Press.

Weiss, R.F. 1988. *Herbal Medicine.* Beaconsfield, England: Beaconsfield Publishers.

Wichtl, M. and N.G. Bisset (eds.). 1994. *Herbal Drugs and Phytopharmaceuticals.* Stuttgart: Medpharm Scientific Publishers.

Wichtl, M. (ed.). 1989. *Teedrogen,* 2th ed. Stuttgart: Wissenschaftliche Verlagsgesellschaft.

Wichtl, M. (ed.). 1997. *Teedrogen,* 4th ed. Stuttgart: Wissenschaftliche Verlagsgesellschaft.

World Health Organization (WHO). 1999. "Radix Glycyrrhizae." *WHO Monographs on Selected Medicinal Plants,* Vol. 1. Geneva: World Health Organization.

Wren, R.C. 1988. *Potter's New Cyclopaedia of Botanical Drugs and Preparations.* Essex: The C.W. Daniel Company Ltd.

Yen, K.Y. 1992. *The Illustrated Chinese Materia Medica—Crude and Prepared.* Taipei: SMC Publishing, Inc.

INDEX

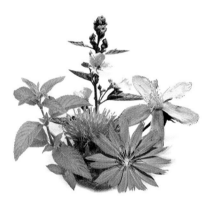